Cognitive-Behavioral Therapies for Trauma

Cognitive-Behavioral Therapies for Trauma

Second Edition

Edited by

Victoria M. Follette
Josef I. Ruzek

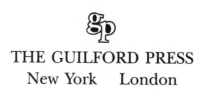

THE GUILFORD PRESS
New York   London

© 2006 The Guilford Press
A Division of Guilford Publications, Inc.
72 Spring Street, New York, NY 10012
www.guilford.com

Printed in the United States of America

This book is printed on acid-free paper.

Last digit is print number: 9 8 7 6 5 4 3 2

Library of Congress Cataloging-in-Publication Data

Cognitive-behavioral therapies for trauma / edited by Victoria M.
   Follette, Josef I. Ruzek.— 2nd ed.
      p. cm.
   Includes bibliographical references and index.
   ISBN-10: 1-59385-247-9 ISBN-13: 978-1-59385-247-4 (hardcover)
   ISBN-10: 1-59385-401-3 ISBN-13: 978-1-59385-401-0 (paperback)
   1. Post-traumatic stress disorder—Treatment. 2. Cognitive
therapy. I. Follette, Victoria M. II. Ruzek, Josef I.
RC552.P67C65 2006
616.85′210651—dc22

                                                    2005032412

To Laura E. Follette
–VMF

To Patty and Alex, with all my love
–JIR

About the Editors

Victoria M. Follette, PhD, is a clinical scientist with a special interest in the etiology and treatment of trauma-related problems. She is Professor of Psychology and Chair of the Department of Psychology at the University of Nevada, Reno. She was named Distinguished Alumna by the Department of Psychology at the University of Memphis, Tennessee, where she received her doctoral degree. Dr. Follette's clinical work is focused on survivors of interpersonal violence, and she examines the use of acceptance-based behavioral therapies in the treatment of this population.

Josef I. Ruzek, PhD, is Associate Director for Education at the National Center for PTSD and a psychologist with the VA Palo Alto Health Care System, Palo Alto, California. He received his doctorate in clinical psychology from the State University of New York at Stony Brook. Dr. Ruzek specializes in early intervention for trauma survivors.

Contributors

Deborah J. Brief, PhD, VA Boston Healthcare System, Boston University School of Medicine, Psychology Service, Boston, Massachusetts

Richard A. Bryant, PhD, School of Psychology, University of New South Wales, Sydney, New South Wales, Australia

Shawn P. Cahill, PhD, Center for the Treatment and Study of Anxiety, Department of Psychiatry, University of Pennsylvania, Philadelphia, Pennsylvania

Marylene Cloitre, PhD, Department of Psychiatry and Child Study Center, Institute for Trauma and Stress, New York University, New York, New York

Jill S. Compton, PhD, Department of Psychiatry and Behavioral Sciences, Duke University Medical Center, Durham, North Carolina

Esther Deblinger, PhD, Department of Psychiatry and Center for Children's Support, School of Osteopathic Medicine, University of Medicine and Dentistry of New Jersey, Stratford, New Jersey

Edna B. Foa, PhD, Center for the Treatment and Study of Anxiety, Department of Psychiatry, University of Pennsylvania, Philadelphia, Pennsylvania

Victoria M. Follette, PhD, Department of Psychology, University of Nevada, Reno, Reno, Nevada

William C. Follette, PhD, Department of Psychology, University of Nevada, Reno, Reno, Nevada

David W. Foy, PhD, Graduate School of Education and Psychology, Pepperdine University, Encino, California

Ellen Frank, PhD, Department of Psychiatry, University of Pittsburgh School of Medicine, Pittsburgh, Pennsylvania

Matthew J. Friedman, MD, PhD, National Center for PTSD, VA Medical Center, White River Junction, Vermont

Steven C. Hayes, PhD, Department of Psychology, University of Nevada, Reno, Reno, Nevada

Terence M. Keane, PhD, National Center for PTSD, VA Boston Healthcare System, Boston University School of Medicine, Boston, Massachusetts

Barbara S. Kohlenberg, PhD, Department of Psychiatry and Behavioral Sciences, University of Nevada, Reno, Nevada

Robert J. Kohlenberg, PhD, Department of Psychology, University of Washington, Seattle, Washington

Edward S. Kubany, PhD, National Center for PTSD, Department of Veterans Affairs, Honolulu, Hawaii

Linnea C. Larson, MA, MPH, Headington Program in International Trauma, Graduate School of Psychology, Fuller Theological Seminary, Pasadena, California

Leah M. Leonard, MA, Department of Psychology, University of Nevada, Reno, Reno, Nevada

Marsha M. Linehan, PhD, Department of Psychology, University of Washington, Seattle, Washington

Candice M. Monson, PhD, Women's Health Sciences Division, National Center for PTSD, VA Boston Healthcare System, Boston, Massachusetts

Lisa M. Najavits, PhD, Department of Psychiatry, Harvard Medical School, Cambridge, Massachusetts; Trauma Research Program (Alcohol and Drug Treatment Center), McLean Hospital, Belmont, Massachusetts

Amy E. Naugle, PhD, Department of Psychology, Western Michigan University, Kalamazoo, Michigan

Elizabeth M. Pratt, PhD, National Center for PTSD, VA Boston Healthcare System, Boston University School of Medicine, Boston, Massachusetts

Tyler C. Ralston, MA, National Center for PTSD, Department of Veterans Affairs, Honolulu, Hawaii

Patricia A. Resick, PhD, Women's Health Sciences Division, National Center for PTSD, VA Boston Healthcare System, Boston, Massachusetts

David S. Riggs, PhD, Center for the Treatment and Study of Anxiety, Department of Psychiatry, University of Pennsylvania, Philadelphia, Pennsylvania

Anna Rosenberg, BA, Adult Anxiety Clinic, Department of Psychology, Temple University, Philadelphia, Pennsylvania

Josef I. Ruzek, PhD, National Center for PTSD, VA Palo Alto Health Care System, Menlo Park, California

Erika Ryan, PhD, New Jersey CARES (Child Abuse Research Education Service) Institute, School of Osteopathic Medicine, University of Medicine and Dentistry of New Jersey, Stratford, New Jersey

Katherine Shear, MD, Department of Psychiatry, University of Pittsburgh School of Medicine, Pittsburgh, Pennsylvania; Bereavement and Grief Program, Western Psychiatric Institute and Clinic, Pittsburgh, Pennsylvania

Jillian C. Shipherd, PhD, Women's Health Sciences Division, National Center for PTSD, VA Boston Healthcare System, Boston, Massachusetts

Amy E. Street, PhD, Women's Health Sciences Division, National Center for PTSD, VA Boston Healthcare System, Boston, Massachusetts

Reena Thakkar-Kolar, PhD, New Jersey CARES (Child Abuse Research Education Service) Institute, School of Osteopathic Medicine, University of Medicine and Dentistry of New Jersey, Stratford, New Jersey

Mavis Tsai, PhD, private practice, Seattle, Washington

Amy W. Wagner, PhD, Department of Psychiatry and Behavioral Sciences, University of Washington, Seattle, Washington

Robyn D. Walser, PhD, National Center for PTSD and Sierra–Pacific Mental Illness Research, Education, and Clinical Centers (MIRECC), VA Palo Alto Health Care System, Menlo Park, California

Preface

This second edition of *Cognitive-Behavioral Therapies for Trauma* assembles contributions from leading developers of cognitive-behavioral[1] therapies applied to trauma-related problems. Cognitive-behavioral treatment approaches, together with the research and theoretical models on which they are based, are increasingly the treatment of choice. Because they are evidence-based helping methods, cognitive-behavioral treatment approaches, in their popularity, are fostering more widespread use of methods that we know are working. Nowhere is this more evident than in the treatment of trauma. In the several practice guidelines for treatment of posttraumatic stress disorder (PTSD) that have been developed since the first edition of this book was published (i.e., Foa, Keane, & Friedman, 2000; VA–DoD Clinical Practice Guideline Working Group, 2003; American Psychiatric Association Work Group on ASD and PTSD, 2004; National Collaborating Centre for Mental Health, 2005), cognitive-behavioral treatments are universally acknowledged to have the most significant empirical support. Cognitive-behavioral treatment approaches figure prominently in the recommendations made in these documents because cognitive-behavioral interventions have been routinely evaluated by reliable and valid assessment tools. Systematic, ongoing assessment of client functioning has always been integral to cognitive-behavioral and behavioral therapies. The empirical tradition of these approaches positions them well in an era where enthusiastic endorsements of treatments are less and less sufficient to justify them.

In addition to reviewing the research evidence supporting many cognitive-behavioral interventions, the 17 chapters in this volume describe and analyze a large range of treatment methodologies that have been applied across many trauma populations and contexts of care. Many of the treatments reviewed in these chapters are complex packages that target not only PTSD but also other trauma-related problems and processes. The complexity of the alternatives the authors offer reflects the fact that treatment providers and

---

[1]For the sake of brevity, the umbrella term "cognitive-behavioral" is used in this text to encompass a range of treatment approaches that have emerged from different behavioral and cognitive therapeutic models.

their clients have an impressive set of pragmatic tools for addressing problems to choose from. In this Preface, we illustrate some of the ways in which cognitive-behavioral interventions can assist providers in their work with traumatized clients, illustrated by the contributions of our chapter authors.

PROMOTING INDIVIDUALIZED ASSESSMENT

Our main rationale for developing this text is the idea that clinicians should base treatment on a detailed assessment of the client's unique individual needs, rather than simply administering a structured treatment package. Cognitive-behavioral assessment of PTSD and other trauma-related problems remains centered on a functional analysis of behavior, outlined in Chapter Two by Follette and Naugle. Their approach is that there is no "average" patient. It is necessary to develop an individualized understanding of the functional relationships among a person's behaviors, life conditions preceding the trauma, and how those factors are maintained after the trauma. For the clinician wrestling with trying to understand a complex human being in a set of complex social environments, these authors' emphasis on identifying important, controllable, and causal factors is critical: what are the specific variables that, when changed, will lead to large improvements in the behaviors of clinical interest, that can be affected by the clinician and client working together, and that, when modified, reliably produce changes in the target problem?

Cognitive-behavioral practitioners also believe that it is important to assess changes in problem behaviors and symptoms and thereby evaluate the effectiveness of their helping efforts. In their review of recent advances in psychological assessment of PTSD in adults, Pratt, Brief, and Keane in Chapter Three conclude that the assessment devices available for evaluating PTSD are comparable to or better than those for other psychological disorders. They identify a variety of measures that are helpful in assessing the effectiveness of treatment, as do most of the chapter authors with regard to their particular interventions.

TOOLS FOR TRAUMA-RELATED PROBLEMS

Cognitive-behavioral treatments are built around a set of fundamental helping procedures that target different sets of problems encountered by trauma survivors. These are (1) *coping skills training*, which focuses on teaching clients to respond effectively to the many situation-specific challenges associated with PTSD and other trauma-related difficulties, and to replace existing maladaptive responses with more effective ones; (2) *prolonged exposure*, which works to reduce conditioned fear responses connected with trauma memories and the stimuli that elicit them; (3) *cognitive therapy*, which assists survivors in modifying ways of thinking that create distress and interfere with recovery; and (4) *acceptance methods*, which recognize that some of the problems of trauma survivors are caused or worsened by avoidance behaviors, therefore encouraging survivors to fully experience and accept their own trauma-related emotions, thoughts, and feelings without trying to avoid them.

A primary feature of most treatments for PTSD is educating clients about the disorder and the rationales for treatment. Treatments focus on providing information and teaching new skills for living. Those who deliver cognitive-behavioral interventions explicitly conceptualize much of what they do as skills training, and as the field has developed, cognitive-behavioral methods have been designed to address a wide and growing array of skills that can be taught by clinicians to their clients. In this book, skills training approaches are outlined across chapters and form large parts of some of the interventions discussed, such as dialectical behavior therapy (DBT) as summarized by Wagner and Linehan in Chapter Six, the skills training in affect and interpersonal regulation (STAIR) treatment described by Cloitre and Rosenberg in Chapter Thirteen, and the Seeking Safety protocol presented by Najavits in Chapter Ten. The book as a whole includes extensive discussion of the client skills sets that are related to distress tolerance, emotion regulation, interpersonal effectiveness, personal safety, and mindfulness. The chapter authors show how cognitive-behavioral skills training technologies can be used to ensure that clients learn, practice, test, and transfer these skills into the real world of their daily lives.

Central to approaches that focus on reduction of posttraumatic fear reactions is exposure therapy. Prolonged exposure (PE) treatment is the most well-validated psychosocial treatment for PTSD. As described by Riggs, Cahill, and Foa in Chapter Four, it focuses on reducing trauma-related anxiety by encouraging the client to confront situations, activities, thoughts, and memories that are feared and avoided but that are not inherently dangerous. Treatment incorporates four primary procedures: education about trauma and PTSD, breathing retraining, *in vivo* or "real-world" exposure to feared but safe trauma-related situations that the client normally avoids, and imaginal exposure in which the client repeatedly describes memories of the traumatic event.

Many cognitive-behavioral approaches also emphasize how important to the recovery process it is to deal with distressing trauma-related appraisals and beliefs. Such beliefs are at the core of the difficulty experienced by clients, and this is readily apparent to most treatment providers. Cognitive processing therapy (CPT) represents perhaps the best articulated application of cognitive therapy methods to the problem of PTSD, and is described at length in this book by Shipherd, Street, and Resick in Chapter Five. CPT is built on the testable hypothesis that "an approach that elicits memories of the traumatic event and then directly confronts maladaptive beliefs, faulty attributions, and inaccurate expectations may be more effective than exposure therapy alone." Cognitive therapies also resonate with therapist experience in that they readily expand the range of trauma-related emotions tackled in therapy to include anger, sadness, helplessness, and guilt. The latter emotion often complicates treatment for those with PTSD; in Chapter Eleven of this volume, Kubany and Ralston provide both a cognitive-behavioral conceptualization of trauma-related guilt and a detailed account of cognitive therapy applied to trauma-related guilt and shame.

Acceptance-based interventions are increasingly being integrated into cognitive-behavioral treatments for trauma survivors. These approaches are represented in these pages, on DBT in Chapter Six by Wagner and Linehan and on acceptance and commitment therapy (ACT) in Chapter Seven by Walser and Hayes. DBT stresses the tension between acceptance and change, between accepting clients as they are but also attempting to modify their behavior. Both change-oriented and acceptance-oriented goals are seen as important in this therapy. ACT (which also stands for Accept, Choose, and Take Action) embraces the same two goals as DBT. It emphasizes a conscious abandonment of the mental and emotional change agenda when these change efforts do not work. The client is encouraged to accept thoughts, feelings, memories, and sensations without trying to eliminate or control them; to engage in practical, safe, and valued behaviors that may include changing the situation; and to discriminate between unworkable solutions (e.g., avoiding emotions) and workable solutions (e.g., commitment to behavior change).

Those who have been exposed to traumatic events are at risk for developing many kinds of problems, and if cognitive-behavioral methods are to be widely adopted by a broad range of practitioners, they need to assist clinicians in comprehensively addressing the needs of their clients. This book illustrates the fact that those who are developing cognitive-behavioral treatment have been showing increased attention to significant problems trauma survivors face that are beyond the traditionally identified diagnosis of PTSD. In this text, this attention is reflected in the work of Najavits in extending cognitive-behavioral methods to the treatment of substance abuse concurrent with PTSD, Cloitre and Rosenberg in conceptualizing interventions to reduce risk of revictimization among sexual assault survivors, and by Shear and Frank in Chapter Twelve in their work on complicated grief. It is also shown in Chapter Nine, in Bryant's adaptation and extension of the procedures found effective in management of chronic PTSD to treat acute stress disorder. In the final chapter in this volume, Chapter Seventeen, Ruzek discusses the potential for cognitive-behavioral psychology to inform efforts to prevent development of PTSD and shows how the work of Bryant and others has led cognitive-behavioral practitioners to become increasingly active in developing and testing early interventions with survivors of recent traumas.

ATTENDING TO INTERPERSONAL PROCESSES
IN TREATMENT

Addressing Survivors' Interpersonal Problems

Trauma survivors' problems often show themselves in the survivors' inter-personal interactions. Cognitive-behavioral psychology has, of course, a rich history of attention to the interpersonal context of behavior problems, a focus that is seeing increasing development related to PTSD. In this book, interventions that focus on couples' concerns are described in Chapter Four-teen by Leonard, Follette, and Compton. Deblinger, Thakkar-Kolar, and Ryan in Chapter Sixteen describe interventions that work conjointly with both children and parents in addressing child traumatic experiences. Group psychotherapy, an important component of treatment for many trauma sur-vivors, is reviewed in Chapter Fifteen by Foy and Larsen. The latter authors point to the advantages for trauma survivors—whose experiences so com-monly involve social isolation, social alienation, perceptions of being ostra-cized from the larger society, shame, and diminished feelings for others—of working toward recovery with other survivors.

Working with Challenging Clinical Behaviors

Mental health providers must navigate many difficult situations in their inter-actions with survivors. For example, clients with a history of trauma in the family of origin may have developed a number of maladaptive coping mech-anisms to deal not only with the trauma but also with other invalidating aspects of their environment. In fact, much of what is particularly helpful in cognitive-behavioral interventions goes beyond the core treatment compo-nents outlined in the sections above, and includes procedures that help the therapist both to motivate the client and to avoid or manage difficult clinical situations such as suicidal behavior. These procedures include encouraging the client to take an active role in setting the goals of treatment, presenting persuasive rationales for treatment, assigning and ensuring completion of homework tasks, instructing clients in techniques of self-monitoring, and so on. For example, Najavits emphasizes in her Seeking Safety treatment ways of giving clients control whenever possible, "listening" to client behavior more than words, giving positive and negative feedback to clients, and asking clients about their reactions to treatment. In the same spirit, Wagner and Linehan utilize a number of techniques from DBT to address noncompli-ance, suicidal ideation, and other self-injurious behavior.

Using the Therapeutic Relationship

In their historical perspective on cognitive-behavioral therapies for trauma, Monson and Friedman in Chapter One observe that cognitive-behavioral therapy is often stereotyped as a mechanical form of therapy lacking in a certain type of human contact. But the attention to interpersonal processes that is included in many cognitive-behavioral therapies also extends to the client–therapist relationship. Generally, most of the approaches described in this text emphasize the importance of the therapeutic relationship. In particular, functional analytic psychotherapy (FAP) as described in Chapter Eight by Kohlenberg, Tsai, and Kohlenberg provides an extensive introduction to how providers of cognitive-behavioral treatments can use the therapeutic relationship as a primary component of treatment. This conceptualization, in contrast to the stereotypes of cognitive-behavioral treatments, places the client–therapist relationship at the core of the change process. FAP theory indicates that the therapeutic process is facilitated by a caring, genuine, sensitive, and emotional client–therapist relationship. The therapeutic relationship itself is used to help identify interpersonal stimuli that lead to problems and to provide *in vivo* opportunities to change interpersonal repertoires. Therapists are taught to recognize and address clinically relevant behaviors that occur in session, and to strengthen client improvements within the therapy session itself. DBT similarly posits that a strong relationship characterized by mutual trust, respect, and positive regard will increase the likelihood that the client will engage in efforts to change that are difficult and uncomfortable, and that a strong relationship can be therapy in itself.

RESPONDING TO THE NEEDS OF CLINICIANS

Providing Training and Support for Clinicians

A prime obstacle to the increased use of cognitive-behavioral methods to assist trauma survivors is the fact that most clinicians have not received training in the types of approaches outlined in this book. Awareness of this is leading developers of cognitive-behavioral treatments to explore ways of improving the training of community providers in using their approaches. For example, Riggs, Cahill, and Foa note the lack of opportunities for training in PE, and also acknowledge that conventional training workshops are ineffective in changing the behavior of practitioners; few workshop attendees actually end up using exposure. In response, they have developed two models of training. In the first, experts provide intensive training as well as continued supervision of therapist trainees. In the second model, experts provide intensive initial training, but ongoing supervision of the new practitioners is provided by local supervisors who consult with the experts but over time become experts themselves. Other authors in this book who devote attention to training and supervision issues include Foy and Larson, who consider the requisite therapist skills for conducting cognitive-behavioral trauma groups; and Kohlenberg, Tsai, and Kohlenberg, who discuss issues of clinical supervision in FAP. As outlined by Wagner and Linehan, DBT is notable for its explicit assertion that therapists treating patients with border-line personality disorder need support. Therapist consultation groups are an essential component of DBT: they provide that needed support, as well as development, and can help minimize therapist burnout.

Enabling Integration with Other Treatment Approaches

The point should be made that cognitive-behavioral methods are more likely to be widely used if they have the potential to be integrated with other approaches. Disseminating cognitive-behavioral approaches does not mean that they should replace the other approaches. Rather, they would be a com-plement to methods they are used in conjunction with, perhaps addressing aspects of the problem not dealt with well by the principal orientation. In the present volume, many of the authors speak to the capacity for integration of their approaches with other treatments. Walser and Hayes state that if research indicates that a client's problems would be better treated by a dif-ferent approach, that latter treatment should be implemented first or inte-grated into the course of ACT. DBT and Seeking Safety are designed to be frontline stages of treatment for individuals with PTSD, so as to get the client stabilized prior to introducing exposure treatment. Najavits has explored how to integrate trauma processing therapy with Seeking Safety. Kubany and Ralston introduce a variety of ways to understand and challenge trauma-related guilt. Awareness of the role of guilt, and Kubany and Ralston's inter-ventions, would be combined with other treatments not designed to system-atically address guilt. An element that Monson and Friedman touch on is that psychopharmacological treatments can either help or impede a concur-rent cognitive-behavioral treatment. Complicated grief treatment (CGT), described in this volume by Shear and Frank, illustrates well the capacity for integration of cognitive-behavioral treatments with those based on other the-oretical orientations. Shear and Frank created CGT by mixing interpersonal therapy—an existing short-term, present-oriented treatment for grief—with cognitive-behavioral methods for treatment of PTSD, as well as with cogni-tive strategies for dealing with the distress of separation.

PROMOTING INDIVIDUALIZED TREATMENT

The question of how cognitive-behavioral treatment should be packaged for delivery by clinicians and programs is an important one. Many of the treat-ments described in this book are broken down into a series of steps, so that clinicians can provide the treatments and apply them effectively. This does not mean that one must slavishly follow the steps of treatment. Indeed, such structured cognitive-behavioral treatments are flexible, provide therapists with options, and rely heavily on therapist and client decision making. Just as "assessment" is really a process of coming to understand a unique individual, so too treatment must reach beyond "cookbook" applications and formulate a cognitive-behavioral approach that fits the individual client. We hope that readers of this book will become familiar with a host of cognitive-behavioral interventions.

In fact, some of the contributors to this book refer to the limitations of step-based, or "manualized," treatments and they propose alternatives. Leonard, Follette, and Compton identify two major potential problems in delivering formalized, prepackaged treatment techniques to survivor couples: (1) use of prepackaged techniques may not sufficiently encourage therapists to *not* lose sight of the individual or couple, and (2) treatments based on a manual do not prepare therapists to cope with problems outside the manual's scope. These authors argue that treatment manuals may lead therapists to believe that they understand a person based on his or her initial presentation or diagnosis, but then they fail to assess clients on a continuing basis. In the worst case, treatment providers are concerned with getting back on the protocol rather than listening to the couple. As an alternative to treatment packages that either are overly formulaic or could be misused that way in the wrong hands, Leonard, Follette, and Compton recommend the development of a "principle-based" intervention for couples that relies on helping principles rather than particular techniques or structures. Similarly, Wagner and Linehan consider DBT to be a principle-driven (not protocol-driven) intervention.

CONCLUSION

Cognitive-behavioral approaches to helping trauma survivors continue to evolve, with treatment methods remaining a work in progress. A number of limitations remain in the current evidence base, but despite this, the chapters in this book provide a significant argument that cognitive-behavioral approaches taken as a whole constitute a powerful form of treatment. They provide the clinician with a substantial and growing set of treatment concepts and tools, address a wide range of trauma-related problems and populations, and consider the interpersonal context of treatment. They reflect the complexity of the individual, and increasingly they take into account the perspective and needs of treatment providers in the field. The contributors to this text are working to develop comprehensive treatment approaches based on the foundation of science. We believe that in doing so, they are providing an invaluable service to the many people who will survive a traumatic experience.

REFERENCES

American Psychiatric Association Work Group on ASD and PTSD. (2004). *Practice guideline for the treatment of patients with acute stress disorder and posttraumatic stress disorder*. Washington, DC: American Psychiatric Association.

Foa, E. B., Keane, T. M., & Friedman, M. J. (2000). *Effective treatments for PTSD: Practice guidelines from the International Society for Traumatic Stress Studies.* New York: Guilford Press.

National Collaborating Centre for Mental Health. (2005). *Post-traumatic stress disorder: The management of PTSD in adults and children in primary and secondary care.* London: National Institute for Clinical Excellence.

VA–DoD Clinical Practice Guideline Working Group, Veterans Health Administration, Department of Veterans Affairs and Health Affairs, Department of Defense. (2003). *Management of post-traumatic stress* (Publication No. 10Q-CPG/PTSD-04). Washington, DC: Office of Quality and Performance.

Contents

CHAPTER ONE

Back to the Future of Understanding Trauma
Implications for Cognitive-Behavioral Therapies for Trauma

Candice M. Monson
Matthew J. Friedman

Cognitive-behavioral therapy (CBT) for trauma represents a broad class of therapies unified by a shared emphasis on observable outcomes, symptom amelioration, time-limited and goal-oriented intervention, and an expectation that patients will assume an active role in getting better. An additional strength of CBT applied to trauma is its adherence to evidence-based conceptualization of patients' posttraumatic psychopathology. We assert that increased understanding of the nature of posttraumatic reactions can translate into enhanced effectiveness and innovations in CBT for trauma. Here we trace the evolving history of understanding posttraumatic pathology, and with an appreciation of this past, offer a vision of upcoming achievements and challenges in the application of CBT for trauma.

POSTTRAUMATIC REACTIONS: LONG RECOGNIZED BUT VARIABLY LABELED

Documented human history is replete with descriptions of individual reactions to traumatic events. For example, a survivor of the Great Fire of London in the 1600s wrote in his diary 6 months after his exposure, "it is strange to think how to this very day I cannot sleep a night without great terrors of the fire; and this very night could not sleep to almost two in the morning through great terrors of the fire" (quoted in Saigh & Bremner, 1999, p. 1). There has been remarkable consistency in the description of such posttraumatic reactions throughout the centuries, whether written by poets and novelists or clinicians and scientists. Despite this general agreement on observable phenomenology, many different causal mechanisms and diagnostic labels have been proposed. Indeed, the theoretical etiology of these reactions as organic versus psychological as well as the diagnostic classification of traumatic reactions have evolved over time.

Historical Conceptualizations

When the scientific approach to psychopathology emerged in the 19th century, the zeitgeist was to determine organic pathogeneses, such as lesions of the nervous system, as the major cause of nervous disorders. Posttraumatic reactions were no exception to this theoretical organic orientation. Some of the most detailed writings and elaborated conceptualizations of traumatic reactions are found in the literature on combatants.

Starting with the Civil War, American conceptualizations of posttraumatic reactions were understood mostly as somatic/physiological reactions, usually affecting the cardiovascular system. According to Hyams, Wignell, and Roswell (1996), proposed somatic/physiological diagnoses were Da Costa syndrome/irritable heart (Civil War); soldier's heart, neurocirculatory asthenia, and shell shock (World War I); and effort syndrome (World War II). Attributing these reactions to organic causes had a number of sociopolitical implications: Soldiers could avoid the stigma and sense of personal failure associated with mental disorders, and the military could ignore the need for psychological interventions.

Although there is only a smattering of accounts of the psychological sequelae of natural and technological disasters during the late 19th century, it is known that civilian traumas were also attributed to organic causes. For example, "Railway spine" was considered to be the result of railroad accidents that produced theoretical, but usually unobservable, physical lesions or insults to the brain, spinal cord, or peripheral nervous system. This condition is representative of the tendency to attribute otherwise unexplainable physical disabilities to abnormal central nervous system mechanisms. Indeed, an English surgeon, John Erichsen (1882), cautioned against confusing (what he assumed to be) the organically caused symptoms of railway spine with hysteria, the prevailing diagnosis of the times (van der Kolk, Weisaeth, & van der Hart, 1996). When physical injuries could not be found in these patients, their symptoms were attributed to subtle forms of neurological damage and a general functional disturbance of the nervous balance or tone. The German neurologist Herman Oppenheim (1915) is credited with coining the term "traumatic neurosis." He proposed that functional problems were a result of subtle molecular changes in the central nervous system following exposure to trauma.

Posttraumatic reactions were not left out of Kraepelin's (1896) efforts in the 1800s to classify and organize mental disorders. He developed a common label for these multiple nervous and psychic phenomena: "schreck-neuroses," or fright neuroses. Schreckneuroses were believed to result from severe emotional upheaval or sudden fright, and to have neurological under-pinnings. The symptoms of schreckneuroses were observed after serious accidents and injuries, particularly fires, railway derailments or collisions (Saigh & Bremner, 1999).

Sigmund Freud rebelled against the primary focus on organic explana-tions for psychopathology in vogue during that period. Because of his influ-ence, psychological etiologies began to be proposed for understanding and treating psychopathology, in general, and posttraumatic reactions, in partic-ular. Freud theorized that, because traumatic events overwhelm the psyche, traumatized individuals must engage extremely primitive defense mecha-nisms such as dissociation, repression, and denial. Catharsis and abreaction, involving high levels of emotional expression, were considered the necessary treatment for countering these primitive defenses (Freud, 1950). Other con-temporaneous psychological conceptualizations of combat trauma included nostalgia (Civil War), battle fatigue/combat exhaustion/operational fatigue (World War I), and war/traumatic neurosis (World War II) (Hyams et al., 1996).

Although Freud stood strong against the winds of the medical and scien-tific culture pertaining to organic versus psychological explanations of psy-chopathology, he unfortunately wavered in the winds of Victorian culture regarding childhood sexual abuse. His emphasis on the internal workings of individuals—psychosexual drives and early developmental processes—to the exclusion of external stressors such as childhood sexual abuse was a serious oversight from our modern perspective (see Pendergrast, 1999, for more thorough review of this debate). Freud's legacy is also found in the recovered memory versus false memory debate that erupted in the early 1990s. His notion of the primitive defenses involved in traumatization, and especially repression, has been the foundation of claims regarding recovered memo-ries of sexual abuse. Although the potential for psychogenic amnesia of trau-matic events cannot be completely ruled out, the past 15 years of scientific evidence questions the veracity of such memories and the possible iatrogenic effects of psychotherapy in creating them (Brewin, 2003).

Freud's contemporary, Pierre Janet, was also instrumental in bringing a psychological approach to posttraumatic reactions, and his writings include some precursor elements of CBT. Indeed, cognitive-behavioral theories of traumatic reactions find their roots in Janet's writings about the categoriza-tion and integration of memories. He contended that people develop mean-ing schemes based on past experiences that prepare them to cope with sub-sequent challenges. When people experience "vehement emotions" in response to frightening experiences, their minds are not capable of integrat-ing the events with existing cognitive schemes. When the memories cannot be integrated into personal awareness, something akin to dissociation occurs. Janet also introduced the notion of patients experiencing a "phobia of memory" that prevents the integration of traumatic events. The memory traces linger as long as they are not translated into a personal narrative. In his conception of trauma, synthesis and integration are the goals of treatment, which was in contrast to the psychoanalytic goals of catharsis and abreaction prevalent at the time (Janet, 1907).

Abram Kardiner, a psychoanalyst who treated World War I veterans, was an early proponent of uniting these organic and psychological conceptual streams. He proposed that veterans who experienced an enduring clinical syndrome resulting from war-zone exposure suffered from a "physioneurosis." This label denotes both physiological and psychological components of trauma reactions and the complex biobehavioral clinical picture exhibited by these veterans. In that regard, Kardiner anticipated, by almost 40 years, many of the symptoms included in the first formal diagnosis of posttraumatic stress disorder (PTSD). Because of this insight, which contradicted prevailing psychoanalytic doctrine, Kardiner might be considered the father of psychobiological theory, research, and practice concerning trauma. As a therapist he acknowledged the changes in self-concept that can occur after trauma exposure, and he was a proponent of psychotherapy to ameliorate both psychological and physiological trauma sequelae (Kardiner, 1941).

Kardiner's work was rediscovered by Lawrence Kolb (1987), who theorized that fear conditioning in the limbic system, especially the amygdala, was responsible for the stable psychological and physiological abnormalities found in posttraumatic reactions. Since Kolb's work, there has been an explosion of basic and translational research documenting psychobiological alterations in trauma patients and thereby providing a rationale for pharmacological interventions (Charney, 2004; Friedman, 2003; Friedman, Charney, & Deutch, 1995; Yehuda & McFarlane, 1997).

Diagnostic Evolution

Our evolving conception of posttraumatic reactions is exemplified by sequential revisions of the *Diagnostic and Statistical Manual of Mental Disorders* (DSM) with regard to both diagnostic categories and PTSD diagnostic criteria across the DSM revisions. To account for the war-related psychopathology discussed above, the first edition of the DSM (DSM-I; American Psychiatric Association [APA], 1952) included the diagnosis "gross stress reaction." This diagnosis was seen as appropriate for cases involving exposure to "severe, physical demands or extreme stress, such as in combat or civilian catastrophe" (p. 40). Like other disorders in the DSM-I, diagnostic criteria delineating the disorder were not specified. Bucking the prevailing notion of the times that those who developed this reaction were characterologically weak, the DSM-I noted that the diagnosis often applied to "previously more or less 'normal' persons who experience intolerable stress" (p. 40). Unfortunately, gross stress reaction was diluted in the second edition of the DSM (DSM-II; APA, 1968) to "transient situational disturbance." Although there was a continued emphasis on the "overwhelming" nature of an environmental stressor(s) over individual diatheses in causing the reaction, the focus was exclusively on "transient fear associated with military combat and manifested by trembling, running and hiding" (p. 48). There was no diagnostic acknowledgment that such symptoms might characterize a chronic, rather than an acute and naturally resolving, condition.

Influential writings in the 1970s and 1980s about the clinical presentations of sexual assault and domestic violence victims led to the "rape trauma syndrome" and "battered women syndrome" designations (Burgess & Holmstrom, 1974; Walker, 1984). These newly recognized conditions, in tandem with research on the mental health of World War II prisoners of war, survivors of the Nazi Holocaust, and returning Vietnam veterans, led to greater realization of the generalizability of reactions to life-threatening stressors. During this time, the PTSD diagnosis was unveiled as an anxiety disorder in the third edition of the DSM (DSM-III; APA, 1980). Criteria for the traumatic stressor and specific symptoms were organized into three clusters. Accounting for the range of potentially traumatic events, the stressor criterion was described as something "generally beyond the realm of normal human experience that would evoke significant symptoms of distress in most people" (p. 236). The DSM-III revision (DSM-III-R; APA, 1987) resulted in few changes in the stressor definition and symptom inclusion and organization, but did delineate age-specific features.

The fourth revision of the DSM (DSM-IV; APA, 1994) and its text revision (DSM-IV-TR; APA, 2000) excluded the provision that the traumatic stressor be generally outside the range of normal human experience. This change reflects the empirical evidence that the experience of a stressor capable of producing PTSD is actually quite common. In fact, 75% or more of people will experience such a stressor in their lifetime (Breslau, 2002). More importantly, in the DSM-IV the nature of the individual's reaction to a traumatic stressor was taken into account. The nomothetic standard that the experience would evoke significant symptoms of distress in most people was replaced with an idiographic, subjective criterion. According to the DSM-IV, individuals who have been "traumatized" must have had an overwhelming emotional reaction, defined as "intense fear, helplessness or horror" (p. 428) when confronted by an extremely stressful experience. The operational definition of stressful experiences was also expanded to include observing or receiving information about the traumatic events suffered by others. Although some of the symptom clusters were rearranged and diagnostic thresholds were adjusted, the greatest changes in the symptom criteria were the requirements of additional functional impairment and 1–month of symptom duration.

As described by Brewin (2003) in his more complete discussion of the controversy surrounding diagnosis of posttraumatic reactions, "skeptics" of the PTSD diagnosis assert that the diagnosis is a sociopolitical invention that has been created in a litigious Western society that seeks to place blame and identify victims and perpetrators. Skeptics argue that PTSD is not found in non-Westernized cultures and contend that normal human reactions to a stressful event only become pathological when diagnoses are applied to them. At their worst, these opponents propose that diagnosing posttraumatic reactions has iatrogenic effects on those who are diagnosed.

These criticisms have been countered by empirical data showing that individuals manifest ongoing trauma-related reactions when there are no identifiable secondary gain issues, and after any of these potential gains has been resolved (e.g., disability compensation, civil or criminal lawsuits; Bryant & Harvey, 2003). Furthermore, evidence has accumulated that PTSD is readily identifiable in traditional, nonindustrialized cultures, although it remains controversial whether more culture-specific idioms of posttraumatic distress might provide a better diagnostic characterization of such syndromes (de Jong, 2002; Green et al., 2003; Marsella, Friedman, Gerrity, & Monsour, 1996).

Prospective studies reveal that a large majority (i.e., 94%) of traumatized individuals will manifest symptoms consistent with a PTSD diagnosis or other mental health problems (e.g., depression, panic, anxiety) in the immediate aftermath of trauma. However, by 3 to 6 months, most individuals' symptoms have resolved (Foa & Riggs, 1995; Kessler, Sonnega, Bromet, Hughes, & Nelson, 1995; Marsella et al., 1996; Norris, Murphy, Baker, & Perilla, 2003; Schlenger et al., 2002). Thus it is important to emphasize that there is a significant amount of "normal" distress that follows exposure to traumatic events that should not be construed as pathological. These data have led several researchers to offer the conceptualization of PTSD as a disorder of "nonrecovery" from trauma exposure (e.g., Rothbaum, Foa, Riggs, Murdock, & Walsh, 1992; Shalev, 1997). It is the persistence and severity of symptoms and the functional impairments that merit diagnosis. Epidemiological studies also argue against the notion of a naturally remitting course for those who do not recover from traumatic events and develop PTSD, given that approximately one-third of affected individuals continue to suffer from the disorder 10 years after their trauma exposure (Kessler et al., 1995). Biological investigations, including psychophysiological, neurohormonal, and neuroimaging studies, contradict the notion that all traumatic reactions are part of a normal stress adaptation process (Yehuda & McFarlane, 1997).

It is important to acknowledge the criticisms leveled against the diagnosis of posttraumatic reactions because they have important implications for deciding whether or not, and when, to provide intervention following traumatic events. From our perspective, there are definitely pathological posttraumatic reactions that call for intervention. We contend that the challenges of treating trauma with CBT are not related to uncertainty regarding the pathological conditions that can develop in response to traumatic exposure, but rather concern the nature and clinical phenomenology of such reactions for treatment.

ANTICIPATED CHALLENGES AND ACHIEVEMENTS

As we previously noted, a scientifically grounded conceptualization of patients' problems is the first step to effective CBT for trauma. Historical review of the understanding of posttraumatic reactions illuminates several important opportunities for the future of CBT for trauma. Translational research and continued interface between science and practice will further the conceptualization of traumatic reactions in order to improve CBT of them. In general, developers and practitioners of CBT for trauma looking toward the future should capitalize on the evidence that the sequelae of trauma are wide-ranging, multidimensional, and multidetermined.

Several factor-analytic studies since DSM-IV was published have raised questions about the nature and processes underlying PTSD (Foa, Riggs, & Gershuny, 1995; King, Leskin, King, & Weathers, 1998). These studies reveal that, contrary to the DSM-IV, there appear to be four, not three, clusters of PTSD symptoms. Symptoms of effortful avoidance and emotional numbing, included together in the DSM-IV, appear to have different properties, functions, and possible etiologies, according to these studies. Moreover, memory loss, a symptom included in the DSM-IV's avoidance/numbing cluster, does not appear to be associated with the overall construct of PTSD or the symptom clusters. Interestingly, the most conclusive of these studies (King et al., 1998) does not support the notion that PTSD is an overarching, unitary disorder comprised of four symptom clusters. Rather, PTSD appears to be best conceptualized as a heterogeneous disorder with correlated, but separate, symptom manifestations. Recent typology efforts also support this heterogeneity in PTSD presentation (Miller, Greif, & Smith, 2003).

Another important classification consideration on the horizon is whether or not acute stress disorder (ASD) and PTSD should be classified as anxiety disorders. Evidence supporting abandonment of the anxiety disorder placement indicates that a myriad of emotions, including guilt, shame, disgust, anger, and sadness, have been implicated in preventing recovery from posttraumatic symptoms (Resick, 2001). Moreover, Pitman (1993) has argued that the pathophysiology of arousal in posttraumatic reaction is not simply anxiety. The *International Statistical Classification of Diseases, Injury, and Causes of Death–10th Edition* (ICD-10; World Health Organization [WHO], 1992) does not classify PTSD as an anxiety disorder; rather, it is categorized within the spectrum of "reactions to severe stress, and adjustment disorders," with the common denominator of stress-related precipitation. A recent taxometric study buttresses the dimensional versus categorical system of trauma-related diagnoses (Ruscio, Ruscio, & Keane, 2002).

A spectrum of stress disorders, with specifiers beyond "acute," "chronic," and "delayed onset" currently used for PTSD, could more fully describe the phenomenology of trauma survivors and have important treatment ramifications. Like other major DSM-IV disorder classes (e.g., mood, psychotic), there could be a range of disorders with various symptom constellations and specifiers. An SD as well as the dissociative disorders, could be placed in this class. PTSD specifiers such as "prominent dissociation," "prominent emotional numbing," and "prominent anger" could have important theoretical and treatment implications. Additionally, age-related features and presentations of these stress reactions are important. There may even be room for chronic stress reactions to nontraumatic stressors.

It is important to remember that previous statistical approaches to organizing the core features of posttraumatic reactions are limited by the items that are included in the statistical analyses. The DSM-IV PTSD Work Group restricted criteria to "essential features" for making the PTSD diagnosis. However, this approach risks the danger of missing characteristics that have important clinical and treatment relevance. We suggest that, in addition to moving beyond anxiety-based symptom presentations and to enhance recovery among survivors of traumatic stress, CBT for trauma consider and address other frequently observed serious psychological, emotional, and interpersonal problems. Regardless of the diagnostic scheme used, the epidemiological and taxometric findings argue for distinct assessment of, and multicomponent treatment for, the multidimensional nature of posttraumatic pathology (Flack, Litz, Weathers, & Beaudreau, 2002; Keane & Kaloupek, 2002).

In spite of having several very efficacious CBTs for trauma-related pathology (described in this book), it is important to realize that about 50% of the patients in efficacy studies maintain their trauma-related diagnoses at the end of treatment and at follow-up periods (Zayfert, Becker, & Gillock, 2002). This symptom maintenance may be related, in part, to our current conceptualization of trauma sequelae and to the fact that the current evidence-based treatments, in isolation, address some specific aspects of trauma better than others. For example, some treatment studies reveal that avoidance and numbing symptoms, and especially emotional numbing, may be less responsive to our current CBT treatments (e.g., Glynn et al., 1999; Keane & Kaloupek, 1982). There is also some early evidence that different CBTs may be better at addressing the different emotional disturbances resulting from traumatization (e.g., Resick, Nishith, Weaver, Astin, & Feuer, 2002).

In this vein, efforts to determine predictors of treatment response to CBT for trauma may help address diagnostic dilemmas and ultimately improve treatment planning and outcomes. We recommend that future studies consider predictors beyond those that have been traditionally investigated (e.g., PTSD severity, anger, substance abuse), and develop theoretically driven models that can be tested. Following from our recommendations about broadening the range of trauma symptoms to consider, interpersonal functioning, social support, affective regulation, and self-efficacy might be considered. Biological markers may even be useful to consider in the future, as the psychobiological findings become more robust and are shown to correspond with CBT treatment response.

In the last decade the field of CBT for trauma has seen a series of head-to-head trials designed to determine the treatment "winner." These trials have resulted in many more "ties" than declared winners. We anticipate that the next generation of dismantling, combination therapy, and effectiveness studies will reveal very intriguing findings about the key ingredients of efficacious treatment, as well as the limits and challenges to using these treatments in clinical settings. Given that many patients simultaneously receive two or more treatments in clinical practice (e.g., Rosen et al., 2004), studies that determine how best to time or integrate treatments for greater efficacy will be valuable. The possibility for psychopharmacological treatments to potentiate or possibly interfere with CBT for trauma should also be investigated. Like others (Foa, Rothbaum, & Furr, 2003), we call for more combination studies aimed at addressing nonresponse or partial response to treatment, in lieu of the rates of non- and partial response found in previous studies.

An additional factor to investigate with regard to treatment timing and sequencing relates to the co-occurring diagnoses often given to traumatized individuals. Determining the best sequence or combination of treatments to treat these disorders is very important for the future of CBT for trauma. As an example, many prior PTSD treatment studies have excluded patients with comorbid substance dependence, suggesting that these issues should be addressed prior to a course of CBT for PTSD. There have been a few developing efforts to provide serial or integrative trauma and substance abuse treatment (Coffey, Dansky, & Brady, 2003; Najavits, 2002). Depression, personality disorders, anger problems, self-harming behavior, and relationship dysfunction are other frequently co-occurring diagnoses or clinical issues to address. Researchers have designed several treatments to specifically address these problems in tandem with PTSD treatment (Chemtob, Novaco, Hamada, & Gross, 1997; Cloitre, Koenen, Cohen, & Han, 2002; Monson, Schnurr, Stevens, & Guthrie, 2004). However, other researchers have argued that the existing CBTs for PTSD should be undertaken first, because effective treatment for PTSD can remedy many of these co-occurring issues (e.g., Cahill, Rauch, Hembree, & Foa, 2003). These are questions in need of further empirical investigation.

The cognitive-behavioral framework has an important role in informing prevention and early-intervention efforts. Because this area has been wrought with controversy, leading with a strong theoretical grounding for these interventions will be crucial. In addition, the caricature of CBT is that it is a mechanical and technical venture devoid of any humanity. A solid therapeutic relationship is essential to all forms of psychotherapy. Treatment process studies that pinpoint specific dimensions of the therapeutic relationship that are detrimental or facilitative of trauma recovery are essential (Cloitre, Stovall-McClough, Miranda, & Chemtob, 2004).

There are a number of intriguing questions to be answered with regard to the effectiveness, versus efficacy, of CBT for trauma. Most of the outcome studies to date have been undertaken in outpatient research clinics. Ongoing efforts to transport these best practices into clinical settings, and likewise, to use the clinical experiences to inform research, will be invaluable.

Although several CBTs for trauma with solid evidence bases are available, there remains a need for innovative treatments that can help the significant number of patients who do not respond to our current treatments. Understanding of the nature and treatment of trauma is a continuously evolving process. We have come a long way in conceptualizing the aftereffects of trauma and in developing elegant, theoretically driven CBTs that work. We look forward to the advancements that will be made in the next generation of CBT for trauma.

ACKNOWLEDGMENTS

This research was supported by a Clinical Research Career Development Award to Candice M. Monson from the Department of Veterans Affairs (VA) Cooperative Studies Program and by the VA National Center for Posttraumatic Stress Disorder.

REFERENCES

American Psychiatric Association. (1952). *Diagnostic and statistical manual of mental disorders*. Washington, DC: Author.

American Psychiatric Association. (1968). *Diagnostic and statistical manual of mental disorders* (2nd ed.). Washington, DC: Author.

American Psychiatric Association. (1980). *Diagnostic and statistical manual of mental disorders* (3rd ed.). Washington, DC: Author.

American Psychiatric Association. (1987). *Diagnostic and statistical manual of mental disorders* (3rd ed., rev.). Washington, DC: Author.

American Psychiatric Association. (1994). *Diagnostic and statistical manual of mental disorders* (4th ed.). Washington, DC: Author.

American Psychiatric Association. (2000). *Diagnostic and statistical manual of mental disorders* (4th ed., text rev.). Washington, DC: Author.

Breslau, N. (2002). Epidemiologic studies of trauma, posttraumatic stress disorder, and other psychiatric disorders. *Canadian Journal of Psychiatry, 47*, 923–929.

Brewin, C. R. (2003). *Posttraumatic stress disorder: Malady or myth?* New Haven, CT: Yale University Press.

Bryant, R. A., & Harvey, A. G. (2003). The influence of litigation on maintenance of posttraumatic stress disorder. *Journal of Nervous and Mental Disease, 191*(3), 191–193.

Burgess, A. W., & Holmstrom, L. L. (1974). Rape trauma syndrome. *American Journal of Psychiatry, 131*(9), 981–986.

Cahill, S. P., Rauch, S. M., Hembree, E. A., & Foa, E. B. (2003). Effect of cognitive-behavioral treatments for PTSD on anger. *Journal of Cognitive Psychotherapy, 17*(3), 113–131.

Charney, D. S. (2004). Psychobiological mechanisms of resilience and vulnerability:

Implications for successful adaptation to extreme stress. *American Journal of Psychiatry, 161*(2), 195–216.

Chemtob, C. M., Novaco, R. W., Hamada, R. S., & Gross, D. M. (1997). Cognitive-behavioral treatment for severe anger in posttraumatic stress disorder. *Journal of Consulting and Clinical Psychology, 65,* 184–189.

Cloitre, M., Koenen, K. C., Cohen, L. R., & Han, H. (2002). Skills training in affective and interpersonal regulation followed by exposure: A phase based treatment for PTSD related to childhood abuse. *Journal of Consulting and Clinical Psychology, 70*(5), 1067–1074.

Cloitre, M., Stovall-McClough, K., Miranda, R., & Chemtob, C. M. (2004). Therapeutic alliance, negative mood regulation, and treatment outcome in child abuse-related posttraumatic stress disorder. *Journal of Consulting and Clinical Psychology, 72,* 411–416.

Coffey, S. F., Dansky, B. S., & Brady, K. T. (2003). Exposure-based, trauma-focused therapy for comorbid posttraumatic stress disorder-substance use disorder. In P. C. Ouimette & P. J. Brown (Eds.), *Trauma and substance abuse: Causes, consequences, and treatment of comorbid disorders* (pp. 127–146). Washington, DC: American Psychological Association.

de Jong, J. T. V. M. (2002). *Trauma, war, and violence: Public mental health in socio-cultural context.* New York: Kluwer Academic/Plenum.

Erichsen, J. E. (1882). *On concussion of the spine, nervous shock, and other obscure injuries of the nervous system in their clinical and medico-legal aspects.* New York: Gham.

Flack, W. F., Jr., Litz, B. T., Weathers, F. W., & Beaudreau, S. A. (2002). Assessment and diagnosis of PTSD in adults: A comprehensive psychological approach. In M. B. Williams & J. F. Sommer (Eds.), *Simple and complex posttraumatic stress disorder: Strategies for comprehensive treatment in clinical practice* (pp. 9–22). Binghamton, NY: Haworth.

Foa, E. B., & Riggs, D. S. (1995). Posttraumatic stress disorder following assault: Theoretical considerations and empirical findings. *Current Directions in Psychological Science, 4*(2), 61–65.

Foa, E. B., Riggs, D. S., & Gershuny, B. S. (1995). Arousal, numbing, and intrusion: Symptom structure of PTSD following assault. *American Journal of Psychiatry, 152*(1), 116–120.

Foa, E. B., Rothbaum, B. O., & Furr, J. M. (2003). Augmenting exposure therapy with other CBT procedures. *Psychiatric Annals, 33,* 47–53.

Freud, S. (1950). Psycho-analysis and war neuroses. *International Psycho-analytical Library, 37,* 83–87.

Friedman, M. J. (2003). Pharmacologic management of posttraumatic stress disorder. *Primary Psychiatry, 10,* 66–68, 71–73.

Friedman, M. J., Charney, D. S., & Deutch, A. Y. (1995). *Neurobiological and clinical consequences of stress: From normal adaptation to posttraumatic stress disorder.* Philadelphia: Lippincott-Raven.

Glynn, S. M., Eth, S., Randolph, E. T., Foy, D. W., Urbaitis, M., Boxer, L., et al. (1999). A test of behavioral family therapy to augment exposure for combat-related posttraumatic stress disorder. *Journal of Consulting and Clinical Psychology, 67,* 243–251.

Green, B. L., Friedman, M. J., de Jong, J. T. V. M., Solomon, S. D., Keane, T. M., Fairbank, J. A., et al. (2003). *Trauma interventions in war and peace: Prevention, practice, and policy.* New York: Kluwer Academic/Plenum.

Hyams, K. C., Wignall, F. S., & Roswell, R. (1996). War syndromes and their evaluation: From the U.S. Civil War to the Persian Gulf War. *Annals of Internal Medicine, 125,* 398–405.

Janet, P. (1907). *The major symptoms of hysteria: Fifteen lectures given in the medical school of Harvard University.* New York: Macmillan.

Kardiner, A. (1941). *The traumatic neuroses of war.* New York: Hoeber.

Keane, T. M., & Kaloupek, D. G. (1982). Imaginal flooding in the treatment of a posttraumatic stress disorder. *Journal of Consulting and Clinical Psychology, 50,* 138–140.

Keane, T. M., & Kaloupek, D. G. (2002). Diagnosis, assessment, and monitoring outcomes in PTSD. In R. Yehuda (Ed.), *Treating trauma survivors with PTSD* (pp. 21–42). Washington, DC: American Psychiatric Press.

Kessler, R. C., Sonnega, A., Bromet, E., Hughes, M., & Nelson, C. B. (1995). Posttraumatic stress disorder in the National Comorbidity Survey. *Archives of General Psychiatry, 52,* 1048–1060.

King, D. W., Leskin, G. A., King, L. A., & Weathers, F. W. (1998). Confirmatory factor analysis of the clinician-administered PTSD scale: Evidence for the dimensionality of posttraumatic stress disorder. *Psychological Assessment, 10,* 90–96.

Kolb, L. C. (1987). A neuropsychological hypothesis explaining posttraumatic stress disorders. *American Journal of Psychiatry, 144*(8), 989–995.

Kraepelin, E. (1896). *Psychiatrie.* Oxford, UK: Barth.

Marsella, A. J., Friedman, M. J., Gerrity, E. T., & Monsour, R. (1996). *Ethnocultural aspects of posttraumatic stress disorder: Issues, research, and clinical implications.* Washington, DC: American Psychological Association.

Miller, M. W., Greif, J. L., & Smith, A. A. (2003). Multidimensional personality questionnaire profiles of veterans with traumatic combat exposure: Externalizing and internalizing subtypes. *Psychological Assessment, 15,* 205–215.

Monson, C. M., Schnurr, P. P., Stevens, S. P., & Guthrie, K. A. (2004). Cognitive-behavioral couple's treatment for posttraumatic stress disorder: Initial findings. *Journal of Traumatic Stress, 17,* 341–344.

Najavits, L. M. (2002). *Seeking Safety: A treatment manual for PTSD and substance abuse.* New York: Guilford Press.

Norris, F. H., Murphy, A. D., Baker, C. K., & Perilla, J. L. (2003). Severity, timing, and duration of reactions to trauma in the population: An example from Mexico. *Biological Psychiatry, 53*(9), 769–778.

Oppenheim, H. (1915). *Der krieg und die traumatischen neurosen* [The war and the traumatic neuroses]. *Berliner Klinische Wochenschrift, 52,* 257–261.

Pendergrast, M. (1999). From Mesmer to memories: A historical, scientific look at the recovered memories controversy. In S. Taub (Ed.), *Recovered memories of child sexual abuse: Psychological, social, and legal perspectives on a contemporary mental health controversy* (pp. 40–55). Springfield, IL: Thomas.

Pitman, R. K. (1993). Biological findings in PTSD: Implications for DSM-IV. In J. R. T. Davidson & E. B. Foa (Eds.), *PTSD: DSM-IV and beyond* (pp. 173–189). Washington, DC: American Psychiatric Press.

Resick, P. A. (2001). Cognitive therapy for posttraumatic stress disorder. *Journal of Cognitive Psychotherapy, 15,* 321–329.

Resick, P. A., Nishith, P., Weaver, T. L., Astin, M. C., & Feuer, C. A. (2002). A comparison of cognitive processing therapy with prolonged exposure and a waiting condition for the treatment of chronic posttraumatic stress disorder in female rape victims. *Journal of Consulting and Clinical Psychology, 70*(4), 867–879.

Rosen, C. S., Chow, H. C., Finney, J. F., Greenbaum, M. A., Moos, R. H., Sheikh, J. I., et al. (2004). Practice guidelines and VA practice patterns for treating posttraumatic stress disorder. *Journal of Traumatic Stress, 17*, 213–222.

Rothbaum, B. O., Foa, E. B., Riggs, D. S., Murdock, T. B., & Walsh, W. (1992). A prospective examination of posttraumatic stress disorder in rape victims. *Journal of Traumatic Stress, 5*, 455–475.

Ruscio, A. M., Ruscio, J., & Keane, T. M. (2002). The latent structure of posttraumatic stress disorder: A taxometric investigation of reactions to extreme stress. *Journal of Abnormal Psychology, 111*, 290–301.

Saigh, P. A., & Bremner, J. D. (1999). The history of posttraumatic stress disorder. In P. A. Saigh & J. D. Bremner (Eds.), *Posttraumatic stress disorder: A comprehensive text* (pp. 1–17). Boston: Allyn & Bacon.

Schlenger, W. E., Caddell, J. M., Ebert, L., Jordan, B. K., Rourke, K. M., Wilson, D., et al. (2002). Psychological reactions to terrorist attacks: Findings from the National Study of Americans' Reactions to September 11. *Journal of the American Medical Association, 288*, 581–588.

Shalev, A. Y. (1997). Acute to chronic: Etiology and pathophysiology of PTSD. In C. S. Fullerton & R. J. Ursano (Eds.), *Posttraumatic stress disorder* (pp. 209–240). Washington, DC: American Psychiatric Press.

van der Kolk, B. A., Weisaeth, L., & van der Hart, O. (1996). History of trauma in psychiatry. In B. A. van der Kolk, A. C. McFarlane, & L. Weisaeth (Eds.), *Traumatic stress: The effects of overwhelming experience on mind, body, and society* (pp. 47–74). New York: Guilford Press.

Walker, L. A. (1984). Battered women, psychology, and public policy. *American Psychologist, 39*, 1178–1182.

World Health Organization. (1992). *International statistical classification of diseases and related health problems* (10th rev. ed.). Geneva, Switzerland: Author.

Yehuda, R., & McFarlane, A. C. (1997). *Psychobiology of posttraumatic stress disorder.* New York: New York Academy of Sciences.

Zayfert, C., Becker, C. B., & Gillock, K. G. (2002). Managing obstacles to the utilization of exposure therapy with PTSD patients. In L. Van de Creek & T. L. Jackson (Eds.), *Innovations in clinical practice: A source book* (pp. 201–222). Sarasota, FL: Professional Resource Press.

PART ONE
Assessment

CHAPTER TWO

Functional Analytic Clinical Assessment in Trauma Treatment

William C. Follette
Amy E. Naugle

Assessment serves a variety of functions. In Chapter 3 of this volume, Pratt, Brief, and Keane provide a review of assessment procedures for the diagnosis of posttraumatic stress disorder (PTSD) as well as scales for assessing treatment outcome. One purpose of assigning a diagnostic label is its implication that a particular treatment will lead to a useful outcome, when properly applied to the appropriate person. If that useful outcome were always the case, then assessment for the purpose of diagnosis, along with an evaluation of treatment integrity, would be all that were necessary. Although much of this volume addresses how to treat patients who have experienced significant traumatic stressors, there is no treatment that is completely guaranteed to alleviate all of the symptoms a patient might report. This chapter focuses on the application of behavioral principles to assess areas of functioning that might need to be considered as treatment planning and implementation proceeds.

Since the establishment of the diagnosis of PTSD in the DSM-III and subsequent updates (American Psychiatric Association, 1980, 1987, 1994, 2000), a considerable volume of literature has been published that describes clinical problems that may be likely to co-occur with PTSD. At the level of diagnostic labels, PTSD is noted to co-occur with depression, anxiety, phobia, and panic disorders perhaps in part because of symptom overlap in diagnostic criteria (Davidson & Foa, 1991). A variety of other diagnostic labels are also associated with PTSD, including substance abuse and Axis II cluster B disorders, such as borderline personality disorders with impulsivity (Foa, Davidson, Frances, & Anxiety Disorders Association of America, 1999).

Treatment guidelines include cognitive therapy to address unrealistic assumptions, thoughts, and beliefs; anxiety management and stress inoculation techniques, including relaxation training; and imaginal or *in vivo* exposure (Foa et al., 1999). The same guideline document describes a variety of adjunct medication treatments for more complex cases (Foa et al., 1999).

The experience of trauma exposure is not rare; however, the trauma responses of avoidance and arousal spontaneously extinguish in the majority of people exposed (Breslau, Davis, Andreski, & Peterson, 1991; Breslau et al., 1998). It has been argued that those who experience PTSD have flatter generalization gradients and do not respond to cues of safety (Foa, Steketee, & Rothbaum, 1989; Foa, Zinbarg, & Rothbaum, 1992; Rothbaum & Davis, 2003). Rothbaum and Davis describe the conditions that are likely to produce more or less successful outcomes in response to exposure-based treatments.

PTSD is not a response to a traumatic event that occurs in isolation; other factors might serve to ameliorate, maintain, or exacerbate symptoms and course. The purpose of this chapter is to complement what is known about the treatment of PTSD by calling attention to a more complete analysis of variables that are potentially clinically important to consider when treating PTSD.

For the purposes of this chapter, it is assumed that an evidenced-based intervention treatment for PTSD is already being provided. A primary assumption behind applying an empirically supported treatment for PTSD in a specific case is that a significant proportion of variance in outcome can be accounted for by the mechanism(s) presumed to be affected by the treatment protocol (Haynes, Kaholokula, & Nelson, 1999). The effect size for any particular patient will vary depending on whether those mechanisms of change targeted by an empirically supported treatment are the same mechanisms as those controlling symptoms in a specific patient. For any specific patient, it is likely that common as well as unique factors will influence the presenting problems and outcomes, and the unique factors could well account for the major portion of outcome variance.

Because PTSD is one of the few diagnostic categories in the DSM for which the etiology of the disorder is specified, one might presume that a very homogeneous set of causal factors is present and therefore that each individual patient will respond predictably to treatment. However, patients with PTSD may report a complex set of symptoms that still qualify for the diagnosis. As mentioned earlier, PTSD has a high rate of comorbidity; this comorbidity makes the causal analysis of a particular patient's problems even more difficult. One goal of this chapter is to describe a method that can identify additional (or even alternative) causal factors that, when properly addressed, produce the largest benefits for patients.

FUNCTIONAL ANALYTIC CLINICAL ASSESSMENT

The Purpose of Functional Analysis

The purpose of functional analytic clinical assessment is to identify factors that, when addressed, will lead to an individualized understanding of the relationship between behaviors and their antecedent conditions and maintaining effects. A functional analysis is a process that identifies causal relationships between observable, manipulable variables and clinically important target behaviors. In any particular patient there may be a number of variables that are affecting the frequency and severity of a clinical problem. Haynes and O'Brien (1990) have suggested limiting the vast universe of factors to be considered to those that are important, controllable, and causal. By "important" they mean, the identification of a variable that, when altered, leads to a large change in the target behavior or the behavior of clinical interest. Because most behaviors are multiply determined, it is conceivable that therapists could waste valuable time and patient goodwill by attending to many small sources of influence that, when targeted in treatment, simply do not effect enough benefit for clients. Simply stated, when looking for sources of influence over a particular behavior, choose the ones that get you "the biggest bang for the buck."

The second heuristic to which to attend is to select controllable variables for study. "Controllable" here means to attend to a variable about which the therapist and the patient can do something. For example, the therapist cannot change the patient's age, but the therapist, could, in principle, change the patient's social repertoire in a way that increases his or her access to social reinforcement. This issue is particularly important in the treatment of PTSD when the patient would like more than anything to erase the traumatic stressor that seemingly caused all his or her problems in the first place. Of course, the event itself cannot be changed, but many of its consequences can be changed in the present.

The last criterion Haynes and O'Brien suggest is to identify causal variables. "Causal" in this context is not so much a notion of ultimate causality as a reference to those variables that, when changed, reliably precede and produce change in the targeted clinical problem. If the therapist can identify unique functional relationships that ameliorate specific individual problems for individual patients, then the therapist will also observe additional treatment effects to those derived by administering a protocol-driven treatment plan that is designed for the hypothetical "average patient." For example, for a rape victim, a sexual encounter with a new romanitic partner may seemingly cause anxiety and distress. In fact, it is not the current romantic encouter that is the ultimate cause of symptoms—the rape is. However, from a clinical standpoint, the current sexual stimuli such as touch, smells, and arousal can serve as cues for when and what desensitization strategies should be applied.

A Functional Analysis Is Not Always Stable

The identification of important clinical functional relationships between stimuli and responses can greatly enhance therapy outcome. However, therapists must keep certain qualifications in mind when conducting a functional analysis (see Haynes & O'Brien, 1990, pp. 651–653). A functional analysis of a clinical problem rarely exhausts all possible sources of influence. Identifying how one causal variable affects a target behavior does not prove, or even imply, that other causal relationships do not exist between other potentially important variables and the target behavior. It is quite possible that many sets of independent variables exist. Another caveat is that a functional relationship that exists at one point in time may not function in the same way at another point in time. Emotional distancing following a traumatic event may be caused by high levels of distressing arousal immediately following the trauma. This same distancing may be maintained at a later time because of marital distress that occurred subsequently. This phenomenon is referred to as "functional autonomy"—that is, the notion that behaviors that come into existence under the control of one reinforcer can be maintained at a different point in time or set of circumstances because of an entirely different set of reinforcers. A third point to remember about an apparent functional relationship is that it likely to exist under some circumstances but not others (Johnston & Pennypacker, 1980). A patient may avoid talking about the traumatic stressor with some people because doing so with these particular individuals arouses feelings of distress, guilt, or stigmatization. The same patient may be quite willing to discuss the stressor with others who respond more instrumentally.

A functional analytic case conceptualization is never perfect. It "is always hypothesized, probabilistic, and incomplete" (Haynes, Leisen, & Blaine, 1997, p. 337). One generally starts the analysis by referring to the research on empirical relationships that have been identified in experimental or clinical settings. This information provides guidance as to where and how to gather data to generate working hypotheses. These data include in-session behavioral observations, observations of interactions between the patient and others, structured role-playing tasks, self-report data, and reports from significant collaterals. Given the qualifiers on the robustness of hypothesized functional relationships, it is not unusual to gather conflicting data—perhaps because, as noted, a causal relationship may exist under one set of observational conditions, but not others. Reports from collaterals may be inconsistent because they are reporting on observations that were true in the past but are no longer accurate. Patients, collaterals, and clinicians are all prone to making a variety of heuristic errors that add inaccuracy to observational reporting, thus complicating case formulation (Arnoult & Anderson, 1988; Kahneman, Slovic, & Tversky, 1982; Turk & Salovey, 1988).

As mentioned previously, the intended result of a functional analytic case conceptualization is the identification of important, controllable, and causal variables that, if altered, would lead to useful change for the patient. Ideally, the therapist would identify alterable variables that would result in the largest changes first. However, without an empirical trial, the therapist cannot know if the selected variable is the most important change; he or she can only select a variable and then observe the effect. If the hypothesized relationship does not result in a change in the target behavior, the functional analysis should be reevaluated and modified in light of these new data. On other occasions, the clinician may believe that he or she knows an important functional relationship but not have the technology available to create the necessary conditions to produce change. For example, say a therapist hypothesizes that a comorbid depression that was initially the result of a traumatic stressor is being maintained by a distressful marital relationship. The patient's spouse may now be quite willing to address relationship problems, but the patient is not. At present, there is relatively little research or clinical evidence that clinicians can alter motivation in this type of situation. Such an analysis would fail the controllability criterion described above. If new treatment technology were to emerge that could effectively alter motivation to change in marital relationships, then this variable might well be a good place to start an intervention.

Analysis of the Behavior in Context

One of the fundamental issues in functional understanding of clinical interventions is to appreciate the proper unit and level of analysis of a behavioral problem. In the case of PTSD it can be tempting to see the problem as residing in the relationship between the patient and the traumatic stressor. In fact, because there is considerable variability in how patients respond to stressors, we must infer that there are other factors that affect course and outcome. From a behavior analytic perspective it is important to appreciate that examining behavior in isolation misses the point. The only meaningful unit of analysis is the behavior in context. By "context" we mean that not only must the patient's responses to the characteristics of the stressor be considered, but they must be considered in light of the patient's history prior to the stressor, along with how the people, institutions, and agencies that are part of the patient's environment purposefully or inadvertently reinforce (or punish) the patient's responses. The *behavior in context* is the proper unit of analysis; to study one part of the context independently of all others will lose the meaning of the behavior. A behavior is only interpretable when considered in the context of its antecedents and consequences.

Functional Classes

One useful idea to understand is that behaviors that vary in topography (how they appear) but share the same common effect on the environment all form a functional class. One of the problems for clinicians working with complex cases is to make sense out of the litany of problems that each patient reports on any given day. On different days a patient might come to therapy angry, suicidal, crying about a distressed relationship, or highly distracted. Each of these behaviors looks very different from the others; that is, the behaviors vary in their *topography* or form. However, from a functional analytic perspective, we would have to determine whether they were distinct behaviors or whether they all functioned similarly. In this case, it may be that the topographically distinct behaviors all function to distract the therapist from talking about interpersonal closeness. All the behaviors in the class are negatively reinforced by having the therapist change topics to discuss the topography of the behaviors. If the therapist notices this shared function among these behaviors, he or she can begin to respond to all of them similarly and more usefully, rather than being distracted by trying to orient to each specific behavior as if it required a completely different therapist response.

FUNCTIONAL PROBLEMS IN PTSD

The point of describing what is entailed in a conceptual understanding of a functional analytic case conceptualization is to notice the idiographic nature of the assessment process for the purpose of identifying additional sources of information of variance in problem behaviors to improve clinical outcome. There are many sources about how to conduct and even quantify a functional analysis (e. g., Follette, Naugle, & Linnerooth, 2000; Hawkins, 1986; Hayes, Nelson, & Jarret, 1987; Haynes, 1992, 1998; Haynes & O'Brien, 2000; Haynes & Williams, 2003; Johnston & Pennypacker, 1980; Kanfer & Grimm, 1977; Kanfer & Saslow, 1969; Naugle & Follette, 1998; Nelson & Hayes, 1986). As mentioned above, reviewing the scientific literature about likely sources of control in a particular clinical situation is a typical starting point. In this section we present a few of the symptoms of PTSD and consider them as target behaviors that are the focus of treatment.

In applying an evidence-based intervention, we presume that many of these symptoms are interrelated and may well remit when the nomothetic treatment protocol is utilized. However, that may not, and often does not, happen. There are certainly unique sources of variance not addressed by standard treatment protocols that would improve treatment outcome if properly identified and addressed.

Most of the symptoms of PTSD described under criteria B, C, and D in the DSM-IV (American Psychiatric Association, 1994) are easily thought of as reactions to stress. From a functional analytic perspective these reactions are themselves behaviors that function in a complex context. As behaviors they can be reinforced or punished by others and therefore become more or less likely to occur in the same or similar circumstances. These same behaviors can serve as discriminative stimuli or signs to others in the patient's environment. A discriminative stimulus indicates that certain behaviors are likely to be differentially reinforced or punished in the presence of that particular stimulus. For example, tears could indicate that comforting comments may be reinforcing to the patient. Additionally, these same behaviors can serve as reinforcers or punishers in response to someone else's behavior, thereby making the other person's behavior more or less likely to occur. For example, the sampe tearful response following an expression of intimacy may make intimacy less likely. In a social context, the stress reactions listed in criteria B, C, and D for PTSD can serve multiple functions at the same time, thereby affecting, and being affected by, many others simultaneously. It would be nice if all the consequences of these interdependencies disappeared as a result of, for example, a successful exposure treatment. However, the stress reaction behaviors have created effects of their own that may not be related to the original traumatic event.

Let us consider an analysis of symptoms 5 and 6 from criterion C as target behaviors: feeling of detachment or estrangement from others, and restricted range of affect. These behaviors are part of the numbing phenomena said to characterize PTSD. Presumably the numbing is functionally useful to the patient in that it is an avoidance strategy whose purpose is to control otherwise highly negative feelings. Without disagreeing that these numbing responses are adaptive in the short run, let us further hypothesize about how these target behaviors might arise and be maintained in a way that could lead to an improved outcome if addressed from a functional perspective. The analysis might begin with an explanation of what would lead to a feeling of closeness—the opposite of estrangement and restricted affect. The therapist might begin by taking a behavioral history of the patient's close relationships and find that they were characterized by shared expressions of feelings, wants, and needs, and physical or emotional intimacy. In the case of a couple, for example, the dyad has a common history expressing and reinforcing all of the above.

The expression of these feelings, wants, and needs entails two important verbal behavioral repertoires that Skinner referred to as the ability to tact and mand (1945, 1957). A "tact" is a label for a state condition, or event (including private events such as feelings) that is reinforced by the understanding of the listener (or the "verbal community," as Skinner called it). A "mand" is a request for something that is reinforced by the verbal community by providing whatever the speaker specified. An example of a simple tact would be "I am hungry." The tact is reinforced by the speaker being understood by the listener. An example of a mand would be "Give me a sandwich." The mand would be reinforced by getting the sandwich. Although there are many nuances, let us use these verbal operants to further some additional hypotheses about the maintenance of the numbing behaviors described in criteria C.

Consider this scenario: A married woman experienced a rape. In addition to the initial avoidance behaviors that frequently occur immediately after such a trauma, there is a substantial change in the communication between her and her husband. The husband may be reluctant to ask the question "How do you feel?" because he finds any discussion of what happened to his wife to be extremely aversive. It may remind him of a failure to protect his family, whether the feeling is sensible or not. This change in husband-initiated conversation may be a contributing variable to her feeling distant from intimate relations. Note that in this example, the husband's decrease in inquiries about feelings is only a function of the wife being present. Nothing she has done, other than be a stimulus in his presence, has led to this change in his behavior. This fact in itself could lead to a sense of distancing in the relationship—and yet the patient has done nothing except be present.

But suppose the husband does engage in a conversation:

HUSBAND: How do you feel? [This is a mand to the victim to reply with a statement of feelings. The wife now runs into an important deficit in her own behavioral repertoire: Namely, she may have no verbal repertoire to label her feelings accurately. She has no experience with the private events she is currently experiencing, so she is not likely to have a learning history from interacting with others so that her verbal behavior would be shaped to describe her feelings.]

WIFE: I don't know. [The husband's mand has not been reinforced, which could lead to a decreased likelihood of further inquiry into her feelings, making her feel more distanced.]

HUSBAND: But I really want to know [how you feel]. [This is a repeated mand.]

WIFE: Well, I guess I feel ashamed. [This is a tact, probably used for the first time in this dyad under these circumstances and probably not completely accurate. In fact, there probably is no well understood label to apply.]

HUSBAND: Ashamed? You have no reason to be ashamed. It wasn't your fault. [In what might have been intended to be a supportive comment, the husband has certainly not reinforced the spouse's tact. Therefore, she is not feeling understood.]

WIFE: Well, maybe guilty that I should have done something to prevent it. [This is another attempt to tact her private experience.]

HUSBAND: There is no reason for you to feel guilty, Honey. There was nothing you could have done. [Again, the husband does not reinforce her talking about her feelings by any indication that he understands them. Although his responses may be intended to be soothing or supportive, they function to make it less likely that she will try to describe her important personal feelings.]

Because intimacy is partially characterized by the sharing of feelings and mutual understanding, exchanges such as this one are likely to decrease her efforts to talk about her feelings. If this pattern were to continue, it seems likely that she would feel more distant from her husband, with whom she formerly felt intimate. One of the mechanisms for this feeling of estrangement is the lack of intimate communication. An additional consequence of the victim's decreased conversations with her husband may be the self-perception of restricted affect because she is verbalizing less affective content (Bem, 1978).

The point of the above analysis is not to suggest that these symptoms of numbing do not have other causes or functions. It is simply to point out that a behavior that has one initial cause may be maintained or increased by influences not directly related to the trauma itself but rather to a change in communication behavior with important people in the individual's environment. Spousal communication could be concomitantly addressed while other kinds of interventions were occurring if this hypothesis seemed plausible. One reason why this case example was chosen was because the victim described feelings of guilt. Whether the tact was understood by the husband is not the only issue that is important. Empirically, there is evidence that feelings of guilt by trauma survivors is a contributing factor in the development of PTSD, especially in the absence of social support (e.g., Kubany et al., 1996; Ullman & Filipas, 2001). Identifying this source of control over portions of the numbing response could explain a significant amount of outcome response. Note how a successful exposure or anxiety management treatment protocol might not target this spousal interaction at all.

Another symptom of PTSD is the avoidance of thoughts, feelings, or conversations associated with the trauma. Avoidance is a high-probability response to trauma for which exposure based interventions could be useful. An additional functional analysis of the victim's social environment might identify other factors that could lead to the maintenance of avoidance of thoughts or conversations associated with trauma. Stigmatization is often one unfortunate consequence of traumatic victimization. However, a functional analysis of stigmatization might yield a more useful understanding of the discriminative stimulus functions of the patient. If we were to collect reports from collaterals in the patient's environment, we might discover that other women who are important in the patient's social network have shown negative reactions to the patient when she starts to discuss anything related to the trauma. Keeping in mind that behaviors are generally multiply determined, we would have to investigate several hypotheses. One possible determinant of the friends' negative reactions is the fact that her experience is evidence that none of them is immune from this kind of victimization. She elicits vague feelings of uneasiness that escalate when the topic of the trauma is mentioned. These subtle social contingencies could make the patient less likely to want to discuss or process the event. In fact, if we observed interactions between this patient and her friends, we might see the friends actively punish the conversation or at least obviously change topics to help manage their own discomfort. The patient then becomes unwilling to engage in conversation about the event not because it is necessarily aversive to her so much as it is aversive to her friends, who have no repertoire for either discussing the topic or soothing their own discomfort at being vulnerable.

There are many other potential reasons a patient may appear to be numb that are not directly related to the traumatic event, but are rather under the control of social processes that must be addressed to achieve maximum treatment effects. Here, a last functional example reveals what we consider to be a discrimination deficit on the part of the client. In this instance the client may have some repertoire for describing (tacting) her feelings. However, she may not properly discriminate with whom to share these feelings. In given social interaction, the person with whom the patient is interacting would or would not be a good candidate for providing socially meaningful reinforcement. It is up to the patient to make that discrimination. Failure to recognize with whom it is appropriate to seek support can lead to ineffective interactions that eventually extinguish all support-seeking behavior or even lead to punishing interactions in which support is not only not forthcoming, but criticism comes instead. The latter might be the case if one discloses a traumatic event to someone who is too young to understand the event or might even be negatively impacted by it.

The point of the general description of a functional analytic case assessment is to call attention to the fact that whereas there are likely common causal factors that will be addressed by standardized treatment, there are many other sources of causal influence that, when they are not considered, may explain large differences in treatment outcome. The obvious etiology of PTSD does not explain the vastly different responses to treatment. This treatment response variability requires us to look more thoroughly for causal factors on which we can intervene. These factors are most frequently found in the posttrauma environment.

IDENTIFYING FUNCTIONAL VARIABLES THAT INTERACT WITH TREATMENTS

So far we have discussed sources of variance that could extend the effects of a nomothetically derived evidence-based intervention by identifying additional factors that cause or maintain symptoms that are not part of the immediate posttraumatic response. Now let us consider observable factors that might directly compete with active treatment components of an evidenced-based intervention.

Let us take two examples. One empirically supported treatment principle for PTSD is the use of cognitive therapy, whose techniques include identifying dysfunctional cognitions and gathering and evaluating evidence for and against those cognitions. Presumably, examining this evidence will lead the patient to a more realistic and functional set of beliefs and cognitions. If that intervention did not achieve the anticipated results—and assuming that the treatment was delivered competently—then we are left considering whether there are other important causal factors that could be identified by a functional analysis. In addition to the kinds of analyses already described, we can also consider the existence of competing contingencies. Are there salient contingencies operating in the patient's environment that compete with the goals of therapy? While the therapist is diligently helping the patient identify dysfunctional beliefs and encouraging him or her to test them in the real world, there may be people in the patient's environment who are reinforcing the opposite behavior. If this is the case, the assessment issue, becomes, what is controlling the therapy-interfering behavior of these other people? Interviews, diaries, and journals may help generate hypotheses. A child who realizes his mother is vulnerable may cling to her, preventing her from doing exploratory homework. The child may even subtly support the mother's avoidance behavior. A spouse who initially worried about the victim's safety may now actually prefer a more dependent partner, and, like the child, may undermine treatment compliance.

As a second example, in an exposure-based treatment that is producing poorer outcomes than might be expected, it is important to functionally analyze what environmental contingencies might be competing with therapy tasks and goals. If the therapist had constructed an *in vivo* desensitization hierarchy with the patient, and the patient reports doing the *in vivo* exposure homework, why might the treatment not being working? Relying on theory to help guide the assessment, we recall that PTSD patients generally have very broad networks of stimuli that can produce aversive conditioned responses that might be of a larger magnitude than expected. For example, an element on the exposure hierarchy might be intimate touching with the spouse. Each time the patient reaches this level of the hierarchy, she experiences a resurgence of anxiety that interferes with extinction. A careful analysis of the reactions to this activity on the hierarchy might reveal that though the spouse is being as sensitive as possible during the task, the spouse may possess some subtle physical characteristic of the perpetrator. It might be difficult to elicit this information from the patient, because the patient does not have verbal access to what is bothersome about the task or because she tries to complete the task, believing it crucial to her spouse, but cannot reduce her anxiety sufficiently for extinction to occur. In fact, spontaneous recovery of the conditioned response could even occur at that point. We present these examples to demonstrate that a functional analysis can and should be applied to identify additional sources of control over behavior change that compete with successful treatment implementation.

THINKING OUTSIDE THE BLACK BOX

We mentioned earlier that behavior had to be considered in context to be properly understood. At that point "context" meant considering the behavior in terms of the patient's history and the antecedents and consequences of his or her behavior. Context actually entails even more. At a psychological level, a patient is changed by every new experience that contributes to his or her history. Treatment itself can be thought of as adding to the person's history to change the impact of the traumatic event. Behavior theory long ago rejected any implied dualism between body and behavior. Behavior exists in a biological milieu. Behavior and biology cannot be separated and still retain sensible meaning. Therefore, one other source of behavioral variance to consider is how neurophysiological changes associated with traumatic experiences can alter the patient's interactions with the world. It is well beyond the scope of this chapter to try to resolve all of the interesting, though often conflicting, neurophysiological and neuroanatomical changes that are sometimes attributable to traumatic experiences, especially when experienced by the young. However, many functional and sometimes structural changes have been noted that may involve memory impairment: changes in the hippocampus that could affect declarative memory, possible frontal lobe changes, and even changes in amygdaloid regions. Because of a variety of methodological and measurement problems, it is not known the extent to which these changes are due to PTSD alone or in combination with comorbid conditions, are transient, or even reach clinical significance (cf. Brandes et al., 2002; Bustamante, Mellman, David, & Fins, 2001; Danckwerts & Leathem, 2003; Neylan et al., 2004). However, some of the clinical changes observed in PTSD could be influenced by a biologically changed person who interacts differently with his or her environment, thereby adding to the sense of loss of control and estrangement. These findings are still speculative as to their duration, cause, and significance. Yet a complete functional analysis of target behaviors to be addressed during an intervention requires a consideration of these emerging data as additional changes that might contribute to altered relationships between the patient and his or her environment. There is convincing evidence that these changes, if substantiated, could be the target of therapy to restore pretrauma levels of functioning, at least in adults.

Once again, the issue that would remain important to assess is not just the topography of the trauma response but the stimulus functions the patient presents to others. Whether or not memory disturbances are related to trauma or other comorbid conditions, memory or emotion regulation functions that are altered from what significant people in the environment are used to expecting, can produce distressing interactions that exacerbate symptoms or change the way in which people respond to the patient.

Certainly the immediate reactions of a patient to a traumatic event are appropriately the focus of evidence-based treatments. What we have described thus far is the notion that there are social consequences to these reactions that are far reaching and can lead to problems of their own (e.g., Soloman, 1989). We have further suggested that these reactions can produce or exacerbate some of the symptoms that are the basis for making the PTSD diagnosis.

HOW TO EVALUATE THE FUNCTIONAL ANALYSIS

How do we know if an important, causal, and controllable variable has been identified? There are two ways to answer this question. First, a useful functional analysis has treatment utility if it leads the therapist to do something differently from what was planned (Hayes et al., 1987), *and* a differential treatment effect is then observed (Nelson, Hayes, Jarrett, Sigmon, & McKnight, 1987). The second way of knowing whether an important functional relationship has been identified is to manipulate the variable and observe its effect in the clinical setting. There are many methods of conducting single-subject design studies that are applicable in clinical settings (e.g., Haynes & O'Brien, 2000; Haynes & Williams, 2003; Kazdin, 1982). Because of well-known heuristic biases that affect the interpretation of clinical findings (Turk & Salovey, 1988), it is important to gather data on whether a putative functional relationship actually matters. Having just referred to a variety of technical solutions for examining single-subject studies in the clinical setting, it is still possible to make use of simple strategies that can shed light on the utility of an analysis.

Simple data gathering procedures and ethical strategies are necessary in a clinical setting. The therapist does not want to provide ineffective treatment, nor does he or she wish to add to the client's stress unreasonably. Having said that, it is indeed ethical to inform the patient of deviations from evidenced-based interventions and collect data to test whether these changes are benefiting the patient.

There are different strategies that provide higher- or lower-quality data about the utility of making a clinical change based on a hypothesized functional relationship. A weak but simple procedure that can provide probative data about whether the analysis is correct is an A–B within-patient design. *A* and *B* refer to two different treatment conditions. *A* is usually some baseline or steady-state condition, and *B* is a different treatment condition. Assume that an evidenced-based intervention is being used and that the patient has either not progressed or has progressed but stabilized at some less-than-optimal level of symptom state. For example, say that the therapist has been gathering data on family functioning, and a stable, significant degree of estrangement remains. These estrangement data constitute a steady state or treatment phase we can call *A*. The therapist then changes treatment on the basis of a presumed functional relationship that addresses problems beyond the standard protocol. This new treatment element is the *B* phase. If the functional relationship (e.g., see the above discussion of tacts and mands) has an effect, then an improvement in estrangement rating should occur during the *B* phase. However, a change in estrangement also could have occurred by chance just when *B* was implemented. If no change is observed, then the absence of change is evidence the analysis is incorrect or incomplete.

A more stringent demonstration of control over estrangement would require a reversal design, or an A–B–A–B. As is implied by the name, in this type of data gathering strategy, if the first B produced a useful effect, then the baseline or steady-state condition, A, is reinstated with the expectation that estrangement would then increase. A second implementation of B and a corresponding improvement in estrangement reduces the likelihood that the relationship between treatment element B and estrangement were random. The ethical problem is obvious. The second A period would be expected to be associated with a worsening of symptoms. This is difficult for both patients and therapists to undergo. However, there is a real value to knowing with greater certainty which factors will help maintain improvement and increase generalization. Sometimes treatment B cannot be undone. For example, once a patient has learned a skill, that skill cannot be taken away in the reversal portion of the treatment. It would be like teaching someone to ski and then saying, "Now pretend you don't know how to ski."

An alternative form of testing an hypothesis regarding behavior change is a multiple baseline design. In this design steady-state data are gathered and then a change strategy is implemented sequentially in different settings in the patient's life. Staying with the estrangement example, after gathering the baseline data, the therapist could teach the spouse how to better interact so that the patient could learn to tact and mand. The patient could gather data about communications with the spouse and in another setting, such as with the patient's parents. We would expect improvement in one setting (with the spouse) but not the other (with the parents) because the intervention has only been implemented in the one setting with the spouse. The estrangement problem with the parents should remain at baseline. Next, the same intervention could be introduced to the parents, and now the estrangement should change in that setting. This logic can be applied to multiple settings; estrangement should change independently in each setting only when the treatment is implemented in that setting. This is a more elegant demonstration of control. In reality, some cross-communication could eventually occur which would lead to improvements in settings not yet targeted for intervention. However, multiple baseline designs are convenient and avoid the reversal problem described above.

One other design that is very convenient and natural to use is the alternating treatment design. This type of design can be used within a single session or across multiple sessions to gather evidence about the utility of a hypothesized functional relationship. In this design the therapist uses one type of intervention in one session and a different type in another session. If the therapist is gathering some kind of clinically relevant data, he or she can do a simple comparison of how the patient responds to each intervention. If there are no differences in how the patient responds, there is no evidence that the change in therapy procedure works, though the reasons for the failure could be complicated to interpret.

Employing these simple designs to test a functional analysis is useful because functional analyses are dynamic, often starting out incomplete and becoming more refined as data are gathered. As cautioned above, a functional relationship is limited in the domains it can influence and is limited in the time it is useful. Once one clinical problem is resolved, another may emerge that requires a whole new analysis. It is this idiographic procedure that can produce individualized treatment plans that can greatly supplement the evidenced-based treatment of individuals with PTSD.

REFERENCES

American Psychiatric Association. (1980). *Diagnostic and statistical manual of mental disorders* (3rd ed.). Washington, DC: Author.

American Psychiatric Association. (1987). *Diagnostic and statistical manual of mental disorders* (3rd ed., rev.). Washington, DC: Author.

American Psychiatric Association. (1994). *Diagnostic and statistical manual of mental disorders* (4th ed.). Washington, DC: Author.

American Psychiatric Association. (2000). *Diagnostic and statistical manual of mental disorders* (4th ed., text rev.). Washington, DC: Author.

Arnoult, L. H., & Anderson, C. A. (1988). Identifying and reducing causal reasoning biases in clinical practice. In D. C. Turk & P. Salovey (Eds.), *Reasoning, inference, and judgment in clinical psychology* (pp. 209–232). New York: Free Press.

Bem, D. J. (1978). Self-perception theory. In L. Berkowitz (Ed.), *Cognitive theories in social psychology* (pp. 221–282). New York: Academic Press.

Brandes, D., Ben-Schachar, G., Gilboa, A., Bonne, O., Freedman, S., & Shalev, A. Y. (2002). PTSD symptoms and cognitive performance in recent trauma survivors. *Psychiatry Research, 110*, 231–238.

Breslau, N., Davis, G. C., Andreski, P., & Peterson, E. (1991). Traumatic events and posttraumatic stress disorder in an urban population of young adults. *Archives of General Psychiatry, 48*, 218–222.

Breslau, N., Kessler, R. C., Chilcoat, H. D., Schultz, L. R., Davis, G. C., & Andreski, P. (1998). Trauma and posttraumatic stress disorder in the community: The 1996 Detroit Area Survey of Trauma. *Archives of General Psychiatry, 55*, 626–631.

Bustamante, V., Mellman, T. A., David, D., & Fins, A. I. (2001). Cognitive functioning and the early development of PTSD. *Journal of Traumatic Stress, 14*, 791–797.

Danckwerts, A., & Leathem, J. (2003). Questioning the link between PTSD and cognitive dysfunction. *Neuropsychology Review, 13*, 221–235.

Davidson, J. R. T., & Foa, E. B. (1991). Diagnostic issues in possttraumatic stress disorder: Considerations for the DSM-IV. *Journal of Abnormal Psychology, 100*, 346–355.

Foa, E. B., Davidson, J. R. T., Frances, A., & Anxiety Disorders Association of America. (1999). The expert consensus guideline series: Treatment of posttraumatic stress disorder. *Journal of Clinical Psychiatry, 60* (Suppl. 16), 4–76.

Foa, E. B., Steketee, G., & Rothbaum, B. (1989). Behavioral/cognitive conceptualizations of post-traumatic stress disorder. *Behavior Therapy, 20*, 155–176.

Foa, E. B., Zinbarg, R., & Rothbaum, B. (1992). Uncontrollability and unpredictability in post-traumatic stress disorder: An animal model. *Psychological Bulletin, 112*, 218–238.

Follette, W. C., Naugle, A. E., & Linnerooth, P. J. N. (2000). Functional alternatives to traditional assessment and diagnosis. In M. J. Dougher (Ed.), *Clinical behavior analysis* (pp. 99–125). Reno, NV: Context Press.

Hawkins, R. P. (1986). Selection of target behaviors. In R. O. Nelson & S. C. Hayes (Eds.), *Conceptual foundations of behavioral assessment* (pp. 331–385). New York: Guilford Press.

Hayes, S. C., Nelson, R. O., & Jarret, R. (1987). Treatment utility of assessment: A functional approach to evaluating quality of assessment. *American Psychologist, 42*, 963–974.

Haynes, S. N. (1992). *Models of causality in psychopathology: Toward dynamic, synthetic and nonlinear models of behavior disorders.* New York: Macmillan.

Haynes, S. N. (1998). The assessment–treatment relationship and functional analysis in behavior therapy. *European Journal of Psychological Assessment, 14*, 26–35.

Haynes, S. N., Kaholokula, J. K., & Nelson, K. (1999). The idiographic application of nomothetic empirically based treatments. *Clinical Psychology: Science and Practice, 6*, 456–461.

Haynes, S. N., Leisen, M. B., & Blaine, D. D. (1997). Design of individualized behavioral treatment programs using functional analytic clinical case models. *Psychological Assessment, 9*, 334–348.

Haynes, S. N., & O'Brien, W. H. (1990). Functional analysis in behavior therapy. *Clinical Psychology Review, 10*, 649–668.

Haynes, S. N., & O'Brien, W. H. (2000). *Principles and practice of behavioral assessment.* New York: Plenum Press.

Haynes, S. N., & Williams, A. E. (2003). Case formulation and design of behavioral treatment programs: Matching treatment mechanisms to causal variables for behavior problems. *European Journal of Psychological Assessment, 19*, 164–174.

Johnston, J. M., & Pennypacker, H. S. (1980). *Strategies and tactics of human behavioral research.* Hillsdale, NJ: Erlbaum.

Kahneman, D., Slovic, P., & Tversky, A. (1982). *Judgment under uncertainty: Heuristics and biases.* New York: Cambridge University Press.

Kanfer, F. H., & Grimm, L. G. (1977). Behavioral analysis: Selecting target behaviors in the interview. *Behavior Modification, 1*, 7–28.

Kanfer, F. H., & Saslow, G. (1969). Behavioral diagnosis. In C. M. Franks (Ed.), *Behavior therapy: Appraisal and status* (pp. 417–444). New York: McGraw-Hill.

Kazdin, A. E. (1982). *Single case research designs: Methods for clinical and applied settings.* New York: Oxford University Press.

Kubany, E. S., Haynes, S. N., Abueg, F. R., Manke, F. P., Brennan, J. M., & Stahura, C. (1996). Development and validation of the trauma-related guilt inventory (TRGI). *Psychological Assessment, 8*, 428–444.

Naugle, A. E., & Follette, W. C. (1998). A functional analysis of trauma symptoms. In V. M. Follette, J. I. Ruzek, & F. R. Abueg (Eds.), *Cognitive-behavioral therapies for trauma* (pp. 48–73). New York: Guilford Press.

Nelson, R. O., & Hayes, S. C. (Eds.). (1986). *Conceptual foundations of behavioral assessment.* New York: Guilford Press.

Nelson, R. O., Hayes, S. C., Jarrett, R. B., Sigmon, S. T., & McKnight, D. L. (1987). The treatment utility of response class assessment in heterosexual difficulties. *Psychological Reports, 61*, 816–818.

Neylan, T. C., Lenoci, M., Rothlind, J., Metzler, T. J., Schuff, N., Du, A.-T., et al.

(2004). Attention, learning, and memory in posttraumatic stress disorder. *Journal of Traumatic Stress, 17,* 41–46.

Rothbaum, B. O., & Davis, M. (2003). Applying learning principles to the treatment of post-trauma reactions. *Annals of the New York Academy of Sciences, 1008,* 112–121.

Skinner, B. F. (1945). The operational analysis of psychological terms. *Psychological Review, 52,* 270–277.

Skinner, B. F. (1957). *Verbal behavior.* New York: Appleton-Century-Crofts.

Soloman, Z. (1989). PTSD and social functioning: A three year prospective study. *Social Psychiatry and Psychiatric Epidemiology, 24,* 127–133.

Turk, D. C., & Salovey, P. (Eds.). (1988). *Reasoning, inference, and judgment in clinical psychology.* New York: Free Press.

Ullman, S. E., & Filipas, H. H. (2001). Predictors of PTSD symptom severity and social reactions in sexual assault victims. *Journal of Traumatic Stress, 14,* 369–389.

CHAPTER THREE

Recent Advances in Psychological Assessment of Adults with Posttraumatic Stress Disorder

Elizabeth M. Pratt
Deborah J. Brief
Terence M. Keane

Originally conceptualized in the DSM-III (American Psychiatric Association, 1980) as relatively rare, traumatic events and posttraumatic stress disorder (PTSD) are now viewed as common across the world. As interest in PTSD grows internationally, so does the need for sensitive and specific diagnostic interviews, questionnaires, and psychological tests. As progress is made in understanding the impact of trauma on psychological functioning, the consistent use of standardized psychological measures will permit cross-study comparisons, meaningful meta-analyses, the specification of conclusions regarding public policy based on sound empirical methods, and the more expeditious use of evidence-based clinical protocols for treatment. The purpose of this chapter is to discuss the various methods for assessing PTSD in a wide variety of settings. Understanding the optimal methods for assessing the presence of PTSD, related psychiatric conditions, treatment outcome, and the monitoring of progress in real time are a few of the important topics we address.

ASSESSMENT OF PTSD

Increasingly, clinicians have come to recognize that a substantial portion of their patients have experienced traumatic events and may require treatment for PTSD. Additionally, patients who seek treatment for medical or psychiatric disorders other than PTSD may have a presentation that is complicated by the presence of PTSD. Thus clinicians are interested in the proper assessment and evaluation of patients with PTSD.

Clearly, PTSD is assessed for many different reasons, and the goals of a particular assessment will determine the methods selected by the professional. The objective of many mental health clinicians is a diagnostic evaluation that includes a differential diagnosis and other information that is helpful in treatment planning. Other practitioners may be involved in forensic evaluations for which diagnostic accuracy is of paramount importance. Researchers involved in epidemiological studies may be interested in the rate of occurrence of PTSD and its associated risk factors and comorbidity. In addition, researchers may be interested in which assessments offer the highest levels of diagnostic accuracy when examining the biological and psychological indicators of the disorder, as in case–control studies. Different clinical and research situations require different solutions, depending upon the particular assessment goals of the professional. For this reason, we present a general overview of the means by which a clinician can evaluate the quality of measures.

Recommendations from the National Institute of Mental Health–National Center for PTSD Conference

In November 1995, 45 clinicians and researchers from around the world met in Boston, Massachusetts, in conjunction with the annual meeting of the International Society for Traumatic Stress Studies, to discuss and debate various approaches to the assessment of PTSD (Keane, Solomon, Maser, & Gerrity, 1995b). Although their task was to provide guidance for conducting clinical research in the field, their recommendations relate to the development of standards for assessing PTSD in many different settings and for a variety of purposes. The conference participants reached consensus on several parameters of the assessment process. Those relevant to the selection of measures to assess PTSD and symptom severity are described below.

1. Clinician-administered structured diagnostic interviews provide valuable clinical information. The clinician should evaluate their quality, using the psychometric properties of reliability, validity, and clinical utility as a guideline.
2. Structured diagnostic interviews that provide both a dichotomous and continuous rating of PTSD symptoms are preferred.
3. The dimensions of symptom frequency, intensity, and duration of a particular episode should be assessed. Levels of distress, as articulated by the patient regarding his or her symptom, are important to identify.
4. Ratings of impairment and disability secondary to the symptom complex provide important information regarding the severity of the condition.

5. Measures that evaluate both the components of the traumatic event (i.e., A1) and the severity of thr reaction to that event (i.e., A2) are essential.

6. Instruments whose reliability and validity studies contain information regarding instrument performance across gender, racial, and ethnic groups are preferred, especially evaluating males and females of different cultures and races.

7. Self-report instruments for PTSD should meet the standards for psychometric instruments established by the American Psychological Association's "Standards for Educational and Psychological Tests."

8. The events identified as key to review when examining for the presence of traumatic events include war-zone stressors, sexual assault in childhood or adulthood, robberies, accidents, technological disasters, natural disasters or hazardous exposures, sudden death of a loved one, life-threatening illnesses, and witnessing or experiencing violence. In general, the committee recommended that "in depth questions need to be asked about event occurrences, perceived life threat, harm, injuries, frequency, duration, and age."

9. The committee also recommended that comorbidity be closely examined because response to treatment can vary depending upon the presence of additional psychological conditions. The committee recommended a full assessment of Axis I disorders using a structured clinical interview, such as the Structured Clinical Interview for the DSM (First, Spitzer, Williams, & Gibbon, 2000) or something comparable in scope and efficiency.

10. Finally, the committee recommended that "in evaluating stressors, careful behaviorally-anchored terminology should be used, avoiding jargon such as abuse, rape, etc., terms which are inherently imprecise and not universally understood in the same way within and across cultures."

Selection of Assessment Measures

Since the inclusion of PTSD in the diagnostic nomenclature of the American Psychiatric Association in 1980, excellent progress has been made in developing high-quality measures to assess trauma symptoms in adults (Keane & Barlow, 2002; Keane, Weathers, & Foa, 2000). The assessment and diagnosis of PTSD may require a range of different approaches, such as a clinician-administered structured diagnostic interview for PTSD and/or related comorbidity, self-report psychological tests and questionnaires, and/or psychophysiological measures. The clinician may also want to review medical records and check with multiple informants regarding the patient's behavior and experiences. We have referred to this approach as a multimethod assessment of PTSD (Keane, Fairbank, Caddell, Zimering, & Bender, 1995). When faced with a choice of measures, clinicians and researchers are encouraged to evaluate the quality of the measure, using as a guideline the psychometric properties of each instrument. Standards for evaluating these measures are briefly described below.

Psychometric Theory and Principles

The quality of psychological assessment is primarily determined by evaluating the presence of the psychometric characteristics of reliability and validity. "Reliability" refers to the consistency or replicability of test scores. Reliability data are reported in terms of the consistency of test results over time (i.e., test–retest reliability), over different interviewers or raters (i.e., inter-rater reliability), or over the many items comprising a particular test (internal consistency). For continuous measures, reliability is reported as a simple correlation coefficient that can vary between 0 and 1 (referred to as "Cronbach's alpha" when internal consistency is evaluated). For dichotomous measures such as diagnostic interviews (indicating the presence or absence of a disorder), reliability is reported as a kappa coefficient (Cohen, 1960) between 0 and 1 and is interpreted as the percent agreement above chance (Keane & Kaloupek, 2002; Keane et al., 2000).

"Validity" refers to the extent to which evidence exists to support the various inferences, interpretations, conclusions, or decisions that will be made on the basis of a test. "Content validity" represents the extent to which a test provides coverage of the domain of symptoms of a condition. The better the coverage of key symptoms, the better the content validity. "Criterion-related validity" refers to evidence that the test can predict some variable or criterion of interest (e.g., response to an intervention). The criterion may be measured either at the same time the test is administered (concurrent) or at some point after the test is administered (predictive). Finally, "construct validity" refers to evidence that the test measures the construct of interest (e.g., PTSD). This is often demonstrated by showing that the test correlates strongly with other measures of the same construct but not with measures of other constructs (Keane & Kaloupek, 2002; Keane, Kimble, Kaufman, & Kaloupek, in press; Keane et al., 2000).

Diagnostic instruments in the field of mental health are usually evaluated on the basis of their diagnostic utility, a type of criterion-related validity pertaining to a test's capacity to predict diagnostic status (Kraemer, 1992). There are three steps in determining the diagnostic utility of a given instrument. First, a "gold standard" is selected. In psychological research this gold standard is ordinarily a diagnosis that is made on the basis of a clinical interview, but may also be a composite based on several sources of information. Second, both the gold standard and the newly developed test are administered to the experimental group of participants. Finally, cutoff scores are examined to determine their diagnostic utility—that is, in other words, their ability to predict the diagnosis provided by the gold standard. Optimal cutoff scores for the test are those that predict the greatest number of cases and non-cases from the original sample (Keane et al., 2000; Weathers, Keane, King, & King, 1996).

All measures of psychological disorders are imperfect (Gerardi, Keane, & Penk, 1989). Two measures of the error contained within a test are false positives and false negatives. A false positive occurs when a patient falls above the cutoff but does not have the disorder. A false negative occurs when a patient falls below the given cutoff but does have the disorder. Diagnostic utility is often described in terms of a test's sensitivity and specificity. "Sensitivity" is the measure of a test's true positive rate, or the probability that those with the disorder will score above a given cutoff score. "Specificity" is the true negative rate of a test, or the probability that those without the disorder will score below the cutoff for the test. Sensitivity is low if the test yields too many false negatives, whereas specificity is low if the test yields too many false positives (Keane et al., 2000).

Types of Assessment Measures

Structured Diagnostic Interviews

Clinician-administered structured diagnostic interviews are considered extremely valuable tools for assessing PTSD symptomatology (Keane et al., 1995). Although it is standard practice in clinical research settings to employ structured diagnostic interviews, the use of these types of interviews in the clinical setting is less common, with perhaps the single exception of clinical forensic practice (Keane, 1995; Keane, Buckley, & Miller, 2003). In general, the infrequency of use may be due to time and cost burdens, as well as the need for specialized training to master the administration of many of these interviews. Nonetheless, it has been suggested that increased use of structured diagnostic interviews for PTSD in clinical settings may well improve diagnostic accuracy and aid in treatment planning (Litz & Weathers, 1994).

Several structured interviews are available that were developed for the assessment of PTSD either as modules of comprehensive diagnostic assessment tools or as independent PTSD measures. These are described below.

STRUCTURED CLINICAL INTERVIEW FOR THE DSM-IV

The Structured Clinical Interview for the DSM-IV (SCID-IV; First et al., 2000) is designed to assess a broad range of psychiatric conditions on Axes I and II. It is divided into separate modules corresponding to DSM-IV diagnostic criteria (American Psychiatric Association, 1994); each module provides the interviewer with specific prompts and follow-up inquiries intended to be read verbatim to respondents. Symptom presence is rated on a 3-point confidence scale based on the interviewer's interpretation of the individual's responses to the questions. To assess PTSD, respondents are asked to frame symptoms in terms of their "worst trauma experience." The SCID is intended for use only by clinicians and highly trained interviewers.

Although the administration of the full SCID-IV can be time consuming, the modular structure allows clinicians to limit their assessment to conditions that are frequently comorbid with PTSD. Within the context of a trauma clinic, it is recommended that modules for anxiety disorders, mood disorders, and substance use disorders be administered. Administration of the psychotic screen will also help to rule out conditions that require a different set of interventions (Keane & Barlow, 2002).

The SCID-PTSD module is considered psychometrically sound. Keane et al. (1998) examined the interrater reliability of the SCID by asking a second interviewer to listen to audiotapes of an initial interview. They found a kappa of .68 and agreement across lifetime, current, and never PTSD of 78%. Similarly, in a sample of patients who were reinterviewed within a week by a different clinician, they found a kappa of .66 and diagnostic agreement of 78%. McFall, Smith, Roszell, Tarver, and Malas (1990b) reported evidence of convergent validity, finding significant correlations between the number of SCID-PTSD items endorsed and other measures of PTSD (e.g., Mississippi Scale [.65; Keane, Caddell, & Taylor, 1988] and MMPI-PTSD Scale [.46; Keane, Malloy, & Fairbank, 1984]). The SCID-PTSD module also yielded substantial sensitivity (.81) and specificity (.98) and a robust kappa (.82) in one clinical sample against a composite PTSD diagnosis (Kulka et al., 1988), indicating good diagnostic utility.

Disadvantages to the SCID have been described previously. First, the scoring algorithm of the SCID permits only a dichotomous rating (e.g., presence or absence of a PTSD diagnosis), which has limitations. Most clinicians agree that psychological symptoms occur in a dimensional rather than dichotomous fashion (Keane, et al., 2000). Another disadvantage of the SCID is that it does not assess for the frequency or severity of symptoms. Third, by assessing symptoms in response to the "worst event" experienced, important information may be lost regarding the effects of other traumatic events (Cusack, Falsetti, & de Arellano, 2002). Finally, the trauma screen of the SCID may miss significant traumatic events (Falsetti et al., 1996).

CLINICIAN ADMINISTERED PTSD SCALE

Developed by the National Center for PTSD (Blake et al., 1990), the Clinician Administered PTSD Scale (CAPS) is currently one of the most widely used structured interviews for diagnosing and measuring the severity of PTSD (Weathers, Keane, & Davidson, 2001). The CAPS assesses all DSM-IV diagnostic criteria for PTSD, including criteria A (exposure), B–D (core symptom clusters), E (chronology), and F (functional impairment), as well as associated symptoms of guilt and dissociation. An important feature of the CAPS is that it contains separate ratings for the frequency and intensity of each symptom, which can be summed to create a severity score for each symptom. This permits flexibility in scoring and analyses. The CAPS also promotes uniform administration and scoring through carefully phrased prompt questions and explicit rating scale anchors with clear behavioral referents. Once trained, interviewers are able to ask their own follow-up questions and use their clinical judgment in arriving at the best ratings.

Similar to the SCID, flexibility is built into the administration of the CAPS. Interviewers can administer only subscales for the 17 core symptoms, all DSM-IV criteria (American Psychiatric Association, 1994), and/or add subscales for the associated symptoms. If administered in its entirety, the CAPS takes approximately 1 hour, but the time for administration is cut in half if only the 17 core symptoms are assessed.

Weathers et al. (2001) extensively reviewed the psychometric studies conducted on the CAPS; Weathers, Ruscio, and Keane (1999) also examined the reliability and validity data of the CAPS across five samples of male Vietnam veterans, collected at the National Center for PTSD. Robust estimates were found for interrater reliability over a 2- to 3-day interval for each of the three symptom clusters (.86–.87 for frequency, .86–.92 for intensity, and .88–.91 for severity) and all 17 symptoms (.91 for total frequency, .91 for total intensity, and .92 for total severity). Test–retest reliability for a CAPS-based PTSD diagnosis was also high (kappa = .89 in one sample and 1.00 in a second sample). Thus the data indicate that trained and calibrated raters can achieve a high degree of consistency in using the CAPS to rate PTSD symptom severity and diagnose PTSD. Weathers et al. (1999) also found high internal consistency across all 17 items in a research sample (alphas of .93 for frequency and .94 for intensity and severity) and a clinical sample (alphas of .85 for frequency, .86 for intensity, and .87 for severity), which supports the use of the CAPS in both research and clinical settings.

Strong evidence for validity of the CAPS was also provided by Weathers et al. (1999), who found that the CAPS total severity score correlated highly with other measures of PTSD (Mississippi Scale =.91; MMPI-PTSD Scale = .77; the number of PTSD symptoms endorsed on the SCID = .89; and the PTSD Checklist [PCL] = .94). As expected, correlations with measures of antisocial personality disorder were low (.14–.33). Weathers et al. (1999) also found strong evidence for the diagnostic utility of the CAPS, using three CAPS scoring rules for predicting a SCID-based PTSD diagnosis. The rule having the closest correspondence to the SCID yielded a sensitivity of .91, specificity of .84, and efficiency of .88, with a kappa of .75, indicating good diagnostic utility (see Weathers et al., 1999, for a detailed discussion of different scoring rules and their implications).

The CAPS has now been used successfully with a wide variety of trauma populations (e.g., combat veterans, victims of rape, crime, motor vehicle accidents, incest, the Holocaust, torture, and cancer), has served as the primary diagnostic or outcome measure in more than 200 empirical studies on PTSD, and has been translated into at least 12 languages (Weathers et al., 2001). Thus the existing data strongly support its continued use in both clinical and research settings.

PTSD SYMPTOM SCALE INTERVIEW

Developed by Foa, Riggs, Dancu, and Rothbaum (1993), the PTSD Symptom Scale Interview (PSS-I) is a structured interview designed to assess symptoms of PTSD in individuals with a known trauma history. Using a Likert scale, interviewers rate the severity of 17 symptoms corresponding to the DSM-III-R (American Psychiatric Association, 1987) criteria for PTSD. One limitation of the PSS-I is that it measures symptoms over the past 2 weeks, rather than 1 month, which the DSM criteria specify as necessary for a diagnosis of PTSD (Cusack et al., 2002). According to the authors, the PSS-I can be administered by lay interviewers who are trained to recognize the clinical picture presented by traumatized individuals.

The PSS-I was originally tested in a sample of women with a history of rape and nonsexual assault (Foa et al., 1993) and found to have strong psychometric properties. Foa et al. reported high internal consistency (Cronbach alphas = .85 for full scale, .65–.71 for subscales), test–retest reliability over a 1-month period (.80), and interrater agreement for a PTSD diagnosis (kappa = .91, 95% agreement). With respect to validity, the PSS-I was significantly correlated with other measures of traumatic stress (e.g., .69, Impact of Event Scale [IES] Intrusion score [Horowitz, Wilner, & Alvarez, 1979]; .67, Rape Aftermath Symptom Test total score [RAST; Kilpatrick, 1988]) and demonstrated good diagnostic utility when compared to a SCID-PTSD diagnosis (sensitivity = .88; specificity = .96). The PSS-I appears to possess many strong features that warrant its consideration for clinical and research use, especially with sexual assault survivors.

STRUCTURED INTERVIEW FOR PTSD

Originally developed by Davidson, Smith, and Kudler (1989), the Structured Interview for PTSD (SIP) is designed to diagnose PTSD and measure symptom severity. It includes 17 items focused on the DSM-IV (1994) criteria for PTSD as well as two items focused on survivor and behavior guilt. Each item is rated by the interviewer on a Likert scale. There are initial probe questions and follow-up questions to promote a more thorough understanding of the respondent's symptom experiences. It can be administered by clinicians or appropriately trained paraprofessionals. The SIP takes 10–30 minutes to administer, depending upon the level of symptomatology present.

Psychometric data for the SIP is good. In a sample of combat veterans, Davidson et al. (1989) reported high interrater reliability (.97–.99) on total SIP scores and perfect agreement on the presence or absence of PTSD across raters. High alpha coefficients have also been reported (.94 for the veteran sample [Davidson et al., 1989] and .80 for PTSD patients enrolled in a clinical trial [Davidson, Malik, & Travers, 1997]). In the veteran sample, test–retest reliability for the total SIP score was .71 over a 2-week period. With respect to validity, the SIP was significantly correlated with other measures of PTSD, but not with measures of combat exposure (.49–.67; Davidson et al., 1989, 1997, as cited in Orsillo, 2001, p. 291). Davidson et al. (1989) compared the SIP scores of current and remitted SCID-defined PTSD cases and reported good sensitivity (.96) and specificity (.80) against the SCID. At a cutoff score of 25, the SIP correctly classified 94% of cases relative to a structured clinical interview (Davidson et al., 1997). Overall, the SIP appears to be a sound instrument

TREATMENT OUTCOME PTSD SCALE

Derived from the 19-item SIP, the Treatment Outcome PTSD Scale (TOP-8) was designed as a brief interview to assess core symptoms of PTSD in treatment outcome studies (Davidson & Colket, 1997). Item selection was drawn from a sample of patients with chronic PTSD who were taking part in a clinical trial for pharmacological treatment. The interview includes eight items reflecting symptoms that are thought to occur most frequently in PTSD and demonstrate the most change in response to treatment. Using a Likert scale, interviewers rate how much each symptom has "troubled the person" during the past week. It takes 5–10 minutes to administer.

Initial data on the TOP-8 scale indicate that it has good psychometric properties, including high internal consistency (Cronbach alpha = .73), test–retest reliability (.88; Connor & Davidson, 1999), and interrater reliability (.96; Davidson & Colket, 1997). Evidence for convergent validity has also been provided (e.g., correlations of .91 with the Davidson Trauma Scale [Davidson, Book et al., 1997], .89 with the IES, and .98 with the SIP).

According to Davidson and Colket (1997), the advantages of the TOP-8 are that it takes less time than many other structured interviews, eliminates items reflective of symptoms that are rare or unlikely to change, and may reduce counter- or therapeutic effects of lengthy interviews. They acknowledge its disadvantages of eliminating clinically important or distressing symptoms and offering less ability to explore properties of treatment.

Unfortunately, the methodological strategies used to construct and validate the scale are not commonly accepted in the psychometric literature. The results of the preliminary studies might be a function of these idiosyncratic methods, the specific nature of the small samples employed, or the fact that the scale was derived entirely retrospectively rather than prospectively. Thus replications using additional methods are necessary before endorsing the shortened version of the SIP. The authors appropriately recommend that clinicians and researchers may want to use this interview only in conjunction with other clinical measures.

ANXIETY DISORDERS INTERVIEW SCHEDULE–REVISED

Originally developed by DiNardo, O'Brien, Barlow, Waddell, and Blanchard (1983), the Anxiety Disorders Interview Schedule (ADIS) was designed to permit differential diagnoses among the DSM-III (American Psychiatric Association, 1980) anxiety disorder categories and to provide detailed symptom ratings. The interview was revised to fit DSM-III-R (American Psychiatric Association, 1987) (ADIS-R; DiNardo & Barlow, 1988) and more recently DSM-IV (American Psychiatric Association, 1994) criteria (ADIS-IV; DiNardo, Brown, & Barlow, 1994). The ADIS-IV also includes an assessment of mood disorders, substance use disorders, and selected somatoform disorders, a diagnostic time line, and a dimensional assessment of the key and associated features of the disorders. The provision of a dimensional as well as a categorical assessment allows the clinician to describe subthreshold manifestations of each disorder and offers more possibilities for analyses. The ADIS has been translated into numerous languages and used in over 150 clinical and research settings around the world. It is recommended only for trained, experienced interviewers.

Psychometric studies on the ADIS-PTSD module provide mixed results. Originally tested in a small sample of Vietnam combat veterans, the ADIS-PTSD module yielded strong sensitivity (1.0) and specificity (.91), and 93% agreement with interview-determined diagnoses (Blanchard, Gerardi, Kolb, & Barlow, 1986). DiNardo, Moras, Barlow, Rapee, and Brown (1993) tested the reliability of the ADIS-R in a community sample recruited from an anxiety disorders clinic and found only fair agreement between two independent raters when PTSD was the principal diagnosis or an additional diagnosis (kappa = .55). In a test of the ADIS-IV, the interrater reliability across two interviews given 10 days apart was also fair for current diagnoses (kappa = .59; Brown, DiNardo, Lehman, & Campbell, 2001) but slightly improved for lifetime diagnoses (kappa = .61). Additional reliability and validity data on the ADIS-IV are needed to ensure its continued use in clinical and research settings.

PTSD-INTERVIEW

Developed by Watson, Juba, Manifold, Kucala, and Anderson (1991), the PTSD-Interview (PTSD-I) is a diagnostic interview based on the DSM-III-R (American Psychiatric Association, 1987) that differs in administrative format from most other interviews. Patients are given a copy of the scale to read along with the interviewer and are asked to provide a rating (based on a Likert scale) for each of the symptoms. This format shares much in common with self-report questionnaires yet deviates from the other diagnostic scales in that it does not allow clinicians to make ratings of their own, based on their expertise and experience. The PTSD-I yields both dichotomous and continuous information.

Psychometric data on the PTSD-I is excellent. Watson et al. (1991) administered the PTSD-I to a sample of veteran outpatients and found high test–retest reliability (.95) for the PTSD-I total score over a 1-week interval and high interrater reliability for a PTSD diagnosis (kappa = .61, 87% agreement). A high alpha coefficient (.92) indicated good internal consistency. With regard to validity, the total score of the PTSD-I has been shown to correlate highly with other measures of PTSD (e.g., PTSD section of the Diagnostic Interview Schedule [DIS; Robins & Helzer, 1985] = .94, Watson et al., 1991; and the IES =.85, Wilson, Tinker, Becker, & Gillette, 1994). Compared to the DIS-PTSD scale, Watson et al. found that the PTSD-I yielded a sensitivity of .89, specificity of .94, and overall efficiency of .92, indicating good diagnostic utility.

Self-Report PTSD Questionnaires

Numerous self-report measures have been developed as a method of obtaining information on PTSD. For the most part, self-report measures are used as continuous measures of PTSD to reflect symptom severity; in several cases, however, specific cutoff scores have been developed to provide a diagnosis of PTSD. These measures are generally more time and cost efficient than structured interviews and can be especially valuable when used as screens for PTSD or in conjunction with structured interviews. The data also support the use of self-report questionnaires alone in clinical and research settings when administering a structured interview is not feasible or practical. Many of the measures can be used interchangeably, because the findings appear to be robust for the minor variations in methods and approaches involved. In selecting a particular instrument, the clinician is encouraged to examine the data for the population on which that instrument is to be employed. In so doing, the clinician is likely to maximize the accuracy and efficiency of the test employed (Keane & Barlow, 2002).

IMPACT OF EVENT SCALE–REVISED

Developed by Horowitz et al. (1979), the IES is one of the most widely used self-report measures to assess psychological responses to a traumatic stressor. The initial 15-item questionnaire, which focused only on intrusion and avoidance symptoms, was derived from a model of traumatic stress developed by Horowitz (1976). Since the publication of the DSM-IV (American Psychiatric Association, 1994), a revised 22-item version of the scale (IES-R; Weiss & Marmar, 1997) was developed that includes items on hyperarousal symptoms and flashback experiences. Thus the IES-R more closely parallels DSM-IV criteria for PTSD. To complete the measure, respondents rate (on a Likert scale) "how distressed or bothered" they were by each symptom during the past week since a traumatic event. The IES has been translated into several languages and has been used with many different trauma populations. It takes approximately 10 minutes to complete.

Data on the psychometric properties of the revised IES-R are preliminary. In two studies that incorporated four samples of emergency workers and earthquake survivors, Weiss and Marmar (1997) reported satisfactory internal consistency for each of the subscales (alphas = .87–.92 for Intrusion, .84–.86 for Avoidance, and .79–.90 for Hyperarousal). Test–retest reliability data from two samples yielded a range of reliability coefficients for the subscales (Intrusion = .57–.94, Avoidance = .51–.89, and Hyperarousal = .59–.92). Weiss and Marmar suggest that the shorter interval between assessments and the greater recency of the traumatic event contributed to higher coefficients of stability for one sample.

Convergent and discriminant validity data are not yet available for the IES-R. There were many questions raised about the validity of the original scale, in part because it did not assess all DSM criteria for PTSD (see Weathers et al., 1996; Joseph, 2000). Although it now more closely parallels the DSM-IV (1994), items measuring numbing are considered limited by some investigators (Foa, Cashman, Jaycox, & Perry, 1997). In a review of psychometric studies on the IES, Sundin and Horowitz (2002) report a range of correlations between the IES subscales and other self-report measures (e.g., .31–.46 on SCL-90 [Symptom Checklist] PTSD items; Arata, Saunders, & Kilpatrick, 1991) and diagnostic interviews (e.g., .32–.49 for SCID—McFall et al., 1990b; .75–.79 for CAPS—Neal et al., 1994). Neal et al. (1994) reported high sensitivity (.89) and specificity (.88) for the original scale when compared to a CAPS diagnosis. Additional studies with the revised instrument are clearly needed to establish its reliability and validity and ensure its continued use in clinics and research settings.

MISSISSIPPI SCALE FOR COMBAT-RELATED PTSD

Developed by Keane et al. (1988), the 35-item Mississippi Scale is widely used to assess combat-related PTSD symptoms. The scale items were selected from an initial pool of 200 items generated by experts to closely match the DSM-III (American Psychiatric Association, 1980) criteria for the disorder. The Mississippi Scale has been updated and now assesses the presence of symptoms reflecting the DSM-IV (1994) criteria for PTSD and several associated features. Respondents are asked to rate, on a Likert scale, the severity of symptoms over the time period occurring "since the event." The Mississippi Scale yields a continuous score of symptom severity as well as diagnostic information. It is available in several languages and takes 10–15 minutes to administer.

The Mississippi Scale has excellent psychometric properties. In Vietnam veterans seeking treatment, Keane et al. (1988) reported high internal consistency (alpha = .94) and test–retest reliability (.97) over a 1-week time interval. In a subsequent validation study, the authors found substantial sensitivity (.93) and specificity (.89) with a cutoff of 107, and an overall hit rate of 90% when the scale was used to differentiate between a PTSD group and two non-PTSD comparison groups.

McFall, Smith, Mackay, and Tarver (1990a) replicated these findings and further demonstrated that PTSD patients with and without substance use disorders did not differ on the Mississippi Scale. Given the high comorbidity between PTSD and substance use disorders, the authors felt it was important to demonstrate that the test assesses PTSD symptoms rather than effects associated with alcohol and drug use. McFall et al. (1990a) also obtained information on convergent validity, finding significant correlations between the Mississippi Scale and other measures of PTSD, including the total number of SCID-PTSD symptoms (.57), total IES score (.46), and degree of traumatic combat exposure (.40; Vietnam-Era Stress Inventory, Wilson & Krauss, 1984). These findings suggest that the Mississippi Scale is a valuable self-report tool in settings where assessment of combat-related PTSD is needed.

KEANE PTSD SCALE OF THE MMPI-2

Originally derived from the MMPI Form R (Keane et al., 1984), the Keane PTSD Scale (PK) now consists of 46 items empirically drawn from the MMPI-2 (Lyons & Keane, 1992). The items are answered in a true/false format. The scale is typically administered as part of the full MMPI-2 but can be useful as a stand-alone scale. The embedded and stand-alone versions are highly correlated (.90; Herman, Weathers, Litz, & Keane, 1996). The PK Scale yields a total score that reflects the presence or absence of PTSD. The stand-alone scale takes 15 minutes to administer.

Psychometric data on the embedded and stand-alone versions of the PK Scale are excellent. Herman et al. (1996) reported evidence from a veteran sample of strong internal consistency of the embedded and stand-alone versions of the MMPI-2 PTSD Scale (alphas ranging from .95 to .96), and high test–retest reliability coefficients for the stand-alone version over 2 to 3 days (.95). With regard to validity, the embedded and stand-alone versions of the MMPI-2 PTSD scale were correlated with other self-report measures of PTSD, including the Mississippi Scale (.81–.85), IES (.65–.71), and PCL (.77–.83), and a diagnostic interview (CAPS; .77 to .80). The embedded and stand-alone versions differed slightly in their optimally efficient cutoff score (26 vs. 24, respectively), but both demonstrated good sensitivity (.72 for embedded, .82 for stand-alone), specificity (.82 for embedded, .76 for stand-alone), and efficiency (.76 for embedded, .80 for stand-alone) compared to a CAPS diagnosis.

More research is needed to determine the generalizability of the findings on veterans with other populations, as well as the optimal cutoff scores (Foa et al., 1997; Watson, Kucala, & Manifold, 1986). Although only a few studies have been conducted on the PK in nonveteran populations, the data presented appear to be promising (Koretzky & Peck, 1990; Neal et al., 1994). The PK may be particularly useful in the area of forensic psychology, where the MMPI-2 is frequently employed because of its validity indexes.

POSTTRAUMATIC STRESS DIAGNOSTIC SCALE

Developed by Foa et al. (1997), the Posttraumatic Stress Diagnostic Scale (PDS) is a 49-item scale designed to measure DSM-IV (American Psychiatric Association, 1994) PTSD criteria and symptom severity. The PDS is a revised version of an earlier self-report scale based on the DSM-III-R (American Psychiatric Association, 1987), referred to as the PTSD Symptom Scale–Self-Report Version (PSS-SR; Foa et al., 1993). The PDS reviews trauma exposure and identifies the most distressing trauma. It also assesses criterion A-2 (physical threat or helplessness), criteria B–D (intensity and frequency of all 17 symptoms), and Criterion F (functional impairment). This scale has been used with several populations, including combat veterans, accident victims, and sexual and nonsexual assault survivors. The PDS can be administered in 10–15 minutes.

The psychometric properties of the PDS were evaluated among 264 volunteers recruited from several PTSD treatment centers as well as from nontreatment-seeking populations at high risk for trauma (Foa, et al., 1997). Investigators reported high internal consistency for the PTSD total score (alpha = .92) and subscales (alphas = .78–.84) and satisfactory test–retest reliability coefficients for the total PDS score and for the symptom cluster scores (.77–.85). With regard to validity, the PDS total score correlated highly with other scales that measure traumatic responses (IES Intrusion = .80 and Avoidance = .66; RAST = .81). In addition, the measure yielded substantial sensitivity (.89), specificity (.75), and high levels of diagnostic agreement with a SCID diagnosis (kappa = .65, 82% agreement). Based on these data, the authors have recommended the PDS as an effective and efficient screening tool for PTSD.

PTSD CHECKLIST

Developed by researchers at the National Center for PTSD (Weathers et al., 1993), the PTSD Checklist (PCL) is a 17-item self-report measure of PTSD symptomatology. Different scoring procedures may be used to yield either a continuous measure of PTSD symptom severity or a dichotomous indicator of diagnostic status. Furthermore, dichotomous scoring methods include either an overall cutoff score or a symptom cluster scoring approach. The original scale was based on the DSM-III-R criteria for PTSD; the PCL has been updated to assess the 17 diagnostic criteria outlined in the DSM-IV (American Psychiatric Association, 1994). Respondents are asked to rate, on a Likert scale, "how much each problem has bothered them" during the past month. The time frame can be adjusted, as needed, to suit the goals of the assessment. There is a civilian (PCL-C) and a military version (PCL-M) of the measure. On the civilian version reexperiencing and avoidance symptoms apply to any lifetime stressful event, whereas on the PCL-M, reexperiencing and avoidance symptoms apply only to stressful events that are military-related. The PCL has been used extensively in both research and clinical settings and takes 5–10 minutes to administer. If needed, a 17-item Life Events Checklist, developed as a companion to the CAPS and aimed at identifying exposure to potentially traumatic experiences (thereby establishing criteria A for the diagnosis), can be used with the PCL.

The PCL was originally validated in a sample of Vietnam and Persian Gulf War veterans and found to have strong psychometric properties (Weathers, Litz, Herman, Huska, & Keane, 1993). Keen, Kutter, Niles, and Krinsley (2004) examined the psychometric properties of the updated PCL in veterans with both combat and noncombat traumas and found evidence for high internal consistency (alpha = .96 for all 17 symptoms). Test–retest reliability was not examined, but the original study suggested that reliability was robust (.96) over a 2- to 3-day interval, and other investigators have documented adequate test–retest reliability of this measure over a 2-week time frame (Ruggiero, Del Ben, Scotti, & Rabalais, 2003).

With respect to validity, Keen et al. (2004) found that the scale was highly correlated with other measures of PTSD, including the Mississippi Scale (.90) and CAPS (total symptom severity = .79). Using a slightly higher cutoff score (i.e., 60) than Weathers et al. (1993) used, Keen et al. also found that the PCL had a sensitivity of .56, a specificity of .92, and overall efficiency of .84 when compared to the CAPS, indicating good diagnostic power.

Several studies now offer evidence for the reliability and validity of the PCL in nonveteran samples, although there are discrepancies reported in the optimal cutoff score to obtain the highest level of diagnostic efficiency. The possible reasons for these discrepancies (e.g., gender, recency of trauma, severity of trauma, and treatment-seeking status; Manne, DuHamel, Gallelli, Sorgen, & Redd, 1998) warrant further investigation. In addition, there is evidence that different scoring options for the PCL (e.g., an absolute cutoff score vs. symptom cluster scoring) yield differences in sensitivity, specificity, and diagnostic efficiency. Keen et al. (2004) suggest that the selection of a scoring routine may depend on the goal of the assessment; for example, symptom cluster scoring was associated with higher sensitivity and may be preferable when the goal is to identify all possible cases of PTSD, whereas the cutoff method was associated with higher specificity and may be preferable for research or when clinical resources are limited.

LOS ANGELES SYMPTOM CHECKLIST

Developed by King, King, Leskin, and Foy (1995), the Los Angeles Symptom Checklist (LASC) is a 43-item scale that diagnoses PTSD and describes symptom severity. The original scale, referred to as the PTSD Symptom Checklist (Foy, Sipprelle, Rueger, & Carroll, 1984), was designed to closely adhere to DSM-III (American Psychiatric Association, 1980) criteria and has now been updated to correspond to the DSM-IV (American Psychiatric Association, 1994). The LASC includes an assessment of B, C, and D criteria (17 items). Respondents are asked to rate, on a Likert scale, "how much of a problem" each symptom is for them. There is also a global assessment of distress and adjustment problems related to trauma exposure. No time frame is established for rating symptoms. Originally validated on a veteran sample, the LACS has now been used to assess trauma symptoms in several other traumatized groups (see King et al., 1995 for details). It takes approximately 15 minutes to administer.

Psychometric data on the LASC are strong. King et al. (1995) combined data from 10 studies that used the LACS with clinical samples derived from a diverse set of populations (i.e., Vietnam veterans, battered women, adult survivors of childhood abuse, maritally distressed women, psychiatric outpatients, and high-risk adolescents). Evidence was provided for high internal consistency among veterans (alpha = .94 for 17 items measuring PTSD and .94 for the 43-item index) and women (alpha = .89 for 17-item index and .93 for 43-item index). With regard to test–retest reliability over a 2-week period, the 17-item set yielded a coefficient of .94, and the 43-item set yielded a coefficient of .90, suggesting stability in responses over time. With respect to validity, LASC scores correlate to varying degrees with measures of combat exposure (.51 for Combat Exposure Scale; Foy et al., 1984) and traumatic stress (e.g., 38 for Intrusion and .48 for Avoidance subscales on the IES; Astin, Lawrence, & Foy, 1993). Using only the 17-item PTSD severity index, King et al. found a sensitivity of .74, specificity of .77, and an overall hit rate of 76% compared to a SCID diagnosis. Using a diagnostic categorization scheme, the sensitivity was .78, specificity was .82, and the overall hit rate was 80% compared to the SCID. Thus the results obtained by using either scoring scheme provide an acceptable level of precision in classifying patients with and without PTSD.

DISTRESSING EVENT QUESTIONNAIRE

Developed by Kubany, Leisen, Kaplan, and Kelly (2000), the Distressing Event Questionnaire (DEQ) provides dichotomous and continuous information. It does not assess criterion A-1 (occurrence of the traumatic event) but has three items that assess criterion A-2 (presence of intense fear, helplessness, and horror at the time of the event) and 17 items that assess the DSM-IV (American Psychiatric Association, 1994) diagnostic symptoms of PTSD (criteria B–D). Respondents are asked to indicate, on a Likert scale, "the degree to which they experienced each of the symptoms" within the last month. Additional items focus on chronology (criterion E), distress and functional impairment (criterion F), and associated features of guilt, anger, and unresolved grief. The DEQ takes 5–7 minutes to complete.

Kubany et al. (2000) conducted a series of studies to evaluate the psychometric properties of the DEQ, and the results are excellent. Samples included male Vietnam combat veterans and women with mixed trauma histories (including incest, rape, partner abuse, prostitution, and sexual abuse). In the initial study they found high internal consistency (alpha = .93 for total score and .88–.91 across symptom clusters). In a second study they reported high test–retest reliability (.83–.94) over an average of 10 days using a variety of scoring methods. The third and largest study provided evidence for construct validity. The DEQ total scale score was highly correlated with the

CAPS (.82–.90) and Modified PTSD Symptom Scale (.86–.94; Falsetti, Resnick, Resick, & Kilpatrick, 1993). Furthermore, using the CAPS as a criterion measure, an optimal cutoff score of 26 yielded a sensitivity of .87, specificity of .85, and diagnostic efficiency of .86 in the veteran sample. For women, a cutoff score of 18 yielded a sensitivity of .98, specificity of .58, and overall efficiency of .90. A particular strength of this scale is that it was able to correctly classify PTSD in a high percentage of men and women despite differences in trauma exposure and ethnicities.

Psychophysiological Measures

Over the past 10 years, research on biologically based measures of PTSD has established a foundation for a psychobiological description of PTSD (Orr, Metzger, Miller, & Kaloupek, 2004). Much of the work found that PTSD alters a wide range of physiological functions (Yehuda, 1997), and some researchers assert that PTSD may affect structural components of the brain (particularly the hippocampus; Bremner et al., 1995). Overall, the most consistent finding in this area is that psychophysiological reactivity to trauma-specific cues is elevated in individuals with PTSD, but not in trauma-exposed individuals without PTSD (for reviews see Orr et al., 2004; Prins, Kaloupek, & Keane, 1995).

As an extension of these findings, a number of studies has attempted to identify and classify cases of PTSD on the basis of psychophysiological reactivity to trauma-related cues (Blanchard, Kolb, & Prins, 1991; Malloy, Fairbank, & Keane, 1983; Pitman, Orr, Forgue, de Jong, & Claiborne, 1987). A psychophysiological assessment usually involves presenting individuals with standardized stimuli (e.g., combat photos, noises, odors) or personalized cues (e.g., taped scripts of traumatic experiences) related to their trauma. Measurements are taken of one or more physiological indices (e.g., blood pressure, heart rate, muscle tension, or skin conductance level), subjective responses (e.g., arousal and distress), and behavior (e.g., startle response, averting gaze, crying). Because no one psychophysiological index is error-free, convergent measures are recommended.

The capacity of psychophysiological indices to identify and classify cases of PTSD on the basis of reactivity to trauma cues has been documented, with sensitivity values ranging from 60 to 90% and specificity values falling between 80 and 100% (Keane et al., 1998; Orr et al., 2004). Furthermore, these findings were replicated in individuals exposed to a range of traumatic events (e.g., motor vehicle accidents, combat, sexual assault, and terrorism).

Although psychophysiological assessment can provide unique and accurate information, widespread use of this approach is not anticipated. Psychophysiological assessment can be expensive in terms of time and patient burden, and requires specialized training on the part of the clinician. In many situations, more time- and cost-efficient methods of assessment, such as the diagnostic interview or self-report measures, are adequate. Nonetheless, in cases where diagnostic accuracy is of the utmost importance (e.g., in forensic evaluations), it may be wise to employ this assessment strategy (cf. Keane, 1995; Prins et al., 1995). The availability of portable systems to conduct this type of measurement makes this technique increasingly feasible.

Another biological system of great interest for the assessment of PTSD is the hypothalamic–pituitary–adrenocortical axis. In particular, indices of cortisol and norepinephrine, and their ratio, appear important in terms of their ability to improve assessment of PTSD, above and beyond the use of diagnostic interviews and self-report measures (Yehuda, Giller, Levengood, Southwick, & Siever, 1995). Further research will help to determine how much benefit is achieved by adding these biological measures.

Special Issues in Assessment of PTSD

Cultural Issues

Several clinicians highlight the importance of considering the different populations on which an assessment instrument for PTSD was validated when selecting a measure. The need to develop instruments that are culturally sensitive has been of great interest for many years as a result of documentation of ethnocultural-specific responses to traumatic events. For example, several researchers have provided evidence of differences between people from ethnic minorities and European Americans in the severity of PTSD symptoms experienced following a traumatic event (e.g., Frueh, Brady, & Arellano, 1998; Green, Grace, Lindy, & Leonard, 1990; Kulka et al., 1990). The need for culturally sensitive instruments is further emphasized by the growing awareness among scholars that developing countries have a higher prevalence of PTSD than industrialized nations (De Girolamo & McFarlane, 1996).

To date, the psychological assessment of PTSD has developed primarily within the context of Western, developed, and industrialized countries. Thus PTSD assessment may be limited by a lack of culturally sensitive measures and by the tremendous diversity among the cultural groups of interest (Marsella, Friedman, Gerrity, & Scurfield, 1996). However, progress in developing culturally sensitive measures has been made.

A good example of a measure that possesses culturally relevant features is the Harvard Trauma Questionnaire (HTQ; Mollica et al., 1992), which has been widely used in refugee samples. The HTQ assesses a range of potentially traumatic events and trauma-related symptoms. The assessment of trauma includes many types of events to which refugees from war-torn countries may have been exposed, including torture, brainwashing, and deprivation of food or water. Originally developed in English, the HTQ has been translated and validated in Vietnamese, Laotian, and Khmer versions. In addition, the HTQ possesses linguistic equivalence across the many cultures and languages with which it has been used. Thus far, Mollica et al. have reported good reliability (test–retest = .89; interrater = .93; coefficient alpha = .96) for the HTQ (Cusack et al., 2002). Future research will need to document the reliability and validity of new instruments on a wider range of populations and develop additional instruments that have the culturally sensitive characteristics exemplified in the HTQ.

Comorbidity in PTSD

High rates of comorbidity are common in PTSD across diverse samples (e.g., males, females, veterans, sexual assault victims, crime victims, the general population), traumatic events (e.g., military, combat, rape, physical assault, childhood sexual abuse, violence), and patient and nonpatient status (help-seeking patients vs. community-based groups; Keane & Kaloupek, 1997; Kessler et al., 1994; Kessler, Sonnega, Bromet, Hughes, & Nelson, 1995). The most commonly diagnosed comorbid disorders are substance use disorders, mood disorders (e.g., major depressive disorder and dysthymia), and anxiety disorders (e.g., panic and phobias). Unlike other forms of depression seen in the absence of PTSD, when combined with PTSD depression often seems unremitting and in many cases appears as a "double depression" (i.e., major depressive episodes combined with longstanding dysthymia). In many cases, substance abuse may be secondary to PTSD and represent an effort to self-medicate symptoms. The co-occurrence of other disorders with PTSD is likely to complicate an individual's clinical presentation, compromise functioning across multiple domains, and negatively affect treatment outcomes (e.g., Brown, Stout, & Mueller, 1996; Ouimette, Finney, & Moos, 1999). Thus careful consideration of the onset of each disorder may be important to assess in order to arrive at the most appropriate treatment plan for an individual.

MONITORING OUTCOMES IN PTSD TREATMENT

Monitoring the outcome of psychological treatment is essential to help providers demonstrate the effectiveness of their treatments to patients and payers—something that has been in demand since the growth of managed care companies in the 1990s. Keane and Kaloupek (1982) presented the first empirical evidence that cognitive-behavioral treatments for PTSD had promise. Using a single-subject design, they employed subjective units of distress (SUDs) ratings (0–10) within treatment sessions to monitor changes in the presentation of traumatic memories in a prolonged exposure treatment paradigm. Between sessions, they utilized the Spielberger's State Anxiety Inventory (Spielberger, Gorsuch, Lushene, Vagg, & Jacobs, 1983) to monitor levels of anxiety and distress throughout the course of the 19 treatment sessions.

Currently, the use of sound psychometric instruments has become an important part of monitoring outcomes of PTSD treatment, regardless of whether the intervention is psychopharmacological, psychological, or a combination of the two (Keane & Kaloupek, 2002). Psychological tests and questionnaires often possess many virtues, including test–retest reliability, internal consistency, and indicators of validity. Moreover, they frequently present normative information against which an individual's performance can be compared to either the general population or target populations of interest (cf. Kraemer, 1992). For all these reasons, psychological tests or questionnaires with sound psychometric properties are warranted for consideration when clinicians are deciding how best to monitor the outcomes of their interventions (Keane & Kaloupek, 2002).

Fairbank and Keane (1982) also demonstrated the benefits of psychophysiological measurement in monitoring outcomes. They designed a study to evaluate the treatment of combat veterans with PTSD, using a multiple baseline design across traumatic memories. Measures to monitor change included SUDs ratings and heart rate and skin conductance response. Systematic improvement was observed in the treatment of traumatic memories, as evidenced by changes in SUDS ratings, heart rate, and number of skin conductance responses. Although this form of monitoring is intensive, it suggests that the level of change incorporates physiological domains and thus is a rigorous assessment of the impact of the treatment provided. Clinicians are also encouraged to consider outcomes at several levels, including the symptom level, the individual level, the system level, and the social and contextual levels. All are important and can provide valuable information for both clinician and patient (Keane & Kaloupek, 1997; Keane & Kaloupek, 2002). There are numerous measures available to measure psychopathology; clinicians are encouraged to select the measures that are most appropriate for their circumstances and settings. Use of these measures at intervals (e.g., daily, weekly, monthly, quarterly) during the course of treatment will provide knowledge of the patient's status and communicate to the clinician the extent to which the patient is changing in the desired directions.

There are also a number of measures available to monitor a wider range of outcomes in other areas of an individual's life. For example, two increasingly popular measures of functioning across multiple domains, including physical and psychiatric functioning, are the SF-36 Health Survey (Ware & Kosinski, 2001) and the Behavior and Symptom Identification Scale (BASIS-32) (Eisen, Wilcox, Leff, Schaefer, & Culhane, 1999). Instruments are also available to measure patient and services satisfaction (Atkisson & Greenfield, 1999) as well as the dimensions of marital satisfaction and quality of life (e.g. Frisch, Cornell, Villañueva, & Retzlaff, 1992). Selection of the most appropriate measure of outcome is fundamentally a clinical decision that needs to rest with the provider in consultation with the patient.

SUMMARY

Assessment of traumatic events and PTSD is a topic of growing interest and concern in the mental health field (Wilson & Keane, 1997, 2004). Since the inclusion of PTSD in the DSM-III (American Psychiatric Association, 1980), there has been considerable progress in understanding and evaluating the psychological consequences of exposure to traumatic events. Conceptual models of PTSD assessment have evolved (Keane, Wolfe, & Taylor, 1987; Sutker, Uddo-Crane, & Allain, 1991), psychological tests have been developed (Foa et al., 1997; Norris & Riad, 1997), diagnostic interviews have been validated (Davidson et al., 1989; Foa et al., 1993; Weathers et al., 2001), and subscales of existing tests have been created to assess PTSD (i.e., MMPI-2, Keane et al., 1984). We can rightly conclude that the assessment devices available to evaluate PTSD are comparable to, or better than, those available for any disorder in the DSM. Moreover, multiple instruments are now available that cover the range of clinical needs. The psychometric data examining the reliability and validity of these instruments are nothing short of outstanding.

Clearly, the assessment of PTSD in clinical settings focuses on more than the presence, absence, and severity of PTSD. A comprehensive assessment strategy would purport to gather information about an individual's family history, life context, symptoms, beliefs, strengths, weaknesses, support system, and coping abilities (Newman, Kaloupek, & Keane, 1996). This comprehensive information would assist in the development of an effective treatment plan for the patient. The primary purpose of this review has been to examine the quality of a range of different instruments used to diagnose and assess PTSD (of course, the comprehensive assessment of a patient certainly needs to include indices of social, interpersonal, and occupational functioning). Finally, a satisfactory assessment ultimately relies upon the clinical and interpersonal skills of the clinician, because many topics related to trauma are inherently difficult for patients to disclose to others.

The present review is not intended to provide a comprehensive analysis of the psychometric properties of all instruments available for the assessment of PTSD. The intent of the review has been to provide a heuristic structure that clinicians might employ when selecting a particular instrument for their clinical purposes. By carefully examining the psychometric properties of an instrument, the clinician can make an informed decision about the appropriateness of a particular instrument for the task at hand. Instruments that provide a full utility analysis (e.g., sensitivity, specificity, hit rate) greatly assist clinicians in making their final judgments. Finally, instruments that are developed and evaluated on multiple trauma populations, across genders, and with different racial, cultural, and age groups are highly desirable; these are the fundamental objectives for future research.

REFERENCES

American Psychiatric Association. (1980). *Diagnostic and statistical manual of mental disorders* (3rd ed.). Washington, DC: Author.

American Psychiatric Association. (1987). *Diagnostic and statistical manual of mental disorders* (3rd ed., rev.). Washington, DC: Author.

American Psychiatric Association. (1994). *Diagnostic and statistical manual of mental disorders* (4th edition). Washington, DC: Author.

Arata, C. M., Saunders, B. E., & Kilpatrick, D. G. (1991). Concurrent validity of a crime-related post-traumatic stress disorder scale for women within the Symptom Checklist-90–Revised. *Violence and Victims, 6,* 191–199.

Astin, M. C., Lawrence, K. J., & Foy, D. W. (1993). Posttraumatic stress disorder among battered women: Risk and resiliency factors. *Violence and Victims, 8,* 17–28.

Atkisson, C. C., & Greenfield, T. K. (1999). The UCSF Client Satisfaction Scales. In M. E. Maruish (Ed.), *The use of psychological testing for treatment planning and outcomes assessment* (2nd ed., pp. 1333–1346). Mahwah, NJ: Erlbaum.

Blake, D. D., Weathers, F. W., Nagy, L. M., Kaloupek, D. G., Charney, D. S., & Keane, T. M. (1990). *The Clinician Administered PTSD Scale-IV.* Boston: National Center for PTSD, Behavioral Sciences Division.

Blanchard, E. B., Gerardi, R. J., Kolb, L. C., & Barlow, D. H. (1986). The utility of the Anxiety Disorders Interview Schedule (ADIS) in the diagnosis of post-traumatic stress disorder (PTSD) in Vietnam veterans. *Behaviour Research and Therapy, 24,* 577–580.

Blanchard, E. B., Kolb, L. C., & Prins, A. (1991). Psychophysiological responses in the diagnosis of posttraumatic stress disorder in Vietnam veterans. *Journal of Nervous and Mental Disease, 179,* 97–101.

Bremner, J. D., Randall, T. M., Scott, T. M., Bronen, R. A., Seibyl, J. P., Southwick, S. M. et al. (1995). MRI-based measures of hippocampal volume in patients with combat-related PTSD. *American Journal of Psychiatry, 152,* 973–981.

Brown, P. J., Stout, R. L., & Mueller, T. (1996). Posttraumatic stress disorder and substance abuse relapse among women: A pilot study. *Psychology of Addictive Behaviors, 10,* 124–128.

Brown, T. A., DiNardo, P. A., Lehman, C. L., & Campbell, L. A. (2001). Reliability of DSM-IV anxiety and mood disorders: Implications for the classification of emotional disorders. *Journal of Abnormal Psychology, 110,* 49–58.

Cohen, J. (1960). A coefficient of agreement for nominal scales. *Educational and Psychological Measurement, 20,* 37–46.

Connor, K. M., & Davidson, J. R. T. (1999). Further psychometric assessment of the TOP-8: A brief interview-based measure of PTSD. *Depression and Anxiety, 9,* 135–137.

Cusack, K., Falsetti, S., & de Arellano, M. (2002). Gender considerations in the psychometric assessment of PTSD. In R. Kimerling, P. Ouimette, & J. Wolfe (Eds.), *Gender and PTSD* (pp. 150–176). New York: Guilford Press.

Davidson, J. R. T., Book, S. W., Colket, J. T., Tupler, L. A., Roth, S., Hertzberg, M., et al. (1997). Assessment of a new self-rating scale for post-traumatic stress disorder. *Psychological Medicine, 27,* 153–160.

Davidson, J. R. T., & Colket, J. T. (1997). The eight-item treatment-outcome post-traumatic stress disorder scale: A brief measure to assess treatment outcome in post-traumatic stress disorder. *International Clinical Psychopharmacology, 12,* 41–45.

Davidson, J. R. T., Malik, M. A., & Travers, J. (1997). Structured Interview for PTSD (SIP): Psychometric validation for DSM-IV criteria. *Depression and Anxiety, 5,* 127–129.

Davidson, J. R. T., Smith, R., & Kudler, H. (1989). Validity and reliability of the DSM-III criteria for posttraumatic stress disorder: Experience with a structured interview. *Journal of Nervous and Mental Disease, 177,* 336–341.

De Girolamo, G., & McFarlane, A. C. (1996). Epidemiology of posttraumatic stress disorder among victims of intentional violence: A review of the literature. In F. L. Mak & C. C. Nadelson (Eds.), *International Review of Psychiatry* (Vol. 2, pp. 93–119). Washington, DC: American Psychiatric Press.

DiNardo, P. A., & Barlow, D. H. (1988). *Anxiety Disorder Interview Schedule–Revised (ADIS-R).* Albany, NY: Graywind.

DiNardo, P. A., Brown, T. A., & Barlow, D. H. (1994). *Anxiety Disorders Interview Schedule for DSM-IV–Lifetime version (ADIS-IV-L).* San Antonio, TX: Psychological Corporation.

DiNardo, P. A., Moras, K., Barlow, D. H., Rapee, R. M., & Brown, T. A. (1993). Reliability of DSM-III-R anxiety disorder categories: Using the Anxiety Disorders Interview Schedule—Revised (ADIS-R). *Archives of General Psychiatry, 50,* 251–256.

DiNardo, P. A., O'Brien, G. T., Barlow, D. H., Waddell, M. T., & Blanchard, E. B. (1983). Reliability of DSM-III anxiety disorder categories using a new structured interview. *Archives of General Psychiatry, 40,* 1070–1074.

Eisen, S. V., Wilcox, M., Leff, H. S., Schaefer, E., & Culhane, M. A. (1999). Assessing behavioral health outcomes in outpatient programs: Reliability and validity of the BASIS-32. *Journal of Behavioral Health Services and Research, 26,* 5–17.

Fairbank, J. A., & Keane, T. M. (1982). Flooding for combat-related stress disorders: Assessment of anxiety reduction across traumatic memories. *Behavior Therapy, 13,* 499–510.

Falsetti, S. A., Johnson, M. R., Ware, M. R., Emmanuel, N. J., Mintzer, O., Book, S., Ballenger, J. C., & Lydiard, R. B. (1996, March). *Beyond PTSD: Prevalence of trauma in an anxiety disorders sample.* Paper presented at the 16th annual conference of the Anxiety Disorders Association of America, Orlando, FL.

Falsetti, S. A., Resnick, H. S., Resick, P. A., & Kilpatrick, D. G. (1993). The Modified PTSD Symptom Scale: A brief self-report measure of posttraumatic stress disorder. *Behavior Therapist, 16,* 161–162.

First, M., Spitzer, R., Williams, J., & Gibbon, M. (2000). Structured Clinical Interview for DSM-IV Axis I disorders (SCID-I). In *American Psychiatric Association handbook of psychiatric measures* (pp. 49–53). Washington, DC: American Psychiatric Press.

Foa, E. B., Cashman, L., Jaycox, L., & Perry, K. (1997). The validation of a self-report measure of posttraumatic stress disorder: The Posttraumatic Diagnostic Scale. *Psychological Assessment, 9,* 445–451.

Foa, E. B., Riggs, D. S., Dancu, C. V., & Rothbaum, B. O. (1993). Reliability and validity of a brief instrument for assessing post-traumatic stress disorder. *Journal of Traumatic Stress, 6,* 459–474.

Foy, D. W., Sipprelle, R. C., Rueger, D. B., & Carroll, E. M. (1984). Etiology of post-traumatic stress syndrome in Vietnam veterans: Analysis of premilitary, military, and combat exposure influences. *Journal of Consulting and Clinical Psychology, 52,* 79–87.

Frisch, M. B., Cornell, J., Villañueva, M., & Retzlaff, P. J. (1992). Clinical validation of the Quality of Life Inventory: A measure of life satisfaction for use in treatment planning and outcome assessment. *Psychological Assessment, 4,* 92–101.

Frueh, B. C., Brady, K. L., & Arellano, M. A. (1998). Racial differences in combat-related PTSD: Empirical findings and conceptual issues. *Clinical Psychology Review, 18,* 287–305.

Gerardi, R., Keane, T. M., & Penk, W. E. (1989). Utility: Sensitivity and specificity in developing diagnostic tests of combat-related post-traumatic stress disorder (PTSD). *Journal of Clinical Psychology, 45,* 691–703.

Green, B. L., Grace, M. C., Lindy, J. D., & Leonard, A. C. (1990). Race differences in response to combat stress. *Journal of Traumatic Stress, 3,* 379–393.

Herman, D. S., Weathers, F. W., Litz, B. T., & Keane, T. M. (1996). Psychometric properties of the embedded and stand-alone versions of the MMPI-2 Keane PTSD Scale. *Assessment, 3,* 437–442.

Horowitz, M. J. (1976). *Stress response syndromes.* Northvale, NJ: Aronson.

Horowitz, M. J., Wilner, N., & Alvarez, W. (1979). Impact of Event Scale: A measure of subjective stress. *Psychosomatic Medicine, 41,* 209–218.

Joseph, S. (2000). Psychometric evaluation of Horowitz's Impact of Event Scale: A review. *Journal of Traumatic Stress, 13,* 101–113.

Keane, T. M. (1995). Guidelines for the forensic psychological assessment of post-traumatic stress disorder claimants. In R. I. Simon (Ed.), *Posttraumatic stress disorder in litigation: Guidelines for forensic assessment* (pp. 99–115). Washington, DC: American Psychiatric Press.

Keane, T. M., & Barlow, D. H. (2002). Posttraumatic stress disorder. In D. H. Barlow (Ed.), *Anxiety and its disorders: The nature and treatment of anxiety and panic* (2nd ed., pp. 418–453). New York: Guilford Press.

Keane, T. M., Buckley, T., & Miller, M. (2003). Guidelines for the forensic psychological assessment of posttraumatic stress disorder claimants. In R. I. Simon (Ed.), *Posttraumatic stress disorder in litigation: Guidelines for forensic assessment* (2nd ed., pp. 119–140). Washington, DC: American Psychiatric Association Press.

Keane, T. M., Caddell, J. M., & Taylor, K. L. (1988). Mississippi Scale for combat-related posttraumatic stress disorder: Three studies in reliability and validity. *Journal of Consulting and Clinical Psychology, 56,* 85–90.

Keane, T. M., Fairbank, J. A., Caddell, J. M., Zimering, R. T., & Bender, M. E. (1995). A behavioral approach to assessing and treating post-traumatic stress disorder in Vietnam veterans. In C. R. Figley (Ed.), *Trauma and its wake* (pp. 257–294). New York: Brunner/Mazel.

Keane, T. M., & Kaloupek, D. G. (1982). Imaginal flooding in the treatment of posttraumatic stress disorder. *Journal of Consulting and Clinical Psychology, 50,* 138–140.

Keane, T. M., & Kaloupek, D. G. (1997). Comorbid psychiatric disorders in PTSD: Implications for research. *Annals of the New York Academy of Sciences, 821,* 24–34.

Keane, T. M., & Kaloupek, D. G. (2002). Posttraumatic stress disorder: Diagnosis, assessment, and monitoring outcomes. In R. Yehuda (Ed.) *Treating trauma survivors with PTSD* (pp. 21–42). Washington, DC: American Psychiatric Press.

Keane, T. M., Kimble, M. O., Kaufman, M., & Kaloupek, D. G. (in press). Diagnosis and assessment of posttraumatic stress disorder in adults. *Journal of Interpersonal Violence.*

Keane, T. M., Kolb, L. C, Kaloupek, D. G., Orr, S. P., Blanchard, E. B., Thomas, R. G., Hsieh, F. Y., & Lavori, P. W. (1998). Utility of psychophysiology measurement in the diagnosis of posttraumatic stress disorder: Results from a Department of Veterans Affairs cooperative study. *Journal of Consulting and Clinical Psychology, 66,* 914–923.

Keane, T. M., Malloy, P. F., & Fairbank, J. A. (1984). Empirical development of an MMPI subscale for the assessment of combat-related posttraumatic stress disorder. *Journal of Consulting and Clinical Psychology, 52,* 888–891.

Keane, T. M., Solomon, S., Maser, J., & Gerrity, E. (1995b, November). *Assessment of PTSD.* National Institute of Mental Health–National Center for PTSD Consensus Conference on Assessment of PTSD, Boston, MA.

Keane, T. M., Weathers, F. W., & Foa, E. B. (2000). Diagnosis and assessment. In E. B. Foa, T. M. Keane, & M. J. Friedman (Eds.), *Effective treatments for PTSD* (pp. 18–36). New York: Guilford Press.

Keane, T. M., Wolfe, J., & Taylor, K. L. (1987). Post-traumatic stress disorder: Evidence for diagnostic validity and methods for psychological assessment. *Journal of Clinical Psychology, 43,* 32–43.

Keen, S. M., Kutter, C. J., Niles, B. L., & Krinsley, K. E. (2004). Psychometric properties of the PTSD Checklist in a sample of male veterans. *Manuscript submitted for publication.*

Kessler, R. C., McGonagle, K. A., Zhao, S., Nelson, C. B., Hughes, M., Eshleman, S., Wittchen H. U., & Kendler, K. S. (1994). Lifetime and 12–month prevalence of DSM-III-R psychiatric disorders in the United States: Results from the National Comorbidity Survey. *Archives of General Psychiatry, 51,* 8–19.

Kessler, R. C., Sonnega, A., Bromet, E., Hughes, M., & Nelson, C. B. (1995). Posttraumatic stress disorder in the National Comorbidity Survey. *Archives of General Psychiatry, 52,* 1048–1060.

Kilpatrick, D. G. (1988). Rape aftermath symptom test. In M. Hersen & A. S. Bellack (Eds.), *Dictionary of behavioral assessment techniques* (pp. 658–669). Oxford, UK: Pergamon Press.

King, L. A., King, D. W., Leskin, G., & Foy, D. (1995). The Los Angeles Symptom Checklist: A self-report measure of posttraumatic stress disorder. *Assessment, 2,* 1–17.

Koretzky, M. B., & Peck, A. H. (1990). Validation and cross-validation of the PTSD subscale of the MMPI with civilian trauma victims. *Journal of Clinical Psychology, 46,* 296–300.

Kraemer, H. C. (1992). *Evaluating medical tests: Objective and quantitative guidelines.* Newbury Park, CA: Sage.

Kubany, E. S., Leisen, M. B., Kaplan, A. S., & Kelly, M. P. (2000). Validation of a brief measure of posttraumatic stress disorder: The Distressing Event Questionnaire (DEQ). *Psychological Assessment, 12,* 197–209.

Kulka, R. A., Schlenger, W. E., Fairbank, J. A., Hough, R. L., Jordan, B. K., Marmar, C. R., & Weiss, D. S. (1988). *National Vietnam Veterans Readjustment Study (NVVRS): Design, current status, and initial PTSD prevalence estimates.* Research Triangle Park, NC: Research Triangle Park Institute.

Kulka, R. A., Schlenger, W. E., Fairbank, J. A., Jordan, B. K., Hough, R. L., Marmar, CR., & Weiss, D. S. (1990). *Trauma and the Vietnam war generation: Report of find-*

ings from the National Vietnam Veterans Readjustment Study. New York: Brunner/ Mazel.

Litz, B. T., & Weathers, F. (1994). The diagnosis and assessment of post-traumatic stress disorder in adults. In M. B. Williams & J. F. Sommer (Eds.), *The handbook of post-traumatic therapy* (pp. 20–37). Westport, CT: Greenwood Press.

Lyons, J. A., & Keane, T. M. (1992). Keane PTSD scale: MMPI and MMPI-2 update. *Journal of Traumatic Stress, 5,* 111–117.

Malloy, P. F., Fairbank, J. A., & Keane, T. M. (1983). Validation of a multimethod assessment of posttraumatic stress disorders in Vietnam veterans. *Journal of Consulting and Clinical Psychology, 51,* 488–494.

Manne, S. L., DuHamel, K., Gallelli, K., Sorgen, K., & Redd, W. H. (1998). Posttraumatic stress disorder among mothers of pediatric cancer survivors: Diagnosis, comorbidity, and utility of the PTSD Checklist as a screening instrument. *Journal of Pediatric Psychology, 23,* 357–366.

Marsella, A. J., Friedman, M. J., Gerrity, E. T., & Scurfield, R. M. (Eds.). (1996). *Ethnocultural aspects of posttraumatic stress disorder*. Washington, DC: American Psychological Association.

McFall, M. E., Smith, D. E., Mackay, P. W., & Tarver, D. J. (1990a). Reliability and validity of Mississippi Scale for combat-related posttraumatic stress disorder. *Journal of Consulting and Clinical Psychology, 2,* 114–121.

McFall, M. E., Smith, D., Roszell, D. K., Tarver, D. J., & Malas, K. L. (1990b). Convergent validity of measures of PTSD in Vietnam combat veterans. *American Journal of Psychiatry, 147,* 645–648.

Mollica, R. F., Caspi-Yavin, Y., Bollini, P., Truong, T., Tor, S., & Lavelle, J. (1992). The Harvard Trauma Questionnaire: Validating a cross-cultural instrument for measuring torture, trauma, and posttraumatic stress disorder in Indochinese refugees. *Journal of Nervous and Mental Disease, 180,* 111–116.

Neal, L. A., Busuttil, W., Rollins, J., Herepath, R., Strike, P., & Turnbull, G. (1994). Convergent validity of measures of post-traumatic stress disorder in a mixed military and civilian population. *Journal of Traumatic Stress, 7,* 447–455.

Newman, E., Kaloupek, D. G., & Keane, T. M. (1996). Assessment of PTSD in clinical and research settings. In B. A. van der Kolk, A. C. McFarlane, & L. Weisaeth (Eds.), *Traumatic stress: The effects of overwhelming experience on mind, body, and society* (pp. 242–275). New York: Guilford Press.

Norris, F. H., & Riad, J. K. (1997). Standardized self-report measures of civilian trauma and posttraumatic stress disorder. In J. P. Wilson & T. M. Keane (Eds.) *Assessing psychological trauma and PTSD* (pp. 7–42). New York: Guilford Press.

Orr, S. P., Metzger, L., Miller, M., & Kaloupek, D. G. (2004). Psychophysiological assessment of PTSD. In J. P. Wilson & T. M. Keane (Eds.), *Assessing psychological trauma and PTSD* (2nd ed., pp. 289–343). New York: Guilford Press.

Orsillo, S. M. (2001). Measures for acute stress disorder and posttraumatic stress disorder. In M. M. Antony, S. M. Orsillo, & L. Roemer (Eds.), *Practitioner's guide to empirically based measures of anxiety* (pp. 255–307). New York: Kluwer Academic/ Plenum.

Ouimette, P. C., Finney, J. W., & Moos, R. H. (1999). Two-year posttreatment functioning and coping of substance abuse patients with posttraumatic stress disorder. *Psychology of Addictive Behaviors, 13,* 105–114.

Pitman, R. K., Orr, S. P, Forgue, D. F., de Jong, J. B., & Claiborne, J. M. (1987).

Psychophysiological assessment of posttraumatic stress disorder imagery in Vietnam combat veterans. *Archives of General Psychiatry, 44,* 970–975.

Prins, A., Kaloupek, D. G., & Keane, T. M. (1995). Psychophysiological evidence for autonomic arousal and startle in traumatized adult populations. In M. J. Friedman, D. Charney, & A. Deutch (Eds.), *Neurobiological and clinical consequences of stress: From normal adaptation to PTSD.* New York: Raven Press.

Robins, L. H., & Helzer, J. E. (1985). *Diagnostic Interview Schedule (DIS Version III-A).* St. Louis, MO: Washington University, Department of Psychiatry.

Ruggiero, K. J., Del Ben, K., Scotti, J. R., & Rabalais, A. E. (2003). Psychometric properties of the PTSD Checklist—Civilian Version. *Journal of Traumatic Stress, 16,* 495–502.

Spielberger, C. S., Gorsuch, R. L., Lushene, R., Vagg, P. R., & Jacobs, G. A. (1983). *Manual for the State–Trait Anxiety Inventory (Form Y).* Palo Alto, CA: Mind Garden.

Sundin, E. C., & Horowitz, M. J. (2002). Impact of Event Scale: Psychometric properties. *British Journal of Psychiatry, 180,* 205–209.

Sutker, P. B., Uddo-Crane, M., & Allain, A. N. (1991). Clinical and research assessment of posttraumatic stress disorder: A conceptual overview. *Psychological Assessment: A Journal of Consulting and Clinical Psychology, 3,* 520–530.

Ware, J. E., & Kosinski, M. (2001). *SF-36 Physical and Mental Health Summary Scales: A manual for users of version 1* (2nd ed.). Lincoln, RI: QualityMetric.

Watson, C. G., Juba, M. P., Manifold, V., Kucala, T., & Anderson, P. E. D. (1991). The PTSD interview: Rationale, description, reliability, and concurrent validity of a DSM-III based technique. *Journal of Clinical Psychology, 47,* 179–188.

Watson, C. G., Kucala, T., & Manifold, V. (1986). A cross-validation of the Keane and Penk MMPI scales as measure of posttraumatic stress disorder. *Journal of Clinical Psychology, 42,* 727–732.

Weathers, F. W., Keane, T. M., & Davidson, J. R. T. (2001). The Clinician Administered PTSD Scale (CAPS): A review of the first ten years of research. *Depression and Anxiety, 13,* 132–156.

Weathers, F. W., Keane, T. M., King, L. A., & King, D. W. (1996). Psychometric theory in the development of posttraumatic stress disorder assessment tools. In J. P. Wilson & T. M. Keane (Eds.), *Assessing psychological trauma and PTSD* (pp. 98–135). New York: Guilford Press.

Weathers, F. W., Litz, B. T., Herman, D. S., Huska, J. A., & Keane, T. M. (1993, October). *The PTSD Checklist (PCL): Reliability, validity, and diagnostic utility.* Poster presented at the 9th annual meeting of the International Society for Traumatic Stress Studies, San Antonio, TX.

Weathers, F. W., Ruscio, A. M., & Keane, T. M. (1999). Psychometric properties of nine scoring rules for the Clinician-Administered PTSD scale (CAPS). *Psychological Assessment, 11,* 124–133.

Weiss, D., & Marmar, C. (1997). The Impact of Event Scale—Revised. In J. P. Wilson & T. M. Keane (Eds.), *Assessing psychological trauma and PTSD* (pp. 399–411). New York: Guilford Press.

Wilson, J. P., & Keane, T. M. (Eds.). (1997). *Assessing psychological trauma and PTSD.* New York: Guilford Press.

Wilson, J. P., & Keane, T. M. (2004) *Assessing psychological trauma and PTSD* (2nd ed.). New York: Guilford Press.

Wilson, J. P., & Krauss, G. E. (1984, September). *The Vietnam Era Stress Inventory: A scale to measure war stress and post-traumatic stress disorder among Vietnam veterans.* Paper presented at the Third National Conference on Post-Traumatic Stress Disorder, Baltimore, MD.

Wilson, S. A., Tinker, R. H., Becker, L. A., & Gillette, C. S. (1994, November). *Using the PTSD-I as an outcome measure.* Poster presented at the annual meeting of the International Society for Traumatic Stress Studies, Chicago, IL.

Yehuda, R. (1997). Sensitization of the hypothalamic–pituitary–adrenal axis in PTSD. In R. Yehuda & A. McFarlane (Eds.), *Psychobiology of posttraumatic stress disorder* (pp. 57–75). New York: Annals of the New York Academy of Sciences.

Yehuda, R., Giller, E., Levengood, R. A., Southwick, S., & Siever, L. J. (1995). Hypothalamic–pituitary–adrenal alterations in PTSD. In M. Friedman, D. Charney, & A. Deutch (Eds.) *Neurobiological and clinical adaptations to stress: From normal adaptations to PTSD.* New York: Raven Press.

PART TWO
Interventions

CHAPTER FOUR

Prolonged Exposure Treatment of Posttraumatic Stress Disorder

David S. Riggs
Shawn P. Cahill
Edna B. Foa

Posttraumatic stress disorder (PTSD) is an anxiety disorder that develops in some individuals following exposure to a traumatic event such as combat, sexual or physical assault, a serious accident, or the witnessing of someone being injured or killed (American Psychiatric Association, 1994). The classification of PTSD as an anxiety disorder reflects the longstanding recognition that anxious arousal plays a prominent role in people who experience pathological responses to trauma. However, research and theory into the nature of PTSD have documented that pathological reactions to trauma incorporate many emotions other than anxiety. Accordingly, in addition to reducing trauma-related anxiety and avoidance, treatments for PTSD are expected to modify other negative emotions such as guilt, shame, depression, and general anxiety.

Anxiety has played an especially important role in the development of many treatment programs that target PTSD. These programs tend to focus on reducing or managing anxiety in PTSD patients. In particular, exposure therapy—a form of treatment that encourages clients to recall their traumatic memories and confront traumatic reminders—owes a great deal to the conceptualization of PTSD as an anxiety disorder (although, as noted above, other emotions are also targeted). The term "exposure therapy" is used here to refer to a general treatment strategy for reducing anxiety that involves confronting situations, activities, thoughts, and memories that are feared and avoided even though they are not inherently harmful. Prolonged exposure (PE), a specific treatment protocol that has been developed and evaluated as a treatment for PTSD (Foa, Rothbaum, Ruggs, & Murdock, 1991; Foa et al., 1999; Foa & Rothbaum, 1998), has adopted techniques that are used in exposure therapies for other anxiety disorders, such as obsessive–compulsive disorder, panic disorder, and phobias.

In the present chapter we examine the theoretical underpinnings of PE for PTSD as well as the empirical support for its efficacy in treating trauma survivors. We then discuss concerns that have been raised about exposure therapy and summarize research findings relevant to these concerns. Finally, we describe recent attempts to disseminate PE to clinicians who regularly provide mental health services to trauma survivors.

PE FOR PTSD

Description of PE

PE is described in detail in Foa and Rothbaum (1998), so here we provide only a shorter overview. PE is delivered in an individual format and typically consists of 9–12 sessions, each lasting about 90 minutes. The treatment incorporates four procedures: (1) psychoeducation about trauma, reactions to trauma, and PTSD; (2) breathing retraining; (3) *in vivo* exposure to the feared (but now safe) trauma-related situations that the client avoids; and (4) imaginal exposure that consists of repeatedly recounting memories of the traumatic event. At the end of each imaginal exposure session the client and therapist process the thoughts and feelings that emerged during the imaginal exposure or as a result of recounting the trauma. Finally, each session ends with a homework assignment that includes *in vivo* exercises and listening to tape recordings of the imaginal exposure exercise conducted in that session.

The first session of PE is devoted to laying the groundwork for the program. The therapist provides a description of the treatment and each of the procedures that will be used. The therapist also provides the client with a model for understanding the persistence of PTSD symptoms. The model emphasizes the role of avoidance and negative beliefs about the world and the self in impeding recovery and thus maintaining PTSD symptoms (Foa & Riggs, 1993; Foa & Rothbuam, 1998). Following the overall rationale for the treatment and a general description of the PE procedures, the therapist collects information about the patient's traumatic experience, using a semi-structured interview format to elicit details about the trauma and the patient's reactions during and after the trauma. (This information may also be collected in a less structured format.) At the end of the session, the patient is trained to use controlled breathing to manage anxiety. Setting a pattern for all sessions, this session ends with a homework assignment. For the first session, the homework consists of practicing controlled breathing (3 × 10 minutes each day), reading a handout that outlines the rationale for PE, and listening to an audiotape of the session.

The second PE session focuses on two treatment components. First, the therapist continues to educate the client about trauma and PTSD by discussing reactions that are commonly reported by people who have experienced trauma. Second, the therapist introduces *in vivo* exposure. In addition to providing a framework for understanding the patient's symptoms and normalizing the reaction to the trauma, the discussion of common reactions provides an opportunity for the patient to identify specific difficulties that he or she has experienced. Once this discussion is completed, the therapist provides a detailed rationale and description of the *in vivo* exposure procedure. Together the client and therapist construct the hierarchy by identifying situations that the patient avoids and rating each situation on a subjective distress scale. This hierarchy will guide the *in vivo* exercises through the balance of the program. Homework assignments for the second session consist of (1) reading a handout that describes the common reactions to trauma discussed in the session; (2) listening to the tape of the treatment session; (3) continuing the breathing exercises; and (4) completing one or more *in vivo* exposure exercises. Typically, the *in vivo* exposure assignments in this session involve confronting situations or objects that will elicit anxiety but will not overwhelm the patient—that is, items on the hierarchy that the patient rated as moderately distressing. The therapist also reviews the instructions for *in vivo* exposure and explains in detail how the particular exercise will be conducted.

The third session introduces imaginal exposure, in which the patient is asked to recount the identified index trauma. The session begins with a review of the client's homework and continues with the therapist's expansion of the rationale for the imaginal exposure exercises. The patient is then guided through approximately 45 minutes of imaginal exposure to a single traumatic event (when the client has experienced multiple traumas, he or she is asked to recount the event that causes the most distress at the time of treatment). The patient is asked to close his or her eyes, imagine the traumatic event as vividly as possible, and recount it aloud in the present tense. If recounting of the trauma does not fill the allotted 45 minutes (as is usually the case), the client is asked to return to the beginning of the memory and repeat the procedure until 45 minutes has elapsed. Following the recounting, the therapist and patient spend time discussing the patient's reactions to the exposure exercise, with particular emphasis on thoughts and emotions that arose during the recounting. We refer to this as "processing" the trauma memory. The time allotted to processing also helps the patient to calm any distress remaining from the exposure. Homework assigned for this session includes (1) daily *in vivo* exercises; (2) listening to the imaginal exposure audiotape daily while imagining the trauma as vividly as possible; (3) listening to the audiotape of the session at least one time; and (4) continuing the breathing practice.

With the exception of the last session, the rest of the PE sessions follow the same format. First, the therapist reviews the previous week's homework, and then the client completes an imaginal exposure exercise lasting 30–45 minutes. This is followed by a 15- to 20-minute processing of the imaginal exposure and homework assignment. Homework for these sessions includes daily *in vivo* exercises selected from the hierarchy and daily listening to the imaginal exposure audiotape from the preceding session. Beginning around session six or seven, the focus of the imaginal exposure exercise is shifted from the entire traumatic event to the particular aspects that are associated with the greatest distress during the recounting. Patients are asked to focus their recounting on these "hot spots," one at a time, describing the event and their thoughts and emotions in as much detail as possible. Patients are asked to repeat this "hot spot" as many times as necessary to fill the 30- to 45-minute imaginal exposure.

The format of the final session is similar to the previous sessions, except that the imaginal exposure exercise is usually shortened to 20–30 minutes, and the discussion of the client's reactions is focused on progress achieved during treatment and the application of what the client has learned to other aspects of his or her life. In the course of this discussion, the therapist asks the client to re-rate the items on the *in vivo* hierarchy to identify progress and any items that remain problematic. The therapist briefly discusses issues related to relapse prevention, such as the potential for PTSD symptoms to increase temporarily and the utility of the techniques used in treatment to address stressful situations that arise in the future.

Facilitating PE Treatment

PE requires that patients overcome their natural tendency to avoid thinking and talking about the traumas that they experienced. The challenge for patients is the fact that avoidance has been the primary strategy they have used to cope with their trauma-related distress. Many of the procedures incorporated into the PE program, including the structure imposed by using a manualized treatment, provide a foundation for encouraging clients to overcome their avoidance in order to experience the exposure exercises. In addition to specific aspects of the PE program, numerous nonspecific factors can facilitate treatment. Basic therapeutic skills, such as empathy and active listening, are invaluable. Perhaps most important is the therapist's ability to convey confidence in the effectiveness of the therapy, the client's ability to complete the treatment program, and expertise in conducting the treatment.

It is important to form a strong therapeutic alliance with the client during the first two sessions of PE. This may be quite challenging with survivors of interpersonal traumas, such as rape or physical assault, for whom trusting another individual may be particularly difficult and frightening. Several aspects of the PE program are designed to foster this alliance. Among them are (1) providing a clear description of the therapy and the rationale for the procedures employed during PE; (2) conveying empathy for the difficulties of abandoning avoidance strategies; (3) communicating caring for the patient; (4) acknowledging the challenge presented by PE; and (5) recognizing the patient's courage in electing to participate in the treatment program. More generally, it is important for the therapist to take a strong empathic, nonjudgmental stance throughout treatment to foster communication. The therapist should work actively to build the alliance with the patient. For example, the therapist should use the patient's own experience to illustrate concepts such as common reactions to trauma or *in vivo* exercises, and convey a strong commitment to apply PE in a way that takes into account the client's unique experience. It is also extremely important to foster a sense of collaboration between therapist and patient throughout treatment. The therapist and patient should work together to select the situations to be used in the *in vivo* exercises and which aspects of the trauma memory to be included during imaginal exposure. The essence of the collaboration is that the therapist makes recommendations based on his or her experience in treating others with PTSD while taking into consideration the patient's unique presentation and needs.

As noted above, an important aspect of PE is the therapist's explanation of the rationale for the treatment and how the treatment addresses the factors that maintain PTSD. Similarly, it is crucial that the patient understands how *in vivo* and imaginal exposure will help him or her overcome chronic symptoms and related problems. If patients do not have a firm understanding of why they are asked to engage in exposure exercises, they may not comply with treatment demands. Therapists should also praise clients freely for engaging in and completing exposure exercises, especially very difficult assignments. It is important to remember that the structure of PE provides ample flexibility to accommodate the specific needs of patients. Although a detailed description of how to incorporate a flexible approach to exposure lies beyond the scope of this chapter (see Foa & Rothbaum, 1998; Hembree et al., 2003b), it is important to note that PE does not require that therapists abandon basic therapeutic skills. On the contrary, the techniques included in PE must be presented in a manner that reflects caring and respect for the individual experience of the patient and addresses his or her individual needs.

THE THEORETICAL FOUNDATIONS FOR PE

PE is founded on Foa and Kozak's (1986) theory of emotional processing that explains the pathological underpinnings of anxiety disorders and their treatment by exposure therapy. At its core, the emotional processing theory of exposure therapy rests on two basic propositions: (1) anxiety disorders reflect the existence of pathological fear structures in memory, which are activated when information represented in the structures is encountered; and (2) successful treatment modifies the pathological elements of the fear structure, such that information that used to evoke anxiety symptoms no longer does so. The process of modifying the pathological elements of the fear structure is called emotional processing. Foa and Kozak further proposed that for therapy to successfully modify the fear structure, the fear structure must be activated and corrective information must be incorporated in to it.

Fear Structures of Anxiety Disorders

A fear structure is represented as a network of interconnecting elements that contain information about (1) the feared stimuli, (2) verbal, physiological, and behavioral responses, and (3) the meaning of stimulus and response elements in the structure. The structure serves as a blueprint for escaping or avoiding danger; as such, it supports adaptive behavior when a person is faced with a realistically threatening situation. However, a fear structure may become maladaptive when (1) associations among stimulus elements do not accurately represent the world; (2) physiological and escape/avoidance responses are evoked by harmless stimuli; (3) excessive and easily triggered response elements interfere with other adaptive behavior; and (4) harmless stimulus and response elements are erroneously interpreted as dangerous.

The Fear Structure of PTSD

Foa, Steketee, and Rothbaum (1989) proposed that a traumatic event is represented in memory as a fear structure that is characterized by a large number of harmless stimulus elements erroneously associated with the meaning of danger. These erroneous associations are reflected in the perception of the world as entirely dangerous. In a further development of emotional theory for PTSD, Foa and Jaycox (1999) suggested that the physiological and behavioral responses that occurred during and after the event, including the PTSD symptoms themselves, are interpreted as signs of personal incompetence, leading survivors to the erroneous perception about themselves as entirely incompetent. The erroneous cognitions about the world and the self underlie PTSD symptoms, which in turn reinforce the erroneous cognitions in a vicious cycle (for a more detailed discussion, see Foa & Rothbaum, 1998). PTSD symptoms are further maintained by cognitive and behavioral avoidance strategies that prevent exposure to corrective information and the incorporation of such information into fear structure. For example, by avoiding safe reminders of the trauma, the person does not have the opportunity to disconfirm the belief that feared consequences will occur (e.g., being assaulted again, not being able to cope with the distress produced by the situation). Overcoming the tendency to avoid trauma-related stimuli and countering the erroneous cognitions are seen as critical mechanisms of natural recovery from trauma as well as recovery through therapy.

Emotional Processing Theory of Natural Recovery

Although a necessary condition for the development of PTSD, exposure to trauma per se does not inevitably lead to chronic PTSD. Prospective studies of traumatized individuals indicate that PTSD symptoms, general anxiety, depression, and disruption in social functioning are common immediately after the traumatic event. Over the subsequent weeks and months, the majority of individuals recover naturally, with symptoms declining most rapidly during the 1- to 3-month period immediately following the trauma. This pattern of natural recovery has been documented for female rape victims (Atkeson, Calhoun, Resick, & Ellis, 1982; Calhoun, Atkeson, & Resick, 1982; Resick, Calhoun, Atkeson, & Ellis, 1981; Rothbaum, Foa, Riggs, Murdock, & Walsh, 1992), male and female victims of nonsexual assault (Riggs, Rothbaum, & Foa, 1995), and victims of motor vehicle accidents (Harvey & Bryant, 1998).

Foa and Cahill (2001) suggested that, over time, trauma survivors encounter situations that include trauma-relevant stimuli and activate their trauma memory structures. The activation of the trauma structure is reflected in reexperiencing symptoms such as intrusive thoughts, flashbacks, and emotional distress. Because these situations are safe and the feared consequence (e.g., repeated trauma) does not occur, the trauma-related associations are repeatedly disconfirmed, resulting in changes in the fear structure and corresponding reductions in PTSD symptom severity. Corrective information is also provided through experiences such as talking about the trauma with friends and confidants.

A significant minority of trauma victims does not recover naturally after the trauma. For these individuals, PTSD becomes a chronic condition that may last for many years (Kessler, Sonnega, Bromet, Hughes, & Nelson, 1995). Within the framework of emotional processing theory, the development of chronic PTSD is conceptualized as a failure to adequately process the traumatic memory. According to Foa and Kozak (1986), this failure is due to inadequate activation of the fear structure in the wake of the trauma and/or the unavailability of corrective information. Survivors with chronic PTSD appear to access their trauma memory structure quite easily, as evidenced by reexperiencing symptoms (Foa et al., 1989). Therefore, the most likely reason for the development of chronic PTSD is the failure to incorporate corrective information into the fear structure. Foa and Cahill (2001) suggest that the absence of corrective information is due to extensive use of avoidance strategies to manage distress. Avoidance limits activation of the fear structure and the availability of corrective information, thereby hindering natural recovery. The goal of treatment is to help patients overcome their tendency to avoid and encourage them to fully activate the trauma fear structure in order to incorporate corrective information about the world and themselves into it.

Modification of Fear Structures in PE

As noted above, Foa and Kozak (1986) proposed that, for emotional process-ing to occur, a fear network must be activated and information that is not compatible with it must be introduced and incorporated. Within the frame-work of PE, activating the fear network is accomplished through *in vivo* and imaginal exposure exercises. Successful activation of the trauma-related fear structure is indicated by fear responses such as physiological arousal, self-reports of distress, emotionally expressive behavior, and escape/avoidance behavior. The introduction of new, incompatible information occurs in sev-eral ways. Foa and Jaycox (1999) have summarized six different mechanisms or sources of information that are thought to be relevant to improvement in PTSD.

1. Blocking further negative reinforcement of cognitive avoidance of trauma-related thoughts and feelings.
2. Helping clients realize that remembering the trauma, although emo-tionally upsetting, is not dangerous.
3. Promoting habituation of anxiety to the trauma memory and thereby correcting erroneous beliefs that anxiety will not diminish without engaging avoidance or escape strategies.
4. Helping clients to differentiate the traumatic event from other (simi-lar) nontraumatic events, thereby allowing them to view the trauma as a specific occurrence rather than an indication that the entire world is dangerous and that the self is completely incompetent.
5. Altering clients' perceptions of their symptoms as further evidence of their incompetence to indications of personal mastery and cour-age. In other words, clients learn that they can tolerate their symp-toms and that having them does not lead to going crazy or losing control. As a result, individuals may come to see themselves as trau-ma *survivors* rather than trauma *victims*.
6. Helping clients to more accurately evaluate aspects of the event that are contrary to beliefs about danger and self-incompetence that may otherwise be overshadowed by the more salient threat-related ele-ments of the memory. For example, an individual feeling guilty about not having done more to resist an assailant may come to the realization that, had he or she resisted more, he or she may have been assaulted all the more severely.

EFFICACY OF EXPOSURE THERAPY FOR PTSD

Over the past 15 years many studies have found cognitive-behavioral therapy (CBT) effective in reducing PTSD, making CBT the most empirically vali-dated approach among the psychosocial treatments for PTSD (for reviews, see Foa & Meadows, 1997; Foa & Rothbaum, 1998; Harvey, Bryant, & Tarrier, 2003). The CBT programs that have been empirically examined include prolonged exposure (PE), stress inoculation training (SIT), cognitive therapy (CT), and eye movement desensitization and reprocessing (EMDR). There are more studies demonstrating the efficacy of exposure therapy (including PE) than of any other treatment for PTSD (Foa & Rothbaum, 1998; Rothbaum, Meadows, Resick, & Foy, 2000), and PE has been shown effective in treating PTSD associated with a wide variety of traumas. When directly compared, PE produces results as good as or better than other CBT approaches (CT, SIT, EMDR) or PE combined with components of the other treatments (see discussion below).

Studies of Exposure Therapy

A number of programs based on exposure therapy have been used to treat PTSD. Among the variations of exposure therapy, the PE protocol has been the most extensively studied and has been found to be highly effective. Like PE, some other exposure therapy programs include both imaginal confrontation with the traumatic memories and *in vivo* exposure to trauma reminders (e.g., Marks, Lovell, Noshirvani, Livanou, & Thrasher, 1998), however, some programs rely exclusively on imaginal exposure to the trauma memory (Bryant et al., 2003a; Cloitre, Koenen, Cohen, & Han, 2002; Tarrier et al., 1999). Even among programs that include both imaginal and *in vivo* exposure, there are differences in the specific application of the techniques. For example, PE utilizes both components from the beginning of treatment; in contrast, Marks et al. (1998) introduced imaginal exposure in the first half of the program and *in vivo* exposure in later sessions. Finally, exposure therapy programs differ in the extent to which they include other treatment components. For example, Foa et al. (1999) limited PE to exposure plus psychoeducation, training in controlled breathing, and discussion of the exposure experience (called "processing"). In comparison, Blanchard et al. (2003) combined exposure with psychoeducation, progressive muscle relaxation, monitoring of thoughts and CT, and behavioral activation strategies.

Variants of exposure therapy, either alone or in combination with other CBT approaches, have been found effective in samples of female survivors of rape (e.g., Foa et al., 1991, 1999, 2002a; Resick, Nishith, Weaver, Astin, & Feuer, 2002; Rothbaum, 2002) and physical assault (Foa et al., 1999, 2002a); domestic violence (Kubany, Hill, & Owens, 2003; Kubany et al., 2004); physical and sexual abuse in childhood (Cloitre et al., 2002; Echeburua, Corral, Zubizarreta, & Sarasua 1997; Foa et al., 2002a); male and female survivors of motor vehicle accidents (Blanchard et al., 2003; Fecteau & Nicki, 1999); refugees (Otto et al., 2003; Paunovik & Ost, 2001); and mixed trauma samples (Bryant et al., 2003a; Marks et al., 1998; Power et al., 2002; Tarrier et al., 1999; Taylor et al., 2003) comprised primarily of physical and sexual assault victims and survivors of motor vehicle accidents. Below we outline the empirical support for PE and other forms of exposure therapy.

Studies of PE

The efficacy of PE has been investigated in six separate studies. In the first of these, Foa et al. (1991) compared rape survivors treated with PE to a waiting-list control group, a group receiving supportive counseling, and another treated with SIT (Meichenbaum, 1977; Veronen & Kilpatrick, 1983). SIT is a CBT package that teaches clients several anxiety management strategies and encourages them to apply these strategies in their daily life. At the end of nine treatment sessions, women in the PE and SIT groups showed significant improvement, whereas those who received supportive counseling or were placed on the waiting list did not. The SIT group showed the most improvement on PTSD symptoms immediately after treatment. However, the PE group continued to improve over the follow-up period, such that at follow-up, the PE group tended to be superior to the other groups on symptoms of PTSD, depression, and anxiety.

Foa et al. (1999) extended this research by examining the effects of PE alone, SIT alone, the combination of PE and SIT, and a waiting-list condition. All three active treatments produced significant improvement compared to the waiting-list condition. Contrary to expectations, though, there was no evidence that combining PE and SIT improved outcome. Also, this study did not replicate the superiority of SIT at posttreatment found in the earlier study. Instead, at both posttreatment and follow-up assessments, PE was found superior to SIT on some measures, whereas on other measures the two treatments did not differ.

In a third study examining the efficacy of PE, Foa and her colleagues (2002a) compared PE presented alone to a program that combined PE and cognitive restructuring (CR) and to a waiting-list condition. The researchers hypothesized that cognitive restructuring represented the most important ingredient of SIT and that focusing on this skill and reducing the complexity of the combined treatment might prove more effective in treating PTSD. Results indicated that PE and PE/CR were highly and equally effective at reducing PTSD, depression, and anxiety compared to the waiting list. As in the earlier study, combined treatment was not superior to PE alone. The treatment gains of both groups were maintained during follow-up. Similar results were reported by Paunovic and Ost (2001), who also compared PE with PE plus CR and found that both treatments produced significant improvement, but PE/CR was not superior to PE alone.

Resick et al. (2002) compared PE with cognitive processing therapy (CPT), a form of cognitive therapy specifically developed for rape survivors (Resick & Schnicke, 1992), and a waiting-list condition. In addition to the cognitive therapy techniques that form the core of CPT, this program includes an exposure component of repeatedly writing and reading the trauma narrative. Resick et al. (2002) found that, compared to the waiting-list condition, both PE and CPT produced large improvement in PTSD symptoms and depression, and the gains were maintained through 9 months of follow-up. There were no significant differences between groups on these measures, but CPT appeared to have a slight advantage over PE on measures of guilt.

Rothbaum (2002) compared a group of survivors treated with PE to a waiting-list group and a group treated with EMDR (Shapiro, 1989, 1995). EMDR combines elements of brief, repeated imaginal exposure, a form of CR, and therapist-induced rapid eye movements or other laterally alternating stimuli (e.g., finger tapping) that occurs during exposure to the trauma-related imagery. Results indicated that, compared to the waiting-list condition, both treatments produced significant improvement in PTSD, depression, and anxiety, and the two active treatments did not differ at the posttreatment assessment. However, the PE group was superior to the EMDR group on several measures taken at a 6-month follow-up assessment.

In sum, studies of PE have consistently found it to be a highly effective treatment for PTSD and associated anxiety and depression. When directly compared, PE has been found to be as or more effective than relaxation, SIT, CT, and EMDR. Moreover, treatments that have combined PE with SIT or CR, although very effective, have not yielded better results than PE alone.

Variations on a Theme: Studies of Other Exposure Protocols

Civilian Samples

Several recent studies compared exposure therapy protocols other than PE with alternative CBT interventions. Marks et al. (1998) compared exposure, CR, and their combination with a relaxation control group. Like PE, the exposure therapy used in this study included imaginal and *in vivo* exercises. However, whereas the two modalities are administered simultaneously in PE, the program examined by Marks et al. (1998) presented the modalities sequentially; the first five sessions were limited to imaginal exposure and corresponding homework, and the remaining five sessions focused on in-session, therapist-assisted *in vivo* exposure and corresponding homework. Immediately after treatment, the exposure, cognitive restructuring, and combined interventions were superior to relaxation, and they retained their superiority at follow-up. Comparisons among the three interventions failed to reveal any consistent pattern of superior performance for one treatment over the others. Notably, like the Foa et al. (2002a) study, the combined exposure plus CR group was not better than the groups that received either treatment alone.

Taylor et al. (2003) utilized an eight-session variation of the Marks et al. (1998) exposure therapy protocol (four sessions of imaginal exposure followed by four sessions of *in vivo* exposure) compared to EMDR and relaxation. All three groups showed significant improvement in PTSD symptoms at the end of treatment. The exposure therapy group was significantly more improved than the group that received relaxation training. In contrast, the EMDR group did not differ from either the relaxation group or the exposure therapy group.

Power and colleagues (2002) utilized Marks et al.'s (1998) combined treatment protocol (imaginal and *in vivo* exposure plus CR), offering patients up to 10 sessions over 10 weeks of exposure therapy or EMDR or wait list. Both active treatments resulted in significant reductions in PTSD severity, anxiety, depression, and functional impairment, and both treatments were superior to the waiting-list condition, which showed very little change. Few differences were observed between the two active treatments, except that EMDR required, on average, fewer sessions (4.2 vs. 6.4) and achieved greater reduction in depression scores.

Devilly and Spence (1999) compared a CBT intervention, called trauma treatment protocol (combines imaginal and *in vivo* exposure with elements of SIT), and additional CT techniques to EMDR. Both treatments produced significant improvements from pre- to posttreatment. However, the trauma treatment protocol was found to be superior to EMDR both immediately after treatment and at the 3-month follow-up assessment. Whereas individuals treated with the trauma treatment protocol maintained their treatment gains at the follow-up assessment, individuals treated with EMDR displayed evidence of relapse on several measures.

Lee, Gavriel, Drummond, Richards, and Greenwald (2002) compared the combination of imaginal and *in vivo* exposure plus SIT with EMDR. All participants completed a 6-week waiting-list phase before beginning active treatment. Very little change in PTSD symptoms was observed during the waiting-list period, followed by significant reductions after completion of either active treatment. There were no differences between groups at posttreatment. However, at follow-up results slightly favored EMDR due to further gains obtained during follow-up in the EMDR condition, compared to no additional improvement in the exposure therapy plus SIT condition.

Echeburua et al. (1997) compared a group of survivors treated with six sessions of combined gradual exposure and CR to a group of survivors treated with Bernstein and Borkovec's (1973) protocol for progressive relaxation training. Although both groups displayed significant improvement on measures of PTSD, fear, and depression, improvement was significantly greater in the exposure condition than the relaxation condition. This group difference was maintained at each of the 3-, 6-, and 12-month follow-up assessments.

Tarrier et al. (1999) compared an exposure therapy that included only imaginal exposure to CT. Both groups improved significantly from pre- to posttreatment on measures of PTSD, depression, and anxiety, and these improvements persisted through follow-up. There were no differences observed between the two treatment groups at either posttreatment or follow-up.

Bryant, Moulds, Guthrie, Dang, and Nixon (2003a) compared eight sessions of imaginal exposure, either alone or combined with CR, with supportive counseling. Both immediately after treatment and at follow-up, each of the exposure therapy groups was superior to supportive counseling on measures of PTSD symptoms, anxiety, depression, and trauma-related cognitions. Slightly superior results were obtained in the imaginal exposure plus CR condition, compared to imaginal exposure alone, on one measure of trauma-related reexperiencing symptoms (posttreatment and at follow-up) and on trauma-related cognitions (follow-up only).

Cloitre and her colleagues (2002) examined the efficacy of a treatment that sequentially combined skills training in affect and interpersonal regulation (STAIR) followed by imaginal exposure for treating PTSD. Their sample consisted of a group of women who had been sexually abused as children. Compared to a waiting-list condition, the combined treatment was highly effective in reducing PTSD symptoms, depression, and anxiety as well as improving affect regulation and interpersonal functioning. Cloitre et al. (2002) hypothesized that preliminary treatment with STAIR would facilitate their patients' ability to participate in, and benefit from, the imaginal exposure component of the treatment. However, as we have noted elsewhere (Cahill, Zoelner, Feen, & Riggs, 2004), the design of this study precludes any strong conclusions about whether the addition of STAIR enhanced treatment compliance or outcome (for a rejoinder, see Cloitre, Storall-McClough, & Levitt, 2004).

Fecteau and Nicki (1999) provided four sessions of CBT that combined education, breathing retraining, imaginal and *in vivo* exposure, and CR for PTSD following a recent motor vehicle accident. Compared to a waiting-list group, this brief CBT program resulted in significant reductions in PTSD symptoms, anxiety, depression, and heart-rate reactivity in response to script-driven imagery of the participants' accidents.

Blanchard et al. (2003) examined a CBT program that combined exposure therapy (i.e., exposure to the memory of the trauma by writing a trauma narrative and reading it repeatedly), *in vivo* exposure, relaxation training, and behavioral activation for the treatment of PTSD associated with automobile accidents. At posttreatment, the CBT program was superior to supportive psychotherapy and a waiting-list group on measures of PTSD, depression, and anxiety. At a 3-month follow-up assessment, the CBT group continued to show less severe symptoms than did the supportive counseling group.

Kubany and his colleagues (Kubany et al., 2003, 2004) used a CT focused on guilt-related issues in combination with limited exposure to treat women with PTSD and guilt related to domestic violence. Additional aspects of the intervention included psychoeducation about PTSD and related issues, managing unwanted contact with the abuser, self-advocacy, decision making, and anger management. Compared to a waiting-list condition, this cognitive-behavioral treatment program was very effective in reducing symptoms of PTSD, depression, and guilt and in improving self-esteem (Kubany et al., 2004).

In summary, several CBT interventions that incorporate exposure techniques have been found to be effective in the amelioration of PTSD in civilian samples.

Veteran Samples

There are no studies of PE per se in treating combat veterans with PTSD; however, several studies have examined other forms of exposure therapy in this population. The initial trials of exposure therapy for PTSD were conducted using samples of veterans with combat-related PTSD. In the first of these studies, Keane, Fairbank, Caddell, and Zimering (1989) compared Vietnam veterans treated with 14–16 90-minute sessions of imaginal exposure (which they called implosive or flooding therapy; see Lyons & Keane, 1989) to a waiting-list control group. Veterans in both groups were maintained on whatever psychiatric mediations that had been prescribed prior to participation in the study. Results indicated that, compared to those on the waiting-list, participants treated with exposure displayed significantly more improvement on PTSD reexperiencing symptoms, state-anxiety (but not trait-anxiety), and depression. Treatment did not appear to have an effect on the emotional numbing and social avoidance associated with PTSD.

Two additional studies of veteran samples soon followed. Cooper and Clum (1989) compared veterans receiving standard VA outpatient treatment supplemented with imaginal exposure to a group receiving standard treatment alone. Veterans in the imaginal exposure group received up to 14 90-minute individual sessions with the exposure therapist, though the maximum number of sessions devoted to conducting exposure was 9. Results indicated that augmenting standard care with imaginal exposure improved outcome on state-anxiety (but not trait-anxiety), subjective anxiety in response to a slide show of trauma-related images and sounds, and sleep disturbance. Unlike Keane et al. (1989), Cooper and Clum (1989) did not find a significant effect of treatment on depression. Boudewyns and Hyer (1990; see also Boudewyns, Hyer, Woods, Harrison, & McCranie, 1990) compared veterans treated with specialized VA inpatient care supplemented with 10–12 50-minute sessions of imaginal exposure to a group whose inpatient treatment was supplemented with "more conventional individual psychotherapy" (Boudewyns et al., 1990, p. 361). No group differences were found immediately after treatment. However, veterans whose treatment was supplemented with imaginal exposure showed greater gains on the Veterans Adjustment Scale at a 3-month follow-up assessment.

More recently, Glynn, et al. (1999) compared veterans treated with 13–14 90-minute sessions of imaginal exposure plus CR with a standard care control group and a third group that received the imaginal exposure plus CR intervention supplemented by 16–18 additional sessions of behavioral family therapy. All of the veterans were allowed to remain on previously prescribed psychiatric medications. The various dependent variables in this study were factor analyzed and yielded a positive symptoms factor (i.e., reexperiencing, hyperarousal) and negative symptoms factor (i.e., avoidance, emotional numbing). Results revealed that, compared to the waiting-list condition, treatment with imaginal exposure plus CR resulted in significant improvement on the positive symptoms but not the negative symptoms. Contrary to expectations, adding behavioral family therapy did not enhance outcome.

In sum, although PE has not been tested directly in samples of combat veterans, studies using variations of exposure therapy with veterans have consistently revealed significant benefits for this treatment approach. However, the magnitude of the improvement has been somewhat limited. Furthermore, the benefits of exposure treatment appear to be greater for symptoms of intrusion and arousal than for avoidance and numbing. These studies represent very strict tests of exposure therapy. In all of the trials, exposure was compared to other treatments focused on PTSD symptoms: either a continuation of treatment that the veterans were already receiving or focused PTSD interventions. An important consideration in evaluating the results of these studies is the well-recognized reality that there are incentives for veterans to emphasize their symptoms and to minimize treatment gains (e.g., gaining or losing service-connected disability compensation; for additional discussion, see Frueh, Hamner, Cahill, Gold, & Hamlin, 2000). It should also be noted that the exposure interventions in these studies emphasized imaginal exposure, to the relative neglect of *in vivo* exposure. It is possible that the results of exposure therapy with this population, particularly on measures of avoidance and withdrawal, could be improved with *in vivo* exposure to social situations. Finally, no studies with veteran populations have compared PE alone with PE combined with another treatment approach. The only study (Glynn et al., 1999) that attempted to augment exposure therapy with other behavioral interventions found that adding behavioral family therapy did not produce any further gains.

CONCERNS ABOUT EXPOSURE THERAPY

Therapists often raise concerns that the emotional arousal experienced by trauma survivors undergoing exposure therapy may be extremely distressing and even damaging. Indeed, several clinical researchers have expressed reservations about the safety of exposure therapy in the treatment of at least some populations with PTSD (e.g., Cloitre et al., 2002; Kilpatrick & Best, 1984; Pitman et al., 1991). Two potential safety issues, in particular, have gained attention in the literature: (1) exposure therapy may exacerbate the very PTSD symptoms that it is designed to ameliorate; and (2) although

PTSD symptoms may be alleviated, other psychological symptoms (e.g., drinking, depression, guilt) may worsen.

For years, the primary evidence for the dangerousness of exposure therapy has been a paper by Pitman et al. (1991) that described six cases of combat veterans whose PTSD symptoms worsened after treatment by imaginal exposure. However, the study from which the case series was obtained did not include a control condition; therefore it is unknown how many veterans would have experienced an acute exacerbation of their symptoms during the study period had they not received treatment. Moreover, in the full sample, fear and physiological arousal as well as guilt, sadness, and anger were decreased after exposure therapy (Pitman et al., 1996).

More recently, Tarrier et al. (1999) conducted a randomized controlled trial comparing imaginal exposure with CT and reported that overall, the two treatments produced comparable outcomes on measures of PTSD prevalence and severity, anxiety, and depression. However, significantly more participants in the imaginal exposure group (31%) than in the CT condition (9%) exhibited "symptom worsening" at posttreatment. Taken at face value, these data would seem to support concerns about the safety of exposure therapy in the treatment of PTSD. However, several considerations lend doubt to this conclusion. First, the operational definition of "symptom worsening" was a posttreatment PTSD severity score that was greater than the corresponding pretreatment score by 1 or more points; the mean increase in PTSD severity scores was not reported. Given that an increase of just 1 point is within the measurement error of the instrument (CAPS), this definition may not reflect actual symptom worsening (for an extended discussion, see Devilly & Foa, 2001). Second, Tarrier et al. did not include a waiting-list condition; therefore it is not possible to determine whether the rates of "symptom worsening" observed in the imaginal exposure condition represented an increase, decrease, or no difference from what would have been observed if treatment had been withheld. Third, the group differences were not apparent on measures of depression and anxiety, areas of psychopathology that are correlated with PTSD. Finally, the group differences that were found on the PTSD measure at posttreatment were not found at the follow-up assessment.

Subsequent research has failed to support the safety concerns about exposure therapy raised by Pitman et al. (1991) and Tarrier et al. (1999). Taylor et al. (2003) investigated symptom worsening following treatment in a study comparing a group treated with imaginal plus *in vivo* exposure to a group treated with EMDR and a group treated with relaxation training. Rates of symptoms worsening were uniformly low across all three conditions (0%, 7%, and 7%, respectively). Similarly, Gillespie, Duffy, Hackman, and Clark (2002) administered a treatment that combined exposure and CR and found no symptom worsening. Cloitre et al. (2002) investigated the efficacy of a treatment involving sequentially combined skills training in affect and interpersonal regulation (STAIR), based on principles of dialectical behavior therapy (DBT; Linehan, 1993), compared with imaginal exposure, to treat PTSD in female victims of childhood abuse. Applying the Tarrier et al. definition of "symptom worsening," Cloitre et al. reported that 4.5% of patients receiving STAIR/imaginal exposure had some increase in PTSD severity following treatment, compared to 25% in the waiting-list group. Although limitations on the design of this study preclude conclusions about whether or not the low rate of symptom worsening can be attributed to treatment with STAIR prior to administering exposure, the results do illustrate that treatment with exposure therapy does not result in symptom worsening.

Cahill, Riggs, Rauch, and Foa (2003b) analyzed data from the Foa et al. (1999) study of PE versus SIT versus PE/SIT versus waiting list and our recently completed study comparing PE alone to PE with CR (PE/CR) versus waiting list (Foa et al., 2002a). Of 162 participants who completed one of the active treatments, only one (0.6%) showed symptom worsening, defined as an increase in PTSD severity by 1 or more points on the PTSD Symptom Scale–Interview (PSS-I), the primary outcome measure. In the waiting-list condition, 3 out of 39 participants (7.7%) showed symptom worsening. Cahill et al. (2003b) also investigated symptom worsening on self-report measures of depression and anxiety. Only 6 out of 159 participants receiving active treatment (3.8%) showed an increase on depression, compared to 11 out of 36 waiting-list participants (30.6%). For general anxiety, the corresponding numbers were 12 out of 159 active treatment participants (7.5%) and 13 out of 34 waiting-list participants (38.2%). Combining across measures, there was a total of 16 out of 159 active treatment participants (10.1%) who showed worsening on one or more measures, compared to 20 out of 35 waiting-list participants (57.1%). Across the active treatments, rates of symptom worsening on at least one of the three measures were 6.8% for PE alone, 6.8% for PE/CR, 10.5% for SIT alone, and 27.3% for PE/SIT.

In summary, the results from the studies described above suggest that the rates of symptom worsening associated with exposure treatments are generally very low and that exposure therapy is not associated with a greater risk of symptom worsening than other forms of treatment. Indeed, results from the studies that included waiting-list controls would suggest that, if anything, withholding treatment rather than providing active treatments is associated with greater symptom worsening.

Another often-expressed concern is that the emotional distress associated with exposure therapy leads to high rates of dropout from treatment (Cloitre et al., 2002). Again, there is no empirical evidence for this concern. In a recent meta-analytic study, Hembree et al. (2003a) found no difference in the dropout rates from exposure therapy alone (20.5%), SIT or CT alone (22.1%), exposure therapy combined with SIT or CT (26.9%) or EMDR (18.9%), though active treatment did have higher dropout rates than did control conditions (11.4%). Overall, participants tolerate exposure therapy at least as well as other forms of CBT.

SPECIAL CONSIDERATION
IN THE IMPLEMENTATION OF PE

Prolonged or Multiple Traumas

It is not unusual for PTSD patients to report multiple traumatic experiences. Others report repeated or prolonged traumas in which they experienced similar assaults on more than one occasion (e.g., multiple assaults at the hands of an intimate partner; childhood sexual abuse). The presence of multiple or repeated traumas raises the question of which trauma should be the target for imaginal exposure. Often therapists ask, "Where do we start?" and "must we conduct imaginal exposure to all of the events?" The answer to the second question appears to be "no." Our clinical experience indicates that the gains made in response to imaginal exposure and processing of the most distressing memory (or perhaps the two most distressing memories) generalizes such that the distress associated with memories of the other events lessens without direct exposure exercises. This finding is important because within a 10- to 12-session treatment program, only two or, at most, three memories can be submitted to imaginal exposure. Consequently, the therapist and patient need to identify the most distressing traumatic event. In the case of multiple distinct traumatic events, we ask the client to identify which of the various events is most upsetting at the present time in terms of reexperiencing symptoms, or which memory causes the most disruption in their life. In the case of repeated or prolonged trauma, the therapist needs to identify a single incident that stands out in the patient's memory as the worst, as judged by the degree of intrusive thoughts, flashbacks, or nightmares. The specific memory with which treatment begins is selected by a consensus between the client and the therapist. If memories that are not targeted with exposure continue to prompt distress, additional imaginal exposure to these memories will need to be conducted.

Avoidance

In the overall rationale for PE provided in first treatment session, avoidance is described as a major factor in maintaining posttrauma disturbances, with exposure exercises designed to counter it. This rationale makes sense to clients who can identify many situations that they have been avoiding, and they realize that avoidance prevents them from finding out that these situations are not inherently dangerous. Nonetheless, avoidance is probably the most common impediment to compliance with PE treatment. When avoidance hinders exposure exercises, the therapist should validate the client's fear and urge to avoid but, at the same time, remind him or her that although avoidance reduces anxiety in the short term, in the long run it serves to maintain it. In other words, the therapist should review the rationale for treatment to help the patient overcome his or her avoidance.

It is not unusual for patients' avoidance to intensify several sessions into treatment, when they have to confront their most distressing memories and most feared situations. Some patients may have experienced benefits from PE, but their remaining symptoms may lead them to question the efficacy of the treatment. Others may actually feel worse than they did when they entered treatment, although such exacerbations are temporary, do not result in significant dropout from treatment, and are not predictive of worse outcome (Foa et al., 2002b). For those patients, reiterating the rationale, although important, may not be sufficient to overcome the tendency to avoid. In these cases it can be helpful to review the reasons that the patient sought treatment for PTSD in the first place (i.e., the many ways in which PTSD interferes with life satisfaction) and to review the progress that he or she has already made. Therapists should reinforce patients for efforts that they do make toward completing the exposure exercises. Addressing the negative consequence of avoidance and at the same time validating the client's fear of, and concerns about, exposure will help him or her to renew the struggle against avoidance.

The therapist may also find it helpful to examine possible obstacles that prevent the patient from completing the exposure exercises and provide encouragement to overcome them. It may be necessary to modify the *in vivo* hierarchy and introduce a more gradual progression. Alternatively, specific *in vivo* exercises may need to be modified in a way that will help the patient to complete them. For example, a client who finds it difficult to complete an exposure exercise of shopping at a mall because of transportation limitations may substitute this exercise with an exposure to crowds (the actual feared situation) at a more convenient location. Similarly, there may be practical problems in completing imaginal homework exercises (e.g., no place with privacy in which to listen to tapes). The therapist should work with clients to identify such problems so that they do not become easy excuses for not completing the exercise.

Anger

It has been our clinical impression that the experience and expression of intense anger during imaginal exposure may interfere with the emotional processing of fear and thereby limit reductions in PTSD symptoms. In support of this impression, Foa, Riggs, Massie, and Yarczower (1995) found that high levels of anger prior to treatment are associated with less fear arousal during imaginal exposure, which in turn is associated with poorer outcome. Therefore, to optimize the gains from PE it is important for the client to focus his or her attention and narrative on the fear- rather than the anger-eliciting aspects of the event. However, it is also important to validate the survivor's anger. When a client focuses primarily on anger, we first validate these feeling as an appropriate response to trauma and as a symptom of PTSD. We then explain that the focus on anger may prevent him or her from fully engaging the fear associated with the traumatic memory, although it may be less distressing to feel angry than to feel frightened. Indeed, some therapists have suggested that anger serves as a way of avoiding the fear associated with the memory. In most cases, clients agree readily with this observation and are able to refocus on the fear-related aspects of the memory. This shift can be further reinforced by reviewing the treatment rationale and explaining the importance of focusing on fear and anxiety. Support for the value of shifting away from anger and maintaining the focus of treatment on anxiety is provided by Cahill, Rauch, Hembree, and Foa (2003a), who found that treatments that targeted PTSD also resulted in a significant reduction in anger. The effect of PTSD treatment on anger was particularly notable among patients with extremely high anger scores prior to treatment. Anger scores at posttreatment did not differ between patients who started treatment with extremely high levels of anger and those who did not. Moreover, average posttreatment anger scores in both groups of patients were within the "normal" range, based on the normative sample.

Maintaining the Focus of Treatment on PTSD

Clients with chronic PTSD often face multiple life stressors that lead to impaired general functioning. In addition, individuals with chronic PTSD often have comorbid psychiatric and medical problems (e.g., Davidson, Hughes, Blazer, & George, 1991; Kessler et al., 1995). Therefore, crises during treatment are not unusual, especially if early or multiple traumatic experiences have interfered with the development of healthy coping skills. Poorly modulated affect, self-destructive impulse-control problems (e.g., alcohol binges, substance abuse, risky behaviors), numerous conflicts with family members or others, and severe depression with suicidal ideation are common comorbid conditions with PTSD. These problems require attention but can potentially disrupt the focus on treatment of PTSD. If careful pretreatment assessment has determined that chronic PTSD is the client's primary problem, our goal is to maintain the focus on PTSD with periodic reassessment of other problem areas, as needed.

If the client's mood or behavior raises concern about his or her personal safety or the safety of others, the need to focus on this issue and reduce the imminent risk may require temporary cessation of PE. However, if a crisis does not include imminent risk, the therapist should explain to the client that completing the treatment, and thereby decreasing PTSD symptoms and other problems, is likely the best course of action. When appropriate, the therapist may point out the links between the external crisis and the PTSD symptoms and help the patient realize that these situations will improve as the client's ability to manage distress improves and PTSD symptoms decrease. In maintaining the focus of therapy on PTSD symptoms, the therapist should remind the client of the overall goal (i.e., to recover from PTSD), but should not discount the significance of the more immediate crisis. It is also helpful to put the crisis and therapy into chronological perspective. Reminding the client that treatment is brief (9–12 sessions) and determining whether the crisis truly needs to be dealt with prior to the end of treatment (e.g., for safety purposes) can serve to bring the focus back to the goals of treatment. By reaching an agreement at the beginning of the program that crises should be addressed but that the focus of treatment must remain on the PTSD, the therapist will be better able to refocus the client when the need arises.

DISSEMINATION OF PE FOR PTSD

Despite the demonstrated efficacy of PE and other exposure therapies for PTSD, clinicians have been slow to adopt the techniques into their practice. Becker, Zayfert, and Anderson (2004) surveyed a large sample of psychologists about whether they treated patients with PTSD and, if so, whether they were trained in the use of imaginal exposure and whether they used it with their patients. Although 63% of the sample reported having treated more than 11 patients with PTSD, only 27% of the sample were trained in the use of imaginal exposure for PTSD and even fewer (9%) reported regularly using imaginal exposure with their patients suffering from PTSD. Thus few therapists who see patients with PTSD are trained in the use of exposure therapy, and even fewer use it. What are the reasons for this low utilization rate?

Becker et al. (2004) found that the commonest reason for not using exposure therapy to treat PTSD was lack of training (60%). The next two commonest reasons were resistance to using manualized treatments (25%) and fears that patients would decompensate from the treatment (22%). As discussed above, although safety concerns have been raised, there is no empirical support for the conclusion that PE carries increased risk compared to other CBT treatments for PTSD or, more importantly, compared to the risk of withholding or delaying treatment. We have been aware of the limitations in adoption of PE resulting from the lack of training opportunities and clinicians' negative attitudes toward manualized treatments and have made several efforts to address these problems.

Over the last several years we have trained many professionals from various disciplines in workshops lasting from 2 hours to 5 days. Clinicians commonly report that they are attracted by the efficacy and efficiency of exposure therapy and are interested in using it with patients who have PTSD. However, they are also worried about being able to properly implement it without further assistance, and we strongly believe that few of these clinicians actually end up using PE in their practices. Although an extended workshop (e.g., 3–5 days) may be adequate for training clinicians who have a background in CBT and experience in utilizing exposure therapy with other disorders (e.g., phobias, panic disorder, obsessive–compulsive disorder), therapists trained in other models of psychotherapy (e.g., psychodynamic,

Rogerian) may find that applying PE requires them to think about and work with patients in an entirely new way. PE, like other CBT treatment programs, differs from traditional therapies in several important ways. For example, CBT programs focus on reducing specific symptoms, whereas other types of therapies may focus on processes such as the therapist–patient relationship or seek to understand the historical causes of the problems. These traditional therapies are often less structured, and the agenda is driven by what the patient wants to talk about from session to session. By contrast, the CBT therapist exerts a major influence in each therapy session because many CBT programs, including PE, follow detailed protocols that specify the content and the techniques to be utilized in each session. Thus non-CBT therapists need to learn not only the specifics of how to conduct imaginal and *in vivo* exposure, but also how to take an active role in setting the therapeutic agenda, keeping the focus of treatment on PTSD, instructing patients in doing home exercises, and so on.

Based on our own work and a review of the literature, two dissemination models have emerged. In the first model experts provide intensive training as well as continued supervision of the therapists who administer the treatment. In the second model experts provide the intensive initial training of the therapists, but ongoing supervision of the therapists and initial training new therapists are provided by local supervisors who consult with the experts but, over time, become experts themselves.

Model I: Intensive Initial Training of Therapists Plus Ongoing Expert Supervision

As described above, we recently completed a study (Foa et al., 2002a) in which we trained community-based clinicians to use PE to treat rape survivors with PTSD. In this 6-year study we trained therapists with master's degrees in social work or counseling, using a training model in which an initial workshop was followed with ongoing supervision provided by expert PE therapists. All of the community therapists had substantial experience in working with survivors of sexual assault, but none of them had prior training in CBT, nor had they any experience with conducting research or delivering manualized interventions. Indeed, some of them expressed reservations about the ethics of doing research with rape victims and were initially reluctant to use manualized treatments with their patients. Of note, they were not opposed to using exposure therapy with rape survivors and readily accepted the idea that confronting painful memories, images, and feelings promotes healing.

In the first step of dissemination, Center for the Treatment and Study of Anxiety (CTSA) experts provided the community therapists with a 5-day intensive workshop that included an introduction to the theory and efficacy data supporting the use of PE in the treatment of PTSD as well as instruction in the administration of PE techniques. Much of the time was spent teaching and practicing how to deliver the overall rationale for the treatment, rationales for imaginal and *in vivo* exposure, and how to implement the two forms of exposure. Additional time was allocated to discussing ways to manage patients who present with too little or too much emotional engagement while completing imaginal exposure exercises. Training included detailed instructions of "how to do it," watching excerpts from videotapes of expert therapists demonstrating each aspect of PE, and role plays in small groups. Intensive training was devoted to cognitive restructuring (CR), conducted by Dr. David M. Clark of Oxford, England, and the CTSA experts. This training in how to implement CR was tailored to working with trauma survivors and began with a detailed theoretical presentation of the profound impact trauma has on survivors' thoughts and beliefs about the self, others, and the world.

After the initial training, each therapist then completed at least two training cases under supervision by a CTSA supervisor. Supervision consisted of weekly 3-hour meetings on the premises of the community sites. All therapists working in the study attended the supervision sessions, in which each ongoing case was discussed and videotapes of that week's therapy sessions were viewed. For the first 2 years of the study, the CTSA experts conducted 2-day booster workshops every 6 months, in which therapists from both the community clinic and the CTSA presented cases and videotapes of therapy sessions. Throughout the 6-year study, CTSA supervisors continued to provide weekly supervision to the therapists.

Participants were recruited through the CTSA and the community agency and were randomly assigned to PE, PE/CR, or waiting-list (WL) conditions at each location. Like the community therapists, CTSA therapists participated in weekly supervision meetings that included discussion about ongoing cases and the viewing of videotapes of therapy sessions. Indeed, the supervision established at the community agency was modeled after our standard supervision practices at the CTSA. As noted in the section on the efficacy of PE, the results from this study revealed that both treatments resulted in greater reductions in symptoms of PTSD, anxiety, and depression than the WL condition and that both treatments were equally effective. More importantly, no differences in treatment outcome were found between patients who were treated at the CTSA and those who were treated at the community agency. We are currently conducting additional dissemination studies to determine how well community therapists can continue to use PE as expert supervision is withdrawn.

Currently, a multisite study comparing PE to present-centered therapy (PCT) is being conducted within the Cooperative Studies Program of the Veterans Administration (Principal investigators: Paula P. Schnurr, PhD; Matthew J. Friedman, MD, PhD; and Charles C. Engel, MD, MPH) that utilizes a similar training model. Therapists were initially trained at an intensive 5-day workshop structured like that of the Foa et al. (2002a) study. Therapists then completed an average of two training cases under weekly expert supervision before treating actual study cases, also under expert supervision. Because therapists in this study are located throughout the United States, supervision was conducted long distance rather than in person. Supervisors viewed videotapes and provided written feedback and individual telephone consultation on a weekly basis. No data are yet available on the outcome of this study, but supervisors report that most of the therapists trained to conduct PE are doing an excellent job. However, it is important to note that most of the therapists and supervisors agreed that ongoing supervision was important for the therapists to feel comfortable with the techniques.

In another application of this model, several members of the CTSA conducted a 4-day workshop to train a group of New York City therapists in the use of PE for individuals suffering significant symptoms of PTSD after the September 11 attacks on the World Trade Center. In collaboration with the Mount Sinai School of Medicine, the efficacy of a brief course of PE (four sessions) was compared to that of supportive counseling. The therapy sessions were video- or audiotaped and supervisors from the CTSA reviewed each tape and provided therapists with weekly supervision through telephone calls and frequent trips (every 2 or 3 weeks) to New York for direct group supervision, in which videotapes of therapy sessions were viewed and discussed. Although data analyses have not been completed, the supervisors indicated that therapists were able to conduct PE appropriately with trauma survivors and that both brief interventions seemed to be quite effective in alleviating PSTD and depression.

In summary, the existing evidence suggests that, for PE, a dissemination model that includes an intensive workshop over several days and ongoing supervision by experts can be quite effective. Indeed, it has been heartening to witness the natural ripple effect that our work has had in the Philadelphia rape-treatment community. Based on the study of PE versus PE/CR, PE has been adopted as one of the primary treatment interventions for survivors of rape and childhood sexual abuse at the collaborating clinic. Moreover, the therapists who were originally trained by CTSA clinicians for that study are now training other community clinicians in the use of PE. These trained therapists also took the initiative to have the PE manual translated into Spanish and then used the translated manual to train local Latino community therapists so that Spanish-speaking clients could also benefit from this treatment. Similarly, our experience training VA therapists in the ongoing study is that once therapists become familiar and comfortable with PE, they begin to use the techniques with traumatized patients who are not in the research protocol. Although it has been gratifying to see how therapists in these studies have enthusiastically adopted PE, this method of dissemination can be expensive because of the intensive, ongoing expert supervision that is involved.

Model II: Intensive Initial Training of Therapists Plus Local Supervision

A second model of treatment dissemination aims to reduce the involvement of external experts by creating local expertise. In this model community clinicians train in expert clinics for various lengths of time with the expectation that they will go back to their communities to train and supervise local clinicians in the delivery of PE. At the same time, experts provide workshops to introduce PE techniques to broader groups of community therapists, who then acquire supervision from the local experts. To our knowledge, no systematic evaluation of this dissemination approach has been conducted.

An example of dissemination conducted using this model is a series of efforts made by clinicians at the CTSA over the last several years to train therapists in Israel to deliver PE. CTSA experts have delivered 3- to 5-day workshops on PE to clinicians in Israel whose work focuses on trauma-related distress and PTSD. A number of the clinicians who have attended these workshops have traveled to the United States for additional training (lasting 2–3 weeks) at the CTSA, focused on the observation of experts using PE and acquisition of experience in supervising therapists in the use of PE. Subsequently, supervision groups have formed in Israel led by one or more of the clinicians who received the additional training at the CTSA. The supervision groups meet regularly, viewing tapes and discussing patients' treatment plans and progress. Although we remain available for consultation to the supervisors on an as-needed basis, our involvement as consultants at this point has been very limited.

Although there has not been a systematic examination of the efficacy of these dissemination efforts, results from the first 10 patients treated in one of the supervision groups were presented at the Annual Meeting of the Israeli Psychiatric Association (Nacasch et al., 2003). All patients were male; most had chronic combat-related PTSD, some of them suffering from PTSD symptoms for 30 years, despite years of psychiatric treatment that had produced no or little improvement. After 10–12 sessions of PE, the mean reduction of symptoms was 58%. The outcome was quite impressive and is comparable to that of our clinic and at community clinics where we have provided direct supervision. Thus, although our experience with this second dissemination method is more limited, preliminary results suggest that PE can be successfully disseminated using local supervisors.

CONCLUSION

Working with clients who have chronic PTSD can be extremely rewarding for therapists. The availability of effective treatments for PTSD, including PE, allows mental health professionals to positively impact the disrupted lives of sufferers in a short period of time. As would be expected given the prominent role of fear and anxiety in the presentation of PTSD, treatments based on the principles of exposure therapy have proven particularly effective and efficient at treating PTSD, as they have with other anxiety disorders. However, PTSD symptoms themselves and comorbid disorders may hinder some clients' ability to engage in, and benefit from, the therapy. It is common for clients with PTSD to attend therapy irregularly, to drop out prematurely, or to take long, unofficial breaks from treatment. Many struggle with avoidance and are reluctant to complete exposure exercises. Other clients may have difficulty tolerating anxiety or engaging the traumatic memory.

A strong, collaborative, therapeutic relationship is essential to help clients overcome these hurdles. Therapists must utilize their basic clinical skills, particularly empathic, active listening, to foster such a relationship. Furthermore, specific aspects of the PE protocol, such as ensuring the client's understanding of what is being done and why by explaining the techniques and sharing the rationale for each one, are designed to further this collaborative relationship. Beyond simply needing a collaborative relationship in which to conduct PE, the treatment requires joint decision making by the therapist and client about treatment focus, pace, and homework assignments. Helping the client to be and feel in control of this process is imperative and can itself be therapeutic, because many clients with PTSD feel out of control of most of their lives—even (or especially) their own thoughts, feelings, and behavior. In addition to facilitating a collaborative relationship in the treatment program, the PE therapist should express confidence in the client's ability to recover and should actively praise the client's effort, courage, and coping resources.

Numerous studies have shown PE to be effective in treating PTSD in survivors of a variety of traumatic events. Further, when directly compared, PE produces reductions in PTSD at least as large as other CBT treatments, and adding other CBT techniques to PE appears to produce little additional gain to that achieved with PE alone. Despite the overwhelming empirical support for PE, there has been some hesitancy among practitioners to adopt this approach to treating PTSD. Some of this reticence arises from concerns about the safety of PE—concerns that have arisen without substantial evidence. In addition, efforts to disseminate PE have been slow to manifest. However, all evidence available to date supports the conclusion that PE can be successfully disseminated to practitioners in the field.

REFERENCES

American Psychiatric Association. (1994). *Diagnostic and statistical manual of mental disorders* (4th ed.). Washington, DC: Author.

Atkeson, B. M., Calhoun, K. S., Resick, P. A., & Ellis, E. M. (1982). Victims of rape: Repeated assessment of depressive symptoms. *Journal of Consulting and Clinical Psychology, 50*(1), 96–102.

Becker, C. B., Zayfert, C., & Anderson, E. (2004). A survey of psychologists' attitudes towards and utilization of exposure therapy for PTSD. *Behaviour Research and Therapy, 42*(3), 277–292.

Bernstein, D. A., & Borkovec, T. D. (1973). *Progressive relaxation training: A manual for the helping professions.* Champaign, IL: Research Press.

Blanchard, E. B., Hickling, E. J., Devineni, T., Veazey, C. H., Galovski, T. E., Mundy, E., et al. (2003). A controlled evaluation of cognitive behavioral therapy for post-traumatic stress in motor vehicle accident survivors. *Behaviour Research and Therapy, 41*(1), 79–96.

Boudewyns, P. A., & Hyer, L. (1990). Physiological response to combat memories and preliminary treatment outcome in Vietnam veterans: PTSD patients treated with direct therapeutic exposure. *Behavior Therapy, 21*(1), 63–87.

Boudewyns, P. A., Hyer, L., Woods, M. G., Harrison, W. R., McCranie, E. (1990). PTSD among Vietnam veterans: An early look at treatment outcome using direct therapeutic exposure. *Journal of Traumatic Stress, 3*(3), 359–368.

Bryant, R. A., Moulds, M. L., Guthrie, R. M., Dang, S. T., & Nixon, R. D. V. (2003a). Imaginal exposure alone and imaginal exposure with cognitive restructuring in treatment of posttraumatic stress disorder. *Journal of Consulting and Clinical Psychology, 71,* 706–712.

Bryant, R. A., Moulds, M., Guthrie, R., & Nixon, R. D. V. (2003b). Treating acute stress disorder following mild traumatic brain injury. *American Journal of Psychiatry, 160*(3), 585–587.

Cahill, S. P., Rauch, S. A., Hembree, E. A., & Foa, E. B. (2003a). Effect of cognitive-behavioral treatments for PTSD on anger. *Journal of Cognitive Psychotherapy, 17,* 113–131.

Cahill, S. P., Riggs, D. S., Rauch, S. A. M., & Foa, E. B. (2003b, March). *Does prolonged exposure therapy for PTSD make people worse?* Convention proceedings of the 23rd annual meeting of the Anxiety Disorders Association of America, Silver Springs, MD.

Cahill, S. P., Zoellner, L. A., Feeny, N. C., & Riggs, D. S. (2004). Sequential treatment for child abuse-related PTSD: Methodological comment on Cloitre et al. (2002). *Journal of Consulting and Clinical Psychology, 72,* 543–548.

Calhoun, K. S., Atkeson, B. M., & Resick, P. A. (1982). A longitudinal examination of fear reactions in victims of rape. *Journal of Consulting and Clinical Psychology, 29*(6), 655–661.

Cloitre, M., Koenen, K. C., Cohen, L. R., & Han, H. (2002). Skills training in affective and interpersonal regulation followed by exposure: A phase-based treatment for PTSD related to childhood abuse. *Journal of Consulting and Clinical Psychology, 70*(5), 1067–1074.

Cloitre, M., Stovall-McClough, C., & Levitt, J. T. (2004). Treating life-impairing problems beyond PTSD: Reply to Cahill, Zoellner, Feeny, and Riggs (2004). *Journal of Consulting and Clinical Psychology, 72*(3), 549–551.

Cooper, N. A., & Clum, G. A. (1989). Imaginal flooding as a supplementary treatment for PTSD in combat veterans: A controlled study. *Behavior Therapy, 20*(3), 381–391.

Davidson, J. R., Hughes, D., Blazer, D. G., & George, L. K. (1991). Post-traumatic stress disorder in the community: An epidemiological study. *Psychological Medicine, 21*(3), 713–721.

Devilly, G. J., & Foa, E. B. (2001). The investigation of exposure and cognitive therapy: Comment on Tarrier et al. (1999). *Journal of Consulting and Clinical Psychology, 69*(1), 114–116.

Devilly, G. J., & Spence, S. H. (1999). The relative efficacy and treatment distress of EMDR and a cognitive-behavior trauma treatment protocol in the amelioration of posttraumatic stress disorder. *Journal of Anxiety Disorders, 13*(1–2), 131–157.

Echeburua, E., Corral, P. D., Zubizarreta, I., & Sarasua, B. (1997). Psychological treatment of chronic posttraumatic stress disorder in victims of sexual aggression. *Behavior Modification, 21*(4), 433–456.

Fecteau, G., & Nicki, R. (1999). Cognitive behavioural treatment of post traumatic stress disorder after motor vehicle accident. *Behavioural and Cognitive Psychotherapy, 27*, 201–214.

Foa, E. B., & Cahill, S. P. (2001). Psychological therapies: Emotional processing. In N. J. Smelser & P. B. Bates (Eds.), *International encyclopedia of the social and behavioral sciences* (pp. 12,363–12,369). Oxford, UK: Elsevier.

Foa, E. B., Dancu, C. V., Hembree, E. A., Jaycox, L. H., Meadows, E. A., & Street, G. (1999). The efficacy of exposure therapy, stress inoculation training and their combination in ameliorating PTSD for female victims of assault. *Journal of Consulting and Clinical Psychology, 67*, 194–200.

Foa, E. B., Hembree, E. A., Feeny, N. C., & Zoellner, L. A. (2002a, March). Posttraumatic stress disorder treatment for female assault victims. In L. A. Zoellner (Chair), *Recent innovations in posttraumatic stress disorder treatment*. Symposium conducted at the annual convention of the Anxiety Disorders Association of America, Austin, TX.

Foa, E. B., & Jaycox, L. H. (1999). Cognitive-behavioral theory and treatment of posttraumatic stress disorder. In D. Spiegel (Ed.), *Efficacy and cost-effectiveness of psychotherapy* (pp. 23–61). Washington, DC: American Psychiatric Press.

Foa, E. B., & Kozak, M. J. (1986). Emotional processing of fear: Exposure to corrective information. *Psychological Bulletin, 99*, 20–35.

Foa, E. B., & Meadows, E. A. (1997). Psychosocial treatments for post-traumatic stress disorder: A critical review. *Annual Review of Psychology, 48*, 449–480.

Foa, E. B., & Riggs, D. S. (1993). Post-traumatic stress disorder in rape victims. In J. Oldham, M. B. Riba, & A. Tasman (Eds.), *American Psychiatric Press Review of Psychiatry, Vol. 12* (pp. 285–309). Washington, DC: American Psychiatric Press.

Foa, E. B., Riggs, D. S., Massie, E. D., & Yarczower, M. (1995). The impact of fear activation and anger on the efficacy of exposure treatment for posttraumatic stress disorder. *Behavior Therapy, 26*, 487–499.

Foa, E. B., & Rothbaum, B. O. (1998). *Treating the trauma of rape: Cognitive-behavioral therapy for PTSD*. New York: Guilford Press.

Foa, E. B., Rothbaum, B. O., Riggs, D. S., & Murdock, T. B. (1991). Treatment of posttraumatic stress disorder in rape victims: A comparison between cognitive-behavioral procedures and counseling. *Journal of Consulting and Clinical Psychology, 59*, 715–723.

Foa, E. B., Steketee, G., & Rothbaum, B. (1989). Behavioral/cognitive conceptualizations of post-traumatic stress disorder. *Behavior Therapy, 20*, 155–176.

Foa, E. B., Zoellner, L. A.., Feeny, N. C., Hembree, E. A., & Alvarez-Conrad, J. (2002b). Does imaginal exposure exacerbate PTSD symptoms? *Journal of Consulting and Clinical Psychology, 70*, 1022–1028.

Frueh, B. C., Hamner, M. B., Cahill, S. P., Gold, P. B., & Hamlin, K. L. (2000). Apparent symptom overreporting in combat veterans evaluated for PTSD. *Clinical Psychology Review, 20,* 853–885.

Gillespie, K., Duffy, M., Hackmann, A., & Clark, D. M. (2002). Community based cognitive therapy in the treatment of posttraumatic stress disorder following the Omagh bomb. *Behaviour Research and Therapy, 40,* 345–357.

Glynn, S. M., Eth, S., Randolph, E. T., Foy, D. W., Urbaitis, M., Boxer, L., & et al. (1999). A test of behavioral family therapy to augment exposure for combat-related posttraumatic stress disorder. *Journal of Consulting and Clinical Psychology, 67,* 243–251.

Harvey, A. G., & Bryant, R. A. (1998). The relationship between acute stress disorder and posttraumatic stress disorder: A prospective evaluation of motor vehicle accident survivors. *Journal of Consulting and Clinical Psychology, 66,* 507–512.

Harvey, A. G., Bryant, R. A., & Tarrier, N. (2003). Cognitive behaviour therapy for posttraumatic stress disorder. *Clinical Psychology Review, 3,* 501–522.

Hembree, E. A., Foa, E. B., Dorfan, N. M., Street, G. P., Kowalski, J., & Tu, X. (2003a). Do patients drop out prematurely from exposure therapy for PTSD? *Journal of Traumatic Stress, 16*(6), 555–562.

Hembree, E. A., Rauch, S. A. M., & Foa, E. B. (2003b). Beyond the manual: The insider's guide to prolonged exposure for PTSD. *Cognitive and Behavioral Practice, 10,* 22–30.

Keane, T. M., Fairbank, J. A., Caddell, J. M., & Zimering, R. T. (1989). Implosive (flooding) therapy reduces symptoms of PTSD in Vietnam combat veterans. *Behavior Therapy, 20,* 245–260.

Kessler, R. C., Sonnega, A., Bromet, E., Hughes, M., & Nelson, C. B. (1995). Posttraumatic stress disorder in the National Comorbidity Survey. *Archives of General Psychiatry, 52,* 1048–1060.

Kilpatrick, D. G., & Best, C. L., (1984). Some cautionary remarks on treating sexual assault victims with implosion. *Behavior Therapy, 15*(4), 421–423.

Kubany, E. S., Hill, E. E., & Owens, J. A. (2003). Cognitive trauma therapy for battered women with PTSD: preliminary findings. *Journal of Traumatic Stress, 16*(1), 81–91.

Kubany, E. S., Hill, E. E., Owens, J. A., Iannce-Spencer, C., McCaig, M. A., Tremayne, K. J., et al. (2004). Cognitive trauma therapy for battered women with PTSD (CTT-BW). *Journal of Consulting and Clinical Psychology, 72*(1), 3–18.

Lee, C., Gavriel, H., Drummond, P., Richards, J., & Greenwald, R. (2002). Treatment of PTSD: Stress inoculation training with prolonged exposure compared to EMDR. *Journal of Clinical Psychology, 58,* 1071–1089.

Linehan, M. M. (1993). *Cognitive-behavioral treatment of borderline personality disorder.* New York: Guilford Press.

Lyons, J. A., & Keane, T. M. (1989). Implosive therapy in the treatment of combat related PTSD. *Journal of Traumatic Stress, 2,* 137–152.

Marks, I., Lovell, K., Noshirvani, H., Livanou, M., & Thrasher, S. (1998). Treatment of posttraumatic stress disorder by exposure and/or cognitive restructuring. *Archives of General Psychiatry, 55,* 317–325.

Meichenbaum, D. (1977). Cognitive-behavioral modification: An integrative approach. New York: Plenum Press.

Nacasch, N., Cohen-Rapperot, G., Polliack, M., Knobler, H. Y., Zohar, J., & Foa, E. B. (2003, April). *Prolonged exposure therapy for PTSD: The dissemination and the preliminary results of the implementation of the treatment protocol in Israel.* Abstract in the

Proceedings of the 11th Conference of the Israel Psychiatric Association, Haifa, Israel.

Otto, M. W., Hinton, D., Korbly, N. B., Chea, A., Ba, P., Gershuny, B. S., et al. (2003). Treatment of pharmacotherapy-refractory posttraumatic stress disorder among Cambodian refugees: A pilot study of combination treatment with cognitive-behavior therapy vs sertraline alone. *Behaviour Research and Therapy, 41*(11), 1271–1276.

Paunovic, N., & Ost, L. G. (2001). Cognitive-behavior therapy vs exposure therapy in the treatment of PTSD in refugees. *Behaviour Research and Therapy, 39*, 1183–1197.

Pitman, R. K., Altman, B., Greenwald, E., Longpre, R. E., Macklin, M. L., Poire, R. E., et al. (1991). Psychiatric complications during flooding therapy for posttraumatic stress disorder. *Journal of Clinical Psychiatry, 52*, 17–20.

Pitman, R. K., Orr, S. P., Altman, B., Longpre, R. E., Poire, R. E., Macklin, M. L., et al. (1996). Emotional processing and outcome of imaginal flooding therapy in Vietnam veterans with chronic posttraumatic stress disorder. *Comprehensive Psychiatry, 37*, 409–418.

Power, K., McGoldrick, T., Brown, K., Buchanan, R., Sharp, D., Swanson, V., & Karatzias, A. (2002). A controlled comparison of eye movement desensitization and reprocessing versus exposure plus cognitive restructuring versus waiting list in the treatment of post-traumatic stress disorder. *Clinical Psychology and Psychotherapy, 9*, 299–318.

Rachman, S. (1980). Emotional processing. *Behaviour Research and Therapy, 18*, 51–60.

Resick, P. A., Calhoun, K. S., Atkeson, B. M., & Ellis, E. M. (1981). Social adjustment in victims of sexual assault. *Journal of Consulting and Clinical Psychology, 49*, 705–712.

Resick, P. A., Nishith, P., Weaver, T. A., Astin, M.C., & Feuer, C. A. (2002). A comparison of cognitive processing therapy with prolonged exposure and a waiting condition for the treatment of posttraumatic stress disorder in female rape victims. *Journal of Consulting and Clinical Psychology, 70*(4), 867–879.

Resick, P. A., & Schnicke, M. K. (1992). Cognitive processing therapy for sexual assault victims. *Journal of Consulting and Clinical Psychology, 60*(5), 748–756.

Resick, P. A., & Schnicke, M. K. (1993). *Cognitive processing therapy for rape victims: A treatment manual.* Newbury Park, CA: Sage.

Riggs, D. S., Rothbaum, B. O., & Foa, E. B. (1995). A prospective examination of symptoms of posttraumatic stress disorder in victims of nonsexual assault. *Journal of Interpersonal Violence, 10*, 201–214.

Rothbaum, B. O. (2002, March). A controlled study of PE versus EMDR for PTSD rape victims. In L. A. Zoellner (Chair), *Recent innovations in posttraumatic stress disorder treatment.* Symposium conducted at the annual convention of the Anxiety Disorders Association of America, Austin, TX.

Rothbaum, B. O., Foa, E. B., Riggs, D. S., Murdock, T., & Walsh, W. (1992). A prospective examination of post-traumatic stress disorder in rape victims. *Journal of Traumatic Stress, 5*, 455–475.

Rothbaum, B. O., Meadows E. A., Resick, P., & Foy, D. (2000). Cognitive-behavioral therapy. In E. B. Foa, T. M. Keane, & M. J. Friedman (Eds.), *Effective treatments for PTSD: Practice guidelines from the International Society for Traumatic Stress Studies* (pp. 320–325). New York: Guilford Press.

Shapiro, F. (1989). Efficacy of eye movement desensitization procedure in the treatment of traumatic memories. *Journal of Traumatic Stress, 2,* 199–223.

Shapiro, F. (1995). *Eye movement desensitization and reprocessing: Basic principles, protocols, and procedures.* New York: Guilford Press.

Tarrier, N., Pilgrim, H., Sommerfield, C., Faragher, B., Reynolds, M., Graham, E., et al. (1999). A randomized trial of cognitive therapy and imaginal exposure in the treatment of chronic posttraumatic stress disorder. *Journal of Consulting and Clinical Psychology, 67,* 13–18.

Taylor, S., Thordarson, D. S., Maxfield, L., Fedoroff, I. C., Lovell, K., & Ogrodniczuk, J. (2003). Comparative efficacy, speed, and adverse effects of three PTSD treatments: Exposure therapy, EMDR, and relaxation training. *Journal of Consulting and Clinical Psychology, 71,* 330–338.

Veronen, L. J., & Kilpatrick, D. G. (1983). Stress management for rape victims. In D. Meichenbaum & M. E. Jaremko (Eds.), *Stress reduction and prevention* (pp. 341–374). New York: Plenum Press.

CHAPTER FIVE

Cognitive Therapy for Posttraumatic Stress Disorder

Jillian C. Shipherd
Amy E. Street
Patricia A. Resick

The increased media attention on posttraumatic stress disorder (PTSD) in recent years has highlighted both the scientific advances in this area and remaining questions about the pathology and treatment of PTSD. Among psychotherapeutic interventions, several cognitive-behavioral strategies have demonstrated efficacy (e.g., van Etten & Taylor, 1998). Commonly used cognitive-behavioral therapy (CBT) protocols include, but are not limited to, cognitive processing therapy (CPT; Resick & Schnicke, 1993), prolonged exposure (PE; Foa, Rothbaum, Riggs, & Murdock, 1991b; Foa et al., 1999a), and stress inoculation training (SIT; Foa et al., 1991b, 1999a). However, the mechanisms of action in these treatments are not well understood. The relative contributions of cognitive versus behavioral components of treatment have only begun to be explored. Further, the heterogeneity of strategies included under the rubric of "cognitive therapy" often makes it difficult to evaluate the relative utility of this approach. In this chapter we provide an overview of cognitive theories and highlight examples of good clinical practice with one type of cognitive intervention, CPT.

COGNITIVE MODELS OF PTSD

Information-processing theory has been widely used to understand the development and maintenance of anxiety disorders, including PTSD (Lang, 1979, 1985). This theory suggests that emotions, such as fear, are encoded in memory in the form of networks, where representations of anxiety-provoking events are stored. Fear networks are hypothesized to contain three important types of information: (1) information about the feared stimuli or situation; (2) information about the person's response to the feared stimuli or situation; and (3) information about the meaning of the feared stimuli and the consequent response. Foa and Kozak (1986) posited that the fear networks of individuals with PTSD differ from the fear networks of individuals with other anxiety disorders in three ways. First, the fear network of individuals with PTSD is larger because it contains a greater number of erroneous or inaccurate connections between stimulus, response, and meaning elements. Second, the network is more easily activated by stimulus, response, or meaning elements. Third, the affective and physiological response elements of the networks are more intense. Accordingly, for individuals with PTSD, stimuli reminiscent of the traumatic experience activate the fear network and prompt states of high sympathetic arousal (e.g., increased heart rate and blood pressure, sweating, muscle tension), retrieval of fear-related memories (e.g., intrusive memories, dissociative flashbacks), intense feelings of fear and anxiety, and fear-related behavioral acts (e.g., avoidance or escape behaviors, hypervigilant behaviors).

Chemtob, Roitblat, Hamada, Carlson, and Twentyman's (1988) hierarchical cognitive action theory extended information-processing theory by proposing that for individuals with PTSD, these fear networks (or "threat-response structures") are at least weakly activated at all times, guiding their interpretation of ambiguous events as potentially dangerous. More recently, Ehlers and Clark (2000) proposed a cognitive model of the persistence of PTSD that can also be viewed as an extension of earlier information-processing theories. This cognitive model suggests that PTSD becomes chronic when traumatized individuals appraise the traumatic event or its sequelae in a way that leads to a sense of serious, current threat (e.g., "Nowhere is safe"; "If I think about the trauma, I will go mad"). A second factor proposed by this model as causally related to the persistence of PTSD are changes in autobiographical memory similar to those proposed by earlier information-processing theorists (e.g., strong associations between stimulus and response elements in memory; low thresholds for priming memories associated with the traumatic event).

Although these information-processing theories emphasize the role of fear in the development and maintenance of PTSD, empirical evidence suggests that many PTSD symptoms, including intrusive memories and behavioral avoidance, may be prompted by other strong emotion states. For example, in a longitudinal investigation of crime victims, Brewin, Andrews, and Rose (2000) found that, in addition to fear, emotional responses of helplessness and horror experienced within 1 month of the crime were predictive of PTSD status 6 months later. Further, emotions of shame and anger predicted later PTSD status, even after controlling for intense emotions of fear, helplessness, and horror. Similarly, Pitman, Orr, Forgue, Altman, de Jong, and Herz (1990) found that combat veterans with PTSD who listened to individualized traumatic scripts reported experiencing a range of emotions other than fear. In fact, veterans with PTSD were no more likely to report experiencing fear than other emotions.

The range of emotional reactions evident in individuals with PTSD suggests the need for a theory of PTSD that includes factors other than purely fear-based information processing. Several social-cognitive theories have been proposed to explain the wide range of emotional reactions reported by victims of traumatic events. Social-cognitive models suggest that traumatic events can dramatically alter basic beliefs about the world, the self, and other people. Accordingly, these models tend to focus on the process by which trauma survivors integrate traumatic events into their overall conceptual systems, or schemas, either by assimilating the information into existing schemas or by altering existing schemas to accommodate the new information (Hollon & Garber, 1988). For example, Janoff-Bulman (1992) focused primarily on three major assumptions that may be shattered in the face of a traumatic event: (1) personal invulnerability, (2) the world as a meaningful and predictable place, and (3) the self as positive or worthy. Although it has been demonstrated that trauma victims have significantly more negative beliefs in these realms than nonvictims (Janoff-Bulman, 1992), this "shattered assumptions" theory does not account for the increased level of PTSD symptomatology observed in individuals with a history of traumatic events prior to the index trauma (e.g., Nishith, Mechanic, & Resick, 2000), individuals whose assumptions presumably had already been shattered. A second schema-based social-cognitive model (McCann, Sakheim, & Abrahamson, 1988) proposed five major dimensions that may be disrupted by traumatic victimization: safety, trust, power, esteem, and intimacy. McCann and colleagues hypothesize that for each of these dimensions, schemas may be disrupted either in relation to the self or to others. This theory suggests that difficulties with psychological adaptation following a traumatic event may result if previously positive schemas are disrupted by the experience or if previous negative schemas are seemingly confirmed by the experience.

In an attempt to reconcile the information-processing theories with the social-cognitive theories of PTSD, Brewin, Dalgleish and Joseph (1996) proposed a dual representation theory of PTSD. This theory suggests that memories of a traumatic experience are stored in two ways. Some memories of the experience are referred to as "verbally accessible" memories. This term denotes information the individual attended to before, during, and after the traumatic event (e.g., response and meaning elements) that received sufficient conscious processing to be transferred to long-term memory. In theory this information can be deliberately retrieved from memory. Other memories are referred to as "situationally accessed" memories. These memories contain extensive nonconscious information about the traumatic event that cannot be deliberately accessed or easily altered. Dual representation theory also proposes two types of emotional reactions: primary emotions conditioned during the traumatic event (e.g., fear) and secondary emotions that result from the meaning of the traumatic event (e.g., anger, shame, sadness).

Brewin and colleagues suggest that successful emotional processing of a traumatic event (i.e., "completion/integration") requires the activation of both the verbally accessible memories and the situationally accessed memories. During activation of these memory components, resolution of schema conflicts can occur through a conscious search for meaning.

As an extension of these cognitive theories of PTSD, cognitive therapies for PTSD are designed to address cognitive variables as factors that contribute to the development or persistence of PTSD. It is important to note that cognitive therapy is an umbrella term that captures a variety of strategies that are derived from a rich theoretical literature, not simply an added skill included in an otherwise complete treatment. The conceptualization behind these interventions is that an approach that elicits memories of the traumatic event and then directly confronts maladaptive beliefs, faulty attributions, and inaccurate expectations may be more effective than exposure therapy alone. Although imaginal exposure activates the memory structure of the traumatic event and facilitates habituation, it does not provide explicit direction in correcting misattributions or other maladaptive beliefs. Thus, cognitive behavioral therapies for PTSD often supplement exposure with some type of cognitive intervention, most often cognitive restructuring. The technique of cognitive restructuring involves identifying and challenging thoughts that are maladaptive in specific situations. This type of cognitive restructuring is often more present-centered, focusing on "here-and-now" cognitions that impact mood and functioning. In contrast, other types of cognitive interventions may address more general trauma-focused themes, rather than challenging only those thoughts that occur in specific situations. These interventions may examine the traumatic event itself or beliefs about the event. Alternatively, these interventions may address meaning elements of the traumatic events (e.g., tying the event into the meaning of other life events) or underlying dimensions that the trauma impacts (e.g., safety, trust, power, esteem, and intimacy). Further, cognitive therapies can also expand the range of emotion states (beyond fear) that can be targeted in treatment. The inclusion of other emotion states in treatment, including shame, anger, and helplessness, is essential due to their implication in the development and persistence of PTSD.

ASSESSMENT OF COGNITIONS

An extensive review of potential measurements to use to assess cognitions is beyond the scope of this chapter. However, a few measures deserve mention for those readers who are seeking appropriate assessment instruments that are sensitive to changes in cognition anticipated over the course of treatment. Among the commonly used measures of cognition are the Trauma and Attachment Belief Scale (TABS; Pearlman, 2003), the Personal Beliefs and Reactions Scale (PBRS; Mechanic & Resick, 1993), the World Assumptions Scale (WAS; Janoff-Bulman, 1989), and the Posttraumatic Cognitions Inventory (PTCI; Foa, Ehlers, Clark, Tolin, & Orsillo, 1999b).

The TABS is an 84-item measure that identifies disruption in several dimensions that impact interpersonal relationships, including Safety, Trust, Esteem, Intimacy, and Control. Similarly, the PBRS is a 55-item measure developed for use with sexual assault survivors to assess eight dimensions of Safety, Trust, Power, Esteem, Intimacy, Negative Rape Beliefs, Self-Blame, and Undoing (i.e., trying to deny or alter the event as a method of assimilation). Three subscales of the PBRS are predictive of intrusive symptoms of PTSD (Self-Blame, Undoing, and Safety), whereas four scales were predictive of avoidant symptoms of PTSD (Trust, Self-Blame, Undoing, Intimacy), and two scales were predictive of arousal symptoms (Power, Safety; Mechanic & Resick, 1993). The WAS is a 32-item measure that evaluates eight categories of personal beliefs, including Benevolence of the World, Benevolence of People, Justice, Controllability of Life Events, Randomness of Life Events, Self-Worth, Self-Control, and Personal Luck. Three of these subscales appear to discriminate between trauma survivors and nontrauma survivors (Self-Worth, Randomness of Life Events, and Benevolence of the World; Janoff-Bulman, 1989). Finally, the PTCI is a 36-item measure that assesses three cognitive factors: Negative Cognitions about Self, Negative Cognitions about the World, and Self-Blame. This measure has also demonstrated an ability to discriminate between clients with and without PTSD (Foa et al., 1999b). Thus there are ample measures available to assess the trauma-related cognitions that are frequently targeted by cognitive interventions.

OVERVIEW OF CPT

CPT was adapted from basic cognitive techniques explicated by Beck and Emery (1985) and was originally developed for use with rape and crime victims. The first goal of CPT is to address emotions other than fear in clients with PTSD (Resick & Schnicke, 1992). Other strong emotions such as anger, humiliation, shame, and sadness can often result from traumatic events and can also potentially be addressed through exposure. However, it is not assumed that all emotions can be addressed through exposure alone. For example, emotions that are the product of distorted thinking (e.g., guilt and shame stemming from thoughts such as "I should have prevented the event") may not necessarily habituate and therefore may benefit from direct cognitive intervention. Thus a second goal of CPT addresses the content of the meaning elements of the traumatic memory. A final goal is to examine the level of accommodation that has been made for the traumatic memory in relationship to more general schemas regarding one's self and the world (Resick & Schnicke, 1992, 1993). Drawing on the work of cognitive and constructivist theorists, Resick and Schnicke proposed that beliefs about the traumatic event might become distorted (assimilation) in the victim's attempt to maintain old beliefs and schemas about one's self and the world. Although accommodation of the new event into the person's memory and beliefs is desirable, overaccommodation (overgeneralization) may lead to extreme distortions about the safety or trustworthiness of others and/or overly harsh judgments about one's self. Thus a primary goal of this therapy is to develop an appropriate balance in the level of accommodation for the traumatic memory.

A main element of the CPT process is the therapist's coaching and following through with the client in filling out the following forms: the Impact Statement, ABC Sheets (which breaks down the following causal series: event, thought, and resulting feeling), the Challenging Questions Sheet, the Faulty Thinking Patterns Sheet, and the Challenging Beliefs Worksheet. Resick and Schnicke codified the CPT process into a 12-step course of therapy, the outlines of which we present below in the form of a case study, and which integrates the use of these forms. (For the original, blank versions of these forms, and more detailed instructions on their use, refer to Resick & Schnicke, 1993.)

The initial session of CPT is a psychoeducational one in which the symptoms of PTSD are explained within a framework of information-processing theory. After this initial session clients are asked to write the Impact Statement describing what the traumatic event means to them as well as their beliefs about why the event happened. The statement is reviewed in session two with an eye toward identifying problematic beliefs and cognitions ("stuck points"). In this way therapists help clients examine whether the trauma appeared to disrupt or confirm previously held beliefs. Further, therapists begin to examine if clients have overaccommodated the traumatic event in their general beliefs about themselves and the world. This initial psychoeducation provides a basis for the remainder of therapy, in which clients are taught to challenge their self-statements and to modify their extreme beliefs to bring them into balance.

The next two sessions of therapy include exposure to the traumatic memory with a focus on feelings, beliefs, and thoughts that are associated with the traumatic event. Clients are asked to write an account of the event, including thoughts, feelings, and sensory details. Clients read the account to the therapist and reread it daily outside the sessions. After rewriting the account, the therapy moves into the cognitive challenging phase. Using a Socratic style of therapy (i.e., using questions to lead clients to understand their reasoning processes and beliefs), therapists teach clients to ask questions about their assumptions and self-statements in order to begin challenging them. Examples of Socratic questions that lead clients to question their longstanding assumptions might be "I don't understand how it's your fault. How could you have known that it was going to happen?" or "You have said that you should have done something to stop it. What were the options you considered at the time?" Often clients have not thought through the likely outcomes of alternative actions or have fantasies that something they imagine now would have worked at the time. At that point the therapist might ask, "But isn't it possible that you made the best decision under the circumstances and that the other options would have led to a worse outcome?"

The early stages of the cognitive therapy typically focus on the client's self-blame and his or her attempts to undo the event after the fact (assimilation). In the final five sessions the therapy progresses systematically through the common dimensions of cognitive disruption: safety, trust, control, esteem, and intimacy. Overaccommodated beliefs in these dimensions are challenged, in regard to both self and others. Table 5.1 summarizes the 12 sessions of CPT.

A CASE EXAMPLE ILLUSTRATING COMMON OBSTACLES

Sam was a 34-year-old unemployed European American male with a college education. He had a long history of alcohol and drug abuse, starting with his first drink at the age of 8. In addition, Sam had an extensive history of being physically and sexually assaulted. At the time he sought treatment, he had already been abstinent from alcohol and drugs for 6 months, following a more recent traumatic assault. Thus, at his initial assessment, Sam met criteria for PTSD, major depressive disorder, and polysubstance dependence in early full remission. The index event that brought him into treatment this time was the more recent assault, which included a sexual assault. The CPT treatment was initiated, and during the first session, the therapist explained the symptoms of PTSD, gave a rationale for treatment, described the course of the therapy, and explained the first homework assignment, which was for Sam to write an Impact Statement about the meaning of the index assault.

When the rationale for treatment was presented, particular emphasis was placed on the importance of Sam not using alcohol or drugs during the course of therapy; this was characterized as an avoidance strategy that could shut down emotions that might emerge in therapy. Further, Sam and his therapist discussed the role of substances in increasing his risk for revictimization. In particular, Sam recognized that when he had used substances in the past, he would seek out environments that happened to be high crime areas. Sam also acknowledged that when using substances, his ability to extricate himself from dangerous situations or defend himself was reduced. The therapist emphasized that using substances did not cause the traumatic event, and Sam was not to blame for the event, but intoxication may have reduced his ability to escape from the situation. Throughout the course of treatment, the therapist monitored whether Sam had any urges to drink or use drugs. He expressed determination to stay off of substances and insisted that he could do the exposure work of the therapy without relapsing.

Over the course of the first session, it became clear that the identified index trauma might not have been a criterion A stressor and therefore might not be the most appropriate focus for treatment. In CPT (as well as PE),

TABLE 5.1. CPT Session by Session

Session 1: Introduction and education
1. Explain the symptoms of PTSD in terms of cognitive-behavioral theory
2. Five-minute account of the trauma (the worst one identified)
3. Treatment rationale
4. Provide overview of treatment
5. Homework:
   Write an Impact Statement

Session 2: The meaning of the event
1. Review concepts from the first session
2. Have the client read the Impact Statement; begin to identify stuck points
3. Discuss the meaning of the Impact Statement
4. Identify
   a. Assimilation (changing memories to fit beliefs)
   b. Overaccommodation (overgeneralizing beliefs as a result of memories)
   c. Accommodation (changing beliefs to incorporate the trauma)
5. Help identify and see the connections among events, thoughts, and feelings
6. Introduce the ABC Sheet (Figure 5.1, p. 107), to help client with this phase
7. Fill out one ABC Sheet together
8. Homework:
   Complete ABC Sheets to become aware of connection between events, thoughts, feelings, and behavior

Session 3: Identification of thoughts and feelings
1. Review the ABC Sheets, further differentiating between thoughts and feelings
   a. Label thoughts versus feelings
   b. Recognize that changing thoughts can change the intensity of types of feelings
   c. Begin challenging self-blame and guilt with Socratic questions
2. Discuss the ABC Sheet related to trauma (orally, if client has not completed it)
3. Challenge stuck points of self-blame using Socratic questions
4. Homework:
   a. Write a Trauma Account, with sensory details, and read daily
   b. Complete ABC Sheets daily

Session 4: Remembering the trauma
1. Have the client read the Trauma Account aloud; encourage affect
2. Identify stuck points
3. Challenge stuck points of self-blame and other forms of assimilation using Socratic questions
4. Homework:
   a. Rewrite the Trauma Account
   b. Complete ABC Sheets daily

cont.

TABLE 5.1. *cont.*

Session 5: Identification of stuck points

1. Read the second Trauma Account aloud; discuss new details that emerge
2. Involve client in challenging assumptions and conclusions that the client has made after processing affect, with particular focus on self-blame and other forms of assimilation
3. Introduce the Challenging Questions Sheet (Figure 5.2, p. 109), to help the client challenge stuck points
4. Homework:

   Challenge at least one stuck point a day, using the Challenging Questions Sheet

Session 6: Challenging questions

1. Review the Challenging Questions Sheet to address stuck point (start with self-blame, if present)
2. Continue cognitive therapy regarding stuck points
3. Introduce the Faulty Thinking Patterns Sheet (Figure 5.3, p. 111)
4. Homework:

   Notice and record examples of faulty thinking patterns on the Challenging Beliefs Worksheet

Session 7: Faulty thinking patterns

1. Review the Faulty Thinking Patterns Sheet to address trauma-related stuck points
2. Introduce the Challenging Beliefs Worksheet (Figure 5.4, p. 113) with a trauma example
3. Introduce the first of five problem areas: safety issues related to self and others; go over the module on safety
4. Homework:

   Identify stuck points every day, one relating to safety, and challenge them using the Challenging Beliefs Worksheet

Session 8: Safety issues

1. Review the Challenging Beliefs Worksheet to address safety and other relevant stuck points
2. Help the client confront faulty cognitions using the Challenging Beliefs Worksheet and generate alternative beliefs
3. Introduce second of five problem areas: trust issues related to self and others; use the trust module and the Challenging Beliefs Worksheet
4. Homework:

   Client to identify stuck points every day, one relating to trust, and confront them using the Challenging Beliefs Worksheet

Session 9: Trust issues

1. Review the Challenging Beliefs Worksheet to challenge stuck points of trust; generate alternative beliefs
2. Introduce the third of five problem areas: power/control issues related to self and others

3. Homework:

Identify stuck points, one relating to power/control (and other stuck points, as needed); confront them using the Challenging Beliefs Worksheet

Session 10: Power/control issues

1. Discuss the connection between power/control and self-blame; challenge power/control stuck points using the Challenging Beliefs Worksheet

2. Introduce the fourth of five problem areas: esteem issues related to self and others

   a. Review the esteem module in terms of self and others
   b. Explore the client's self-esteem before the traumatic event

3. Introduce the Identifying Assumptions Sheet and determine which assumptions are applicable to client

4. Homework:

   a. Identify stuck points daily, one relating to esteem issues; challenge them using the Challenging Beliefs Worksheet
   b. Confront assumptions checked on the Identifying Assumptions Sheet, using the Challenging Beliefs Worksheet
   c. Practice giving and receiving compliments daily
   d. Do a nice thing for the self at least once per day

Session 11: Esteem issues

1. Discuss the client's reactions to giving and receiving compliments and doing nice things for oneself

2. Help the client identify esteem issues and assumptions; challenge them using the Challenging Beliefs Worksheet

3. Introduce the fifth of five problem areas: intimacy issues related to self and others

4. Homework:

   a. Identify stuck points, one of which relates to intimacy issues; challenge them using the Challenging Beliefs Worksheet
   b. Rewrite the Impact Statement
   c. Continue to give and receive compliments
   d. Continue to do at least one nice thing for the self each day

Session 12: Intimacy issues

1. Help the client identify intimacy issues and assumptions as well as any remaining stuck points; challenge them using the Challenging Beliefs Worksheet

2. Have the client read the new Impact Statement(s)

3. Involve the client in reviewing the course of treatment and his or her progress

4. Help the client identify goals for the future and delineate strategies for meeting them

5. Remind the client that, in a sense, he or she is taking over as his or her own therapist now and should continue to use the skills learned

when selecting the trauma on which to focus, the therapist should attempt to identify the worst trauma with regard to current symptoms and psychosocial impact. This is sometimes difficult; the client might identify the most recent incident as the worst trauma because this incident may be strongly related to current reexperiencing of symptoms and distress. However, the first incident to produce PTSD might, in fact, be a more appropriate target, particularly with regard to the overall impact upon the person's life. This pattern may be most likely when the initial incident is child sexual abuse. In Sam's first session, he began to question whether the recent sexual assault was a true assault because while he was drinking, he had agreed to perform sex in order to obtain drugs. However, he had felt helpless to stop this sexual encounter once it began. Sam made statements such as "It is always the same. I get swept into situations that I don't want to be in but can't stop." The therapist asked Sam what other situations this event reminded him of and if they were always in the context of alcohol and drugs. He stated that as an adult, drugs and alcohol were always involved in these incidents. However, Sam indicated that as a child there had been other situations during which he had felt the same feelings in the absence of drugs or alcohol. When asked about those incidents, he described a series of sexual assaults by adolescent boys that occurred over the course of a year, beginning at age 7. The therapist suggested beginning treatment with those events and focusing the account on the worst of them, which occurred at age 8. Sam agreed. At the second session, Sam read the following Impact Statement:

> The overall feeling of what it means to me to have been assaulted is the feeling that I must be bad or a bad person for something like this to have occurred. I feel it will or could happen again at any time. I feel safe only at home. The world scares me, and I think it unsafe. I feel all people are more powerful than I am, and am scared by most people. I view myself as ugly and stupid. I can't let people get real close to me. I have a hard time communicating with people of authority, so plainly I haven't been able to work. My fiancée and I rarely have sex and sometimes just a hug revolts me and scares me. I feel if I spend too much time out in the world, an event like what happened in my past will take place. I feel hatred and anger toward myself for letting these things happen. I feel guilty that I've caused problems with my family (parents' divorce). I feel dirty most of the time and believe that's how others view me. I don't trust others when they make promises. I find it hard to accept that these events have happened to me.

The therapist reflected that the abuse had had a very large impact in many areas of functioning. She asked whether he was "bad" because of what had happened or was he "bad to begin with." Sam said that he must have been "bad to begin with" to be in a situation in which these traumas could happen. "Good people don't allow such things to happen." The therapist replied, "It sounds like you believe if an 8-year-old boy couldn't prevent this from happening, he must have been 'bad.' This will be an important belief for us to continue to talk about."

The therapist asked a series of Socratic questions to narrow down his statement regarding fear of people in authority so that he could begin to discriminate between different situations (e.g., men and women equally? people of different ages? employers or others in authority?). After they processed his Impact Statement, the therapist taught him about labeling feelings and noticing which thoughts are associated with various feelings, then introduced the concept that changing thoughts can change feelings. Sam was assigned to complete event-thought-feeling ABC Sheets every day until the next session.

At the third session, Sam had a number of worksheets with four or five examples on each. The therapist noticed that he did not discriminate between levels of danger. Because he was scared, a trip to the grocery store during the day felt just as dangerous as being in a drug neighborhood at 4:00 in the morning. The therapist again used Socratic questioning to help him identify this pattern and to begin to question differences in probabilities between the objective danger in different situations. They also worked on an ABC Sheet about the childhood sexual abuse (see Figure 5.1).

The therapist began the process of helping Sam to question the assumptions that he had made about these events. Then Sam was assigned to write his account of the worst incident for homework before the fourth session. He was asked to read the account to himself every day and was encouraged to experience his emotions fully while completing this task. At the next session Sam arrived 20 minutes early, saying that he was afraid that if he did not arrive early, he might not come at all. His account was very brief, and he read it quickly. Sam also admitted that he had experienced urges to drink over the course of the week, but that he had resisted these urges.

A: "Something happens"	B: "I tell myself something"	C: "I feel"
I was abused by two guys.	I must be bad for this to happen.	Angry at myself.
I wasn't given a choice as to when I decided sex was OK for me.	I don't get choices. Things just happen. I have no control.	I feel frustrated, sad, and angry.
I was told bad things about myself and my body.	I am stupid and ugly.	I feel ashamed of myself.

FIGURE 5.1. Sam's ABC Sheet.

The therapist and Sam discussed why he was holding back his emotions in his written descriptions, and Sam described a pervasive sense of guilt about a range of events in his life. In his memory several events were tangled together, and he could not separate what was done to him from what he had done—it was all the same. The process of challenging these beliefs caused Sam to admit that he had perpetrated sexual assaults as well as being the victim. After ascertaining that Sam had not perpetrated any assaults since late adolescence and had no urges to rape, the therapist helped him differentiate situations in which he intended harm and had responsibility from those in which he had no control and was clearly a victim.

At the fifth session Sam reported that he had gone home and spent 10 consecutive hours writing the most recent account of his worst traumatic experience. He cried, felt angry, ashamed, embarrassed, afraid, and guilty; in other words, the whole range of emotions he had been avoiding. After reading his account to the therapist and discussing his emotions, the therapist introduced and explained the concepts of hindsight bias ("I should have known what was going to happen and prevented it") and considering the source ("just because your perpetrator said something about you doesn't make it true"), and explained how children can become sexually reactive when exposed to sexual contact at an early age. The therapist encouraged Sam to continue reading his account every day. In addition, she introduced the "Challenging Questions" (see below) homework, in which he would pick a single thought and answer 12 questions about that thought. Figure 5.2 is one of the homework sheets Sam brought to the sixth session.

After homework sheets were reviewed and the therapist assisted Sam in answering the questions regarding various thoughts (referred to as "stuck points"), the next concepts and homework were assigned. Along with challenging single beliefs, clients are asked to look for patterns of counterproductive thinking. For homework the client is asked to notice examples in day-to-day living (or with regard to the traumas) that represent various categories of faulty thinking (Figure 5.3). The purpose of this exercise is to assist clients in determining which types of dysfunctional thinking are particularly problematic so that they can catch themselves.

Sam also opted to write an account of a different event that was associated with flashbacks and intrusive recollections and had not diminished along with those from the first account. He brought this account to the seventh session, and he and his therapist addressed it along with other homework and new material. Sam also continued working with the Challenging Questions Sheets. During the session, he and his therapist challenged his beliefs regarding anger ("I'll be out of control"), continuing guilt regarding the child abuse ("Why me, if it wasn't my fault?") and his confusion regarding sexual arousal during the abuse. With the therapist's help, Sam recognized that he did not enjoy the abuse and that he was confusing sexual arousal with enjoyment. Differentiating these concepts relieved greatly Sam's

Below is a list of questions to be used in helping you challenge your maladaptive or problematic beliefs. Not all questions will be appropriate for the belief you choose to challenge. Answer as many questions as you can for the belief you have chosen to challenge below.

Belief: I take blame for the abuse and feel I did something bad to cause it.

1. What is the evidence for and against this idea?

   For—I should have walked away or said no. I feel as if I could have done something.

   Against—They would have done what they wanted, regardless of what I said or did.

2. Are you confusing a habit with a fact?

   Yes. I have always told myself that it happened to me because I was bad or did something wrong. I have always told myself, "If only I had done something different," like it was all about what I did or was doing.

3. Are your interpretations of the situation too far removed from reality to be accurate?

   I have distorted the reality of the situation. I have blamed myself for being bad and allowing this to happen to me. In reality, I had no control or power over the situation. The abusers were in total control and they are to blame.

4. Are you thinking in all-or-none terms?

   Yes. I have always used terms such as "bad" and "wrong" and considered the events as my fault. "I was bad," "I did something wrong," is what I've told myself.

5. Are you using words or phrases that are extreme or exaggerated (i.e., "always," "forever," "never," "need," "should," "must," "can't," and "every time")?

   Yes. I used a lot of "shoulds" in my statements when describing the abuse.

6. Are you taking selected examples out of context?

   Yes. I am saying that there was something I could or should of done or changed about myself to have prevented it from happening.

7. Are you making excuses? (e.g., "I'm not afraid. I just don't want to go out"; "Other people expect me to be perfect"; or "I don't want to make the call because I don't have time").

   Yes. I am afraid that I might let this happen again. I make excuses to not go into the world and excuses that if I take blame then nobody else has to deal with it.

8. Is the source of information reliable?

   No. All the sources were straight from the mouths of my abusers. They were only interested in hurting me, and nothing they said was true of me or who I was.

   cont.

FIGURE 5.2. Sam's Challenging Questions Sheet.

9. Are you thinking in terms of certainties instead of probabilities?

Yes. I have never been objective about abuse. It has always made me feel unsafe with others, and when things felt uncomfortable, I always wondered, what is wrong with me?

10. Are you confusing a low probability with a high probability?

The probability of this happening again is low, but I still feel as if it could, and I believe the probability to be higher than it actually is.

11. Are your judgments based on feelings rather than facts?

Yes. I feel guilty so I assume that I did something wrong. That is not the fact at all.

12. Are you focusing on irrelevant factors?

My focus has always been on what I did or could have done—things I had no control over. The abuse took place because the abuser wanted it to, not because of something I did.

FIGURE 5.2. *cont.*

confusion, guilt, and thoughts that he must be "a pervert" to have experienced an erection.

At the seventh session a final worksheet was introduced that incorporated all of the other worksheets. This Challenging Beliefs Worksheet (Figure 5.4, see p. 113) was used throughout the remainder of the therapy and assisted the client in producing alternative thoughts through a process of dismantling counterproductive thoughts. During the remaining five sessions of the therapy, this worksheet was used to explore remaining stuck points and to examine cognitive dimensions that were likely to be disrupted as a result of traumatic events: safety, trust, power/control, esteem, and intimacy. Sam was asked to complete worksheets each day on personally relevant stuck points and to do at least one on each dimension. He was also given a module to read on each topic to stimulate his thoughts about each dimension and possible resolutions to stuck points.

At the eighth session Sam's self-blame and self-loathing had diminished, and he began to express anger at the perpetrators. He also began to express anger at his parents for their neglect and abuse, but focused most of his worksheets on issues of safety and trust. Power and control, the topic introduced in session nine, was a big issue for Sam, as was the topic of trust. Because he felt helpless in most situations and did not trust himself or others, he felt unable to make changes in his life. The worksheets helped Sam to put these constructs on a continuum and to ask himself questions such as "trust with regard to what?" and "control with regard to what?" in order to see trust and control as multidimensional rather than all-or-nothing concepts.

In session 10 Sam brought in a number of worksheets focused on trust and control themes, particularly as they related to his feelings of helplessness and fear when around his father. In Figure 5.4 is a worksheet illustrating Sam's continuing fear of his father and his inability to express anger toward his father for his abuse. The therapist and Sam discussed this fear of his father as a reason why he spent a great deal of time wandering around the neighborhood as a child, increasing his vulnerability to sexual abuse, and as a reason why he was unable to disclose the abuse to his father. As a recovering alcoholic, his father had received a good deal of therapy in the subsequent years and had apologized to Sam for his behavior and neglect. Sam felt some pressure to forgive his father and did not believe he was entitled to

Considering your own stuck points, find examples for each of these patterns. Write in the stuck point under the appropriate pattern and describe how it fits that pattern. Think about how that pattern affects you.

1. Drawing conclusions when evidence is lacking or even contradictory.

2. Exaggerating or minimizing the meaning of an event (you blow things way out of proportion or shrink their importance inappropriately).

3. Disregarding important aspects of a situation.

4. Oversimplifying events or beliefs as good/bad or right/wrong.

5. Overgeneralizing from a single incident (you view a negative event as a never-ending pattern).

6. Mind reading (you assume people are thinking negatively of you when there is no definite evidence for this).

7. Emotional reasoning (you reason based on how you feel).

FIGURE 5.3. Faulty Thinking Patterns Sheet.

feel angry at this point. The therapist reminded Sam that he had been so busy blaming himself all of these years that he had never had an opportunity to experience his justified anger at either the perpetrators or his father. She pointed out that Sam had plenty of time to forgive his father in the future, but this week he should allow himself to feel this emotion (anger) that he had avoided. They reviewed Sam's worksheet about fearing his father and also discussed his concern that if he felt anger, he would "become out of control" (see Figure 5.4).

After session 10 of CPT, clients are asked, in addition to completing worksheets on esteem, to practice giving and receiving compliments and to do at least one nice thing for themselves each day. These exercises serve the multiple purposes of helping clients work on esteem building, reconnect with other people, and think about the subject of esteem. Sam came into session 11 stating that doing nice things for himself helped his depression but that he tended to dismiss compliments as untrue. After challenging the validity of his assumptions about compliments and reviewing other self-esteem worksheets, the focus of treatment shifted to intimacy. He talked about discussions he had had with his father and described how passive he was in his relationship with his fiancée. In session 12 Sam was instructed to complete worksheets on intimacy, continue to practice giving and receiving compliments, continue to do nice things for himself, and finally to rewrite his Impact Statement about what the abuse meant to him now. The second Impact Statement was as follows:

Homework 12

Being assaulted means I was chosen to be a victim of abuse by perpetrators who knew what they were doing. I didn't ask for it to happen. I did nothing to cause it. They took from me my pride, self-esteem, and ability to count on myself and do the best thing for myself. I know that I'm not to blame, but I'm left with guilt and anger toward the world for this happening. The world was unsafe for me, but now I see it is my interpretation of my abuse that makes me see it as unsafe. I lost trust in others that they will treat me kindly. I felt unsafe in the world.

My abusers told me bad things about myself and I believed them and even repeated them to myself. I felt out of control and powerless over my life. I drank and did drugs to try to forget the memories. I hated myself and hurt myself because I couldn't live with the thought of what I believed I had done. But I did nothing. I was a child who was doing child things, not an adult able to make grown-up decisions. They took from me the ability to be close to someone and love someone, but I know I can regain all those abilities I lost to my abuse.

At the final session, aside from reviewing the new worksheets, the therapist and Sam read over his new Impact Statement and compared it to the first one to see how his thinking had changed over the course of therapy. They reviewed his progress in therapy and discussed topics that he still

Column A	Column B	Column C	Column D	Column E	Column F
Situation	Automatic thoughts	Challenging your automatic thoughts	Faulty thinking patterns	Alternative thoughts	Decatastrophizing
Describe the event(s), thought(s), or belief(s) leading to the unpleasant emotion(s).	Write the automatic thought(s) that precede the emotion(s) in Column A Rate belief in each automatic thought below from 0–100%	Use the Challenging Questions Sheet to examine your automatic thought(s) from Column B	Use the Faulty Thinking Patterns Sheet to examine your automatic thought(s) from Column B	What else can you say instead of what you've written in Column B? How else can you interpret the event instead of what you've written in Column B? Rate belief in alternative thought(s) from 0–100%	What's the worst that could ever *realistically* happen? My dad could say very mean things to me again Even if that happened, what could you do? *Consider the source and don't blame self.*
My dad was mean to me when I was young.	I am afraid of him. 90%	For: I am still afraid of him. Against: There is really nothing to be afraid of.	Evidence is lacking that I was bad.	We are both adults, I have nothing to fear.	
	I must have been bad or deserved it. 70%	"Must have been…" is an extreme statement. Source is not reliable This thinking is a habit not a fact	Exaggerating my fear. Reasoning from feelings.	I wasn't bad. My dad was an adult who knew what he was doing. 90%	**Outcome** Rerate belief in automatic thought(s) in Column B from 0–100% 60% / 30%
Emotion(s) Specify sad, angry, etc., and rate the degree to which you feel each emotion from 0–100% Fear 90% Anger 80%					Specify and rate subsequent emotion(s) from 0–100% Fear 30% Anger 50%

FIGURE 5.4. Sam's Challenging Beliefs Worksheet.

113

needed to work on, and the therapist gave Sam sets of worksheets to continue to use on his own. To further evaluate the intervention, Sam was given the Posttraumatic Diagnostic Scale (Foa, Cashman, Jaycox, & Perry, 1997) and the Beck Depression Inventory (Beck, Steer, & Brown, 1996) at pretreatment, every other session during treatment, posttreatment, and at a 6-month follow-up. His scores are in Figure 5.5.

CONCLUSIONS

In this chapter we have provided an overview of the theoretical models that guide cognitive interventions for PTSD, an overview of the experimental literature that highlights the importance of cognitions, and we have reviewed one form of cognitive intervention, CPT. The case description was designed to provide practitioners with a practical perspective of the treatment while highlighting commonly encountered obstacles and potential ways of overcoming them. The literature reviewed supports the conclusion that cognitive interventions for PTSD are effective at reducing PTSD symptomatology. However, the findings from these studies do not clearly support any one theoretical account for understanding PTSD over other theories. Similarly, the mechanism of action in these treatments remains unknown. Further empirical study of cognitive factors relevant to PTSD psychopathology and cognitive therapies is needed in order to elucidate the elements that are critical to successful outcomes. Future studies should continue to be guided by the current theoretical and empirical literature, with an emphasis on examining fac-

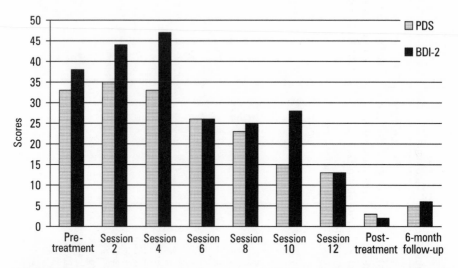

FIGURE 5.5. Sam's scores on the Posttraumatic Diagnostic Scale (PDS) and Beck Depression Inventory–Second Edition (BDI-2) at pretreatment, each treatment session, posttreatment, and 6-month follow-up.

ets of PTSD that could assist in discriminating between the different theoretical conceptualizations.

REFERENCES

Beck, A. T., & Emery, G. (1985). *Anxiety disorders and phobias: A cognitive perspective.* New York: Basic Books.

Beck, A. T., Steer, R. A., & Brown, G. K. (1996). *Manual for the Beck Depression Inventory* (2nd ed.). San Antonio, TX: Psychological Corporation.

Beck, J. G., Freeman, J. B., Shipherd, J. C., Hamblen, J. L., & Lackner, J. M. (2001). Specificity of Stroop interference in patients with pain and PTSD. *Journal of Abnormal Psychology, 110,* 536–543.

Brewin, C. R., Andrews, B., & Rose, S. (2000). Fear, helplessness, and horror in posttraumatic stress disorder: Investigating DSM-IV criterion A2 in victims of violent crime. *Journal of Traumatic Stress, 13*(3), 499–509.

Brewin, C. R., Dalgleish, T., & Joseph, S. (1996). A dual representation theory of posttraumatic stress disorder. *Psychological Review, 103*(4), 670–686.

Chemtob, C., Roitblat, H. L., Hamada, R. S., Carlson, J. G., & Twentyman, C. T. (1988). A cognitive action theory of post-traumatic stress disorder. *Journal of Anxiety Disorders, 2,* 253–275.

Ehlers, A., & Clark, D. M. (2000). A cognitive model of posttraumatic stress disorder. *Behaviour Research and Therapy, 38,* 319–345.

Foa, E. B., Cashman, L., Jaycox, L. H., & Perry, K. J. (1997). The validation of a self-report measure of posttraumatic stress disorder: The Posttraumatic Diagnostic Scale. *Psychological Assessment, 9*(4), 445–451.

Foa, E. B., Dancu, C. V., Hembree, E. A., Jaycox, L. H., Meadows, E. A., & Street, G. P. (1999a). A comparison of exposure therapy, stress inoculation training, and their combination for reducing posttraumatic stress disorder in female assault victims. *Journal of Consulting and Clinical Psychology, 67,* 194–200.

Foa, E. B., Ehlers, A., Clark, D. M., Tolin, D. F., & Orsillo, S. M. (1999b). The Post-traumatic Cognitions Inventory (PTCI): Development and validation. *Psychological Assessment, 11*(3), 303–314.

Foa, E. B., Feske, U., Murdock, T. B., Kozak, M. J., & McCarthy, P. R. (1991a). Processing of threat-related information in rape victims. *Journal of Abnormal Psychology, 100,* 156–162.

Foa, E. B., & Kozak, M. J. (1986). Emotional processing of fear: Exposure to corrective information. *Psychological Bulletin, 99,* 20–35.

Foa, E. B., Rothbaum, B. O., Riggs, D. S., & Murdock, T. B. (1991b). Treatment of post-traumatic stress disorder in rape victims: A comparison between cognitive-behavioral procedures and counseling. *Journal of Consulting and Clinical Psychology, 59,* 715–723.

Hollon, S. D., & Garber, J. (1988). Cognitive therapy. In L. Y. Abramson (Ed.), *Social cognition and clinical psychology: A synthesis* (pp. 204–253). New York: Guilford Press.

Janoff-Bulman, R. (1989). Assumptive worlds and the stress of traumatic events: Applications of the schema construct. *Social Cognition, 7*(2), 113–136.

Janoff-Bulman, R. (1992). *Shattered assumptions: Towards a new psychology of trauma.* New York: Free Press.

Lang, P. J. (1979). A bio-informational theory of emotional imagery. *Psychophysiology*, *16*, 495–512.

Lang, P. J. (1985). The cognitive psychophysiology of emotion: Fear and anxiety. In A. H. Tuma & J. D. Maser (Eds.), *Anxiety and anxiety disorders* (pp. 131–170). Hillsdale, NJ: Erlbaum.

McCann, I. L., Sakheim, D. K., & Abrahamson, D. J. (1988). Trauma and victimization: A model of psychological adaptation. *Counseling Psychologist*, *16*(4), 531–594.

Mechanic, M. B., & Resick, P. A. (1993). *The Personal Beliefs and Reactions Scale: Assessing rape-related cognitive schemata.* Paper presented at the 9th annual meeting of the International Society for Traumatic Stress Studies, San Antonio, Texas.

Nishith, P., Mechanic, M. B., & Resick, P. A. (2000). Prior interpersonal trauma: The contribution to current PTSD symptoms in female rape victims. *Journal of Abnormal Psychology*, *109*(1), 20–25.

Pearlman, L. A. (2003). *Trauma and Attachment Belief Scale*. Los Angeles: Western Psychological Services.

Pitman, R. K., Orr, S. P., Forgue, D. F., Altman, B., de Jong, J. B., & Herz, L. R. (1990). Psychophysiologic responses to combat imagery of Vietnam veterans with posttraumatic stress disorder versus other anxiety disorders. *Journal of Abnormal Psychology*, *99*(1), 49–54.

Resick, P. A., & Schnicke, M. K. (1992). Cognitive processing therapy for sexual assault victims. *Journal of Consulting and Clinical Psychology*, *60*(5), 748–756.

Resick, P. A., & Schnicke, M. K. (1993). *Cognitive processing therapy for rape victims: A treatment manual.* Newbury Park, CA: Sage.

van Etten, M. L., & Taylor, S. (1998). Comparative efficacy of treatments for PTSD: A meta-analysis. *Clinical Psychology and Psychotherapy*, *5*(3), 126–145.

CHAPTER SIX

Applications of Dialectical Behavior Therapy to Posttraumatic Stress Disorder and Related Problems

Amy W. Wagner
Marsha M. Linehan

Dialectical behavior therapy (DBT) was initially developed for the treatment of chronically suicidal individuals who meet criteria for borderline personality disorder (BPD). Because the majority of people with BPD have histories of trauma and meet criteria for posttraumatic stress disorder (PTSD), it seems appropriate to describe DBT in a book on the treatment of trauma. There are two potential applications of DBT to individuals with histories of trauma. One main application is to achieve stabilization prior to initiating exposure-based interventions. DBT is organized into treatment stages; the first stage aims to achieve behavioral control, safety, and connection to the therapist. This aim is consistent with the initial goals of other stage-oriented treatments for trauma and PTSD (e.g., Cloitre, 1998; Keane, Fisher, Krinsley, & Niles, 1994). Perhaps more than other treatments, DBT clearly specifies the manner in which stabilization can be achieved. A second potential application of DBT is to the treatment of specific trauma-related problems. Stage II DBT aims to treat trauma-related problems in individuals with BPD or histories of severe emotion dysregulation, and therefore may be particularly appropriate for individuals with chronic or complex traumatic histories.

This chapter begins with a brief overview of stage I DBT, including its theoretical underpinnings, structure, and strategies (for excellent, in-depth overviews of stage I DBT, see Koerner & Linehan, 2002; Linehan, 1993a; Linehan, Cochran, & Kehrer, 2001). In the remainder of the chapter we present preliminary ideas on stage II DBT, specifically highlighting the application of DBT principles, strategies, and skills to trauma-related problems. The use of informal exposure as a fundamental intervention in stage II is also described. It should be emphasized, however, that no studies have evaluated the efficacy or effectiveness of either stage I or stage II DBT for PTSD or closely associated problems. Throughout the chapter we emphasize the theoretical and empirical support for using DBT with this population and urge readers to proceed as clinical scientists—whether at the level of single case study or controlled trial—with careful attention to assessment, hypothesis-driven interventions, and evaluation of outcomes.

THEORETICAL ORIENTATION

DBT is considered a principle-driven (as opposed to a protocol-driven psychotherapy); therefore, a thorough understanding of the theories upon which it is based is essential for the effective application of the treatment. This point is particularly relevant when considering novel applications of DBT, such as to the treatment of PTSD and related problems. There are three main theories that underlie the treatment: the biosocial theory (of the etiology of BPD), behavioral theory, and the theory of dialectics.

Biosocial Theory

DBT is based, in part, on a biosocial theory of the etiology of BPD. Although the focus of this chapter is on the application of DBT to trauma-related problems, as opposed to BPD specifically, an understanding of this theory may allow for effective treatment matching. Indeed, as discussed in the next section, emerging data suggest that DBT can be applied effectively to other populations to the extent that problems can be conceptualized according to this theory. As implied, the biosocial theory asserts that both biological and environmental influences contribute to the development of BPD. It is a *transactional* theory that emphasizes the reciprocal and (iterative) influence of each component on the other, over time. Biologically, individuals with BPD are theorized to come into the world with a predisposition to emotion vulnerability. Similar to the notion of a sensitive temperament, this vulnerability manifests as the tendency to notice emotional cues in the environment and oneself more readily, react to the cues more strongly, and return more slowly to a baseline emotional state. Recent research supports the presence of these characteristics in adults with BPD (Lynch, 2004) as well as related structural differences in the brains of individuals with BPD (Tebartz van Elst et al., 2003). By *biological* we do not necessarily mean genetic because emerging research also suggests that environmental influences may have permanent effects on brain regions involved in emotional experiencing and modulation (i.e., the limbic system), particularly highly stressful or traumatic experiences (e.g., Yehuda & McFarlane, 1997).

Of course, many children with these characteristics do not develop BPD. The theory holds that individuals with BPD are exposed to environments that chronically and pervasively *invalidate* this emotional vulnerability. Although the term "invalidation" is used colloquially to refer to a range of negative or negating experiences, in this theory it refers to three specific characteristics. First, an invalidating environment (chronically and pervasively) rejects a child's communication of private experiences and self-generated behavior (e.g., by ignoring, punishing, or contradicting such communications). Similar to the processes described by Kohlenberg and Tsai (1991) this rejection can lead to problems with identifying, labeling, and trusting emotional experiences as valid. Children from these environments instead learn to search the environment for cues on how to respond. Second, an invalidating environment punishes emotional displays and reinforces emotional escalations on an intermittent schedule. This pattern can contribute to problems in effectively communicating emotions as well as to oscillations between extreme emotionality and emotional inhibition. Third, an invalidating environment oversimplifies problem solving and goal attainment. As such, children do not learn how to solve problems adequately or tolerate difficult emotions or situations; instead they form unrealistic goals and expectations, hold perfectionistic standards, and respond to failure with high emotionality.

An invalidating environment can occur in many different forms, including direct verbal communications, neglect, physical abuse, and sexual abuse. Although no studies, to date, have examined the prevalence of invalidation, as described above, among individuals with BPD, a growing body of research links childhood invalidation with emotion dysregulation in children (e.g., Eisenberg, Fabes, & Murphy, 1996; Eisenberg et al., 2001) and psychological distress in adulthood (Krause, Mendelson, & Lynch, 2003). In addition, many studies report high frequencies of verbal, physical, and sexual abuse and neglect in individuals with BPD (e.g., Soloff, Lynch, & Kelly, 2002; Wagner & Linehan, 1997). Nonetheless, it should be stressed that the biosocial theory does not suggest that abuse per se is required for the development of BPD—instead, it is the experience of invalidation that is requisite (see Wagner & Linehan, 1997, for a description of the ways in which the common characteristics of environments in which childhood sexual abuse occurs overlap considerably with the characteristics of the invalidating environment).

The biosocial theory asserts that the combined influence of emotional vulnerability and the invalidating environment contribute to a pervasive dysfunction of the emotion regulation system. The behaviors characteristic of BPD, therefore, are viewed as resulting from emotion dysregulation, or they function to regulate emotions. The transactional component of the theory suggests that BPD can result from varying levels of invalidation combined with varying levels of emotional vulnerability (e.g., a highly emotionally vulnerable child may experience a typical family as invalidating, whereas an emotionally hardy child may not experience an objectively defined "abusive" family as invalidating). Importantly, the transactional component of the theory is incompatible with the assignment of blame—just as the environment influences the child, so does the child influence the environment. Clinical observations suggest that this nonblaming focus helps both clients and their families develop a nonjudgmental stance—a stance viewed as critical for ultimate change.

The biosocial theory is centrally important to DBT; DBT is a treatment that teaches emotion regulation in the context of a validating environment. We assert that DBT may be appropriate to the treatment of individuals with trauma histories to the extent that problems can be similarly conceptualized as related to emotional vulnerability, invalidation, and emotion dysregulation.

Behavioral Theory

At its core, DBT is a behavioral theory. As such, behavior is conceptualized according to the principles of classical and operant conditioning, observational learning (modeling), and relatedly, the transfer of verbal information. Consistent with other behavioral approaches in this book, DBT conceptualizes "behavior" broadly to include everything that humans do, including thinking, feeling, and overt responding. Emphasis is placed on the function of behavior (overt form) and the context in which behavior occurs. A noteworthy assumption in behavioral theory is that the factors related to the maintenance of behavior may be different from the factors related to the initial development of behavior. As discussed later in the chapter, this point is particularly important in the conceptualization of chronic, longstanding problems, such as those associated with childhood abuse or trauma. In DBT, behavioral theory influences all aspects of the treatment, including the manner in which problems are defined, the ways in which behaviors are assessed, case conceptualization, and the interventions that are used. Broadly speaking, the behavioral conceptualization of BPD within DBT emphasizes capability deficits and motivational factors in the maintenance of problem behaviors. Primary behavioral interventions from this view include skills training, contingency management, exposure, and cognitive restructuring.

The Theory of Dialectics

DBT departs from traditional behavior therapy, in part, by its incorporation of the theory of dialectics. Dialectical theory has its roots in the philosophical assumptions of Marx, Hegel, and others (see Basseches, 1988; Linehan & Schmidt, 1995). In DBT, dialectical theory has implications for both a worldview on the nature of reality and the process of change in psychotherapy. From a dialectical perspective, reality is viewed as interrelated and connected (similar to systems perspectives), comprised of opposing forces (thesis–antithesis), and always changing, rather than static. An extension of this perspective is that seemingly opposite views or events exist simultaneously, therefore tension and conflict are part of reality. Because there is no such thing as ultimate truth, different views can be equally valid, and tension can be useful. Change, according to the theory of dialectics, is continual and occurs through the synthesis of oppositions in the context of tension.

This framework impacts the treatment in DBT in significant ways. Based on the assumption of the interrelated and holistic nature of reality, assessment of behavior necessarily takes into account the full range of possible influences, including environmental, interpersonal, cultural, and physiological/biological factors. Combined with the oppositional nature of reality and the notion of no fixed truth, an important approach to assessment in DBT is to always ask the question "What is being left out?" A holistic perspective suggests that assignment of blame is meaningless, in that there is no one cause of behavior but instead multiple, interrelated influences (similar to the transactional theory of BPD). This concept is particularly helpful for clients who are extremely judgmental of themselves or others, or who have difficulty reconciling (apparently) contradictory beliefs and emotions in response to themselves or others—such as is often the case in individuals with histories of trauma (also see Herman, 1995, for similar views).

A dialectical view also holds assumptions about the nature of change: Change is a continuous process that results from the synthesis of opposing views or events. This notion extends the assumption that tension is natural to the assumption that tension is actually *necessary* to bring about change. Therefore, in DBT, the goal is to use tension as an opportunity for teaching dialectical thinking (e.g., "Both can be true"), for finding synthesis, and ultimately for change. The most fundamental dialectical tension in DBT is between *acceptance* and *change*—typically, between accepting the client as he or she is and striving for different behavior. Ultimate change is achieved by pushing for both in therapy. To be more concrete, in DBT the different treatment strategies are categorized as change-oriented or acceptance-oriented, and effective interventions maximize the balance between both categories of strategies. There are also specific dialectical strategies that, by their nature, contain elements of both acceptance and change and are used throughout DBT (e.g., the use of metaphor, devil's advocate strategy). Although paradoxical, the assumption is that acceptance is necessary for change and that acceptance *is* change. The incorporation of acceptance-based interventions into behavior therapy for the treatment of a wide variety of problems and diagnoses is receiving increasing attention and empirical support (e.g., Hayes, Strosahl, & Wilson, 1999; Roemer & Orsillo, 2002; Segal, Williams, & Teasdale, 2003), attesting to the utility of combining these strategies in psychotherapy more generally.

DESCRIPTION OF EMPIRICAL RESEARCH

Over a decade of research has now accumulated that generally supports the efficacy of stage I DBT for the problems it aims to treat. DBT has been evaluated in seven well-controlled studies across four research groups, and in six additional nonrandomized controlled studies (for excellent, in-depth reviews, see Koerner & Dimeff, 2000; Koerner & Linehan 2000; Lieb, Zanarini, Schmahl, Linehan, & Bohus, 2004). Across studies, DBT has been found to significantly reduce the frequency of parasuicidal behavior, the lethality/medical risk of parasuicidal behavior, psychiatric inpatient days, and treatment dropout. These findings generally held when DBT was evaluated against a nonbehavioral treatment by "psychotherapy experts" in the community (Linehan et al., 2002a). Additionally, Linehan, Tutek, Heard, and Armstrong (1994) report improvements in social and functional adjustment and self-reported anger among those receiving DBT. Although most of these studies have included women diagnosed with BPD and chronic suicidal behavior, similar outcomes have been found for mixed samples of men and women (Turner, 2000).

Linehan and colleagues have developed and evaluated DBT for individuals dually diagnosed with BPD and substance abuse disorders (SUD), also known as DBT-SUD (see Dimeff, Rizvi, Brown, & Linehan, 2000). DBT-SUD differs from standard DBT primarily by expanding the targets of treatment to include substance use behaviors and including additional strategies for treatment retention; it retains the fundamental structure and strategies of DBT and is based on the same theoretical underpinnings. In two randomized controlled trials of women diagnosed with both BPD and substance use disorders, DBT-SUD resulted in significant reductions in drug use (Linehan et al., 1999; Linehan et al., 2002b). In a rigorous comparison of DBT-SUD to an intervention that combined a traditional 12-step program with the validation strategies of DBT, this reduction was comparable across groups; however, DBT-SUD participants continued to show improvement over the course of treatment, whereas those in the comparison group showed a slight increase in drug use at the end of treatment (Linehan et al., 2002b).

Additional adaptations of DBT have recently been developed and evaluated for a range of populations and diagnostic groups, including eating disorders (Palmer et al., 2003; Safer, Telch, & Agras, 2001; Telch, Agras, & Linehan, 2000; Telch, Agras, & Linehan, 2001; Wisniewski & Kelly, 2003) incarcerated men (McCann, Ball, Ghanizadeh, Gallietta, & Froelich, 2002), suicidal adolescents (Miller, 1999; Miller, Wyman, Huppert, Glassman, & Rathus, 2000; Rathus & Miller, 2002), female juvenile offenders (Trupin, Stewart, Beach, & Boesky, 2002), and older adults with depression (Lynch, Morse, Mendelson, & Robins, 2003); preliminary data are encouraging. Although apparently disparate groups, each can be conceptualized according to the combined capability deficit and motivational model that underlies DBT. For example, Telch and colleagues view binge eating behavior as dysfunctional emotion regulation behavior that develops from inadequate emotion regulation skills and is maintained by the emotion regulation function of binge behavior; their application of DBT to binge eating disorders emphasizes teaching emotion regulation skills. In both an uncontrolled, preliminary study (Telch, Agras, & Linehan, 2000) and a larger-scale randomized controlled trial (Telch et al., 2001), DBT for binge eating was found to significantly reduce binge eating episodes. Lynch and colleagues propose a similar conceptualization of depression in older adults. Their adaptation of DBT teaches DBT skills and problem-solving strategies to decrease the behaviors maintaining depression in this population and increase more flexible and functional behaviors. In a randomized controlled pilot study of depressed older adults (Lynch et al., 2003), those who received DBT combined with antidepressant medication demonstrated greater reductions on several key measures of depression than individuals who received antidepressant medication alone.

This review is useful for considering possible applications of DBT to PTSD and related problems. First, a number of the diagnoses and problems mentioned above frequently co-occur with PTSD, such as suicidal behavior, substance use disorders, and eating disorders. Therefore, DBT may be useful for the treatment of these coexisting problems, prior to the instigation of exposure-based treatments for PTSD. DBT has, in fact, been proposed as a first stage of treatment for individuals with PTSD, toward the goal of stabilization prior to exposure (Becker & Zayfert, 2001; Melia & Wagner, 2000). This suggestion is supported by both theory and research that emphasize the ability to effectively regulate emotions (i.e., not engage in dysfunctional behavior in the presence of emotional cues) as requisite for exposure to be effective (see Wagner, 2003). Further, given that a sizable portion of individuals with BPD meet criteria for PTSD as well (up to 50% in the samples used by Linehan), the evidence suggests that these coexisting problems can be treated effectively in those with PTSD diagnoses. Second, many additional problems that are common among people with chronic and severe traumatic experiences can be similarly conceptualized according to the theories upon which DBT is based (e.g., dissociative behavior, shame, chronic depression, anxiety). As such, DBT strategies and skills may be useful for the treatment of these problems.

CLINICAL APPLICATIONS

Assessment Issues

As is true for most cognitive-behavioral and behavioral therapies, DBT views assessment as critical to effective treatment. Here we comment on three categories of assessment that are emphasized in DBT: diagnostic assessment, behavioral (functional) analyses, and self-monitoring.

Although the use of psychiatric diagnoses can be criticized on many grounds (and there is no diagnosis that has generated more controversy than BPD), we advocate the use of psychiatric diagnosis for several reasons. Perhaps most important, diagnosis allows for optimal treatment matching, based on the treatment outcome literature. That is, by knowing clients' psychiatric diagnoses, we can more readily determine which treatment is likely to be most effective based on the existing outcome studies. Diagnosis is similarly important when applying existing treatments to novel populations, which is often the case in clinical practice. Even at the level of case studies, diagnostic assessment allows for the accumulation of information that indicates which treatments are effective for which populations. Psychiatric diagnoses have additional benefits, including the facilitation of communication between providers, billing practices, and client referral and staff recruitment to specialty programs.

The cornerstone of assessment in DBT, as in most cognitive-behavioral therapies, is the behavioral (functional) analysis, which, guided by the theories described above, identifies the contextual, antecedent, organismic (i.e., thoughts, emotions, behavior), and consequent factors that are directly related to the maintenance of problems. This analysis results in identification of targets for treatment based on hypothesized maintenance factors; such hypotheses are then tested through intervention and reformulated based on assessed consequences. Behavioral analyses are particularly critical to the adequate treatment of individuals with multiple problems, such as those with BPD and more chronic and complex PTSD. Our approach is quite consistent with that of Follette and Naugle (Chapter 2, this volume) and we therefore refer the reader there for an excellent description of the process of conducting behavioral analyses as well as the utility of behavioral analyses, for trauma-related problems, specifically. In DBT (both stage I and stage II), behavioral analyses are further guided by the biosocial theory and the theory of dialectics. That is, according to the biosocial theory, both motivational factors (behaviorally defined) and capability (i.e., skills) deficits are theorized to maintain problem behaviors. Based on the theory of dialectics, the analysis would necessarily include assessment of the broader context and wide range of factors (always attempting to answer the question "What is being left out?").

The accuracy of behavioral analyses is dependent on careful monitoring of client behavior. In DBT, self-monitoring primarily occurs through use of the DBT Diary Card. Although there are many effective ways to construct the card, typical features include daily measures of the frequency and intensity of high-priority target behaviors, urges to engage in the behaviors, primary emotions, use of prescription and nonprescription drugs, and use of DBT skills. In stage I DBT the Diary Card is essential for tracking suicidal ideation and behavior and organizing individual therapy sessions (in individual sessions the Diary Card becomes the springboard for conducting behavioral analyses). In stage II DBT the Diary Card is equally useful; however, the categories assessed reflect the targets of stage II, as described below. Self-monitoring is difficult for many clients, particularly individuals with BPD or severe and multiple problems (such as those with chronic and complex PTSD). In our experience, compliance with the Diary Card requires that *ther-*

apists view self-monitoring as essential and make noncompliance a high priority in therapy (see later section on Common Obstacles).

Guidelines for Client Selection

The most important (and obvious) consideration in determining whether a client is a good match for DBT is if the client's problems are the types of problems that DBT aims to treat. As mentioned above, one of the primary reasons we advocate for diagnostic interviewing is that it provides a means of reliably assessing constellations of presenting problems and effectively utilizing the relevant treatment outcome literature. DBT would be recommended to the extent that the client falls into a diagnostic group for which there are data supporting the efficacy/effectiveness of DBT. Again, most studies have been conducted on individuals who meet criteria for BPD with current suicidal behavior, and emerging data support the application of DBT to other diagnostic groups as well.

A related consideration of particular relevance to the application of DBT to novel populations is the extent to which the client's presenting problems can be conceptualized according to theories upon which DBT is based. The existing studies seem to suggest that DBT is effective for clients whose problems can be conceptualized according to the biosocial theory as well as the behavioral theory (which emphasizes motivational factors and skills deficits in the maintenance of problem behavior). Because the problems of many clients with severe trauma histories or PTSD can be conceptualized this way (described further below), DBT may be effective for this population as well.

DBT, as with many behavioral therapies, emphasizes fully orienting clients to the goals and expectations of therapy before it begins. Clients are not considered to be "in" DBT until they agree to the goals and expectations of the treatment; therefore, clients who do not demonstrate a moderate degree of commitment are likely poor candidates for the treatment. Nonetheless, lack of motivation for therapy (and change, in general) is viewed as a central problem for many clients and, as such, a set of strategies exist within DBT to generate and strengthen commitment (e.g., evaluating the pros and cons, devil's advocate, shaping). Emphasis is also placed on eliciting clients' own goals and linking these goals to the goals and targets of DBT. Orienting to the structure and expectations of therapy has been emphasized by others in the treatment of PTSD and trauma-related problems (e.g., Foa & Rothbaum, 1998) as well as exposure-based treatments, in general (e.g., Barlow, 2004).

Several initial therapy sessions are typically spent in the pretreatment phase, and behavioral analyses are used to assess obstacles to commitment. Although for some clients the pretreatment phase can be lengthy, and some clients never commit, for the majority of cases this process is sufficient to obtain the commitment necessary to proceed in DBT. As mentioned above, many studies have shown that DBT is particularly effective at reducing treatment dropout. This achievement may be due, in part, to the emphasis placed on providing orientation and eliciting commitment.

The above considerations for client selection are equally applicable to stage I and stage II DBT. We propose additional criteria for the consideration of beginning clients in stage II DBT (discussed later, in the section "From Stage I to Stage II DBT").

Overview of Treatment Approach

As mentioned, DBT is structured into stages of treatment, and these correspond to stages of disorder. Stage I DBT targets severe behavioral dyscontrol, with the goal of achieving overall behavioral control. Once behavioral control is achieved, it becomes possible to work on other important goals: Stage II targets problems with emotional experiencing (including PTSD-related problems), with the goal of increasing the capacity for normative emotional experiencing (without escalating or blunting); stage III targets remaining problems in living and self-respect, toward the goal of resolving these problems; and stage IV targets the sense of incompleteness, with the goal of increasing the capacity for sustained joy and freedom. Again, most of what has been written on DBT (including Linehan's treatment manuals) and treatment outcome studies, to date, pertain to stage I. As we note, DBT also offers a unique approach to treatment of emotional experiencing problems in stage II.

Brief Overview of Stage I DBT

Stage I DBT specifies targets of treatment that are addressed hierarchically, such that those that are most threatening to the individual or the therapy are addressed first. This hierarchical structure is particularly helpful for achieving change in clients with multiple problems who present with frequent and shifting crises week to week. *Life-threatening behaviors* have the highest priority in DBT, followed by *therapy-interfering behaviors* (i.e., any behaviors that directly interfere with, or disrupt, the therapy), followed by other serious *quality-of-life interfering behaviors* (e.g., substance abuse, severe eating-disordered behavior, severe housing, financial, or vocational problems, severe depression). The actual focus of each therapy session, then, is based on which behaviors have occurred in the previous week or time period since the last session and the level of priority of those behaviors. As mentioned, the Diary Card is the primary tool for assessing this area (information from other sources is often available to the therapist as well, such as his or her own observations, feedback from other treatment providers, etc.). In addition to targeting these behaviors to *decrease*, stage I also targets behaviors to *increase* (i.e., behavioral skills). These desirable behaviors are not addressed hierarchically but instead are taught throughout the treatment.

Standard stage I DBT is further structured according to modes of therapy, which are in place in order to achieve specific functions. For example, the mode of individual therapy functions to address motivational factors that maintain problem behaviors toward improving those factors. The skills group mode functions to increase basic capabilities. Additional modes include telephone consultation (to increase skill generalization) and the therapist consultation group (to increase therapist motivation and capabilities).

Interventions in DBT pull largely from standard behavior therapy problem-solving techniques (e.g., contingency management, exposure). In addition, the theory of dialectics and the biosocial theory highlight the importance of balancing these change-oriented strategies with validation, an acceptance-oriented strategy. Together, problem solving and validation are considered the "core" strategies in DBT. Three additional categories of strategies facilitate maintaining the balance between change and acceptance throughout the treatment: communication strategies (i.e., styles of interacting with the client), case management strategies (i.e., methods of interacting with the client in relation to others in his or her environment, including significant others, outside treatment provides, etc.), and dialectical strategies. DBT strategies and skills most relevant to stage II DBT are described further below.

From Stage I to Stage II DBT

The duration of stage I DBT is determined by the length of time it takes to reach the overarching goal of behavioral control. In the majority of existing outcome studies involving individuals with BPD mentioned above, treatment was provided for a span of 6 months to 1 year. Of note, not all individuals in these studies demonstrated clinically significant change from pre- to post-assessment, and even among those who did, some continued to engage in some degree of high-priority target behaviors. The duration of treatment that is required to achieve behavioral control is likely influenced by a number of factors, including the severity and number of initial problems. For some individuals with uncomplicated PTSD, it seems conceivable that stage I may require considerably less than 1 year, particularly if their pretrauma functioning was fairly high, and they are not engaging in a high number of dysfunctional behaviors.

The transition from stage I would also depend on the definition of "behavioral control" that is used. We have recently made efforts to operationalize this concept and propose three general categories of outcome, rooted primarily in the notion of normative functioning. First, the individual should have a reasonable (immediate) life expectancy, defined as the absence of suicide threats or attempts, nonsuicidal self-injury, and severe, ongoing victimization. Also within this category is the control of behaviors that would threaten the life expectancy of others: the absence of aggravated assaults/physical attacks on others, aggressive threats, and severe neglect of legal dependents. Second, the individual should be able to demonstrate stability and control of action, defined as exhibiting behavioral patterns that are within the normative range for his or her peer group (in a nonprotected environment, such as jail or the hospital), with normative or unavoidable cues present. Finally, the individual should possess a range of behavioral skills (basic capabilities) that are evident across role-appropriate, normative, and productive activities (e.g., relationships, work, school). These criteria are considered a "work in progress" and require further clarification (e.g., "absence" of suicidal behavior needs to be described; "range of behavioral skills" needs further specification) as well as empirical support (i.e., for predictive validity).

Stage II DBT is considered appropriate for individuals who have achieved behavioral control yet continue to exhibit significant problems with emotion regulation and experiencing. Because many individuals with BPD have histories of severe and chronic traumatic experiences, these problems frequently take the form of PTSD and related behaviors. Of course, effective psychotherapies exist for the treatment of PTSD (e.g., Foa & Rothbaum, 1998) and therefore stage II DBT would not be recommended for everyone with PTSD or trauma histories. The biosocial theory of BPD and behavioral theory further inform stage II DBT, including which patients might be appropriate for this stage of treatment. Given the central role of invalidation in the development of BPD, problems related to invalidation more generally (and resulting emotion dysregulation) are targeted in this stage. Therefore, individuals with significant self-invalidation, severe emotion dysregulation, and recent histories of dysfunctional behaviors related to emotion dysregulation are recommended for stage II DBT. In addition, the biosocial theory and behavior theory suggest that problems with emotional experiencing can be maintained by a wide variety of current factors that may vary between individuals and even within an individual across behaviors. Therefore, stage II DBT is designed to assess and treat a full range of maintenance factors and may be appropriate for individuals whose emotional experiencing problems cannot be adequately conceptualized according to the standard cognitive-behavioral theory of acute PTSD (e.g., classically conditioned fear responses that are maintained by avoidance and faulty cognitions).

Stage II DBT

Stage II differs from stage I, in part, by the targets of treatment, which include the following: (1) intrusive symptoms (as in the PTSD diagnosis, including memories of traumatic experiences, nightmares, reliving/flashback experiences, and emotional and physiological distress in response to traumatic cues); (2) avoidance of emotions (and behaviors that function as emotional avoidance); (3) avoidance of situations and experiences (the previous two targets overlap with the avoidance criteria of PTSD, but are broader in that they are not specifically limited to avoidance of trauma-related cues);

(4) emotion dysregulation (both heightened and inhibited emotional experiencing, specifically related to anxiety/fear, anger, sadness, shame/guilt); and (5) self-invalidation. No a priori prioritization exists for stage II targets, as there does in stage I; instead, the prioritization of targets is determined by the level of severity and life disruption caused by the problems (with more severe and disruptive behaviors addressed first), the clients' goals, and the functional relationship between targets (e.g., self-invalidation may lead to high shame reactions; therefore, self-invalidation may be targeted directly, toward the reduction of shame).

Stage II is guided by the same primary principles as stage I (biosocial, behavioral, and dialectical strategies). Self-monitoring retains an important role in stage II DBT, though the Diary Cards are modified to reflect the current targets. No published cards currently exist, in part, because of the wide range of behaviors that may be targeted in this stage; instead, practitioners are encouraged to develop their own cards, based on the specific needs of their clients. It is recommended that high-priority stage I targets and associated urges continue to be monitored in stage II, so that therapists (and clients) are aware of any recurrences. Similarly, the structure of individual sessions is consistent with stage I, in that therapists (1) organize sessions by reference to the Diary Card, (2) conduct behavioral and solution-oriented analyses of targeted behaviors, and (3) continuously balance acceptance and change throughout the treatment.

The importance of behavioral analyses in stage II should not be understated. To reiterate, based on behavioral theory and science, the factors related to the current maintenance of behaviors may be quite different from the factors related to the original development of the behaviors. This is an especially critical assumption when working with clients who have trauma or abuse histories, when it can be easy to jump to the conclusion that, if it appears that current problems are caused by the abuse or trauma, the abuse or trauma must be treated directly. However, in many cases (e.g., when abuse or trauma occurred during early development or chronically over a long period of time), a host of factors may be maintaining current problems that only peripherally relate to the past experiences. From this perspective, effective treatment requires intervening at the level of current maintenance factors. In the absence of empirically supported treatments for individuals with chronic/complex traumatic histories (or problems with emotional experiencing more generally), treatment can be (and it could be argued, should be) guided by empirically supported principles of assessment and change (Rosen & Davison, 2003).

CASE FORMULATION OF STAGE II PROBLEMS

As in stage I, the biosocial, behavioral, and dialectical theories guide stage II. That is, target behaviors are viewed as developing from the combined influences of emotional vulnerability and an invalidating environment, and the maintenance of these behaviors is attributable to some combination of skills deficits, faulty contingencies, classically conditioned responding, and dysfunctional cognitions. Change therefore requires an emphasis on skills training, contingency management, exposure, and cognitive interventions, balanced with an equal emphasis on validation and dialectical strategies. In stage II, however, it is assumed that skills *deficits* play somewhat less of a role in the maintenance of behaviors, because stage I focused heavily on increasing basic capabilities. Instead, the skills focus in stage II is more on the aspects of strengthening and generalization. In addition, given the typical learning history of individuals appropriate for stage II DBT, many target behaviors can be conceptualized as classically conditioned responses (e.g., intrusive memories, dissociative behavior, shame) and, as such, exposure, particularly informal exposure, is a frequently used intervention. Further, many stage II clients continue to have difficulty trusting and validating their perceptions and emotional reactions, particularly in the context of discussing past traumatic experiences or in the process of conducting exposure. Indeed, self-invalidation is defined as a specific target of stage II. Therefore, validation, with an emphasis on strengthening the capacity for self-validation, maintains a central role in stage II. Finally, limitations in the capacity for dialectical thinking appear to contribute to the maintenance of many stage II problems (e.g., self-loathing may relate to an inability to conceptualize the complexity of factors related to past abuse and current functioning); therefore, stage II continues to utilize dialectical strategies with a focus on increasing the capacity for dialectical thinking, specifically. In the remainder of this chapter we expand on those interventions that take a more prominent role in stage II, including advanced skills training, exposure, validation, and dialectical strategies. It is important to stress, however, that all treatment planning in stage II DBT must be based on individualized case formulations.

SKILLS TRAINING IN STAGE II

The four modules of skills that are taught in stage I—mindfulness, distress tolerance, emotion regulation, and interpersonal effectiveness—are strengthened and generalized to new contexts (i.e., situations, interpersonal interactions, internal experiences) in stage II. For the reader unfamiliar with the skills training module of DBT, the single most useful source for learning about and teaching DBT skills is the DBT skills training manual (Linehan, 1993b). A brief overview, with an emphasis on the utility of these skills for stage II, is presented here.

Mindfulness skills are derived from Zen philosophy and are compatible with both Western and Eastern contemplative practices. The primary goals of mindfulness skills are to cultivate awareness of internal and external experiences and to be more present-focused. These goals are particularly salient for clients who become overwhelmed by emotions, avoid emotions, have difficulty recognizing emotions or cues for emotions, or who are very ruminative about the past or future, as is true for many individuals with PTSD or trauma histories. Mindfulness skills may also be useful for increasing aware-ness of danger-related cues, thus decreasing the chances of revictimization. In stage I, mindfulness is frequently practiced on external and sensory expe-riences (e.g., mindfulness of what one sees, hears, smells, tastes, feels physi-cally) and practiced for short periods of time (typically 1–10 minutes). In stage II, as clients gain an increasing capacity to focus their attention and tol-erate internal experiences, mindfulness can be expanded to include aware-ness of thoughts and emotions and practiced for more extended periods of time. The exercises in the skills training manual can be adapted for stage II. In addition, there are many sources of mindfulness practices in popular liter-ature that can be used for this purpose (e.g., Kabat-Zinn, 1995; Thich Nhat Hanh [Hanh, 1999]).

The *distress tolerance* module consists of skills related to getting through a crisis or extremely stressful situation without engaging in behaviors that could make the situation worse. As the label implies, these are not skills for solving life problems but instead for coping with problems when they cannot be solved at that particular moment (or at all). The skills can roughly be grouped into two types: crisis survival skills and acceptance skills. Crisis sur-vival skills are highly utilized in stage I because clients are frequently in crises and these skills are relatively easy to learn and apply. The acceptance skills are also taught and viewed as important in stage I; however, they have partic-ular relevance to stage II DBT. Acceptance skills are based on the assump-tion that pain and suffering are part of life (although, indeed, some people seem to have more than others), and that most suffering comes from an inability to accept this fact. "Acceptance," as used here, refers to having a nonjudgmental stance toward oneself and the situation and not demanding that the situation "should" be any different than it is. In essence, this is apply-ing the ideas of mindfulness to difficult situations and oneself. For individu-als who have experienced difficult or traumatic experiences, acceptance is often the only way out of suffering, given that the past cannot be changed.

Although all the DBT skills aim to treat problems related to emotion dysregulation, the overall goal of the *emotion regulation* module is specifically to reduce and change emotional reactions. In Stage I, considerable attention is spent on learning about emotions—what they are, why we have them, how to recognize them, and how to label them. This type of psychoeducation may be particularly helpful to individuals with PTSD, because PTSD has been associated with difficulties in identifying and communicating emotions (e.g., Zlotnick, Mattia, & Zimmerman, 2001). Clients are also taught how to reduce vulnerability to negative emotions and increase positive emotions. Mindful-ness of emotions is taught next in this module, toward the goal of reducing decreasing emotional suffering. As mentioned above, mindfulness is a diffi-cult skill to learn, so it is emphasized and strengthened in stage II. The ability to stay present with emotional experiences is particularly important for exposure-based interventions in stage II and is thus used in conjunction with this intervention. The final skill taught in this module, "opposite action," is also highly relevant to exposure-based interventions. This skill involves learning to recognize the "action urge" associated with emotions as well as specific skills for behaving in a way opposite to that urge. Opposite action is described later, in the discussion of informal exposure.

The *interpersonal effectiveness* module teaches skills necessary for decreasing interpersonal problems and increasing the ability to form and maintain positive relationships. Similar to assertiveness skills, these skills focus specifically on strategies for asking for what one needs or wants, saying no to unwanted requests, and coping with interpersonal conflicts. Clients are taught how to identify and prioritize goals within interpersonal situations, how to identify factors that interfere with effectiveness, and most importantly, concrete skills for effective interactions. In addition, specific skills are included for maintaining the relationship (when this is important) and maintaining self-respect in the context of an interpersonal interaction. Because interpersonal difficulties are common among individuals with complex traumatic histories and PTSD, these skills have particular relevance for this population. Therefore, in stage II, emphasis is placed on applying interpersonal skills to building positive relationships, increasing intimacy, and reducing the likelihood of revictimization.

There are different options for the *format of skills training* in Stage II. In Stage I it is recommended that skills be taught in a group context, largely because this is more economical but also because it is quite difficult to teach skills in individual therapy when a client is in constant crises that require immediate attention (e.g., suicide threats/attempts). Skills may be more easily incorporated into individual therapy in stage II because crises are less frequent and clients enter this stage with these basic capabilities. Regardless of the mode of skills training, the emphasis in stage II is on skills strengthening and generalization—that is, relearning the skills and applying them to new situations. As such, clients should be encouraged to generate options for skillful behavior prior to being offered options by the therapist. Advanced skills groups have been utilized in some settings for this purpose. Although there currently is no specific format for an advanced skills group, (apparently) effective components include (1) decreasing therapist involvement while increasing client participation in structuring the group and teaching the skills; (2) focusing on day-to-day problems while emphasizing DBT skills as solutions; and (3) increasing in-session practice (e.g., with mindfulness exercises) and between-client interactions (with the explicit goal to strengthen interpersonal skills, distress tolerance, and emotion regulation). Telephone skills coaching, which is heavily utilized in stage I (see Linehan, 1993a), is decreased in stage II in order to increase clients' ability to draw on their existing skill knowledge and apply this to new contexts (i.e., the amount of phone contact should be contingent on the client's current level of knowledge and capabilities). The principle of shaping is important to keep in mind when deciding when telephone coaching would be appropriate in stage II.

EXPOSURE AS A PRIMARY INTERVENTION IN STAGE II DBT

Exposure is used frequently in stage II, both formally and informally. By "formal" exposure we are referring to a structured protocol for treating a particular disorder, such as panic disorder (e.g., Barlow & Craske, 1994) or PTSD (e.g., Foa & Rothbaum, 1998). Formal exposure is appropriate for the treatment of target problems that can be conceptualized similarly to the formulations upon which these treatments are based (e.g., when panic disorder can be conceptualized as a conditioned response to interoceptive cues that is maintained by avoidance; or when PTSD can be conceptualized as overgeneralized conditioned responses that are maintained by cognitions and avoidance). In such cases, these protocols are embedded within the structure of the treatment (this is why DBT is referred to as a principle-driven treatment that includes protocols). Many intrusive and associated avoidant symptoms (e.g., memories of past traumatic experiences) could be effectively treated with a protocol treatment for PTSD.

More typically, however, informal exposure is utilized in stage II. "Informal" exposure involves exposure to a relevant cue without an elaborate step-by-step protocol. Informal exposure is appropriate for the treatment of a target problem that is, in part, maintained by a conditioned response and avoidance, but where other maintaining factors are also present. For example, in a behavioral analysis of binge eating, it might be revealed that the client had a conditioned response to criticism (anxiety), followed by catastrophic beliefs about the relationship ("He will leave me"), and anxiety reduction following the binge episode: Treatment may then include exposure to criticism as well as cognitive interventions and skill building on other ways to reduce anxiety. Informal exposure is also appropriate for conditioned responses that are highly overgeneralized but for which no formal protocols exist (e.g., the treatment of shame). The steps are similar in both informal and formal exposure, though in informal exposure the process is typically shorter in duration. As described by others (e.g., Foa & Rothbaum, 1998), the basic steps in exposure include (1) presenting stimuli that elicit the emotion/reaction, (2) ensuring that the affective response is not reinforced (i.e., corrective information is provided), (3) blocking escape responses and other forms of avoidance, and (4) enhancing the client's sense of control. Exposure is said to "work" when there is a reduction in the emotion or sustained attention to the cue without the client resorting to alternative (dysfunctional) avoidant behavior.

In DBT, the steps of exposure are subsumed under the intervention labeled "opposite to emotion action" or "opposite action," for short. Opposite action expands on exposure in that it includes a step for acting differently (i.e., engaging in new behavior while not engaging in the dysfunctional/avoidant behavior that is targeted for intervention). This step is particularly important for clients who have behavioral deficits in addition to the presence of dysfunctional behavior, such as those with histories of long-term, chronic trauma and invalidation. In other words, the goal of treatment is not only to eliminate dysfunctional behavior but to increase new, functional behavior. This skill is taught to clients in the emotion regulation module (to change or reduce negative emotions) as well as used by therapists with clients to counter classically conditioned responding and/or avoidance. As a technique used by therapists, opposite action has been articulated most fully by Rizvi and Linehan (in press) for the treatment of shame among individuals with BPD, specifically. Preliminary case data for this targeted intervention are quite promising, supporting the applicability of this approach to exposure for complex populations. The components of opposite action (which, again, overlap with the steps of exposure) are the following.

Cue Exposure (Presenting the Stimuli That Elicit the Emotion). "Cue exposure" refers to the process of presenting clients with the events, thoughts, memories, or emotions (i.e., the "cues") that elicit the target behaviors. This presentation can be accomplished imaginally by having the client think about a particular scenario associated with a target behavior, or "live" (*in vivo*) by creating a context or having the client engage in an activity that elicits a targeted response. *Imaginal* cue exposure is typically less arousing for clients and can be a useful starting point for exposure. *In vivo* cue exposure can occur both out of the therapy office (through a behavioral "homework assignment") or in the therapy session. Because many relevant behaviors can occur so (seemingly) automatically (e.g., dissociative behavior, shame), use of in-session emotional reactions can be particularly effective for exposure treatment in stage II. For this reason, having a comprehensive case formulation (i.e., a thorough understanding of treatment targets and the factors related to the maintenance of the targets) is essential to enable therapists to be alert to relevant behaviors as they occur. Relatedly, awareness of target-relevant cues and reactions prevents therapists from unwittingly removing cues, which can often be the tendency in the face of apparently adverse reactions (e.g., in response to dissociation, a therapist may avoid similar topics in the future; in fact, the purposeful presentation of those topics would be a much more effective intervention).

Response Prevention (Block Avoidance). The most common obstacle to effective exposure is avoidance of cues and/or emotional experiencing, and it is essential that therapists block these forms of avoidance during exposure. Of course, many of the target behaviors of stage II DBT function as avoidance and therefore "blocking avoidance" often translates to prevention of the target behavior. For example, if the target behavior is dissociation, the client would be presented with the cue for dissociation (e.g., an angry voice tone, which elicits fear) and taught skills for staying in the moment in the presence of the angry voice tone and the feeling of fear. Common forms of avoidance include missing sessions, not doing homework assignments, refusing to participate in behavioral analyses, and diverting the conversation. Less obvious (but effective) means of avoidance include secondary emotions (e.g., shame about anger, fear of fear). If exposure is focusing on the primary emotion, the secondary emotions should be blocked. Similarly, judgments about emotions or self can function as avoidance. For example, a client may berate him- or herself for feeling very sad about a loss. This judgment is likely inhibiting the experience of loss and should be blocked. Blocking avoidance can usually be accomplished by drawing attention to the avoidance and bringing the client's attention back to the exposure. Finally, because many behaviors typical of stage I DBT can similarly function as avoidance, therapists should stay alert to the possible recurrence of these behaviors in stage II (e.g., parasuicidal behavior, substance use, eating-disordered behavior, extreme therapy-interfering behavior, including missing sessions, not collaborating in sessions). The presence of stage I behaviors necessitates treating those behaviors prior to continuing with stage II targets. However, care should be taken to minimize the reinforcing effects of moving out of stage II and into stage I by moving back to stage II as soon as stage I behaviors are under control.

An effective strategy for countering avoidance is increasing clients' perceived ability to control events and emotions. This sense of increased control can be accomplished by giving the client some control over how session time is used, including when the exposure will occur, and allowing the client to control the pace and intensity of exposure if he or she is feeling overwhelmed. In addition, a client's sense of control can be greatly aided by discussing ahead of time the rationale and procedures of exposure and designing interventions with the client's input.

Opposite Action. "Opposite action" is a behavior that is opposite to the "action urge" of the emotion that is elicited through the cue exposure. Opposite action is based on a wide body of theoretical and empirical literature that suggests that all emotions have an associated action urge (e.g., fear is associated with the urge to withdraw, avoid, or run away; anger is associated with the urge to strike out or yell; shame is associated with the urge to hide); and that engaging in behavior that is opposite to the urge of the emotion will reduce the emotion more quickly (Barlow, 1988). Further, opposite action has the additional function of strengthening more adaptive behavior. In this step, clients are taught skills for identifying the action urges associated with emotions and the options for opposite action. For example, if the emotion is fear, clients may be taught ways of approaching the stimuli that elicit fear (as in typical exposure for fear treatments); if the emotion is shame, clients may be taught methods of using voice tone and body posture (e.g., strong voice tone, sitting up straight) as well as behavior (e.g., doing what one feels shame about repeatedly) as opposed to hiding. As in typical exposure treatments, use of opposite action, as just described, would be predicated on the determination that the emotional reaction was dysfunctional (i.e., just as one would not advocate walking down a dark ally at night to reduce fear of being attacked, the strategy of opposite action in response to fear would not be recommended if there were a realistic threat). In DBT, the concept of "justified" versus "unjustified" emotional reactions is taught to clients as a way of making this distinction across emotions. Opposite action is typically recommended for *un*justified emotional reactions only.

VALIDATION IN STAGE II

The theory of dialectics and the biosocial theory highlight the importance of balancing problem solving, a change-oriented strategy, with validation, an acceptance-oriented strategy, throughout the treatment. Problem solving and validation are considered "core" strategies in DBT, and both are essential components of the treatment. For in-depth discussions of validation in DBT, see Linehan (1993a, 1997). Validation is a communication that affirms what is true, accurate, or valid in a client's beliefs, emotional reactions, and behavior. Validation increases clients' motivation for change (i.e., functions as reinforcement and may reduce arousal), strengthens their abilities to distinguish valid from invalid behavior, and teaches the capacity for self-validation (ultimately decreasing clients' sense of emptiness and increasing a "sense of self"). Although similar to the concept of empathy in psychotherapy, validation is different in a key respect: Whereas empathy can be defined as understanding the world from the clients' perspective (i.e., "standing in their shoes"), validation includes understanding the world from the clients' perspective *and* communicating what is accurate—in their emotions, thoughts, and behavior.

There are different ways of communicating validation, and these are categorized in DBT as *levels* of validation. Levels 1–3 are typical of standard psychotherapeutic listening skills (i.e., unbiased listening, reflecting, and articulating a client's unverbalized emotions, thoughts, or behavior patterns); perhaps different from other psychotherapies, however, these skills are used strategically in DBT to achieve the functions mentioned above.

Level 4 validation refers to validating clients' behavior in terms of their learning history or biological dysfunction. For example, in response to a client who became irate with her boss (and subsequently got fired), a level 4 validation might be the statement "It makes sense to me that you got so extreme; given your history of abuse by your father, I know how sensitive you are to people trying to exert authority over you"; or similarly, "This seems like another example of how your temperament sometimes gets the better of you." Level 4 validation is also used frequently in other psychotherapies. As used in DBT, level 4 validation can be particularly helpful to clients who do not understand the nature of their reactions or are highly judgmental (and invalidating) of their reactions. For this reason, level 4 validation is frequently used in stage II DBT.

Level 5 validation is perhaps more unique to DBT than to other therapies. Level 5 validation is given in accordance with the present context or normative functioning. For example, in the case of the client getting irate, above, after hearing about the interaction the therapist might conclude, "It makes sense to me that you got so angry—it sounds like he was really being unreasonable" (if it did sound that way), or "That sounds like an unbearable situation—I bet a lot of people would get angry with someone like that" (again, *if* a lot of people *would* get angry in that type of situation). The critical consideration with Level 5 validation is whether or not the behavior is, in fact, valid. More typically, a reaction has both valid and invalid aspects, and the task of the therapist is to validate the valid (and not validate the invalid). Expanding on the same example, if the client threatened her boss and she had no alternative employment or financial resources, children to feed, and bills that were due, the therapist might respond, "I can completely understand why you felt so angry, he sounded completely off-base; it seems, though, that you got pretty extreme and lost your job because of it. We should work on how to manage those kinds of feelings so that you don't respond in ways that make your situation worse." Importantly, Level 5 validation does not always "feel good," nor is that the goal of the strategy. For example, I (AW) recently had a frustrating interaction with a client and felt irritated as a result. My client stated that I seemed irritated and I responded that I was, that I found the interaction difficult. This was a Level 5 validation in that I validated her observation of my irritation—yet undoubtedly, this information did not put her in a good mood. More often than not, however, Level 5 validation is experienced positively. Level 5 is particularly helpful for clients who have difficulty trusting and validating their emotional reactions or perceptions, as is the case with clients with BPD, PTSD, and trauma histories. Level 5 validation is therefore quite important in stage II DBT.

Finally, Level 6 validation is referred to as "radical genuineness." Therapists practicing radical genuineness are role-independent in voice tone and manner. Typical to how they act in other relationships, a radically genuine therapist is neither overly sweet nor aloof, and tries not to be affected in any way. Radical genuineness can also be communicated by having accurate expectations (i.e., not treating the client as fragile or ignoring true limitations) and the willingness to be vulnerable with clients (e.g., self-disclose reactions in therapy) when this would be helpful. Radical genuineness communicates that clients are equal, capable, and *valid* human beings. As opposed to the strategic use of the preceding levels of validating, radical genuineness is used throughout DBT.

Whereas validation is utilized frequently by *therapists* in stage I DBT, the task in stage II is to teach *clients* to be validating toward themselves. Levels 1, 4, 5, and 6 are relevant to self-validation. Self-validation at Level 1 (i.e., attentiveness) would translate to a client believing that what he or she has to say or express is relevant and worth paying attention to and acting accordingly. Therefore, therapists should stay alert to and encourage self-generated

behavior (e.g., a client initiating a topic or expressing a request) and reinforce this initiative when possible (directly, with such statements as "that
seems important," or functionally, by focusing on the topic or agreeing with
the request). To increase Levels 4 and 5 of self-validation, therapists should
initially use these types of responses in response to clients' statements and
reactions. Therapists should also stay alert to clients' self-invalidating statements and highlight and counter these when they occur. Over time, clients
can be encouraged to generate their own Level 4 and Level 5 validating statements in response to their own reactions, perceptions, and experiences.
Questions such as "How does your response make sense, given your history?" or "How can you understand your reaction, given what was going on
just then?" or "When you start thinking that (invalidating) way, how can you
restate that to yourself to account for what you know to be valid in your
experience?" can be particularly helpful for generating more self-validating
responses. Focus on in-session invalidation can be quite impactful, because
the client has the opportunity to observe and change his or her response in
the moment. Between-session practice is also recommended. This practice
can be implemented by developing tracking forms (similar to thought
records typical of cognitive therapies), in which clients note instances of self-
invalidation, including the situation and their response (cognitive, emotional, behavioral) and then generate Level 4 and/or Level 5 statements.
Finally, clients should be encouraged to practice radical genuineness (Level
6). Often stage II clients will act in ways discordant with how they are feeling
(e.g., act cheerful when they are in pain) or take on the role of someone else.
These behaviors can reinforce their beliefs that who they and what they feel
are not valid, and can also interfere with interpersonal relationships and intimacy. This pattern can be addressed by highlighting the behavior when it is
observed, and reinforcing more genuine behavior.

DIALECTICAL STRATEGIES IN STAGE II

As mentioned earlier, the theory of dialectics is one of the main guiding
principles in DBT, influencing assumptions about the nature of reality, the
structure of the treatment, assessment, and the timing of interventions.
Stage I DBT includes a set of strategies used by therapists (referred to as dialectical strategies) to facilitate the balance of change and acceptance
throughout the treatment. Importantly, these strategies also promote clients'
capacity for dialectical thinking—that is, the capacity to think noncategor-
ically, to take into account the multidimensional nature of reality, and to
accept the notion of no fixed truth (or the possibility of multiple truths). As
such, these strategies are equally important in stage II DBT because many
individuals with histories of abuse or trauma have difficulty reconciling
apparently contradictory aspects of their experiences (e.g., how a beloved
parent could cause great harm).

The specific dialectical strategies include the following:

- Use of metaphor (a well-constructed metaphor can convey both complete understanding and acceptance and the need for change as well as the complexity of any situation)
- Taking the role of the devil's advocate (in which the therapist argues one half of a polarity in order to generate the other half from the client, thus highlighting how "both can be true")
- Use of extending (taking a client's position even more strongly they he or she is making it, thus leading him or her to argue against the position)
- "Making lemonade out of lemons" (pointing out how something apparently negative can have positive or useful aspects)
- Entering the paradox (pointing out the inherent contradictions in any view, reaction, or situation, thus highlighting how different positions can both be true or untrue)
- Activating "wise mind" (a mindfulness skill that includes the synthesis of rational and emotional frames of mind)
- Allowing natural change (thus challenging the notion that things "should" be a certain way)
- Using dialectical assessment (looking for what is left out).

These strategies are woven throughout the treatment in stage II DBT.

In addition, clients can be explicitly oriented to the theory of dialectics and encouraged to look for dialectical dilemmas and syntheses in their perceptions and reactions. For example, a client may be struggling because she feels both anger and love toward her father, who abused her; she is trying to decide whether she should have a relationship with him or cut off contact with him entirely. In this case, the therapist could point out the polarity (e.g., "This seems like a dialectic") and encourage the client to look for "both–and," as opposed to "either/or," solutions. That is, the client may come to see that she can have both loving and angry feelings toward her father and that there may be alternatives besides either having a close relationship or stopping all contact (e.g., getting together occasionally in the presence of others; going to family therapy together). Attention to dialectical dilemmas that arise in the course of therapy or in the context of the therapeutic relationship can be particularly useful for developing the capacity for dialectical thinking (and for strengthening the relationship). For example, a client wanting more between-session contact than a therapist is willing to provide can be treated as an opportunity to discuss the validity in both viewpoints and possibly generate solutions that are a synthesis of these views. The ultimate goal is to facilitate nonjudgmental and flexible evaluations of self and others. Of course, the ability to notice dialectical tensions and generate dialectical syntheses require that the therapist truly adopt a dialectical worldview. This philosophical shift can be facilitated through independent reading (e.g., Basseches, 1985; Levins & Lewontin, 1987) and participation in a consultation group that promotes dialectical thinking.

EMPHASIS ON THE THERAPEUTIC RELATIONSHIP

The effectiveness of stage I DBT depends on the establishment of a strong and positive therapeutic relationship; this is equally the case in stage II DBT. The relationship in DBT affects therapy in two primary ways: A strong relationship allows the therapist to have a certain amount of influence over the process of therapy (i.e., mutual trust, respect, and positive regard will increase the likelihood that the client will engage in tasks and behaviors that are difficult and uncomfortable); further, a strong relationship can be therapy in itself (i.e., through the development of closeness, trust, and intimacy: the therapist is warm, nonjudgmental, accepting, and compassionate, and the client may learn from this new ways of relating to others, healing from some of the damage of past destructive relationships). Just as in the therapy as a whole, the therapist works to achieve a balance within the relationship between accepting it as it is (and the client as he or she is) and initiating problem-solving activities when difficulties arise. Furthermore, emphasis is placed on generalizing aspects of the therapeutic relationship to the client's relationships outside of therapy. This focus can be useful in helping the client recognize and change recurrent problems as well as develop the capacity for positive and intimate relationships outside of therapy. A relational focus is particularly important for individuals who have suffered interpersonal traumas. Given this emphasis, it is imperative that therapists practicing DBT (either stage I or II) convey comfort and flexibility in discussing interpersonal issues.

CONCLUDING COMMENT ON STAGE II DBT

As has been stated, stage II DBT is in the early phases of development, and efforts to further articulate it are underway by our research group and others. The ideas presented here are preliminary, based on empirically supported principles but not evaluated empirically as a structured treatment for this population. *The need for research in this area cannot be stressed enough.*

COMMON OBSTACLES AND POSSIBLE SOLUTIONS

- *Stage I problems reemerge in Stage II.* Although the stages of DBT are presented linearly, as if clients progress smoothly from one stage to the next, in reality, this is rarely the case. Instead, clients often move back and forth between stages I and II. Given that many dysfunctional behaviors function to regulate emotions (such as parasuicide in individuals with BPD or complex trauma histories), and given that stage II emphasizes emotional experiencing, stage I problems are likely to reemerge during Stage II. When this occurs, it is important to move quickly to the treatment of these higher-priority targets and remain focused on these problems until they have been eliminated. However, just as certain behaviors can function as emotional avoidance, attention to these behaviors may also function as avoidance from the originally eliciting cue. Therefore, this likely contingency should be highlighted and therapy should return to the original focus as soon as possible.

• *Client does not see the relevance of the treatment goals as outlined by DBT.* It is often the case that clients come into treatment (either stage I or II) with their own goals and assumptions about how to achieve them. For example, clients may enter stage I with no intention of reducing self-harm behavior, either because they do not think the behavior is a problem or because they fear they will completely lose control (and even kill themselves) if they cease to engage in the behavior. Or clients may begin therapy with many stage I behaviors, firmly believing that they their early abuse is the cause and needs to be addressed first. Similar obstacles can exist in stage II DBT—for example, although a behavioral analysis may reveal that a client's intense shame is precipitated by current signs of criticism by others, he or she may hold the belief that he or she needs to "process" her childhood sexual abuse first to reduce the response of shame. It is imperative, therefore, that clients' goals and assumptions be fully assessed at the onset of therapy. Clients' willingness to proceed with the goals and targets of DBT can be enhanced by fully orienting them to the rationale for the treatment (goals, targets, and interventions) and linking their goals to the goals and targets of DBT (that is, explicitly stating how DBT will help them achieve their goals).

• *Client does not self-monitor.* Although self-monitoring is considered essential in DBT (and behavioral therapies, in general), it is frequently the case that clients do not complete (or do not fully complete) the DBT Diary Cards. This obstacle can be overcome by viewing it as a problem to be solved (in this case, a "therapy-interfering behavior") and as such, conducting a behavioral analysis of the factors that interfered with completing the card and then problem-solving those factors. In our experience the factors related to not completing cards overlap with problems clients are experiencing in general. Therefore, problem-solving the Diary Card exercise not only increases the likelihood that the card will be completed in the future, it also addresses problems relevant to clients' long-term goals. For example, typical factors that interfere with card completion include disorganization (e.g., losing the card), shame (e.g., when thinking about one's problems), and not seeing the relevance of the exercise. Linking the completion of the Diary Card to clients' larger problems thus increases both the relevance of the exercise and the generalizability of the intervention. Of course, adequate attention to Diary Card noncompliance rests on the degree to which therapists view this type of self-monitoring as essential to the treatment.

• *Working with this population can lead to burnout.* DBT addresses the common problem of therapist burnout when working with difficult-to-treat clients. Much has been written about the high emotional stress and likelihood of "burnout" among therapists who work with BPD, and clients with trauma histories, PTSD. In DBT there is an explicit assumption that "therapists who treat BPD patients need support." Hence an essential component of DBT is the therapist consultation group. We assert that the therapist consultation group is equally important in stage II as in stage I DBT because it functions in both stages to improve therapist capabilities and motivation, to offer a venue for exchange of information among treatment providers, and to provide support. Although there is a wide range of formats used in DBT consultation groups (which may overlap with more traditional consultation groups in many ways), DBT groups can be distinguished from other types of consultation groups, in part, by a set of "agreements" shared among members. These agreements model many principles of the therapy as a whole (e.g., "to accept a dialectical philosophy") as well as its strategies (e.g., "to consult with the patient on how to interact with other therapists and not to tell other therapists how to interact with the patient"), and importantly it provides guidelines for minimizing therapist burnout (e.g., "All therapists are to observe their own limits without fear of judgmental reactions from other consultation group members"). In addition to the agreements, DBT consultation groups are also unique in their emphasis on incorporating the mindfulness skills taught to clients in DBT. Given the range of reactions that therapists can experience when working with traumatized and difficult-to-treat clients, effective treatment requires awareness of their own experience as well as careful attention to the moment-to-moment experiences of the clients. Stated as a DBT assumption about therapy, "Clarity, precision, and compassion are of the utmost importance in the conduct of DBT." Mindfulness skills are practiced by therapists toward this goal.

REFERENCES

Barlow, D. H. (1988). *Anxiety and its disorders: The nature and treatment of anxiety and panic.* New York: Guilford Press.

Barlow, D. H. (2004). *Anxiety and its disorders: The nature and treatment of anxiety and panic* (2nd ed.). New York: Guilford Press.

Barlow, D. H., & Craske, M. G. (1994). *Mastery of your anxiety and panic II: Client workbook.* Boston: Psychological Corporation.

Basseches, M. (1988). *Dialectical thinking and adult development.* Norwood, NJ: Ablex.

Becker, C. B., & Zayfert, C. (2001). Integrating DBT-based techniques and concepts to facilitate exposure treatment for PTSD. *Cognitive and Behavioral Practice, 8,* 107–122.

Cloitre, M. (1998). Sexual revictimization risk factors and prevention. In V. M. Follette, J. I. Ruzek, & F. R. Abueg (Eds.), *Cognitive-behavioral therapies for trauma* (pp. 278–304). New York: Guilford Press.

Dimeff, L., Rizvi, S. L., Brown, M., & Linehan, M. M. (2000). Dialectical behavior therapy for substance abuse: A pilot application to methamphetamine-dependent women with borderline personality disorder. *Cognitive and Behavioral Practice, 7,* 457–468.

Eisenberg, N., Fabes, R. A., & Murphy, B. C. (1996). Parents' reactions to children's negative emotions: Relations to children's social competence and comforting behavior. *Child Development, 67,* 2227-2247.

Eisenberg, N., Losoya, S., Fabes, R. A., Guthrie, I. K., Reiser, M., Murphy, B., Shepard, S. A., Poulin, R., & Padgett, S. J. (2001). Parental socialization of children's dysregulated expression of emotion and externalizing problems. *Journal of Family Psychology, 15,* 183-205.

Foa, E. B., & Rothbaum, B. O. (1998). *Treating the trauma of rape.* New York: Guilford Press.

Hanh, T. N. (1999). *The miracle of mindfulness.* Boston: Beacon Press.

Hayes, S. C., Strosahl, K. D., & Wilson, K. G. (1999). *Acceptance and commitment therapy.* New York: Guilford Press.

Herman, J. L. (1995). Crime and memory. *Bulletin of the American Academy of Psychiatry and the Law, 23,* 5-17.

Kabat-Zinn, J. (1995). *Wherever you go, there you are.* New York: Hyperion.

Keane, T. M., Fisher, L. M., Krinsley, K. E., & Niles, B. L. (1994). Posttraumatic stress disorder. In M. Hersen & R. T. Ammerman (Eds.), *Handbook of prescriptive treatments for adults* (pp. 237-260). New York: Plenum Press.

Koerner, K., & Dimeff, L. A. (2000). Further data on dialectical behavior therapy. *Clinical Psychology: Science and Practice, 7,* 104-112.

Koerner, K., & Linehan, M. M. (2000). Research on dialectical behavior therapy for patients with borderline personality disorder. *Psychiatric Clinics of North America, 23,* 151-167.

Koerner, K., & Linehan, M. M. (2002). Dialectical behavior therapy for borderline personality disorder. In S. G. Hofmann & M. C. Tompson (Eds.), *Treating chronic and severe mental disorders: A handbook of empirically supported interventions* (pp. 317-342). New York: Guilford Press.

Kohlenberg, R. J., & Tsai, M. (1991). *Functional analytic psychotherapy.* New York: Plenum Press.

Krause, E. D., Mendelson, T., & Lynch, T. R. (2003). Childhood emotional invalidation and adult psychological distress: The mediating role of emotional inhibition. *Child Abuse and Neglect, 27,* 199-213.

Levins, R., & Lewontin, R. (1987). *The dialectical biologist.* Cambridge: Harvard University Press.

Lieb, K., Zanarini, M. C., Schmahl, C., Linehan, M. M., & Bohus, M. (2004). Borderline personality disorder. *Lancet, 364,* 453-461.

Linehan, M. M. (1993a). *Cognitive-behavioral treatment of borderline personality disorder.* New York: Guilford Press.

Linehan, M. M. (1993b). *Skills training manual for treating borderline personality disorder.* New York: Guilford Press.

Linehan, M. M. (1997). Validation and psychotherapy. In A. C. Bohart & S. L. Greenberg (Eds.), *Empathy reconsidered: New directions in psychotherapy* (pp. 353-392). Washington, DC: American Psychological Association.

Linehan, M. M., Cochran, B. N., & Kehrer, C. A. (2001). Dialectical behavior therapy for borderline personality disorder. In D. H. Barlow (Ed.), *Clinical handbook of psychological disorders: A step-by-step treatment manual* (3rd ed., pp. 470-522). New York: Guilford Press.

Linehan, M. M., Comtois, K. A., Brown, M., Reynolds, S. K., Welch, S. S., Sayrs, J. H. R., & Korslund, K. E. (2002, November). *DBT versus nonbehavioral treatment by experts in the community: Clinical outcomes.* Symposium conducted at the 36th annual convention of the Association for the Advancement of Behavior Therapy, Reno, NV.

Linehan, M. M., Dimeff, L. A., Reynolds, S. K., Comtois, K. A., Welch, S. S., Heagerty, P., & Kivlahan, D. R. (2002). Dialectal behavior therapy versus comprehensive validation therapy plus 12-step for the treatment of opioid dependent women meeting criteria for borderline personality disorder. *Drug and Alcohol Dependence, 67,* 13–26.

Linehan, M. M., & Schmidt, H. (1995). The dialectics of effective treatment of borderline personality disorder. In W. T. O'Donohue & L. Krasner (Eds.), *Theories of behavior therapy: Exploring behavior change* (pp. 553–584). Washington, DC: American Psychological Association.

Linehan, M. M., Schmidt, H. I., Dimeff, L. A., Craft, J. C., Kanter, J., & Comtois, K. A. (1999). Dialectical behavior therapy for patients with borderline personality disorder and drug-dependence. *American Journal on Addictions, 8,* 279–292.

Linehan, M. M., Tutek, D. A., Heard, H. L., & Armstrong, H. E. (1994). Interpersonal outcome of cognitive behavioral treatment for chronically suicidal borderline patients. *American Journal of Psychiatry, 151,* 1771–1776.

Lynch, T. R. (2004). *Potential mediators and moderators of change: Examples from a dialectical behavior therapy perspective.* Paper presented at the National Institute of Mental Health, International Think Tank for More Effective Treatment of Borderline Personality Disorder, Bethesda, MD.

Lynch, T. R., Morse, J. Q., Mendelson, T., Robins, C. J. (2003). Dialectical behavior therapy for depressed older adults: A randomized pilot study. *American Journal of Geriatric Psychiatry, 11,* 33–45.

McCann, R., Ball, E., Ghanizadeh, H., Gallietta, M., & Froelich, R. (2002, November). *Forensic, correctional, and not-so-civil DBT: More data, more mountains to climb.* Panel conducted at the 36th annual convention of the Association for the Advancement of Behavior Therapy, Reno, NV.

Melia, K., & Wagner, A. W. (2000). The application of dialectical behavior therapy to the treatment of posttraumatic stress disorder. *National Center for Posttraumatic Stress Disorder Clinical Quarterly, 9,* 6–12.

Miller, A. L. (1999). Dialectical behavior therapy: A new treatment approach for suicidal adolescents. *American Journal of Psychotherapy, 53,* 413–417.

Miller, A. L., Wyman, S. E., Huppert, J. D., Glassman, S. L., & Rathus, J. H. (2000). Analysis of behavioral skills utilized by suicidal adolescents receiving dialectical behavior therapy. *Cognitive and Behavioral Practice, 7,* 183–187.

Palmer, R. L., Birchall, H., Damani, S., Gatward, N., McGrain, L., & Parker, L. (2003). A dialectical behavior therapy program for people with an eating disorder and borderline personality disorder: Description and outcome. *International Journal of Eating Disorders, 33,* 281–286.

Rathus, J. H., & Miller, A. L. (2002). Dialectical behavior therapy adapted for suicidal adolescents. *Suicide and Life-Threatening Behavior, 32,* 146–157.

Rizvi, S. L., & Linehan, M. M. (in press). The treatment of maladaptive shame in borderline personality disorder: A pilot study. *Cognitive and Behavioral Practice.*

Roemer, L., & Orsillo, S. M. (2002). Expanding our conceptualization of and treatment for generalized anxiety disorder: Integrating mindfulness/acceptance-based approaches with existing cognitive-behavioral models. *Clinical Psychology: Science and Practice, 9,* 54–68.

Rosen, G. M., & Davison, G. C. (2003). Psychology should list empirically supported principles of change (ESPs) and not credential trademarked therapies or other treatment packages. *Behavior Modification, 27,* 300–312.

Safer, D. L., Telch, C. F., & Agras, W. S. (2001). Dialectical behavior therapy for bulimia nervosa. *American Journal of Psychiatry, 158,* 632–634.

Segal, Z. V., Williams, J. M. G., & Teasdale, J. D. (2003). Mindfulness-based cognitive therapy for depression: A new approach to preventing relapse. *Psychotherapy Research, 13,* 123–125.

Soloff, P. H., Lynch, K. G., & Kelly, T. M. (2002). Childhood abuse as a risk factor for suicidal behavior in borderline personality disorder. *Journal of Personality Disorders, 16,* 201–214.

Tebartz van Elst, L., Hesslinger, B., Thiel, T., Geiger, E., Haegele, K., Lemieux, L., Lieb, K., Bohus, M., Hennig, J., & Ebert, D. (2003). Frontolimbic brain abnormalities in patients with borderline personality disorder: A volumetric magnetic resonance imagine study. *Biological Psychiatry, 54,* 163–171.

Telch, C. F., Agras, W. S., & Linehan, M. M. (2000). Group dialectical behavior therapy for binge-eating disorder: A preliminary, uncontrolled trial. *Behavior Therapy, 31,* 569–582.

Telch, C. F., Agras, W. S., & Linehan, M. M. (2001). Dialectical behavior therapy for binge eating disorder. *Journal of Consulting and Clinical Psychology, 69,* 1061–1065.

Trupin, E. W., Stewart, D. G., Beach, B., & Boesky, L. (2002). Effectiveness of dialectical behaviour therapy program for incarcerated female juvenile offenders. *Child and Adolescent Mental Health, 7,* 121–127.

Turner, R. M. (2000). Naturalistic evaluation of dialectical behavior therapy-oriented treatment for borderline personality disorder. *Cognitive and Behavioral Practice, 7,* 413–419.

Wagner, A. W. (2003). Cognitive-behavioral therapy for PTSD: Applications to injured trauma survivors. *Seminars in Neuropsychiatry, 8,* 175–187.

Wagner, A. W., & Linehan, M. M. (1997). The relationship between childhood sexual abuse and suicidal behaviors in borderline patients. In M. Zanarini (Ed.), *The role of sexual abuse in the etiology of borderline personality d isorder* (pp. 203–223). Washington, DC: American Psychiatric Press.

Wiser, S., & Telch, C. F. (1999). Dialectical behavior therapy for binge-eating disorder. *Journal of Clinical Psychology, 55,* 755–768.

Wisniewski, L., & Kelly, E. (2003). The application of dialectical behavior therapy to the treatment of eating disorders. *Cognitive and Behavioral Practice, 10,* 131–138.

Yehuda, R., & McFarlane, A. C. (Eds.). (1997). *Psychobiology of posttraumatic stress disorder: Annals of the New York Academy of Sciences* (Vol. 821). New York: New York Academy of Sciences.

Zlotnick, C., Mattia, J. I., & Zimmerman, M. (2001). The relationship between posttraumatic stress disorder, childhood trauma and alexithymia in an outpatient sample. *Journal of Traumatic Stress, 14,* 177–188.

CHAPTER SEVEN

Acceptance and Commitment Therapy in the Treatment of Posttraumatic Stress Disorder
Theoretical and Applied Issues

Robyn D. Walser
Steven C. Hayes

Acceptance and commitment therapy (ACT; Hayes, Strosahl, & Wilson, 1999) is a behaviorally based intervention designed to target and reduce experiential avoidance and cognitive entanglement while encouraging clients to make life-enhancing behavioral changes that are in accord with their personal values. Although ACT has been applied to a wide variety of problems, it is well suited to the treatment of trauma. Individuals who have been diagnosed with posttraumatic stress disorder (PTSD) are often disturbed by traumatic memories, nightmares, unwanted thoughts, and painful feelings. They are frequently working to avoid these experiences and the trauma-related situations or cues that elicit them. In addition to the symptoms of PTSD, the painful emotional experience and aftermath of trauma can often lead traumatized individuals to view themselves as "damaged" or "broken" in some important way. These difficult emotions and thoughts are associated with a variety of behavioral problems, from substance abuse to relationship problems.

Although most trauma survivors recover naturally without professional intervention, a small percentage develops problems in living and trauma-associated disorders. The job of the professional is to help these traumatized individuals heal from the effects of the traumatic experiences. The word "heal" comes from a word meaning "whole." In an important sense, the client has come to the therapist to be made "whole" once again. Often clients believe that healing somehow involves forgetting or getting away from past traumas—cutting them out of their lives. Clients may work to avoid all emotional, psychological, and physical experiences associated with the trauma. From an ACT perspective the task is very nearly the opposite. ACT helps clients make room for their difficult memories, feelings, and thoughts as they are directly experienced, and to include these experiences as part of a valued *whole* life.

EXPERIENTIAL AVOIDANCE, COGNITIVE FUSION, AND PTSD

The concept of experiential avoidance offers organization to the functional analysis of trauma-related problems and lends coherence to understanding the sequelae of trauma. Experiential avoidance occurs when an individual is unwilling to experience certain private events, such as negatively evaluated emotional states or thoughts and/or unpleasant physiological arousal, and then takes steps to alter the form or frequency of these events even when there is a behavioral "cost" to doing so (Hayes, Wilson, Gifford, Follette, & Strosahl, 1996). For example, a traumatized individual is engaging in experiential avoidance when he or she drinks alcohol to "drown" feelings of pain. From an ACT perspective, experiential avoidance is natural for human beings as evidenced by the fact that it is built into human language—"Figure out how to get rid of bad things and get rid of them"—but nevertheless it is often destructive. The problems with experiential avoidance as a course of action are the following:

1. If traumatized individuals experience feelings that they "cannot have," then, in one sense, there *is* something wrong; whole parts of their own experience must be denied.
2. Humans are very unsuccessful in deliberately eliminating automatic emotions and thoughts.
3. Many of the methods that can be used to skirt the effects of trauma (e.g., substance use, avoidance of situations that trigger the thought or feeling) are themselves destructive.

On the surface, avoidance maneuvers constitute attempts to be free from painful events. Unfortunately, the very inner state survivors are seeking—a sense of wholeness—can be lost in their efforts to avoid private experience (Walser & Hayes, 1998; Follette, 1994).

ACT theorists (e.g., Hayes et al., 1996) contend that experiential avoidance stems, in part, from human verbal behavior itself (the theory of verbal behavior upon which ACT is based is relational frame theory; see Hayes, Barnes-Holmes, & Roche, 2001). Language, and in particular self-talk, can play a critical role in moderating the damage caused directly by a traumatic event. As aversive experiences are described, categorized, and evaluated, the bidirectional nature of human language makes this process itself aversive (Hayes et al., 1999, 2001). For example, telling the story of a trauma evokes negative emotions and experiences. Furthermore, because verbal behavior can occur under virtually any context, unlike most other forms of behavior, the pain it produces cannot be regulated by avoiding situations per se. Left with seemingly no other alternative, humans attempt to regulate psychological pain not just by avoiding objectively aversive situations, but also by avoiding or suppressing negative private experiences themselves (e.g., trying to forget memories). This network of avoidance can expand almost indefinitely, depending on the different contexts that become directly or indirectly related to the painful private experiences (e.g., sexually traumatized individuals may initially have difficulty with romantic relationships following the trauma, but this circumscribed difficulty can then spread to avoidance of many other social situations).

The verbal aspect of the trauma experience has been addressed in the literature. Appraisals of a traumatic event as uncontrollable, unpredictable, and objectively dangerous help determine subsequent reactions to it (Foa, Zinbarg, & Rothbaum, 1992). Furthermore, individuals often feel the need to explain unusual, unwanted, or unexpected events and make causal attributions about them (Weiner, 1985, 1986). The nature of the individual's explanation will often influence how he or she responds to the event (Brewin, 2003; Shaver & Drown, 1986; Tennen & Affleck, 1990; Weiner, 1986).

Some of the key forms of verbal entanglement are captured in the acronym FEAR—fusion, evaluation, avoidance, and reason-giving (Hayes et al., 1999). "Cognitive fusion" refers to a process in which the regulatory power of verbal/cognitive stimuli dominate over other sources of behavioral influence. In this case, individuals view their thinking as literally reflecting truth, and they respond to their constructions of the world as if they *are* the world. For example, buying into the idea that "Deep down I am broken as a result of my trauma" can lead to a number of responses that are unhealthy. "Defusing" from this construction involves seeing the words for what they are—a set of words put together in a particular way—and then choosing to respond in a way that is healthy. "Evaluation" allows us to compare, make decisions, plan, and problem-solve, but it also allows us to judge, evaluate, and assess in unhealthy or unhelpful ways. For instance, an individual who is suffering as a result of childhood trauma can imagine what life might be like if he or she had not been traumatized. The evaluative result may be extensive and painful, as the person yearns for a different history or attempts to deny what history has led her or him to be—an individual with these kinds of unwanted memories. When these attempts to forget are unsuccessful, additional negative judgments about the self are likely to follow, such as labeling oneself as a "failure." Together fusion and evaluation lead readily to "avoidance," which is harmful for several reasons: It narrows the range of behaviors that can occur, prevents healthy forms of exposure, and strengthens responses that are problematic (e.g., avoidance of intimacy). Moreover, and paradoxically, efforts to change internal private events can be self-amplifying. For example, as we document later in this chapter, deliberate attempts to try *not* to think about something tend to bring the event to mind. A cycle of trying not to remember, followed by remembering, followed by trying not to remember may ensue. "Reason-giving"—giving verbal explanations for behavior (e.g., "I can't be in a relationship because I have PTSD")—further amplifies both avoidance and rigidity, and tends to make treatment more difficult because many important "reasons" are unlikely to change (e.g., if the reason for the action is a bad childhood, then some other childhood would seemingly be needed in order to act differently).

ACT targets experiential avoidance and cognitive fusion through acceptance and "defusion" techniques (i.e., mindfulness techniques, viewing thoughts as thoughts, observing personal emotional experience). Acceptance and defusion can create a new context within which the trauma survivor may view the world and the self. If thoughts are observed and noted rather than believed or disbelieved, and efforts to control private experience are relinquished as a means to mental health, then valued and life-enhancing behavioral change is much more likely.

EMPIRICAL RESEARCH: EXPERIENTIAL AVOIDANCE AND COGNITIVE FUSION

A number of empirical studies including an investigation of experiential avoidance and its impact are relevant to PTSD. We describe several areas of research that underscore the theory of experiential avoidance as a component of pathology. In addition, we discuss specific research related to the use of acceptance-based techniques and ACT in the treatment of stress-related symptoms and PTSD.

Avoidance, Fusion, and Pathology

Many of the problematic behaviors seen in PTSD may be the result of unhealthy avoidance strategies, fed by cognitive fusion. Steps taken to avoid experiential states may include directed thinking, rumination, and worry. These cognitive strategies are ways to distract oneself from current experience and the cognitive material associated with emotional content (Wells & Matthews, 1994). Worry and self-analysis seem to provide control over events but, in fact, have been shown to have minimal constructive benefit (Borkovec, Hazlett-Stevens, & Diaz, 1999) and may only serve to complicate psychological struggle. Numbing oneself to emotional responses or engaging in one type of emotional reaction as a way to avoid another (e.g., using anger to avoid hurt), and removing oneself from situations and personal interactions that elicit certain negative thoughts or emotions are all examples of avoidance maneuvers. A victim of trauma may spend large amounts of energy engaging in a number of these behaviors, avoiding feelings and thoughts associated with the trauma or activities that stimulate memories of the trauma (Shapiro & Dominiak, 1992). Avoidance and numbing are two of the more central aspects in a diagnosis of PTSD (American Psychiatric Association, 1994). Avoidance is not always negative, however. Some forms in some contexts may actually be healthy especially, if it is connected to more active methods of coping that help elaborate healthy repertoires, such as positive distraction. But if this coping process dominates, it may result in emotional numbness to cognitive and emotional material and may lead to prolonged problems.

Suppression

A possible result of suppression, a form of avoidance wherein individuals try to block out or inhibit thoughts or feelings, is the recurrence of intrusive traumatic cognitions (Clark, Ball, & Pape, 1991; Wegner, Shortt, Blake, & Page, 1990), which, as noted earlier in the chapter, may result in a paradoxical effect of amplification. Current research suggests that attempting to avoid or suppress unwanted negative thoughts, emotions, and memories as a means to create psychological health may actually contribute to a magnification of the negative emotional responses and thoughts, and to a longer period of experiencing those events (Wegner & Schneider, 2003; Wenzlaff & Wegner, 2000; Wegner, 1994; Cioffi & Holloway, 1993; Wegner & Zanakos, 1994). This means that suppression presents risks of amplification: Avoidance of thoughts increases their importance (a cognitive fusion process), which then increases their negative impact and induces further efforts to avoid them.

The effects of active suppression of unwanted private experience (e.g., unwanted thoughts or emotions) have been documented in many studies (Cioffi & Holloway, 1993; Clark et al., 1991; Kelly & Kahn, 1994; Muris, Merckelback, van den Hout, & de Jong, 1992; Salkovskis & Campbell, 1994; Walser, 1998; Wegner, 1994; Wegner, et al., 1990). The effects of long-term suppression have also been explored (Trinder & Salkovskis, 1994). These suppression effects, which are generally consistent, are explored briefly below.

Thought suppression studies (Macrae, Bodenhousen, Milne, & Jetten, 1994; Wegner, 1994; Wegner, Schneider, Carter, & White, 1987) indicate that subjects have a difficult time suppressing the unwanted thought and mention the thought frequently during suppression conditions. Subjects also report a conscious, effortful search for anything but the thought; however, these efforts to distract fail. The failure of these efforts may be due to the presence of an unusual sensitivity to the thought throughout periods of attempted suppression (Wegner, 1994). These findings support the notion that we are more likely to think of the very thing we would like to avoid.

Personally relevant intrusive thoughts, or unwanted thoughts that repeatedly come to mind (Edwards & Dickerson, 1987), such as recurring memories, images, evaluations, judgments, and so on, have also been investigated (Rachman & Hodgson, 1980; Salkovskis & Harrison, 1982). For instance, Salkovskis and Campbell (1994) found that suppression causes enhancement of personally relevant, negatively valenced intrusive thoughts. Trinder and Salkovskis (1994) found that subjects who were asked to suppress their negative intrusive thoughts experienced significantly more of those thoughts than subjects who were asked just to monitor their thoughts. In addition, the suppression group recorded significantly more discomfort with the negative intrusions than did subjects in the monitor only group.

Although personally relevant intrusive thoughts are quite common and are thought to occur in about 80% of the population (Rachman & de Silva, 1978), they appear to be particularly problematic for survivors of trauma. The suppression of disclosure about disturbing events, such as past trauma, has been linked to both psychological and physiological problems (Pennebaker, Hughes, & O'Heeron, 1987; Pennebaker & O'Heeron, 1984). Riggs, Dancu, Gershuny, Greenberg, and Foa (1992) have found that female crime victims who "hold in" their anger experience more severe PTSD symptoms. Roemer, Orsillo, Litz, and Wagner (2001) found that strategic withholding of emotions is associated with PTSD. The intrusive experience of emotion seen in PTSD can trigger an opposing process of denial or numbness (Horowitz, 1986), and numbness itself may be used as a way to avoid evocative stimuli (Keane, Fairbank, Caddell, Zimering, & Bender, 1985). This numbing, however, may lead to difficulties in emotional processing and maintenance of PTSD symptomatology (Wagner, Roemer, Orsillo, & Litz, 2003).

It makes sense that a trauma survivor would engage in behaviors to counteract or avoid traumatic thoughts and the emotions that may be associated with them, given the aversiveness of the traumatic event. Furthermore, there is considerable evidence that people attempt to suppress thoughts when they are traumatized (Pennebaker & O'Heeron, 1984; Silver, Boon, & Stones, 1983), obsessed (Rachman & de Silva, 1978), anxious (Wegner et al., 1990), or depressed (Sutherland, Newman, & Rachman, 1982; Wenzlaff & Wegner, 1990). However, as noted earlier, efforts at control of one's mood may paradoxically cause the mood to continue and may also lead to the execution of many maladaptive behaviors, such as alcohol use or binge eating (Herman & Polivy, 1993).

Finally, recycling through a process of suppression, with recurrence of emotion and thought countered by further attempts at suppression, could well produce undesirable internal experience that is fairly robust (Wegner et al., 1990). Suppression of thought and emotion may be a part of the development of such disorders as PTSD, depression, anxiety, and panic. What individuals believe to be the antidote may actually be the venom that produces the very problem, further contributing to their distress. Individuals who use suppression and avoidance may actually be generating an assortment of unwanted consequences and problems because of the strategy.

Research that focuses on self-disclosure of traumatic events—a process of talking openly about the trauma without attempts to suppress—has found that disclosure is associated with lower levels of psychological distress and increased ability to care for oneself (Lepore, Silver, Wortman, & Wayment, 1996; Pennebaker & Harber, 1993). In addition, self-disclosure can elicit the emotions associated with the negative event, thus facilitating a possible decrease in, via exposure to, the negative emotion. In other words, being present to, rather than avoiding, the emotional content of trauma may be the healthier avenue. For example, Bolten, Glenn, Orsillo, Roemer, and Litz (2003) found that self-disclosure is associated with lower levels of PTSD symptom severity. Verbal and emotional processing of the traumatic event has also been theorized to be an effective treatment for PTSD. This type of processing includes a full experiencing of the traumatic memory and associated emotions, followed by habituation to the emotions and thoughts (Foa & Rothbaum, 1998). Emotional engagement, rather than emotional avoidance or numbing, appears to be a key ingredient (Jaycox, Foa, & Morral, 1998). Acceptance of previously avoided experiences may have a powerful impact in moving traumatized individuals toward healthy and valued living.

Acceptance, Defusion, and Mindfulness

Mindfulness is traditionally defined as nonjudgmental awareness of, and contact with, the current moment (Kabat-Zinn, 1990). It involves openness to experience and recognition that thoughts and feelings are passing events that do not need to be acted upon. From an ACT point of view, mindfulness involves four key processes (Hayes, 2004): acceptance of experience, defusion from the literal meaning of thought (e.g., observing the thought as a thought, not as what it says it is), continuous contact with the present moment, and a transcendent sense of self. Mindfulness techniques, which generally foster all of these processes, provide a context in which the client can experience internal private events in the moment—that is, observing them as something the mind does without necessarily treating these events as reality. Practicing mindfulness provides exposure to emotion while simultaneously reducing experiential avoidance and demonstrating that emotional events themselves are not harmful. For example, to be aware of feelings of sadness or anxiety, without attempting to avoid or extinguish them, can help individuals learn more about emotional experience and come to realize that it does not have to rule action. That is, clients can learn to be present to emotions, even negatively evaluated ones, and continue to behave in ways that promote health and relationship.

ACT uses mindfulness techniques and also directly targets components of mindfulness. For example, ACT exercises are used to help distinguish between a person as a continuous process or locus of awareness and what the person is aware of (Hayes, 1994). That is, the person can locate a sense of "I" that observes and can learn to view experience as an ongoing process. Any or all things can be experienced in this moment and may be argued to be limitless and therefore not thing-like. It is a clinically important sense of self because it is not threatened by psychological content: Any content, whether "good" or "bad," is experienced from the point of view of "this moment," and given that experience is an ongoing process, it is continuously changing. Finding and experiencing a sense of self as a context for events, rather than allowing the events to determine the context and outcome, thus supports acceptance, defusion, and other ACT processes.

ACT: CLINICAL APPLICATION

Assessment

Assessment methods focus on the goals of change in ACT: facilitating acceptance, defusion, values, and committed action. We review both clinically useful and research-capable assessment types in this section. We do not address assessment of PTSD per se; for that see Pratt, Brief, and Keane, Chapter 3, this volume.

The Acceptance and Action Questionnaire (AAQ; Hayes, Strosahl, et al., 2004c; Bond & Bunce, 2003) is a self-report measure that attempts to assess several of the key features of ACT and its underlying model. Items focus on experiential control, psychological acceptance, and taking action despite experience of aversive private events. Respondents report the extent to which each statement applies to them with higher scores indicating greater experiential avoidance.

There are three validated versions of the AAQ: a nine-item single-factor scale (Hayes, Bissett, et al., 2004a), a very similar 16-item single-factor scale (Hayes et al., 2004c), and a two-factor 16-item scale (Bond & Bunce, 2003). All versions have adequate psychometric properties. More impressive are their operational characteristics. The AAQ correlates in the expected direction with most measures of psychopathology, including depression, anxiety, overall psychiatric severity, and the like (Hayes et al., 2004c). It also predicts quality of life (Hayes et al., 2004c), flexibility at work (Bond & Bunce, 2003), and response to treatments and challenges of various kinds.

The AAQ has been used in studies of trauma and its effects. Marx and Sloan (2002) have shown that self-report measures of childhood sexual abuse (CSA), experiential avoidance, and emotional expressivity are all significantly related to psychological distress. However, only experiential avoidance mediated the relationship between CSA and current distress. Similarly, Marx and Sloan (2005) showed the same in a population of 185 trauma survivors who were assessed for peritraumatic dissociation, experiential avoidance (using the AAQ), and PTSD symptom severity. Both peritraumatic dissociation and experiential avoidance were significantly related to PTSD symptoms at baseline. After the initial levels of PTSD were taken into account, only experiential avoidance was related to PTSD symptoms both 4 and 8 weeks later.

Existing measures of coping styles can be used in an ACT-consistent fashion. There is a significant relationship between methods of coping and certain forms of symptomatology (Abramsom, Seligman, & Teasdale, 1978; Fondacaro & Moos, 1987), many of which are included in the diagnosis of PTSD. The Ways of Coping Questionnaire (WOC; Folkman & Lazarus, 1988), a widely used research instrument for assessing coping strategies, and the Coping Inventory for Stressful Situations (CISS; Endler & Parker, 1994) are both useful instruments that tap into emotion-focused or avoidant strategies. They assess a wide range of thoughts and behaviors that individuals use to deal with stressful life experiences. Three dominant means of coping with stressful situations have been identified; task-oriented, emotion-oriented (Folkman & Lazarus, 1988), and avoidance-oriented (Endler & Parker, 1994). "Task-oriented coping" refers to the attainment of problem resolution through conscious efforts to solve or modify the situation. "Emotion-oriented coping" is defined by a set of reactions, such as tension and anger, of a self-oriented nature that occurs in response to a problematic event. "Avoidance-oriented coping" involves responses that have the effect of distracting or diverting the individual's attention away from the stressful situation (Turner, King, & Tremblay, 1992).

The Emotional Approach Coping (EAC) scale is an eight-item measure developed to assess two aspects of emotional coping: emotional processing (four items) and emotional expression (four items; Stanton, Kirk, Cameron, & Danoff-Burg, 2000). Items are rated on a 4-point Likert scale (from 1, "I usually don't do this at all," to 4, "I usually do this a lot") to determine how often various emotionally based strategies are used to cope with a stressful situation. Psychometric properties of the EAC are strong (Stanton et al., 2000). The questions on the scale include items such as "I acknowledge my emotions" and "I take time to figure out what I am really feeling." This instrument is short and easy to administer, and it can provide a quick snapshot of the individual's style of emotional processing and expression.

Other instruments that more directly assess avoidance and cognition include the White Bear Suppression Inventory (WBSI; Wegner & Zanakos, 1994) and the Automatic Thoughts Questionnaire (ATQ; Kendall & Hollon, 1980). The WBSI is a self-report instrument designed to assess thought suppression—that is, an individual's reported level of desire or ability to successfully avoid a thought (Wegner & Zanakos, 1994). Respondents report the extent to which each of 15 statements applies to them, using a 5-point Likert scale, with higher scores indicating increased desire to suppress. However, recent studies suggest that the WBSI does not exclusively measure thought suppression, but also addresses the experience of intrusive thoughts. Hence, the WBSI does not seem to measure suppression, per se, but rather the failure to suppress (Rassin, 2003). In a recent study, one factor of the WBSI was interpreted as "unwanted intrusive thoughts," the other as "thought suppression." The full scale's correlation with measures of depression, anxiety, and obsessive–compulsive behaviour was largely due to the unwanted intrusive thoughts factor, rather than the thought suppression factor. Neither factor correlated with self-disclosure. The theoretical meaning of separating thought intrusions from thought suppression may play an important role in assessment and research.

Recently, measures of thought control have also emerged as useful assessment tools. One of these measures, the Thought Control Questionnaire (TCQ; Wells & Davies, 1994), was designed to assess strategies that are used to control unpleasant or unwanted thoughts. Wells and Davies (1994) studied the relationship between the use of different strategies of control and measures of stress vulnerability and psychopathology. In factor analyses of the TCQ the authors found five replicable factors: distraction, social control, worry, punishment, and reappraisal. Associations were also found between assessment of emotional vulnerability and perceptions of weakened control over cognitions and the punishment and worry subscales of the TCQ.

Mindfulness measures may prove useful in assessing level of awareness to current experience and ACT-consistent behavior. The Kentucky Inventory of Mindfulness Skills (KIMS; Baer, Smith, & Cochran, 2004) is a 39-item self-report measure that is designed to assess general tendency toward mindfulness in daily life and includes four areas of mindfulness skills: observing, describing, acting with awareness, and accepting without judgment. The KIMS has been found to have high internal consistency and adequate to good test–retest reliability (Baer et al., 2004).

A second mindfulness measure is the Mindfulness Attention Awareness Scale (MAAS; Brown & Ryan, 2003). This is a recently developed 15-item measure that uses a Likert-style self-report format to assess a single factor of mindfulness. The MAAS items generally focus on the presence or absence of attention to the present moment and include questions such as "I find it difficult to stay focused on what is happening in the present," "I rush through activities without really being attentive to them," and "I do jobs or tasks automatically without being aware of what I am doing." Most of the questions appear to be assessing level of attention to specific tasks. The MAAS has been shown to be a reliable and valid instrument for use in student and adult populations.

One of the most important aspects of assessment in the ACT approach investigates individuals' degree of commitment and action. Individuals who have been diagnosed with PTSD are often not living the lives they would like to be living and are inactive around a number of important values. Assessing how well or poorly clients are functioning in relation to their values in a number of areas lends support to a specific target of intervention when using ACT and lends support to the effectiveness of the treatment. The Valued Living Questionnaire (VLQ; Wilson & Groom, 2002; Wilson &

Murrell, 2004) is a 20-item assessment instrument that evaluates both the importance of a particular value plus the degree to which the value is being practiced in an individual's life. Ten different domains are assessed: Family (other than marriage or parenting), Marriage/couples/intimate relations, Parenting, Friends/social life, Work, Education/training, Recreation/fun, Spirituality, Citizenship/community life, and Physical Self-Care (diet, exercise, sleep). The psychometric properties of the VLQ are currently under investigation; in our experience, it is a useful clinical tool that guides both clinicians and clients with respect to importance of and degree of consistent action with specified values. A second clinical assessment of values is also possible. The Values and Goals Worksheet (see Figure 7.1) includes clients' personal definition of their values, goals related to achieving greater degrees of success in living those values, barriers or reasons the values are not being lived, and current level of success in living particular values.

Guidelines for Client Selection

ACT can be used with a variety of clients and clinical presentations, with no specific limitations to its use. However, it is most useful when applied with clients who are assessed to be emotionally avoidant and/or cognitively fused, have chronic conditions, or who have multiple treatment failures. ACT has been demonstrated to be effective when used in the treatment of PTSD (Follette et al., 1993; Walser, Loew, Westrup, Gregg, & Rogers, 2003a; Walser, Westrup, Rogers, Gregg, & Loew, 2003b; Batten & Hayes, 2005), anxiety and stress (Bond & Bunce, 2000; Twohig & Woods, 2004; Zettle, 2003), substance abuse/dependence (Gifford et al., 2004; Hayes et al., 2002), coping with positive psychotic symptoms (Bach & Hayes, 2002), chronic pain (Dahl, Wilson, & Nilsson, 2004; McCracken, Vowles, & Eccleston, 2004), stigma and prejudice in drug abuse counselors (Hayes et al., 2004a), depression (Folke & Parling, 2004; Zettle & Hayes, 1986; Zettle & Raines, 1989), self-management of diabetes (Gregg, 2004), and a variety of other conditions (see Hayes, Masuda, Bissett, Luoma, & Guerrero, 2004b, for a recent review). There are also effectiveness data for ACT. Strosahl, Hayes, Bergan, and Romano (1998) found that training clinicians in ACT produced better overall clinical outcomes in a general clinical practice in a managed care setting.

When selecting clients for ACT who have experienced trauma or who have already been diagnosed with PTSD, there are a number of points to keep in mind. First, the client must be ready (i.e., able to commit to a number of sessions) and willing to undergo an intensive therapy in which the therapist is quite active in session. Second, if the client has problems that would be better treated by a different approach (according to the literature), this approach needs to be implemented first or integrated into the course of ACT. For example, if the client has borderline personality disorder, dialectical behavior therapy should be implemented initially, with ACT brought in during later stages. Finally, a functional analysis of the case should fit the

Instructions: Below is a list of life areas in which most people have important goals and values. That is, there is usually something important in these areas that most people are trying to achieve in their lives. Values are very subjective, and what may be important to you is not necessarily important to someone else. In each area, please write down the values that you have. Try to describe your values as if no one would ever read this worksheet. This is not a test to see if you have the "correct" values. Try to think in terms of both concrete goals and values that are important to you. In terms of goals, we are not asking what you think you could realistically get, or what you or others think you deserve. We want to know what YOU care about what you would want to work toward in life.

How successful are you in living your values? Use the scale below and write down the number in the column provided.

| Not at all successful = 1 | Somewhat successful = 2 | Moderately successful = 3 | Successful = 4 | Very successful = 5 |

Values	Describe your personal values	List several concrete goals	Reasons that values are not being lived	Success in living out values
Relationships (intimate, marriage, couples, families)				
Friendships/ social relations				
Employment/ education/ training				
Recreation/ citizenship				
Spirituality				
Physical well-being				

FIGURE 7.1. Values and Goals Worksheet.

ACT model (e.g., the presenting issue is one of emotional or experiential avoidance, cognitive fusion, lack of clarity about values, and so on).

Overview of Treatment Approach: Acceptance Theory and Intervention

The following section provides detailed information about how to use ACT in a clinical setting. There are several main goals that are generally presented in order when using ACT. This is not to say, however, that the ACT goals cannot be presented in a different order, or that the ACT therapist cannot choose to emphasize one goal over another, depending on the client's specific issues. ACT is diverse and flexible and allows for a range of concepts to be presented depending on client needs. Here we focus on main goals, using clinical examples of issues related to PTSD and trauma. For a more comprehensive presentation of ACT interventions, see Hayes et al., 1999; Hayes and Strosahl, 2005.

The acronym "ACT," while standing for the name of the therapy, also represents key issues in the approach: Accept, Choose, and Take Action. The premise involves a conscious abandonment of the mental and emotional change agenda when change efforts have not worked, replacing it with emotional and social acceptance—openness to one's own emotions and the experience of others (Hayes, 1994). This form of acceptance is applied to the domain of private subjective events and experiences, not to overt behavior or changeable situations (Greenberg, 1994). For instance, when speaking directly of trauma, the therapist using ACT would not encourage a client to stay engaged and "just accept" an abusive situation. Rather, the client would be encouraged to experience emotional processing while engaging in practical, safe, and valued behavior that may include getting out of the situation. Thus, as the very name suggests, ACT involves a focus on both acceptance *and* change.

The element of choosing or choice relates specifically to the client's ability to recognize a valued direction and engage in the required action. Although in tremendous pain, clients usually have a sense of what is important or what matters in their lives. Frequently, however, these valued goals have been lost or given up due to thoughts, feelings, or states of experience that tell the client that he or she cannot have those valued things until certain thoughts, feelings, or memories change or go away. For instance, the sexual abuse survivor may have the thought that she was damaged by the abuse and therefore is unable to engage in romantic relationships until the "damagedness" goes away. Sometimes the client will be in such pain that the idea of a meaningful, intimate relationship will rarely be contacted. Inside the pain there is a strand that leads back to values and choice; however, because the very pain of "damagedness" implies a desire for intimacy.

There are six essential components of ACT (Hayes, 2004), which are shown graphically in Figure 7.2: (1) acceptance, (2) defusion, (3) self as context, (4) committed action, (5) values, and (6) contact with the present moment. The figure helps note the relationship between these six processes. Defusion and acceptance both involve a release of excessive literalness, or "letting go"; self as context and contact with the present moment both involve verbal and nonverbal aspects of contacting the "here and now" as a conscious human being; values and committed action both involve positive uses of language to choose and complete courses of action ("getting moving in life"). The hexagram in Figure 7.2 can be sliced into two larger sections that define ACT more broadly. The first section (see Figure 7.3) describes

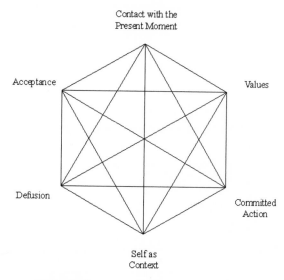

FIGURE 7.2. The ACT model: hexaflex.

the acceptance and mindfulness processes included in ACT, and the second section (see Figure 7.4) describes the commitment and behavior change processes in ACT. The main goal of ACT is to create psychological flexibility: that is, contacting the present moment fully, as a conscious human being with a history, and based on what the situation affords, changing or persist-

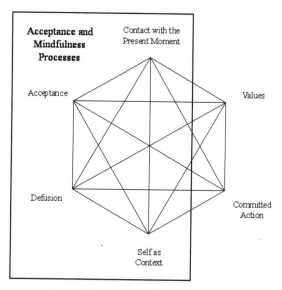

FIGURE 7.3. Acceptance and mindfulness processes of the ACT model.

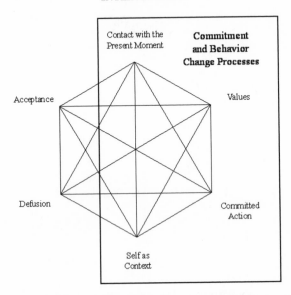

FIGURE 7.4. Commitment and behavior change processes of the ACT model.

ing in behavior in the service of chosen values. This goal is embodied in the following question and is illustrated graphically in Figure 7.5 on top of the hexagram: "Given a distinction between you and the things you are struggling with and trying to change, are you willing to have those things, fully and without defense, as they are, and not as what they say they are, *and* do what takes you in the direction of your chosen values at this time, in this situation? We briefly review the goals of ACT below and show how acceptance might be integrated into a treatment approach for trauma.

The first goal of ACT is to foster a state of *creative hopelessness* (Hayes et al., 1999). This state emerges when clients recognize the unworkability of their efforts to rid themselves of negative emotional content and begin to open up to the possibility of truly new ways of living. Typically clients feel that if they had had a different history (one without sexual abuse, disaster trauma, or war trauma), then their problems would be solved and they would no longer be in emotional turmoil; they would feel better. However, as they repeatedly try this line of thinking as a solution to their discomfort, the behavioral relevance of their painful history is only magnified, and they must search for still more "solutions." In ACT, the solutions the client has been trying are viewed as part of the problem. Metaphors are often used to demonstrate the client's situation:

THERAPIST: Here is a metaphor that will help you understand what I am saying. Imagine you are blindfolded and given a bag of tools and told to run through a large field. So there you are, living your life and running through the field. However, unknown to you, there are large holes in this field, and sooner or later you fall in. Now remember you were blindfolded, so you didn't fall in on purpose; it is not your fault that you fell in. You are not responsible for being in the hole. You want to get out, so you open your bag of tools and find that the only tool is a shovel. So you begin to dig. And you dig. But digging is the thing that makes holes. So you try other things, like figuring out exactly how you fell in the hole, but that doesn't help you get out. Even if you knew every step that you took to get into the hole, it would not help you to get out of it. So you dig differently. You dig fast, you dig slow. You take big scoops, and you take little scoops. And you're still not out. Finally, you think you need to get a "really great shovel," and that is why you are here to see me. Maybe I have a gold-plated shovel. But I don't, and even if I did, I wouldn't give it to you. Shovels don't get people out of holes—they make them.

CLIENT: So what is the solution? Why should I even come here?

THERAPIST: I don't know, but it is not to help you dig your way out. Perhaps we should start with what your experience tells you; that what you have been doing hasn't been working. And what I am going to ask you to consider is that what you have been doing can't work. Until you open up to that reality, that bottom line, you will never let go of the shovel

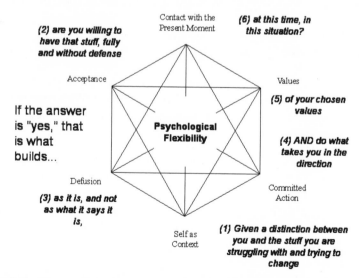

FIGURE 7.5. The "ACT question" as it relates to the ACT model: (1) Given the distinction between you and the things you are struggling with and trying to change, (2) are you willing to have those things, fully and without defense, (3) as they are, and not as what they say they are, (4) *and* do what takes you in the direction (5) of your chosen values (6) at this time, in this situation?

because as far as you know, it's the only thing you've got. But until you let go of it, you can't take hold of anything else.

As a therapist working with trauma survivors, it is very important to take extra care that the client does not feel blamed when working on this goal. When clients are told that they are responsible for their "digging," they can easily misunderstand the message as one of blame. It is important to acknowledge, as the metaphor makes clear, that it is not the client's fault that he or she fell into the hole and that given this circumstance, he or she is responding in the only way he or she knows how. Responsibility is couched as the "ability to respond," an opening up to opportunities to do things differently.

The therapist should always operate from a place of compassion for clients' situations and the struggles in which have been engaging. At this early point in therapy, it also helps to explain to trauma survivors that it is the *agenda* that is not working; the clients themselves, and their lives, can experience all possibilities, based on what they choose to do from here. This point may take some special emphasis in the case of clients who have been diagnosed with chronic PTSD. These individuals often evaluate themselves as hopeless, in the usual sense of that term, and do not yet have the tools to turn this perception into an incentive for positive action. Understanding this perspective comes later in the therapy. At times, when it seems relevant to the situation, we will say that we do have hope for the possibility of a better life for the client. Thus paradoxically the actual emotion most commonly felt in this phase of therapy is relief/hope.

Gaining an understanding that *control of private events is the problem* (Hayes et al., 1999) is the second goal of ACT. Attempts to exert emotional and cognitive control are explored as barriers to successful solutions to clients' problems in living; that is, conscious, purposeful efforts to get rid of, escape, or avoid negative thoughts and feelings actually may be preventing clients from behaving in ways that are consistent with what they value, and may be exacerbating the very events they are trying to control. If a trauma survivor is trying to escape something, a specific memory, perhaps, then (1) that is what the client is doing rather than some other, more productive form of action; and he or she has the added problem that (2) the memories are likely to increase in frequency and negative impact.

This stage of therapy focuses on how efforts to control may not only prove ineffective but may even lead to increased difficulty. One of the metaphors introduced by the therapist that points to this issue is as follows:

"Are you familiar with the Chinese finger trap? This toy is a tube generally made of straw. You place your two index fingers in the tube and then try to pull them out. What happens is that the more you pull, the tighter the straw tube clamps down on your fingers, making it virtually impossible to escape the trap. The more effort you put into escaping, the more uncomfortable you feel—the more trapped you become. Trying to escape negative emotional experience can work like a Chinese finger trap. The harder you try not to have the emotions, the more the emotions "clamp" down on you. Examples of this kind of problem include excessive drinking to escape anxiety. Now you not only have the problem of anxiety, but you also have the problem of excessive drinking and all that that brings with it."

One important note here is that many trauma survivors are triggered by issues related to control, and much of what they are trying to do involves getting back in control of their disrupted or chaotic lives. Many traumas occur under circumstances in which there is loss of a personal sense of control. Therapists hear clients report that they "just want to get their lives back." An important message to give is that ACT therapists are not asking clients to give up control, as it is viewed culturally, but rather they are asking clients to give up control of their internal experience so that they can regain—or gain for the first time—control of their lives.

Distinguishing "I" as content from "I" as context is the third goal (Hayes et al., 1999). In this phase of therapy, the goal is to create a place in which clients can learn to see themselves as context rather than content, which, in turn, defuses the literal content of their self-talk. It is from the position of "I" that clients, and all of us, struggle; that is, it is as if the words that a person says or thinks and the actual person become fused. For example, when thinking "I am bad" from the position of self-as-content, the statement is experienced as an actual truth rather than as just a thought about oneself. From this self-as-content position, the client has to fight against feeling "bad" *in essence*. Now, suppose that "I am bad" could be viewed as a passing thought with which the client did not have to identify; rather, he or she could "deliteralize" or become "de-fused" from the thought. In the ACT approach, this defusion is only likely from an experiential perspective in which "I" is equated with an ongoing awareness (context). Much like a walking mediation, ACT attempts to establish a place from which abandonment of control is not threatening, because the private events are mere content, not "who you are."

There are three aspects of the self that are important to this issue and that can be addressed in ACT sessions. First is the conceptualized self, which is created by our ability to interact verbally with ourselves and others. We can categorize, evaluate, explain, rationalize, and so on. This is what might be called "self as content," a conceptualized self that we create verbally to make sense of ourselves, our history, and our behavior. A problematic issue occurs in this area when we hold the content of this conceptualized self to be literally true. If a person makes the comment "I am messed up because I was abused as a child," the problem to be solved becomes unworkable because no other childhood will occur. Therefore, acceptance of the conceptualized self, held literally, is not desirable.

The second self is the self as a process of knowing. We know about ourselves and can respond to others about our feelings and reactions. This knowing is valuable in terms of socialization and civilization. Through a process of training, we can report when we are hungry or when we are in pain, and so on. We can categorize our own and others' behavior based on this process. When a person's training in this kind of knowledge is deviant, then he or she may not know how to behave in relation to the social environment. For instance, suppose a young boy is sexually abused and his reactions to the abuse are ignored, denied, or reinterpreted. This type of developmental history could set the stage for a person to be unable to know or report to others accurately what he or she is feeling. One can imagine other histories where the process of accurately describing or expressing feelings appropriately is inhibited. Given this kind of history, ACT seeks to reorient the client to a process of knowing that includes both historical and current experience. One can observe oneself or see oneself as a process of ongoing behavior. Helping the client to identify current emotion and thought states is a helpful step toward the goals of mindfulness and acceptance.

The third sense of self is self as context. This is the self in which "I" is the place from which an individual responds verbally. It is the sense of one's own perspective or point of view. This self is consistent and present at all times. If we ask you questions about yourself, you *always* answer from your perspective. The content of your answers will change; however, the context from which you answer does not.

It is not too difficult to help clients experience this sense of connection to self as context. Localizing past memories and events as well as current situations easily puts the client in contact with this sense of "I." The only reasonable thing to do is to engage self as context, because much verbal behavior is based upon it, and we cannot function effectively as nonverbal organisms. It is also this form of self that allows other forms of acceptance. If self as context is always present, various kinds of content may come and go, but a stable sense of "I" will remain. In this state a person may experience pain or horrible memories, but they do not make the person literally those experiences. They too shall pass as new content emerges, but the sense of "I" will remain unchanged.

In the ACT approach, many techniques are used to deliteralize language and establish self as context. These include (1) imagery exercises in which thoughts are allowed to flow as leaves on streams, without being "bought," believed, adopted, or rejected; (2) repeating thoughts rapidly for dozens or hundreds of times; the thought thereby loses its meaning and allows the client to see it for what it is—a sound or thought; (3) use of imagery exercises that turn emotions and thoughts into objects to be viewed and inspected— private experiences are given shapes, sizes, colors, and so on; and (4) extensive use of metaphor. An example of a useful metaphor is the chessboard (adapted from Hayes et al., 1999, pp. 190–191):

"Imagine a chessboard that goes out infinitely in all directions. It's covered with black pieces and white pieces. They work together in teams, as in chess—the white pieces fight against the black pieces. You can think of your thoughts and feelings and beliefs as these pieces; they sort of hang out together in teams too. For example, 'bad' feelings (such as anxiety, depression, and resentment) hang out with 'bad' thoughts and 'bad' memories. Same thing with 'good' ones. Now in the game of chess the goal is to win the war. So it seems that the thing to do is to defeat the team that you don't like or want. So you get upon the pieces that are 'good'—and the battle begins. You work hard to kick the 'bad' pieces off the board. But there is a big problem here—huge pieces of yourself are your own enemy. And what you find as you engage the battle is that the pieces never leave the board; remember, it stretches out infinitely in all directions. So you fight harder. And if you fight hard and long enough, your life becomes a battle to *not* have what this game has to offer. You have the sense that you can't win and you can't stop fighting. If you are focused on the piece level, a move-by-move battle seems the only thing to do. However, there is another place to focus in this game. Do you know what it is? The board level—the board holds all the pieces but it doesn't have to be invested in the battle at all. And notice that the board is not the pieces. You are not your content."

The concept of self as context can prove difficult for some clients. Therapists may encounter clients who report that they have no sense of self. For instance, women who were sexually abused as children (often being revictimized) may have a difficult time locating the sense of self that experiences emotions and thoughts. That is, their sense of self has been so shattered by historical events that they glean who they are only from others or have difficulty viewing themselves as separate entities. The therapist can work with these clients to reestablish a sense of self that is continuous and can observe personal behavior, including thoughts and feelings. At relevant times the therapist can ask "Who is saying this right now?" "Who is this person in the room talking with me? And can that person see that you are talking to me?" The therapist, then, begins to help the client reconnect to that observer self through gentle questioning. It is not too difficult to help clients experience this sense of connection to self as context. Localizing past memories and events and current situations easily puts the client in contact with this sense of "I." It is also this form of self that allows other forms of acceptance. The client may experience difficult memories or pain, but that does not make the client literally those experiences. They too shall pass and new content will be present, but, as noted, the sense of "I" will remain.

There are also clients who are overidentified with their sense of self. For instance, many Vietnam veterans who have chronic PTSD strongly identify themselves as "Vietnam veterans," along with all of the cultural characteristics that accompany that identity. This identity is tightly held and seems to define the individual at nearly all levels of personal existence. Here the ACT therapist can work with the client on the conceptualized self or the self as content. Both self-as-context and deliteralization techniques are useful when addressing this issue.

Letting go of the struggle is the fourth goal of ACT (Hayes et al., 1999). In this stage of therapy the client is encouraged to let go of the agenda of control. This stage is a "willingness move"; that is, the client is asked to be willing to have whatever thoughts, feelings, memories, or bodily sensations that might show up without having to gain control over them. He or she simply experiences them for what they are. Private events are brought into the therapy room and dissembled into component pieces (e.g., thoughts, memories, feelings). The goal is *not* to gain control but to experience without attempts to escape or modify. Many "willingness exercises" are used at this point and generally include imagery and experiential exercises. When working with a trauma survivor in this phase, a great deal of emotional exposure is done.

The fifth goal of ACT is *making a commitment to valued action* and behavior change (Hayes et al., 1999). It is at this point in therapy that clients commit to engaging in actions that are specific to their chosen values and goals. Through previous work, the client has acquired the ability to discriminate between unworkable solutions to a problem (i.e., control and avoidance of emotions) and workable solutions (e.g., commitment to behavior change). The client can begin to lead a valued life and choose directions that support that life. In this phase of therapy with a trauma survivor, the issues turn from making room for one's own history to creating a valued life. For example, concrete steps to develop more productive relationships might be taken, while simultaneously monitoring inner responses to prevent needless struggles with private experiences that might arise.

Common Treatment Obstacles and Possible Solutions

There are three areas in which therapists generally make mistakes when using acceptance-based approaches. First, and specifically with ACT therapy, it is very easy to get caught up in the content of what the client has to say, and therapy can be derailed when this happens. It is critical to maintain a focus on context by asking the client to notice the content and process of his or her private experience on a frequent basis. The therapist should also take notice at those times of her or his own experience, in the sense of being mindful of the ongoing process. This perspective or frame helps create a sense of distance and objectivity toward the content at issue.

A second issue that is particularly crucial in the treatment of trauma survivors pertains to nonacceptance versus acceptance of history. We are not asking clients to accept what has happened to them in an overt behavioral sense. Rather, clients are being asked to embrace those aspects of themselves that they have been trying to cut off. It is not a move in which clients are asked to "like" their history, but a move to hold it for what it is—a memory or thought.

That is, clients' histories can inform them rather than "drive" them. Finally, as stated before, acceptance of private events does not mean acceptance of behavior. Behavior that is harmful or unhealthy is not the kind of acceptance we mean. This distinction should be made clear to the client repeatedly.

Third, the role of personal responsibility in therapy with trauma survivors needs careful attention. As mentioned, it is important to couch responsibility as an "ability to respond," ability to take action. The therapist must be careful not to make the client feel blamed for the trauma when talking about responsibility. Furthermore, if the therapist is not operating from a place of compassion for the client's dilemma, the client can easily be made to feel "wrong" about trying to control his or her private experience. From an ACT standpoint, "right" and "wrong" are also seen as content and not necessarily useful for progress. Essentially, there is only one way for the therapist to participate honestly, and that is to also be experientially willing with respect to their own emotional and psychological content.

Summary

We cannot expunge our private experiences or histories (Hayes, 1994). The difficult part about this reality is that some people have traumatic events that have occurred in their history, and these events may play a negative role in current situations. In addition, as a result of our ability to construct events verbally, we can compare ourselves to an ideal self and imagine that if our history had only been different, we might be able to become that ideal (Hayes, 1994). Trauma survivors often imagine that if their history were different, or if they could change their attitude about their history, they would not currently be experiencing PTSD or trauma-related problems. However, history is additive, and we can only build it from where we are at the moment, and simply having positive psychological reactions to negative experiences does not mean that a difficult psychological history will be removed (Hayes, 1994). The solution is to build a positive history from this moment forward, *with* all of our past experiences in tow. It is a willingness to have all aspects of the self, including the "good" and the "bad." It is an acceptance of private events in conjunction with directed action. Under these conditions, the trauma survivor can begin to live a valued life *with* the history rather than living a life *driven by* the history.

REFERENCES

Abramsom, L. Y., Seligman, M. E. P., & Teasdale, J. (1978). Learned helplessness in humans: Critique and reformulation. *Journal of Abnormal Psychology, 87,* 49–74.

American Psychiatric Association. (1994). *Diagnostic and statistical manual of mental disorders* (4th ed.). Washington, DC: Author.

Anderson, G., Yasenik, L., & Ross, C. A. (1993). Dissociative experiences and disorders among women who identify themselves as sexual abuse survivors. *Child Abuse and Neglect, 17,* 677–686.

Bach, P., & Hayes, S. C. (2002). The use of acceptance and commitment therapy to prevent the rehospitalization of psychotic patients: A randomized controlled trial. *Journal of Consulting and Clinical Psychology, 70*(5), 1129–1139.

Baer, R. A., Smith, G. T., & Cochran, K. B. (2004). Assessment of mindfulness by self-report: The Kentucky Inventory of Mindfulness Skills. *Assessment, 11,* 191–206.

Batten, S. V., & Hayes, S. C. (2005). Acceptance and commitment therapy in the treatment of co-morbid substance abuse and posttraumatic stress disorder: A case study. *Clinical Case Studies.*

Bolten, E. E., Glenn, D. M., Orsillo, S., Roemer, L., & Litz, B. T. (2003). The relationship between self-disclosure and symptoms of posttraumatic stress disorder in peacekeepers deployed to Somalia. *Journal of Traumatic Stress, 16,* 203–210.

Bond, F. W., & Bunce, D. (2000). Mediators of change in emotion-focused and problem-focused worksite stress management interventions. *Journal of Occupational Health Psychology, 5,* 156–163.

Bond, F. W., & Bunce, D. (2003). The role of acceptance and job control in mental health, job satisfaction, and work performance. *Journal of Applied Psychology, 88,* 1057–1067.

Borkovec, T. D., Hazlett-Stevens, H., & Diaz, M. L. (1999). The role of positive beliefs about worry in generalized anxiety disorder and its treatment. *Clinical Psychology and Psychotherapy, 6,* 126–138.

Brewin, C. R. (2003). *Posttraumatic stress disorder: Malady or myth?* New Haven, CT: Yale University Press.

Brown, K. W., & Ryan, R. M. (2003). The benefits of being present: Mindfulness and its role in psychological well-being. *Journal of Personality and Social Psychology, 84,* 822–848.

Cioffi, D., & Holloway, J. (1993). Delayed costs of suppressed pain. *Journal of Personality and Social Psychology, 64,* 274–282.

Clark, D. M., Ball, S., & Pape, D. (1991). An experimental investigation of thought suppression. *Behaviour Research and Therapy, 29,* 253–257.

Dahl, J., Wilson, K. G., & Nilsson, A. (2004). Acceptance and commitment therapy and the treatment for persons at risk for long-term disability resulting from stress and pain symptoms: A preliminary randomized trial. *Behavior Therapy, 35,* 785–801.

Edwards, S., & Dickerson, M. (1987). Intrusive unwanted thoughts: A two-stage model of control. *British Journal of Medical Psychology, 60,* 317–328.

Endler, N. S., & Parker, D. A. (1994). Assessment of multidimensional coping: Task, emotion, and avoidance strategies. *Psychological Assessment, 6,* 50–60.

Foa, E. B., & Rothbaum, B. O. (1998). *Treating the trauma of rape: Cognitive-behavioral therapy for PTSD.* New York: Guilford Press.

Foa, E. B., Zinbarg, R., & Rothbaum, B. O. (1992). Uncontrollability and unpredictability in posttraumatic stress disorder: An animal model. *Psychological Bulletin, 112,* 218–238.

Folke, F., & Parling, T. (2004). *Acceptance and commitment therapy in group format for individuals who are unemployed and on sick leave suffering from depression: A randomized controlled trial.* Unpublished thesis, University of Uppsala, Uppsala, Sweden.

Folkman, S., & Lazarus, R. S. (1988). *Ways of Coping Questionnaire–Research Edition.* Washington, DC: Consulting Psychologists Press.

Follette, V. M. (1994). Survivors of childhood sexual abuse: Treatment using a contextual analysis. In S. C. Hayes, N. S. Jacobson, V. M. Follette, & M. Dougher (Eds.), *Acceptance and change: Content and context in psychotherapy* (pp. 255-268). Reno, NV: Context Press.

Follette, V. M., Pistorello, J., Bechtle, A., Naugle, A. E., Polusny, M., Serafin, J., & Walser, R. D. (1993, June). *Acceptance and commitment therapy with survivors of sexual abuse.* Paper presented at the American Association of Applied and Preventive Psychology (AAAPP), Chicago.

Fondacaro, M. R., & Moos, R. H. (1987). Social support and coping: A longitudinal analysis. *American Journal of Community Psychology, 15,* 653-673.

Gifford, E. V., Kohlenberg, B. S., Hayes, S. C., Antonuccio, D. O., Piasecki, M. M., Rasmussen-Hall, M. L., & Palm, K. M. (2004). Acceptance based treatment for smoking cessation. *Behavior Therapy, 35,* 689-705.

Greenberg, L. (1994). Acceptance in experiential therapy. In S. C. Hayes, N. S. Jacobson, V. M. Follette, & M. J. Dougher (Eds.), *Acceptance and change: Content and context in psychotherapy* (pp. 53-67). Reno, NV: Context Press.

Gregg, J. A. (2004). *A randomized controlled effectiveness trial comparing patient education with and without acceptance and commitment therapy for type 2 diabetes self-management.* Unpublished dissertation, University of Nevada, Reno.

Hayes, S. C. (1994). Content, context, and the types of psychological acceptance. In S. C. Hayes, N. S. Jacobson, V. M. Follette, & M. J. Dougher (Eds.), *Acceptance and change: Content and context in psychotherapy* (pp. 13-32). Reno, NV: Context Press.

Hayes, S. C. (2004). Acceptance and commitment therapy and the new behavior therapies: Mindfulness, acceptance and relationship. In S. C. Hayes, V. M. Follette, & M. Linehan (Eds.), *Mindfulness and acceptance: Expanding the cognitive-behavioral tradition* (pp. 1-29). New York: Guilford Press.

Hayes, S. C., Barnes-Holmes, D., & Roche, B. (2001). *Relational Frame Theory: A post-Skinnerian account of human language and cognition.* New York: Plenum Press.

Hayes, S. C., Bissett, R., Roget, N., Padilla, M., Kohlenberg, B. S., Fisher, G., et al. (2004a). The impact of acceptance and commitment training and multicultural training on the stigmatizing attitudes and professional burnout of substance abuse counselors. *Behavior Therapy.*

Hayes, S. C., Masuda, A., Bissett, R., Luoma, J., & Guerrero, L. F. (2004b). DBT, FAP, and ACT: How empirically oriented are the new behavior therapy technologies? *Behavior Therapy, 35,* 35-54.

Hayes, S. C., & Strosahl, K. D. (2005). *A practical guide to acceptance and commitment therapy.* New York: Plenum Press.

Hayes, S. C., Strosahl, K. D., & Wilson, K. G. (1999). *Acceptance and commitment therapy: An experiential approach to behavior change.* New York: Guilford Press.

Hayes, S. C., Strosahl, K. D., Wilson, K. G., Bissett, R. T., Pistorello, J., Toarmino, D., et al. (2004c). Measuring experiential avoidance: A preliminary test of a working model. *Psychological Record, 54,* 553-578.

Hayes, S. C., Wilson, K. G., Gifford, E., Bissett, R., Batten, S., Piasecki, M., et al. (2002). *The use of acceptance and commitment therapy and 12-step facilitation in the treatment of polysubstance abusing heroin addicts on methadone maintenance: A randomized controlled trial.* Paper presented at the meeting of the Association for Behavior Analysis, Toronto.

Hayes, S. C., Wilson, K. G., Gifford, E. V., Follette, V. M., & Strosahl, K. (1996). Experiential avoidance and behavioral disorders: A functional dimensional approach to diagnosis and treatment. *Journal of Consulting and Clinical Psychology, 64,* 1152–1168.

Herman, C. P., & Polivy, J. (1993). Mental control of eating: Excitatory and inhibitory food thoughts. In D. M. Wegner & J. W. Pennebaker (Eds.), *Handbook of mental control* (pp. 491–505). Englewood Cliffs, NJ: Prentice-Hall.

Horowitz, M. J. (1986). *Stress response syndromes* (2nd ed.). Northvale, NJ: Aronson.

Jaycox, L. H., Foa, E. B., & Morral, A. R. (1998). Influence of emotional engagement and habituation on exposure therapy for PTSD. *Journal of Consulting and Clinical Psychology. 66,* 185–192.

Kabat-Zinn, J. (1990). *Full catastrophe living: Using the wisdom of your body and mind to face stress, pain and illness.* New York: Dell.

Keane, T. M., Fairbank, J. A., Caddell, J. M., Zimering, R. T., & Bender, M. E. (1985). A behavioral approach to treating posttraumatic stress disorder in Vietnam veterans. In C. R. Gigley (Ed.), *Trauma and its wake* (pp. 257–294). New York: Brunner/Mazel.

Kelly, A. E., & Kahn, J. H. (1994). Effects of suppression of personal intrusive thoughts. *Journal of Personality and Social Psychology, 66,* 998–1006.

Kendall, P. C., & Hollon, S. D. (1980). Cognitive self-statements in depression: Development of an Automatic Thoughts Questionnaire. *Cognitive Therapy and Research, 4,* 383–395.

Lepore, S. J., Silver, R. C., Wortman, C. B., & Wayment, A. (1996). Social constraints, intrusive thoughts, and depressive symptoms among bereaved mothers. *Journal of Personality and Social Psychology, 70,* 271–282.

Macrae, C. N., Bodenhausen, G. V., Milne, A. B., & Jetten, J. (1994). Out of mind but back in sight: Stereotypes on the rebound. *Journal of Personality and Social Psychology, 67,* 808–817.

Marx, B. P., & Sloan, D. M. (2002). The role of emotion in the psychological functioning of adult survivors of childhood sexual abuse. *Behavior Therapy, 33,* 563–577.

Marx, B. P., & Sloan, D. M. (2005). Peritraumatic dissociation and experiential avoidance as predictors of posttraumatic stress symptomatology. *Behaviour Research and Therapy, 43,* 569–583.

McCracken, L. M., Vowles, K. E., & Eccleston, C. (2004). Acceptance of chronic pain: Component analysis and a revised assessment method. *Pain, 107,* 159–166.

Muris, P., Merckelback, H., van den Hout, M., & de Jong, P. (1992). Suppression of emotional and neutral material. *Behaviour Research and Therapy, 30,* 639–642.

Pennebaker, J. W., & Harber, K. D. (1993). A social stage model of collective coping: The Loma Prieta earthquake and the Persian Gulf War. *Journal of Social Issues, 49,* 125–145.

Pennebaker, J. W., Hughes, C. F., & O'Heeron, R. C. (1987). The psychophysiology of confession: Linking inhibitory and psychosomatic processes. *Journal of Personality and Social Psychology, 52,* 781–793.

Pennebaker, J. W., & O'Heeron, R. C. (1984). Confiding in others and illness rate among spouses of suicide and accidental-death victims. *Journal of Abnormal Psychology, 93,* 473–476.

Rachman, S., & de Silva, P. (1978). Abnormal and normal obsessions. *Behaviour Research and Therapy, 16,* 233–248.

Rachman, S., & Hodgson, R. J. (1980). *Obsessions and compulsions.* Englewood Cliffs, NJ: Prentice-Hall.

Rassin, E. (2003). The White Bear Suppression Inventory (WBSI) focuses on failing suppression attempts. *European Journal of Personality, 17*, 285–298.

Riggs, D. S., Dancu, C. V., Gershuny, B. S., Greenberg, D., & Foa, E. B. (1992). Anger and posttraumatic stress disorder in female crime victims. *Journal of Traumatic Stress, 5*, 613–625.

Roemer, L., Orsillo, S. M., Litz, B. T., & Wagner, A. W. (2001). A preliminary investigation of the role of strategic withholding of emotions in PTSD. *Journal of Traumatic Stress, 14*, 143–150.

Salkovskis, P. M., & Campbell, P. (1994). Thought suppression induces intrusion in naturally occurring negative intrusive thoughts. *Behaviour Research and Therapy, 32*, 1–8.

Salkovskis, P. M., & Harrison, J. (1982). Abnormal and normal obsessions: A replication. *Behaviour Research and Therapy, 22*, 549–552.

Shapiro, S., & Dominiak, G. M. (1992). *Sexual trauma and psychopathology: Clinical intervention with adult survivors.* New York: Lexington Books.

Shaver, K. G., & Drown, D. (1986). On causality, responsibility, and self-blame: A theoretical note. *Journal of Personality and Social Psychology, 50*, 697–702.

Silver, R. L., Boon, C., & Stones, M. H. (1983). Searching for meaning in misfortune: Making sense of incest. *Journal of Social Issues, 39*, 81–102.

Stanton, A. L., Kirk, S. B., Cameron, C. L., & Danoff-Burg, S. (2000). Coping through emotional approach: Scale construction and validation. *Journal of Personality and Social Psychology, 78*, 1150–1169.

Strosahl, K. D., Hayes, S. C., Bergan, J., & Romano, P. (1998). Assessing the field effectiveness of acceptance and commitment therapy: An example of the manipulated training research method. *Behavior Therapy, 29*, 35–64.

Sutherland, G., Newman, B., & Rachman, S. (1982). Experimental investigations of the relations between mood and intrusive unwanted cognitions. *British Journal of Medical Psychology, 55*, 127–138.

Tennen, H., & Affleck, G. (1990). Blaming others for threatening events. *Psychological Bulletin, 107*, 209–232.

Trimble, M. R. (1981). *Post-traumatic neurosis.* Chichester, UK: Wiley.

Trinder, H., & Salkovskis, P. M. (1994). Personally relevant intrusions outside the laboratory: Long-term suppression increases intrusion. *Behaviour Research and Therapy, 32*, 833–842.

Turner, R. A., King, P. R., & Tremblay, P. F. (1992). Coping styles and depression among psychiatric outpatients. *Personality and Individual Differences, 13*, 1145–1147.

Twohig, M. P., & Woods, D. W. (2004). A preliminary investigation of acceptance and commitment therapy and habit reversal as a treatment for trichotillomania. *Behavior Therapy, 35*, 803–820.

Wagner, A. W., Roemer, L., Orsillo, S. M., & Litz, B. T. (2003). Emotional experiencing in women with posttraumatic stress disorder: Congruence between facial expressivity and self-report. *Journal of Traumatic Stress, 16*, 67–75.

Walser, R. D. (1998). *The effects of acceptance and suppression on thought and emotion.* Unpublished dissertation, University of Nevada, Reno.

Walser, R. D., Loew, D., Westrup, D., Gregg, J., & Rogers, D. (2003a, November). *Acceptance and commitment therapy: Theory and treatment of complex PTSD.* Paper presented at the International Society of Traumatic Stress Studies, Baltimore, MD.

Walser, R. D., Westrup, D., Rogers, D., Gregg, J., & Loew, D. (2003b, November). *Acceptance and commitment therapy for PTSD.* International Society of Traumatic Stress Studies, Chicago..

Wegner, D. M. (1994). Ironic processes of mental control. *Psychological Review, 101,* 34–52.

Wegner, D. M., & Schneider, D. J. (2003). The white bear story. *Psychological Inquiry, 14,* 326–329.

Wegner, D. M., Schneider, D. J., Carter, S., III, & White, L. (1987). Paradoxical effects of thought suppression. *Journal of Personality and Social Psychology, 58,* 409–418.

Wegner, D. M., Shortt, J. W., Blake, A. W., & Page, M. S. (1990). The suppression of exciting thoughts. *Journal of Personality and Social Psychology, 58,* 409–418.

Wegner, D. M., & Zanakos, S. I. (1994). Chronic thought suppression. *Journal of Personality, 62,* 615–640.

Weiner, B. (1985). Spontaneous causal thinking. *Psychological Bulletin, 97,* 74–84.

Weiner, B. (1986). *An attributional theory of motivation and emotion.* New York: Springer Verlag.

Wells, A., & Davies, M. I. (1994). The Thought Control Questionnaire: A measure of individual differences in the control of unwanted thoughts. *Behaviour Research and Therapy, 32,* 871–878.

Wells, A., & Matthews, G. (1994). *Attention and emotion: A clinical perspective.* Hillsdale, NJ: Erlbaum.

Wenzlaff, R. M., & Wegner, D. M. (1990). *How depressed individuals cope with unwanted thoughts.* Unpublished research data.

Wenzlaff, R. M., & Wegner, D. M. (2000). Thought suppression. *Annual Review of Psychology, 51,* 59–91.

Wilson, K. G., & Groom, J. (2002). *The Valued Living Questionnaire.* Available from the first author at Department of Psychology, University of Mississippi, University, MS.

Wilson, K. G., & Murrell, A. R. (2004). Values work in acceptance and commitment therapy: Setting a course for behavioral treatment. In S. C. Hayes, V. M. Follette, & M. Linehan (Eds.), *Mindfulness and acceptance: Expanding the cognitive-behavioral tradition* (pp. 120–151). New York: Guilford Press.

Zettle, R. D. (2003). Acceptance and commitment therapy (ACT) versus systematic desensitization in treatment of mathematics anxiety. *Psychological Record, 5,* 197–215.

Zettle, R. D., & Hayes, S. C. (1986). Dysfunctional control by client verbal behavior: The context of reason giving. *Analysis of Verbal Behavior, 4,* 30–38.

Zettle, R. D., & Raines, J. C. (1989). Group cognitive and contextual therapies in treatment of depression. *Journal of Clinical Psychology, 45,* 438–445.

CHAPTER EIGHT

Functional Analytic Psychotherapy and the Treatment of Complex Posttraumatic Stress Disorder

Barbara S. Kohlenberg
Mavis Tsai
Robert J. Kohlenberg

Functional analytic psychotherapy (FAP; Kohlenberg & Tsai, 1991), a therapy derived from radical behaviorism in which a caring and intimate client–therapist relationship is the core of the therapeutic change process, is designed to promote interpersonal therapeutic opportunities that may be especially effective in treating clients with trauma histories. In this chapter the FAP perspective is applied toward understanding the clinical effects of trauma and how treatment may vary depending on whether the trauma was specific versus interpersonally complex. Also discussed are empirical support for FAP, common complications and pitfalls faced by FAP therapists, and how the relationship between the treating clinician and his or her supervisor or consultant may help shape the creation of meaningful, helpful, client–therapist relationships.

TRAUMA AND INTERPERSONAL EFFECTS

Although the majority of people exposed to trauma appears to be resilient to the experience (Bonanno, 2004), that is not the case for survivors of child-hood abuse because such abuse typically involves repeated trauma at the hands of a trusted caregiver. In fact, for women with symptoms of posttrau-matic stress disorder (PTSD), the most common etiology is childhood sexual or physical abuse (Kessler, Sonnega, Bromet, Hughes, & Nelson, 1995). When trauma involves childhood sexual abuse, the long-term effects may include interpersonal problems, such as marital disruption (Nelson, Wangsgaard, Yorgason, Kessler, & Carter-Vassol, 2002), sexual dysfunction (Tsai, Feldman-Summers, & Edgar, 1978; Merrill, Guimond, Thomsen, & Miller, 2003; Noll, Trickett, & Putnam, 2003), and issues with trust and intimacy (for reviews, see Beitchman et al., 1992). A history of childhood abuse is also believed to increase the severity of traumatic response to interpersonal violence experienced as adults (Kubany et al., 2004). Women with PTSD are overrepresented in substance abuse samples and are considered more difficult to treat than women with substance abuse disorder alone (Najavits, Weiss, Shaw, & Muenz, 1998). In comparison to more circumscribed trauma such as rape, the psychological sequelae of childhood abuse include more pervasive deficits in interpersonal functioning (Archer & Cooper, 1998; Roth, Newman, Pelcovitz, van der Kolk, & Mandel, 1997) that require more intricate treatment considerations (Cloitre, Karestan, Cohen, & Han, 2002; Leahy, Pretty, & Tenebaum, 2003)

THE CAUSES OF THE CLINICAL EFFECTS OF TRAUMA

Before advocating that FAP can be an ideal treatment for complex PTSD, we first turn to a theory of trauma and its treatment implications. A parsimonious way to understand the complexity of trauma and its effects is to utilize the principles of operant and respondent conditioning. This learning account of PTSD (Hyer, 1994) is based on Mowrer's (1960) two-factor theory. Essentially, this theory contends that symptoms or problematic behavior come from two sources. First, as a result of pairing previously neutral stimuli with a highly aversive event, visceral, autonomic responses are now evoked by these previously neutral stimuli. A simple example might be a woman who was attacked by a dog and who now has aversive emotional responses to being near dogs, hearing dogs, or even anticipating the possibility of running into a dog. This woman's emotional responses to dogs and their related stimuli constitute the first set of problems. Then, because of respondent conditioning, this woman would understandably avoid exposure to evocative stimuli, or in the case of this example, dogs. This successful avoidance strategy would result in a decrease in the aversive stimulation caused by approaching dogs. Thus avoidance behavior would be reinforced by the reduction of aversive stimulation. So, at this point, we have a woman who is not only emotionally upset at the sight of a dog, but who has also learned to reduce her upset by avoiding situations that are likely to evoke her negative emotions.

The second set of symptoms would emerge in this woman based on her avoidance behavior. She might begin to develop difficulties because of her avoidance of situations where a dog might be present. This simple avoidance technique could spread such that she would be limited in her ability to go to the home of a loved one who happens to have a friendly dog, or who even lives near a dog. This pattern ultimately could cascade into avoiding many situations that require her presence in order to maintain a meaningful life. Further, the symptoms would likely persist because the avoidance prevents exposure to the evocative stimuli (e.g., dogs) and does not allow extinction to occur. The avoidance would also interfere with the acquisition of more adaptive behavior (e.g., being able to be in the presence of a dog again).

Other kinds of single-event traumas, such as rape, could also fit into this model. That is, the rape plus all of the previously neutral circumstances surrounding it would produce intense emotional arousal, via classical conditioning. The attempts to avoid stimuli that would produce the arousal, such as not approaching any aspect of the situation in which the rape occurred, could also cascade into a secondary set of life problems related to the avoidance strategy employed to reduce the anxiety incurred by the rape trauma.

In this chapter we extend the traditional two-factor theory, developed for discrete forms of trauma exposure, to explain and treat the effects of repeated, interpersonally based trauma. We believe that severe and difficult-to-treat effects of trauma arise from such histories. Thus we distinguish the relatively short-term effects of circumscribed trauma from the longer-term effects of repetitive trauma that occur over an extended period of time.

Short-Term Effects of Circumscribed Trauma and Resilience

The respondent conditioning model provides a reasonable explanation of each of the DSM-IV's diagnostic criteria for PTSD (American Psychiatric Association, 1994; see Kohlenberg & Tsai, 1998, for a complete discussion of DSM-IV, PTSD, and two-factor theory). Of interest here is how a traumatic stimulus (the unconditioned stimulus) can come to elicit responses that are mediated by the autonomic nervous system, and how these responses can be either short-lived or have more long-term, pervasive effects.

When a person experiences a trauma, say a fire in which a beloved pet dies, he or she would understandably experience distress and "increased arousal," as specified in the DSM-IV (American Psychiatric Association, 1994). Because of respondent conditioning, previously neutral stimuli now would elicit conditioned responses (increased arousal). Thus, as a result of the conditioning, the likelihood increases that this person would encounter stimuli that evoke increased arousal during daily life, such as the time of day, the weather, the sounds, and the odors that occurred along with the fire. Other stimuli might involve seeing the pets of others or even having the emotional reaction of love toward an animal. Furthermore, evidence suggests that increased arousal produces a flattened generalization gradient (Sokolov, 1963; Mednick, 1975). That is, as arousal increases, an even wider range of stimuli will evoke conditioned responses (e.g., hearing a noise sounding like one's pet, leaving the house, any stimuli present during the time that one is watching one's house burn). This spreading or spiraling of arousal after traumatic conditioning can be further understood in terms of the concepts of verbal mediation or stimulus equivalence (Dougher,

Auguston, Markham, & Greenway, 1994), or relational frame theory (Hayes, Barnes-Holmes, & Roche, 2001). These approaches provide a conceptual and empirical analysis of how language itself acquires clinically meaningful stimulus properties. Thus our behavioral model is consistent with the DSM-IV's description of increased arousal, as well as with contemporary models of verbal behavior/verbal mediation.

FAP also can help clarify why a single episode of trauma does *not* escalate into the clinical syndrome of PTSD for most people. We know that there is evidence that PTSD is predicted by the level of severity of the experienced grief and distress around a traumatic event (Bonanno & Field, 2001), and that those individuals who are exposed to trauma and show minimal distress are also unlikely to develop PTSD (Bonanno, 2004). Bonanno (2004) further identifies specific factors that appear to buffer the effects of extreme stress, such as hardiness, self-enhancement, repressive coping, and positive emotion and laughter. All of these factors operate, in part, by reducing initial levels of distress related to the traumatic material, generally through social affiliation. Thus Mower's (1960) two-factor theory is also consistent with current theories of resilience to trauma.

TREATMENT FOR CIRCUMSCRIBED PTSD AND EMPIRICAL SUPPORT

The FAP model also underlies current popular treatments for circumscribed PTSD. Exposure is the primary behavioral approach to treating clients with problems resulting from trauma (e.g., Foa & Rothbaum, 1997) and is present in all forms of psychological treatment. From a behavioral point of view, all treatments, even ones not classified as "behavioral," generally expose clients to traumatic material as part of the treatment process, and their treatments would be consistent with an exposure model. The learning principle underlying exposure is extinction. Extinction occurs when the evocative stimulus is presented and then is not followed by an aversive stimulus. Thus, in clinical work, exposure involves presenting the evocative stimulus and making sure that the client does not avoid or escape it. This process of exposure to traumatic material, although potentially healing in its effects, is by necessity emotionally challenging for the client. In fact, clients who initially experience high levels of distress upon imagined contact with their traumas, followed by gradual habituation, tend to show more improvement than those who do not report high levels of initial distress or who do not report habituation to high levels of stress (Jaycox, Foa, & Morral, 1998). If the client avoids or escapes, then the behaviors of avoidance or escape are strengthened (reinforced), and there is no therapeutic progress. Even worse, the problem may be exacerbated.

For example, in using exposure to treat a person suffering from the trauma of a rape, the client would reexperience the emotional arousal present during it (see Riggs, Cahill, & Foa, Chapter 4, this volume). This reexperience could be evoked through imagination, discussion, going to the place where the rape occurred, or any other method that would promote rape-related emotional responding. The emotional arousal would need to be high and sustained; the client would need to remain aroused until that arousal began to decrease. If the client terminated the reexperiencing before the decrease in arousal began, symptoms could even worsen.

Three necessary conditions and one highly desirable one must be met before this kind of exposure-based treatment can begin. First, the evocative stimuli must be known and specifiable. That is, the clinician must know what the evocative stimuli are before a method for exposure can be devised. Second, the client must be cooperative. That is, the client must be willing to talk about the trauma and tolerate a certain amount of anxiety by agreeing to place him- or herself in the presence of the evocative stimuli. Third, the therapist must also be willing to hear about the trauma and potentially experience emotional arousal as a part of the treatment. Finally, it is highly desirable that the evocative stimuli be presented *in vivo*. That is, it is always best when the evocative stimuli be presented in a real form rather than via talk or imagination (Goldfried, 1985).

It is important to note that when exposure treatments are successful, the arousal symptoms that have diminished the person's ability to participate fully in life are greatly attenuated. This does not mean that the sorrow connected with the losses sustained in a trauma is forgotten. The sadness about being raped, attacked by a dog, or losing one's house or beloved pet would naturally linger and would inform life from that point on. The intrusive, uncomfortable, life-interfering aspects of arousal and avoidance, however, would be greatly reduced.

Exposure When the Evocative Stimuli Are Known

In the typical behavioral therapy treatment, the evocative stimuli are easily specified, and thus the presentation of evocative stimuli and the blocking of avoidance responses are straightforward procedures. In order to facilitate the therapeutic blocking of avoidance and to obtain more readily the client's agreement to participate, the therapist may use graded situations (e.g., a hierarchy) in which the client agrees to remain in a related, but less evocative, stimulus situation. According to learning theory, extinction of the conditioned response to the less evocative situation will enable exposure to more evocative ones. Continuing with the above dog attack example, a hierarchy might involve behaviors ranging from talking about dogs, to listening to tapes of dogs barking, to being in the same room as a dog, to going to where the dog attack took place.

A Collaborative Client–Therapist Relationship

As stated above, avoidance is one of the sequelae of traumatic conditioning. If the client were completely avoidant, however, it would be impossible to do exposure treatment because he or she would avoid evocative stimuli. If forced to be physically present with the evocative stimuli, the client would use other forms of avoidance such as "tuning out" or dissociation. In fact, complete avoidance could lead the client to not talk about, or even remember, the traumatic conditioning. In this latter case, the client might seek treatment for problems but would not attribute the symptoms to the trauma or focus on it. A client with total avoidance of traumatization by a fire, for example, might seek treatment for other issues and if asked if he or she had ever experienced a trauma, would not recall the experience and thus would be unable to report it. Thus the "willingness" of the client to tolerate the anxiety and to "remember" and talk about the trauma is necessary for a successful exposure treatment.

Cognitive-behavioral therapists usually treat client cooperation in the therapeutic process as a technical issue that can be addressed by prior negotiation with the client, therapist encouragement, and the use of social contingencies. The establishment of a therapeutic alliance is generally considered a prequisite to potentiating a robust treatment package. That is, the therapist presents an exposure plan and obtains the client's agreement to place him- or herself in the evocative situation and to remain there until extinction takes place.

In Vivo Presentations of Evocative Stimuli

The effectiveness of exposure treatment is greatly enhanced if the evocative stimuli are presented *in vivo*. For example, if the stimuli associated with the original traumatic conditioning included the patient being alone on the block where the dog attack took place, exposure to these actual stimuli will be more effective than talking about them or merely imagining them. As stated by Goldfried (1985), the *in vivo* presentation of evocative stimuli is "more powerful than imagined or described" presentations (p. 71).

SYMPTOMS OF COMPLEX PTSD

The DSM-IV descriptions of PTSD symptoms (American Psychiatric Association, 1994) were developed for problems resulting from circumscribed, physical trauma. The aversive stimuli and the resultant symptoms for such trauma are relatively easy to specify. Furthermore, in order to be diagnosed with PTSD, the trauma has to be remembered. This implies that clients are able to tolerate anxiety to the extent that they are aware of the traumatic conditioning, attribute their PTSD symptoms to the trauma, and seek treatment for these symptoms. Three conditions facilitate the development of hierarchies and the presentation of evocative stimuli, as required for exposure types of treatment: (1) easily described, circumscribed stimuli; (2) a client who is able to tolerate at least some anxiety; and (3) a client whose emotional experience of the trauma is not primarily based in shame and guilt (Meadows & Foa, 1998).

Many clinicians who work with clients who have histories characterized by repetitive trauma and the associated symptoms refer to this syndrome as "complex PTSD" (Herman, 1992a). Although symptoms of complex PTSD involve the same aversive conditioning and avoidance behavior that accounts for DSM-IV PTSD symptoms, they are elaborated and more debilitating because the trauma is generally interpersonal and occurred repeatedly over an extended period of time, usually in childhood (Blake, Albano, & Keane, 1992; Briere, 2002; Herman, 1992a).

These types of traumas have more pervasive and long-lasting negative effects than circumscribed trauma. For example, Terr (1990) reports that circumscribed childhood trauma, such as a kidnapping or sniper attack, can produce specific symptoms that may last for a few years but eventually are resolved without lingering ill effects in adulthood. Bonanno (2004) further describes major circumscribed traumas such as the 9/11 attack on the World Trade Center, in which it was found that among Manhattan residents, PTSD symptoms declined rapidly over time, with PTSD prevalence decreasing to 1.7% 6 months after the trauma. In contrast, repetitive trauma over extended periods of time during childhood produces more complex, pervasive symptoms that usually persist into adulthood (Herman, 1992b). These findings also are found among Holocaust survivors, many of whom suffer from the effects of trauma decades after the prolonged experience (Herman, Russell, & Trocki, 1986; Shmotkin, Blumstein, & Modan, 2003).

Persistent Avoidance of Stimuli Associated with the Trauma

A child who is physically and sexually abused over an extended period of time is, of course, motivated to escape and avoid the pain and humiliation. In contrast to a circumscribed trauma, the direct avoidance of the aversive stimuli would be impossible because the child cannot physically escape or prevent the exposure. When a beloved parent or caretaker is also the perpetrator of the abuse, the trauma is particularly heart-wrenching. Incest creates an association between love, dependence, and the pain of trauma that places the child in a very complicated situation.

In such a complex situation it would be adaptive for the child to isolate his or her relationship to the abuser while the abuse is taking place from the relationship the child has with the same person during other times. This type of perceptual rather than physical avoidance can involve alterations in the "seeing" (perception) or remembering of the event. This response mechanism would be a reasonable option for a child who is unable to physically escape the person who is traumatizing them.

For example, victims may avoid perceptual contact with features of the abuser, the abuse, as well as associated internal stimuli. Effecting a perceptual isolation of the trauma, the child even can be loving or affectionate to the abuser most of the time and thus receive the care, food, and shelter necessary for survival. If this isolation did not happen, then the effects of the trauma would be more intrusive in the daily life of the child (as is the case with short-term adult PTSD), and preclude whatever caretaking might be available. Sometimes a total perceptual avoidance of the abuser and the environment in which it takes place (complete amnesia[1]) is necessary for the child's survival. At times the child may learn to avoid associated internal stimuli. This means that the child would be unable to describe feeling anything at all about the abuse. This kind of avoidance would also allow for the continuation of other, perhaps more nurturing, aspects of the relationship.

The types of avoidance described above could have serious impact on the development of relationship skills involved in ordinary, day-to-day, social interactions as well as those required for intimate relationships, including therapy relationships. Healthy adult functioning involves being able to describe and identify the behavior of others as well as one's own internal reactions. Coping with trauma in a manner that involved externally focused perceptual avoidance could lead to problems such as revictimization. Perceptual avoidance that is directed inward distorts the ability to experience, identify, and describe internal states and may lead to problems of the self and personality disorders (primarily borderline personality disorder; Kohlenberg & Tsai, 1991, Ch. 6; Kohlenberg & Tsai, 1993). Finally, the ability to tolerate the arousal that is required for exposure might also be affected, because the person would simply avoid the exposure experience.

Above all, when a client who has experienced complex trauma enters therapy, it is likely that many of the problems with which he or she struggles will also occur in the context of the therapy. In many ways, the setting of the therapeutic encounter is a very evocative and potent—there is a power differ-

---

[1]Given the notoriety of the "repressed memory controversy," a word is in order about our view of the issues. Our vantage point is a radical behavioral one; thus, we do not believe that there is such a thing as a "memory" that is stored in the mind. Instead, remembering is the behavioral process of seeing, hearing, smelling, touching, and tasting of stimuli that are not currently present in the environment. One implication of viewing memory as the behavior of remembering is that there is no a priori reason for not also accepting the possibility that repression, the behavior of forgetting, also can be developed. Some empirical support for our position is derived from the literature demonstrating that animals can be taught to forget (Maki, 1981). The strength and nature of both remembering and forgetting are the result of our histories. Our view is consistent with both the traditional view that a client may be amnesic for early trauma (repression) as well as the idea that memories may be implanted during therapy by a careless therapist. In either event, remembering can be therapeutic in that avoidance is reduced in the process. For a more complete discussion of this topic, see Kohlenberg and Tsai (1991, Chs. 4 and 6).

ential, potential for emotional intimacy, attachment and dependence possibilities, and potential for harm. Fortunately, each of these possibilities can be viewed as an exposure exercise in which continued aversive stimulation would not occur.

We believe that FAP, as described in the following section, offers a framework that allows for the development of intense, meaningful relationships that can offset the deleterious effects of trauma as well as promote growth for clients struggling with symptoms of complex PTSD.

FAP: AN IDEAL BEHAVIORAL THERAPY FOR COMPLEX PTSD

In theory, the treatment for complex PTSD involves the same exposure-based procedures described for circumscribed PTSD. That is, the evocative stimuli need to be identified and described, the client must be willing to expose him- or herself to these stimuli and not avoid or escape from them, and the stimuli should be presented *in vivo*. Because complex PTSD involves difficult-to-describe evocative stimuli, however, it is difficult to devise an *in vivo* exposure treatment that presents the evocative stimuli but then also blocks avoidance behavior. The stimuli involved in complex PTSD are rarely specific things or events. The situation is further complicated when the client cannot remember details of the trauma, and/or the perpetrator is gone or no longer available. For example, during the original trauma the person might have experienced intense anxiety and fear, and might have responded to these emotions by dissociating. Today, however, when anxiety and fear occur in the client's daily life, the client may continue to dissociate in order to cope with these feelings. It is also possible that the client might avoid situations that evoke anxiety and fear. Either scenario describes a person living life with serious limitations.

The person with complex PTSD may present as an adult who is avoidant of intimacy, does not have a sense of self, and has difficulty trusting others. In this case, even if the evocative stimuli could be specified, such as "becoming comfortable and trusting in a close relationship," it would be unclear how to arrange the *in vivo* presentation of such stimuli in an exposure-based format. Obvious problems exist with an intervention that consists of the therapist encouraging the client to begin an intimate relationship, to become vulnerable in that relationship, and to stay in that relationship even when anxiety or fear intensify—as would be required for an exposure-based treatment. Even if the client did attempt to comply with such instructions, it is doubtful that the outcome would be therapeutic. The "other" in such an exposure-based treatment might not be patient enough to allow extinction to take place, and worse, might act in punishing ways that would reinforce the original trauma.

Such problems can best be dealt with by using the therapeutic relationship as a source for *in vivo* evocative stimuli and thus providing the opportunity to block avoidance. In addition, the treatment of complex PTSD involves the building of interpersonal repertoires that were precluded by the early effects of the trauma, and an establishment of the private control required for emotional responding and development of self (Kohlenberg & Tsai, 1991, 1995).

We believe that FAP can help to produce the conditions that would facilitate the treatment of symptoms of complex PTSD. FAP is a radical behaviorally informed treatment conceptualized by Kohlenberg and Tsai (1991) to account theoretically for the dramatic and pervasive improvements shown by some clients when involved in intense client–therapist relationships, and to delineate the steps therapists can take to facilitate intense and curative relationships. The result is a treatment in which, in contrast to popular misconceptions about radical behaviorism, the client–therapist relationship is at the core of the change process. FAP theory indicates that, in general, the therapeutic process is facilitated by a caring, genuine, sensitive, and emotional client–therapist relationship. It is precisely this type of therapeutic relationship that has the potential for effective treatment of complex PTSD. In the following sections, we describe how FAP provides guidelines for obtaining the type of therapeutic relationship that can (1) lead to identification of the evocative stimuli; (2) provide a venue for presentation of evocative stimuli while blocking avoidance behavior; and (3) provide *in vivo* opportunities to teach the more adaptive repertoires that failed to develop due to traumatic early life conditions. Following this explication of FAP guidelines, we summarize data that support the utility of using FAP with patients who have complex PTSD.

As described below, FAP is based on (1) three types of client behavior that are clinically relevant, and (2) rules or guidelines for therapeutic technique. Client behaviors include the daily life problems that occur during the session, improvements that occur during the session, and client interpretations of their own behavior. Therapist guidelines are rules or methods that are aimed at evoking, noticing, reinforcing, and interpreting client behavior.

Clinically Relevant Behaviors

It is assumed that the client with complex PTSD will bring certain behavioral patterns into the therapist–client relationship. These patterns fall into three types and are referred to as clinically relevant behaviors (CRBs).

CRB1: Client Problems That Occur in Session

CRB1s are related to the client's presenting problems and should decrease in frequency during therapy. For example, a client who suffers from complex PTSD and avoids relationships because they have been hurtful may exhibit these CRB1s: avoids eye contact, answers questions curtly, demands to be taken care of and then fails to come to scheduled appointments, gets angry at the therapist for not having all the answers, cancels several appointments in a row after an making an intimate disclosure.

Patient problems can also involve the thinking, perceiving, feeling, seeing, and remembering that occur during the session. For example, problems known as "disturbances of the self" (see Kohlenberg & Tsai, 1991, for an extensive discussion on how such disturbances are acquired and treated), such as "not knowing who the real me is" and dissociative identity disorder, are translated into behavioral terms (e.g., problems with stimulus control of the response "I") and conceptualized as CRB1. Clients with complex PTSD may be unable to describe how they feel or may not recall an emotional episode that occurred in the session. They may fail to perceive an aspect of the therapist that is associated with past trauma, such as denying the obvious fact that the therapist is pregnant.

CRB2: Client Improvements That Occur in Session

In the early stages of treatment, these behaviors typically are not observed or are minimally discernible. For example, consider a male sexual abuse survivor who feels withdrawn and worthless and has minimized discussion of his abuse. Consider too that he has avoided any direct discussion with the therapist about the therapist's tendency to request that his appointment time be adjusted within a particular day, even though this request made him feel extremely devalued and worthless. Possible CRB2s for him would include expressing his feelings about his abuse, talking about what the therapist does that brings up his feelings of worthlessness, and asking directly for what he needs.

CRB3: Client Interpretations of Behavior

CRB3s consist of client discussions of their own behavior and what seems to cause it; "reason giving" (Hayes, 1987; Zettle & Hayes, 1986) and "interpretations" may be part of this behavior. The best CRB3s include observation and description of self behavior and its associated reinforcing, discriminative, and eliciting stimuli. Learning to describe functional connections helps clients increase their ability to elicit reinforcement in daily life. CRB3s include descriptions of "functional equivalence"—that is, descriptions of similarities between what happens in session and what happens in daily life. Consider a client named Carol who, in response to ongoing childhood abuse, had learned to associate her emotional dependence and self-expression with being physically degraded by caregivers. This person had spent her adult life withholding her deepest feelings in relationships, and for the last few years, had struggled with the issue in therapy. After a course of FAP, in which the expression of deeply held feelings was valued and respected, Carol began taking risks in her relationships and began revealing more of these feelings. Her CRB3 was:

> "The reason I'm talking more openly to people in my life is because I have learned that with you, in our therapy, when I express my vulnerability you will not hurt me, and that you will in fact respond to me in a loving, kind way. Over the years I have learned that my vulnerabilities and deepest desires are respected by you. Even when I expressed to you that you have failed me in certain respects, and even when I was angry that you would not be friends with me outside of therapy, you were respectful and treated me as if what I wanted mattered. Because of these experiences with you, I really feel that I am able to be a whole person with others, handle disappointment appropriately, and not protect my deepest feelings with such vigilance."

Rules of Therapy

For a complete description of the rules of therapy, see Kohlenberg and Tsai, (1991). The FAP therapist is encouraged to follow five strategic rules of therapeutic technique: watch for CRBs, evoke CRBs, reinforce CRB2s, observe the potentially reinforcing effects of therapist behavior in relation to client CRBs, and give interpretations of variables that affect client CRB. Each rule is described below.

Rule 1: Watch for CRBs

This rule forms the core of FAP. The better the therapist is at observing CRBs, the better the outcome. That is, when the therapist can discriminate instances of the problem behavior, chances for shaping improvements will increase. It is also hypothesized that following Rule 1 will lead to increased intensity—stronger emotional reactions—between therapist and client.

From a theoretical viewpoint, the importance of Rule 1 cannot be overemphasized. If this were the only rule that a therapist followed, it alone would likely promote a positive outcome. In other words, a therapist who is skilled at observing instances of CRBs as they occur also is more likely to react naturally to these instances. Thus a therapist following Rule 1 is more likely to naturally reinforce, punish, and extinguish client behaviors in ways that foster the development of behavior that is useful in daily life. Any technique that helps the therapist in the detection of a CRB1 has a place in FAP. Techniques can range from directly asking, "Is the problem that you have with your friends happening here, with us, right now?", to interpretations of in-session behaviors, such as, "I wonder if bringing me a gift today might, in fact, reflect your fear that I do not value you for being you, and that you are doing what you have done for years with your family, which is to give gifts in order to feel accepted, even when it never really works and that you always feel not known by your family."

Rule 2: Evoke CRBs

The ideal client–therapist relationship evokes CRB1s and provides for the development of CRB2s. This kind of relationship usually exists for the client with complex PTSD because the effects of complex PTSD produce problems with intimate relating, and the FAP therapist encourages trust, closeness, and the open expression of feelings in the context of the therapy relationship—which is a structure that involves a power differential. Such a structure often evokes clients' conflicts about, and difficulties in, forming and sustaining intimate relationships. FAP guidelines, at times, can lead therapists to disclose their own private feelings to the client (see Rule 3). These disclosures often consist of presentations that constitute the evocative stimuli that are avoided by clients as a result of complex PTSD. For example, the therapist who says, "I really care about you," might evoke CRB1s (e.g., fear, anxiety, avoidance, feelings of worthlessness) in the client.

Clients' descriptions of what they want from therapy point to the importance of an evocative relationship. As one client stated:

> "I have learned a lot about love from you—that love is not about perfection, that it is about accepting some of the barriers and not always getting what you want. I have learned to love you, even though you make me pay for sessions. Our sessions end when you say they are over, not when I want to leave. Allowing myself to love, even when it is not always perfect, has taught me that I can love even when disappointed. And I feel your love for me, even with clear boundaries. Because of these experiences, I am building a more realistic love relationship with my [significant other]."

Rule 3: Reinforce CRB2s

It is generally advisable to avoid procedures that attempt to specify the form of therapist reaction in advance. Such specification occurs when the therapist attempts to conjure up a reinforcing reaction (e.g., phrases such as "that's terrific" or "great") without referencing the specific client–therapist history.

Therapists can be more naturally reinforcing in many ways (Kohlenberg & Tsai, 1991). One such way is for therapists to observe their spontaneous private reactions to client behavior. Such private reactions are accompanied by dispositions to act in ways that are naturally reinforcing.

To illustrate, consider a client with complex PTSD whose problems partly result from avoidance, which has interfered with the acquisition of intimacy skills. That is, the repetitive early trauma precluded any healthy experiences of intimacy in which the child was reinforced for learning relevant skills. Suppose that at some point in therapy this client behaves in a way that evokes the following private, spontaneous reactions in the therapist: (1) dispositions to act in intimate and caring ways, and (2) private reactions that correspond to "feeling close." Because these responses probably are not apparent to the client, the therapist could describe the private reactions by saying, "I feel especially close to you right now." Without such amplification, these important basic reactions would have little or no reinforcing effects on the client's behavior that evoked them (CRB2).

Rule 4: Observe the Potentially Reinforcing Effects of Therapist Behavior in Relation to Client CRBs

If therapists have been emitting behavior that they think is reinforcing, it would be important for them to actually observe whether they are, in fact, increasing, decreasing, or having no effect on a particular client behavior. Feedback of this type is needed to increase therapist effectiveness. Therapists must become sensitive to the actual (observed) effect of their behavior in session, not what they think it should produce.

Rule 5: Give Interpretations of Variables That Affect Client Behavior

As is the case with most other therapies, interpretations are an important part of FAP. As a general strategy, FAP therapists interpret client behavior in terms of learning histories and functional relationships. For example, a client who stated that she never could be herself and felt like she was always on stage was offered the interpretation that perhaps one reason she felt this way was because, in fact, she was only attended to as a child when she was "performing," and that for various reasons her caregivers were unresponsive and inattentive to her nontheatrical expressions of her needs and desires.

FAP and Empirical Support

FAP involves the application of known behavioral principles to the interactions that occur during the course of psychotherapy. The behavioral principles that FAP draws upon are the same principles that are the cornerstone of all behavioral interventions that characterize applied behavior analysis or behavior therapy.

Research findings suggest that FAP can improve interpersonal functioning (Callahan, Summers, & Weidman, 2003; Kohlenberg, Kanter, Bolling, Parker, & Tsai, 2002). Kohlenberg et al. (2002) compared FAP-enhanced cognitive therapy (FECT) with cognitive therapy (CT) for the treatment of depression. Their findings suggested that FECT was more effective than CT alone in reducing depression, and that FECT was more effective than CT alone in helping patients perform well on measures of interpersonal functioning. Client ratings, interviewer ratings, and blind observers determined that clients who had participated in FECT spontaneously described significantly more relationship improvements than did CT clients at the end of therapy.

Callahan et al. (2003) used FAP in a single-case design to treat a client with features of histrionic and narcissistic personality disorders. According to FAP principles, in-session instances of client problematic behavior and improvements were responded to in a contingent manner. This single case study demonstrated both in-session and daily life improvements in interpersonal functioning. Specifically, behaviors defined as narcissistic and histrionic decreased over treatment, and behaviors in the areas of emotional responding, noticing one's impact on others, and being able to assert one's needs improved. Both of these studies provide evidence that FAP can be an efficacious treatment for interpersonal difficulties, even when these behaviors are part of a constellation of other treatment considerations.

Although the strength of the therapeutic relationship has been appreciated as an important predictor of therapy outcome (Horvath & Symonds, 1991) and has been regarded as a critical factor in therapy for abuse survivors (Briere, 2002; Herman, 1992b), only recently have studies empirically examined the role that the therapeutic alliance plays in trauma therapy with adults abused as children (e.g., Cloitre, Chase Stovall-McClough, Miranda, & Chemtob, 2004; Paivio, Holowaty, & Hall 2004). Paivio et al. (2004) demonstrated that, in a population of adults abused as children, therapist relationship skills independently contributed to outcome, and both therapeutic relationship and emotional processing were identified as being important mechanisms of change. Cloitre, Stovall-McClough, Miranda, and Chemtob (2004) noted that the strength of the therapeutic alliance predicted improvement in symptoms at the end of treatment, and that the effect size of this relationship was much larger (0.47) than what has traditionally been found in previous meta-analyses. Cloitre et al. (2004) further suggests:

> The potent role that the positive therapeutic alliance plays in treatment success may reflect a reversal or reparation of interpersonal disturbances, which undermine success in a variety of tasks including psychotherapy. The results underscore the idea that the therapeutic relationship may be an especially "active" ingredient in the remediation of childhood abuse-related PTSD and a component of treatment that should be highlighted, better understood, and carefully developed for this population. (p. 414)

These findings provide compelling support for the rationale offered by FAP that there is particular value in addressing the interpersonal struggles of trauma survivors, as they occur, in session.

COMPLICATIONS AND OBSTACLES FOR FAP
THERAPISTS IN TREATING COMPLEX PTSD

Trauma-focused treatments can be emotionally difficult for therapists of any theoretical orientation, leading to the potential for vicarious traumatization (Brady, Guy, Poelstra, & Fletcher-Brokaw, 1999) and secondary traumatic stress disorder and compassion fatigue (Figley, 1995). Histories of trauma are also found among mental health professionals, with studies suggesting that about 30% report a history of trauma during childhood (Follette, Polusny, & Milbeck, 1994; Pope & Feldman-Summers, 1992). Although many mental health professionals can be deeply affected by the traumatic material that their clients introduce, therapists are more likely to feel compassion fatigue in their trauma-related clinical work if they themselves have trauma histories (Jenkins & Baird, 2002; Pearlman & Mac Ian, 1995). Such histories, however, do not appear to predict therapist functioning as much as more proximal variables such as consulting with colleagues, getting support and assistance from others, and the use of humor (Follette et al., 1994).

Efforts to understand therapists' and caregivers' reactions to traumatic material and to provide help for them are underway (Cadell, Regehr, & Hemsworth, 2003; Figley, 2002; Follette et al., 1994; Jenkins & Baird, 2002; Holmqvist & Anderson, 2003; Pearlman & Mac Ian, 1995). This new effort is not surprising, given that over 50% or professionals who work with trauma report feeling distressed and 27% report experiencing extreme distress (Meldrum, King, & Spooner, 2002). Working with traumatized clients can be emotionally draining for the therapist. Given that about 30% of therapists also report having experienced trauma during childhood, the questions of if and how these histories contribute to therapeutic process and outcome are frequently explored (Follette et al., 1994; Jenkins & Baird, 2002).

FAP therapists are likely to encounter difficulties and emotional barriers similar to therapists of any other orientation when treating clients with complex PTSD. However, because FAP invites consideration of intense emotional experience that is actually focused on interactions that occur in the here and now of the session, both client and therapist may have stronger reactions than in other types of therapy. Because FAP typically leads to more intense connections between therapists and clients, we will discuss common pitfalls and complications may also arise; these we discuss below.

FAP calls for therapists to notice and at times to facilitate client expressions of feelings, such as love, hate, fear, vulnerability, closeness, and the desire to be physically intimate. Such expressions may evoke strong emotions in the therapist, ranging from discomfort and fear all the way to attraction, intimacy, and love. As therapists work toward reinforcing client improvements, they need to aspire to act in ways that benefit the client; they need to make every effort not to punish, exploit, traumatize or invalidate a client's emotional perspective. Because therapists are also part of the general culture and thus may inadvertently behave in ways that reflect exploitive biases, it is important that they discuss their work with colleagues and (ideally) make audiotapes or videotapes of their sessions for consultation or supervision.

It may be the case that similar issues, perhaps on a different scale, affect both client and therapist. For example, consider the client who has had a history of being overpowered and hurt in interpersonal relationships. Now this client is engaging in behaviors (e.g., relentless phone calls, expressions of anger toward the therapist) that result in the therapist feeling overpowered and hurt. In such a situation, it would be helpful for the therapist to obtain support in order to maintain a therapeutic stance. The therapist might say something to a colleague, such as, "I am feeling very upset, hopeless, and helpless right now. I don't seem to be enough for my client. I feel inadequate, angry, and upset. Will you help me understand my feelings better and develop a perspective that will be helpful to my client?" Thus the therapist risks appearing vulnerable, frightened, and desirous of respect and validation. Ideally, the therapist would emerge with new perceptions that would facilitate continued and effective therapeutic work. These behaviors, engaged by the therapist in the service of maintaining equilibrium and not reacting in a vindictive or unilaterally self-protective manner (such as by withdrawing or terminating therapy), might also be the very same behaviors that would be helpful for this client to generate.

In general, because FAP is so demanding and because it is difficult to take clients further than therapists have gone themselves, FAP therapists need to have done, and to continue to do, their own personal work in terms of healing and growth. In seeking personal support, the following questions may be helpful to focus on:

What are your own issues—the therapist versions of CRB1s and CRB2s—and how do these play out in your therapeutic work?

How do you find the balance between caring too much and caring too little?

How do you handle the situation when what is in the best interest of the client clashes with what is in your own best interest?

How can you keep growing as a therapist and as a person while working with your clients?

When a therapist is clear about his or her own issues, it is easier to focus on the client's needs. For example, while exposure and extinction are an important part of the treatment process, a therapist who proceeds too quickly with a client into the experiencing of traumatic material, while blocking avoidance behaviors, can potentially worsen a client's symptoms. This is because the needs of a client prior to approaching traumatic material may include learning how to handle intense feelings, having good self-care and self-soothing skills, and having a support network in place in the earlier stages of therapy. These skills require knowing how to ask for and receive help, both from the therapist and from others in their lives. Therapists' self-awareness of their own issues, as they pertain to creating loving, caring, and supportive relationships with their clients, is essential to this process. A lack of such awareness in the therapist could result in their own avoidance of the difficulty inherent in building a helping relationship, which could then attenuate the positive effects of therapy. Ultimately, the therapy relationship is a place for clients to learn how to ask for and receive support as they work on therapy goals, which can usually be subsumed under the broader categories of having loving relationships and doing gratifying work in personal development.

Often clients learn what it is like to be in a healthy relationship for the first time in FAP by dealing with issues such as honesty, needs, fears, trust, caring, commitment, acceptance, and boundaries. Client dependence and attachment to the therapist can be a concern. As with any other client behavior, dependence needs to be understood in the context of a client's history. When is dependence healthy, and when does it interfere with the client's daily life? For clients who have never allowed themselves to be dependent on anyone, facilitating their expression of a need for more contact (whether in the form of additional sessions or phone or e-mail interactions) with the therapist is a CRB2. When their needs clash with the therapist's (e.g., to limit work hours), the issue needs to be explored with honesty and caring. Perhaps a compromise can be worked out, perhaps not, but discussing the problem directly models for clients what to do when their needs (invariably) clash with someone else's needs. Therapists should get support through supervision, consultation, or informal contact with colleagues for setting their own boundaries with kindness and honesty. In general, the boundaries of the therapy relationship (relative inaccessibility of the therapist, the power differential, fee for service) serve to foster clients' investment in daily life relationships. As clients heal, the understanding that the therapeutic relationship is a means to an end, not an end in itself, becomes more of a focus. Ideally, as FAP draws to a close, clients have the skills to form other healthy emotionally close relationships.

In sum, the practice of FAP necessitates much more than a solid theoretical understanding of the interventions used. Because FAP is interpersonally focused, therapists need to be willing to use their own emotional experiences of their clients as data. Some therapists prefer to keep an emotional distance from their clients, and whereas such therapists might be extremely effective in providing other modalities of therapy, they are not likely to be effective (or happy) FAP therapists. The proper implementation of FAP requires that therapists work outside of their comfort zones—that they bring to the therapeutic relationship honesty, courage, clarity, self-knowledge, a capacity for intimacy, an acceptance of both positive and negative affect, and the ability to take emotional risks. Thus FAP therapists need to take active steps to get consultation, supervision, and/or personal therapy as needed. Below we describe an example of how FAP clinical supervision can be used as an opportunity to create resilient, meaningful, and effective client–therapist relationships.

FAP Clinical Supervision: Case Example

Clients with complex PTSD have particular difficulties with interpersonal intimacy, as previously described. For example, these clients may struggle with discomfort because of the power differential between client and therapist, worrying that they may be further traumatized or devalued. Conversely, the power differential may actually feel very secure to them; it is seeing the therapist's vulnerability and fallibility that causes difficulty, perhaps working avoidant behavior in response. It may be very difficult for clients to develop trust, to learn to ask for help, to display vulnerabilities as well as strengths, and to develop perspective about emotional turmoil experienced within the relationship.

Therapists may have problems similar to their clients, albeit to a lesser degree, in the presence of the supervisor or consultant. In any supervisory relationship there is a power differential; it can therefore be a challenge to display vulnerabilities as well as strengths, and therapists also may struggle with how to place their emotional reactions to supervision in perspective.

The same framework that facilitates treatment of complex PTSD can also facilitate the development of therapist repertoires that serve to promote effective FAP. Being aware, open, vulnerable, honest, and present are aspects of intimate behavior that we wish to shape in both our clients and our supervisees. Explorations of how these behaviors emerge in supervision and serve to impact psychotherapy would be the focus of clinical supervision.

Supervision can serve to model the kinds of FAP principles and behaviors that occur in session. Typical questions asked of the supervisee may include focusing directly on how the supervisee feels toward the supervisor, asking about the similarities between the client's issues and the therapist's issues, noting and blocking emotional avoidance that is noticed in the psychotherapy as well as that which occurs in the supervisory session. Power differential, being evaluated, wanting to avoid punishment, and wanting more (or less) from the supervisor are all features of supervision that are also features of the therapeutic encounter.

The following description of a supervision session serves to illustrate these principles:

SUPERVISOR: I notice that although we are working well together, I feel that there is a distance between us that may be blocking our work from becoming truly meaningful. I notice that just as your client glossed over what had happened with that flashback, you might have glossed over how you felt when I was late to supervision today.

SUPERVISEE: I know. I look forward to our supervision, and I really want you to see me as a great therapist. I worry that if I expressed my upset to you, you would be uncomfortable—and I mainly want to impress you with my skills.

SUPERVISOR: Can you describe more about how you felt when I was late?

SUPERVISEE: I felt kind of devalued, like you didn't want to be in this supervision, that there were a million things more important than me. And I didn't want to say anything because I worried you would like me even less.

SUPERVISOR: Wow, I didn't know. Can you tell me more about these feelings?

SUPERVISEE: I was really jazzed when you and I started working together. I was hopeful about growing immensely as a therapist. I wanted you to see me as really great, and I wanted there to be great feelings between us. Then I got this very difficult client, and I was afraid that I wouldn't be able to handle the degree of emotion that the client has beneath the surface. I didn't want to reach out to you about my fear. I thought you would think I was a bad therapist. So I thought I would just let it alone—not an unfamiliar pattern for me. I have gotten feedback in the past that I tend to avoid getting into my own fears. It extends way back in my life, and I see that it is interfering with our work and my work with my client.

SUPERVISOR: Right now I feel that we are more connected than usual and that this feels very meaningful. Being late might have reflected some of my feelings of disconnection with you, I am not sure. I also struggle at times with uncomfortable affect, so my own discomfort might have contributed to my not bringing up these problems earlier. I want you to know that I value working with you, and that I also wonder a lot about what is preventing our supervision from growing from good to great supervision. I think that when you express your vulnerabilities and fears, as you just did, I feel so much more connected with you, and I am just pulled to invest more.

SUPERVISEE: So what do we do?

SUPERVISOR: I think we continue to notice that for both of us, a proclivity to avoid discomfort can work to really sabotage our supervision. Let's work on noticing how our level of connection waxes and wanes, and let's address more quickly the emotional avoidance on both of our parts that might contribute to gaps occurring.

SUPERVISEE: OK, and I am aware that this same process can help me while in session with my client.

As this example demonstrates, the principles of FAP can be applied in supervision, just as they can be applied in psychotherapy. A common thread involves the kinds of difficulties that occur in any relationship, particularly when there is a power differential and the potential for hurt, along with the potential for tremendous growth and positive connection.

CONCLUSIONS

Repeated traumatic experiences in childhood typically lead to incredible emotional pain and often profoundly disrupt interpersonal functioning. Unlike discrete trauma, for which exposure therapies are relatively simple to design and administer, complex trauma tends not to link back to a clear set of stimuli that are amenable to traditional exposure procedures. Given that complex trauma can present in the form of being unable to develop and sustain intimate relationships, however, the therapeutic encounter itself may provide the perfect exposure exercise. Typical therapy experiences such as being asked to reveal intimate life details, being invited to trust, having emotional responses when being cared for, and so on, are all potentially evocative for the trauma survivor. These experiences can evoke client behavior in the service of avoiding negative affect, which can also serve to disrupt the creation of an effective, intimate, working relationship with the therapist. In many ways, instances of client avoidance that occur in the session are perfect therapeutic opportunities that allow the therapist to work with the patient toward responding differently to the painful affect generated in the therapy.

FAP (Kohlenberg & Tsai, 1991) offers specific guidelines for noticing in-session behavior that is avoidant and thus may interfere with developing a close relationship, as well as guidelines for shaping new behaviors in the service of promoting the creation of caring, engaged, and emotionally intense therapeutic relationships. Providing interactions such as these can impart both corrective experiences and verbal descriptions of how to respond more effectively in the world, thus promoting the development of healthy relationships outside of therapy as well.

In addition to the therapeutic context, FAP is well suited to guide effective clinical supervision of trauma cases. This kind of supervision would direct the supervisor and the supervisee to be attentive to emotional avoidance in the supervision session, and would promote an analysis of the practicality and function of such avoidance. Parallels are drawn between the supervision and the therapy being supervised. Therapists are encouraged to address emotional avoidance in supervision in the service of promoting vitality both in supervision and in therapy. And, of course, the vitality of emotional engagement is an important aspect of the intimate relationships that we hope to help our clients attain.

It is our strong bias that the most powerful treatment experiences make use of CRBs between therapist and the client. This CRB component is especially important when the client's main emotional wounds come from childhood abuse involving trusted adults whose tasks were to protect and to nurture. Such betrayal is among the deepest wounds that can be endured. Because the therapist–client relationship replicates many essential elements of the parent–child relationship, it has great potential for both harm and healing. We hope that our discussion of the origins and treatment of interpersonal trauma provides a clear conceptual system to aid those who have taken on the noble task of helping to heal the emotional scars of clients who were violated as children.

REFERENCES

American Psychiatric Association. (1994). *Diagnostic and statistical manual of mental disorders* (4th ed.). Washington, DC: Author.

Archer, J. A., & Cooper, S. E. (1998). Counseling and mental health services in college contexts: A handbook of contemporary practices and challenges. San Francisco: Jossey-Bass.

Beitchman, J. H., Zucker, K. J., Hood, J. E., Dacosta, G. A., Akman, D., & Cassavia, E. (1992). A review of the long-term effects of child sexual abuse. *Child Abuse and Neglect, 16,* 101–118.

Blake, D., Albano, A., & Keane, T. (1992). Twenty years of trauma: *Psychological Abstracts* through 1989. *Journal of Traumatic Stress, 5,* 477–484.

Bonanno, G. A. (2004). Loss, trauma, and human resilience. *American Psychologist, 59*(1), 20–28.

Bonanno, G. A., & Field, N. P. (2001). Examining the delayed grief hypothesis across five years of bereavement. *American Behavioral Scientist, 44,* 798–806.

Brady, J. L., Guy, J. D., Poelstra, P. L., & Fletcher-Brokaw, B. (1999). Vicarious traumatization, spirituality, and the treatment of sexual abuse survivors: A National Survey of Women Psychotherapists. *Professional Psychology: Research and Practice, 30*(4), 386–393.

Briere, J. (2002). Treating adult survivors of severe childhood abuse and neglect: Further development of an integrative model. In J. E. B. Myers, L. Berliner, J. Briere, C. T. Hendrix, T. Reid, & C. Jenny (Eds.), *The APSAC handbook on child maltreatment* (2nd ed.).Newbury Park, CA: Sage.

Cadell, S., Regehr, C., & Hemsworth, D. (2003). Factors contributing to posttraumatic growth: A proposed structural equation model. *American Journal of Orthopsychiatry, 73*(3), 279–287.

Callaghan, G. M., Summers, C. J., & Weidman, M. (2003). The treatment of histrionic and narcissistic personality disorder behaviors: A single-subject demonstration of clinical improvement using functional analytic psychotherapy. *Journal of Contemporary Psychotherapy, 33*(4), 321–339.

Cloitre, M., Karestan, C. K., Cohen, L. R., & Han, H. (2002). Skills training in affective and interpersonal regulation followed by exposure: A phase-based treatment for PTSD related to childhood abuse. *Journal of Consulting and Clinical Psychology, 70* 1067–1074.

Cloitre, M., Chase Stovall-McClough, K., Miranda, R., & Chemtob, C. M. (2004). Therapeutic alliance, negative mood regulation, and treatment outcome in child abuse-related posttraumatic stress disorder. *Journal of Consulting and Clinical Psychology, 72*(3), 411–416.

Dougher, M. J., Auguston, E., Markham, M. R., & Greenway, D. E. (1994). The transfer of respondent eliciting and extinction functions through stimulus equivalence classes. *Journal of the Experimental Analysis of Behavior, 62,* 331–351.

Figley, C. R. (1995). *Compassion fatigue: Coping with secondary traumatic stress disorder in those who treat the traumatized.* New York: Brunner/Mazel.

Figley, C. R. (2002). *Treating compassion fatigue.* New York: Brunner/Mazel.

Foa, E. B., & Rothbaum, B. O. (1997). *Treating the trauma of rape.* New York: Guilford Press.

Follette, V. M., Polusny, M. M., & Milbeck, K. (1994). Mental health and law enforcement professionals: Trauma history, psychological symptoms, and impact of providing services to child sexual abuse survivors.

Goldfried, M. G. (1985). *In-vivo* intervention or transference?: In W. Dryden (Ed.), *Therapist's dilemmas* (pp. 71–94). London: Harper & Row.

Hayes, S. C. (1987). A contextual approach to therapeutic change. In N. S. Jacobson (Ed.), *Psychotherapists in clinical practice: Cognitive and behavioral perspectives* (pp. 327–387). New York: Guilford Press.

Hayes, S. C., Barns-Holmes, D., & Roche, B. (2001). *Relational frame theory: A post-Skinnerian account of human language and cognition.* New York: Plenum Press.

Herman, J. (1992a). Complex PTSD: A syndrome in survivors of prolonged and repeated trauma. *Journal of Traumatic Stress, 5,* 377–391.

Herman, J. (1992b). *Trauma and recovery.* New York: Basic Books.

Herman, J., Russell, D., & Trocki, K. (1986). Long-term effects of incestuous abuse in childhood. *American Journal of Psychiatry, 143,* 1293–1296.

Holmqvist, R., & Anderson, K. (2003). Therapists' reactions to treatment of survivors of political torture. *Professional Psychology: Research and Practice, 34*(3), 294–300.

Horvath, A. O., & Symonds, B. D. (1991). Relation between working alliance and outcome in psychotherapy: A meta-analysis. *Journal of Counseling Psychology, 38,* 139–149.

Hyer, L. (1994). *Trauma victim: Theoretical issues and practical suggestions.* Muncie, IN: Accelerated Development.

Jaycox, L. H., Foa, E. B., & Morral, A. R. (1998). Influence of emotional engagement and habituation on exposure therapy for PTSD. *Journal of Consulting and Clinical Psychology, 66*(1), 185–192.

Jenkins, S. R., & Baird, S. (2002). Secondary traumatic stress and vicarious trauma: A validated study. *Journal of Traumatic Stress, 15*(5), 423–432.

Kessler, R. C., Sonnega, A., Bromet, E., Hughes, M., & Nelson, C. B. (1995). Posttraumatic stress disorder in the National Comorbidity Survey. *Archives of General Psychiatry, 53,* 1048–1060.

Kohlenberg, R. J., Kanter, J. W., Bolling, M. Y., Parker, C., & Tsai, M. (2002). Enhancing cognitive therapy for depression with functional analytic psychotherapy: Treatment guidelines and empirical findings. *Cognitive and Behavioral Practice, 9*(3), 213–229.

Kohlenberg, R. J., & Tsai, M. (1991). Functional analytic psychotherapy: Creating intense and curative therapeutic relationships. New York: Plenum Press.

Kohlenberg, R. J., & Tsai, M. (1993). Hidden meaning: A behavioral approach. *Behavior Therapist, 16,* 80–82.

Kohlenberg, R. J., & Tsai, M. (1995). I speak, therefore I am: A behavioral approach to understanding of the self. *Behavior Therapist, 18,* 113–116.

Kohlenberg, R. J., & Tsai, M. (1998). Healing interpersonal trauma with the intimacy of the therapeutic relationship. In V. M. Follette, J. I. Ruzek, & F. R. Abueg (Eds.), *Cognitive-behavioral therapies for trauma* (pp. 305–320). New York: Guilford Press.

Kubany, E. S., Hill, E. E., Owens, J. A., Iannce-Spencer, C., McCaig, M. A., Tremayne, K. J., & Williams, P. L. (2004). Cognitive trauma therapy for battered women with PTSD (CTT-BW). *Journal of Consulting and Clinical Psychology, 72*(1), 3–18.

Leahy, T., Pretty, G., & Tenenbaum, G. (2003). Childhood sexual abuse narratives in clinically and nonclinically distressed adult survivors. *Professional Psychology: Research and Practice. Vol. 34,* 657–665.

Maki, W. S. (1981). Directed forgetting in pigeons. *Animal Learning and Behavior, 8,* 567–574.

Meadows, E. A., & Foa, E. B. (1998). Intrusion, arousal, and avoidance: Sexual trauma survivors. In V. Follette, J. Ruzak, & F. Abueg (Eds.), *Cognitive-behavioral therapies for trauma* (pp. 100–123). New York: Guilford Press.

Mednick, S. A. (1975). Autonomic nervous system recovery and psychopathology. *Scandinavian Journal of Behaviour Therapy, 4,* 55–68.

Meldrum, L., King, R., & Spooner, D. (2002). Compassion fatigue in community mental health case managers. In C. R. Figley (Ed.), *Treating compassion fatigue* (pp. 85–106). New York: Brunner/Routledge.

Merrill, L. L., Guimond, J. M., Thomsen, C. J., & Milner, J. S. (2003). Child sexual abuse and number of sexual partners in young women: The role of abuse severity, coping style, and sexual functioning. *Journal of Consulting and Clinical Psychology, 71*(6), 987–996.

Mowrer, O. H. (1960). *Learning theory and behavior.* New York: Wiley.

Najavits, L. M., Weiss, R. D., Shaw, S. R., & Muenz, L. R. (1998). "Seeking Safety": Outcome of a new cognitive-behavioral psychotherapy for women with posttraumatic stress disorder and substance dependence. *Journal of Traumatic Stress, 11,* 437–456.

Nelson, B. S., Wangsgaard, S., Yorgason, J., Kessler, M., & Carter-Vassol, E. (2002). Single- and dual-trauma couples: Clinical observations of relational characteristics and dynamics. *American Journal of Orthopsychiatry, 72*(1), 58–69.

Noll, J. G., Trickett, P. K., & Putnam, F. W. (2003). A prospective investigation of the impact of childhood sexual abuse on the development of sexuality. *Journal of Consulting and Clinical Psychology, 71*(3), 575–586.

Ozer, E. J., Best, S. R., Lipsey, T. L, & Weiss, D. S. (2003). Predictors of posttraumatic stress disorder and symptoms in adults: A metaanalysis. *Psychological Bulletin, 129,* 52–71.

Paivio, S. C., Holowaty, K. A. M., & Hall, I. E. (2004). The influence of therapist adherence and competence on client reprocessing of child abuse memories. *Psychotherapy: Theory, Research, Practice, Training, 41*(1), 56–68.

Pearlman, L. A., & Mac Ian, P. S. (1995). Vicarious traumatization: An empirical study of the effects of trauma work on trauma therapists. *Professional Psychology: Research and Practice, 26*(6), 558–565.

Pope, K. S., & Feldman-Summers, S. (1992). National survey of psychologists' sexual and physical abuse history and their evaluation of training and competence in these areas. *Professional Psychology: Research and Practice, 23,* 353–361.

Roth, S., Newman, E., Pelcovitz, D., van der Kolk, B., & Mandel, F. (1997). Complex PTSD in victims exposed to sexual and physical abuse: Results from the DSM-IV field trial for posttraumatic stress disorder. *Journal of Traumatic Stress*, *10*, 539–555.

Shmotkin, D., Blumstein, T., & Modan, B. (2003). Tracing long-term effects of early trauma: A broad-scope view of Holocaust survivors in late life. *Journal of Consulting and Clinical Psychology*, *71*(2), 223–234.

Sokolov, Y. N. (1963). *Perception and the conditioned reflex* (S. W. Wadenfeld, Trans.). Oxford, UK: Pergamon Press.

Terr, L. C. (1990). *Too scared to cry: Psychic trauma in childhood*. New York: HarperCollins.

Tsai, M., Feldman-Summers, S., & Edgar, M. (1979). Childhood molestation: Variables related to differential impacts on psychosexual functioning in adult women. *Journal of Abnormal Psychology*, *88*(4), 407–417.

Zettle, R. D., & Hayes, S. C. (1986). Dysfunctional control by client verbal behavior: The context of reason giving. *Analysis of Verbal Behavior*, *4*, 30–38.

PART THREE
Specialized Populations and Delivery Considerations

CHAPTER NINE

Cognitive-Behavioral Therapy for Acute Stress Disorder

Richard A. Bryant

The persistent distress that can be suffered by many trauma survivors has led to unprecedented attention on creating ways to prevent this distress. Much of this attention has focused on early interventions with people who are high risk for developing long-term disorders. This chapter reviews recent developments in the early identification of people who are high risk for posttraumatic stress disorder (PTSD). The chapter initially addresses the utility of the acute stress disorder (ASD) diagnosis as a marker of people who require early intervention. The review then proceeds to outline the major developments in assessment and treatment of people with ASD, and provides practical guidelines for managing people in the acute phase after trauma.

THE COURSE OF ACUTE STRESS REACTIONS

Across the literature, there are reports of high rates of emotional numbing (Feinstein, 1989; Noyes, Hoenk, Kuperman, & Slymen, 1977), reduced awareness of one's environment (Berah, Jones, & Valent, 1984; Hillman, 1981), derealization (Cardeña & Spiegel, 1993; Noyes & Kletti, 1977; Sloan, 1988; Freinkel, Koopman, & Spiegel, 1994), depersonalization (Noyes et al., 1977; Cardeña & Spiegel, 1993; Sloan, 1988; Freinkel et al., 1994), intrusive thoughts (Feinstein, 1989; Cardeña & Spiegel, 1993; Sloan, 1988), avoidance behaviors (Cardeña & Spiegel, 1993; North, Smith, McCool, & Lightcap, 1989; Bryant & Harvey, 1996), insomnia (Feinstein, 1989; Cardeña & Spiegel, 1993; Sloan, 1988), concentration deficits (Cardeña & Spiegel, 1993; North et al., 1989), irritability (Sloan, 1988), and autonomic arousal (Feinstein, 1989; Sloan, 1988) in the weeks after a traumatic experience.

Despite the high prevalence of acute stress reactions, it appears that most of these stress responses are transient. For example, whereas 94% of rape victims displayed sufficient PTSD symptoms 2 weeks posttrauma to meet DSM-IV criteria (excluding the 1 month time requirement; American Psychiatric Association, 1994), this rate had dropped to 47% 11 weeks later (Rothbaum, Foa, Riggs, Murdock, & Walsh, 1992). In another study 70% of women and 50% of men were diagnosed with PTSD at an average of 19 days after an assault; the rate of PTSD at 4-month follow-up had dropped to 21% for women and 0% for men (Riggs, Rothbaum, & Foa, 1995). Similarly, half of a sample of individuals who met criteria for PTSD shortly after a motor vehicle accident had remitted by 6 months, and two-thirds had remitted by 1-year posttrauma (Blanchard et al., 1996). There is also evidence that most stress responses after the terrorist attacks of September 11 may have been temporary reactions. Galea et al. (2002) surveyed residents of New York City to gauge their response to the terrorist attacks. Five to eight weeks after the attacks, 7.5% of a random sample of adults living south of 110th Street in Manhattan had developed PTSD, and of those living south of Canal Street, 20% had PTSD. In February 2002, Galea's group did a study on another group of adults living south of 110th Street and found that only 1.7% of the sample had PTSD related to the attacks (Galea et al., 2003). The available evidence suggests that the normative response to trauma is to initially experience a range of PTSD symptoms, which remit in the following months.

ACUTE STRESS DISORDER

In 1994 the fourth edition of the *Diagnostic and Statistical Manual of Mental Disorders* (DSM-IV; American Psychiatric Association, 1994) introduced the ASD diagnosis to describe stress reactions in the initial month following a trauma. It was felt that because DSM-IV stipulated that PTSD could only be recognized at least 1 month after a trauma, there was a need to describe reactions occurring in the initial month. A second goal was to identify people who would develop PTSD shortly after trauma exposure (Koopman, Classen, Cardeña, & Spiegel, 1995). The DSM-IV stipulates that ASD can occur after a fearful response to experiencing or witnessing a threatening event (cluster A). The requisite symptoms to meet criteria for ASD include three dissociative symptoms (cluster B), one reexperiencing symptom (cluster C), marked avoidance (cluster D), marked anxiety or increased arousal (cluster E), and evidence of significant distress or impairment (cluster F). The disturbance must last for a minimum of 2 days and a maximum of 4 weeks (cluster G), after which time a diagnosis of PTSD should be considered. The primary difference between the criteria for ASD and PTSD is the time frame and the former's emphasis on dissociative reactions to the trauma. ASD refers to symptoms manifested during the period from 2 days to 4 weeks posttrauma, whereas PTSD can only be diagnosed 4 weeks posttrauma. The diagnosis of ASD requires that the individual has at least three of the following: (1) a subjective sense of numbing or detachment, (2) reduced awareness of his or her surroundings, (3) derealization, (4) depersonalization, or (5) dissociative amnesia.

The ASD diagnosis was largely influenced by the notion that dissociative reactions are a crucial mechanism in posttraumatic adjustment. Expressing this view much earlier, Janet (1907) proposed that traumatic experiences that were incongruent with existing cognitive schemas led to dissociated awareness. He argued that although this splitting of traumatic memories from awareness led to a reduction in distress, there was a loss of mental functioning because mental resources were not available for other processes. This perspective has received much attention in recent years (van der Kolk & van der Hart, 1989; Nemiah, 1989) and represents the basis for the pivotal role of dissociation in the ASD diagnosis.

DOES ASD PREDICT PTSD?

There are now 12 prospective studies of adults that have assessed the relationship between ASD in the initial month posttrauma and development of subsequent PTSD (Brewin, Andrews, Rose, & Kirk, 1999; Bryant & Harvey, 1998; Creamer, O'Donnell, & Pattison, 2004; Difede et al., 2002; Harvey & Bryant, 1998, 1999, 2000; Holeva, Tarrier, & Wells, 2001; Kangas, Henry, & Bryant, 2005; Murray, Ehlers, & Mayou, 2002; Schnyder, Moergeli, Klaghofer, & Buddeberg, 2001; Staab, Grieger, Fullerton, & Ursano, 1996). In terms of people who meet criteria for ASD, some studies have found that approximately three-quarters of trauma survivors who display ASD subsequently develop PTSD (Brewin et al., 1999; Bryant & Harvey, 1998; Difede et al., 2002; Harvey & Bryant, 1998, 1999, 2000; Holeva et al., 2001; Kangas et al., 2005; Murray et al., 2002). Compared to the expected remission of most people who display initial posttraumatic stress reactions, these studies indicate that the ASD diagnosis is performing reasonably well in predicting people who will develop PTSD. However, the utility of the ASD diagnosis is less encouraging when we consider the proportion of people who eventually developed PTSD and who initially displayed ASD. In most studies the minority of people who eventually developed PTSD initially met criteria for ASD. That is, whereas the majority of people who develop ASD are at high risk for developing subsequent PTSD, many people develop PTSD who do not initially meet ASD criteria. It appears that a major reason for this discrepancy between high risk for PTSD and unfulfilled ASD criteria is the requirement of three dissociative symptoms. In one study, 60% of people who met all ASD criteria except for the dissociation cluster met PTSD criteria 6 months later (Harvey & Bryant, 1998), and 75% of these people still had PTSD 2 years later (Harvey & Bryant, 1999). This pattern suggests that emphasizing dissociation as a critical factor in predicting subsequent PTSD leads to a neglect of other acute stress reactions that also represent a risk for development of chronic PTSD.

IMPLICATIONS FOR ASSESSING ASD

There have been numerous criticisms of the ASD diagnosis (see Koopman, 2000; Simeon & Guralnik, 2000; Butler, 2000; Bryant & Harvey, 2000; Harvey & Bryant, 2002; Keane, Kaufman, & Kimble, 2001; Marshall, Spitzer, & Liebowitz, 2000; Spiegel, Classen, Cardeña, 2000). First, the new ASD diagnosis was introduced with very little evidence to support its inclusion. Whereas inclusion of other diagnoses in the DSM-IV required satisfaction of a number of standards (including literature reviews, statistical analyses of established datasets, and field trials), the ASD diagnosis did not undergo this rigorous scrutiny (Bryant, 2000). Second, the emphasis on dissociation as a necessary response to trauma was criticized on the grounds that there was insufficient evidence to warrant assigning such a pivotal role in acute trauma response to this construct (Bryant & Harvey, 1997; Keane et al., 2001; Marshall et al., 2000). As noted above, the available evidence suggests that the requirement of dissociation leads to oversight of many high-risk people. Third, some objected to the notion that the primary role of the ASD diagnosis was to predict another diagnosis (McNally, 2003). Fourth, there was concern that the diagnosis may pathologize transient reactions (Marshall, Spitzer, & Liebowitz, 1999). Fifth, it was argued that distinguishing between two diagnoses (ASD and PTSD) that have comparable symptoms on the basis of the duration of these symptoms is not justified (Marshall et al., 1999). These criticisms raise questions about the utility of the ASD diagnosis to identify people in the acute phase who are at high risk for subsequent PTSD. Although the data are mixed at this point, it appears that people who satisfy the ASD criteria are at high risk for PTSD and require therapeutic intervention. Additionally, people who display intense acute stress reactions, although lacking dissociative responses, are also at high risk and should be identified as candidates for early intervention. To further increase the accuracy of early identification of people who are at high risk for PTSD, recent attention has also focused on acute cognitive and biological factors that appear to be associated with development of later PTSD.

COGNITIVE MECHANISMS OF ASD

Current models posit that psychopathological responses may be mediated by two core cognitive factors: (1) maladaptive appraisals of the trauma and its aftermath, and (2) disturbances in autobiographical memory that involve impaired retrieval and strong associative memory (Ehlers & Clark, 2000). Consistent with this approach is evidence that people with ASD exaggerate both the probability of future negative events occurring and the adverse effects of these events (Warda & Bryant, 1998a). Moreover, ASD participants display cognitive biases for events related to external harm, somatic sensations, and social concerns (Smith & Bryant, 2000). Experimental studies indicate that ASD individuals respond to a hyperventilation task with more dysfunctional interpretations about their reactions than non-ASD individuals (Nixon & Bryant, 2003). There is also evidence that catastrophic appraisals about self in the period after trauma exposure predict subsequent PTSD (Ehlers, Mayou, & Bryant, 1998b; Engelhard, van den Hout, Arntz, & McNally, 2002). Relatedly, the nature of attributions about the trauma shortly after the event apparently influences longer-term functioning. Prospective studies indicate that attributing responsibility to another person (Delahanty et al., 1997) and attributions of shame (Andrews, Brewin, Rose, & Kirk, 2000) in the acute phase are associated with later PTSD.

There is also evidence that people with ASD may manage trauma-related information differently from other trauma survivors. Specifically, individuals with ASD tend to avoid aversive information. One study employed a directed forgetting paradigm that required ASD, non-ASD, and non-trauma-exposed control participants to read a series of trauma-related, positive, or neutral words. After each presentation participants were instructed to either remember or forget the word (Moulds & Bryant, 2002). The finding that ASD participants recalled fewer trauma-related to-be-forgotten words than non-ASD participants suggests that they have an aptitude for forgetting aversive material. In a similar study that employed the list method form of directed forgetting, which indexes retrieval patterns, ASD participants displayed poorer recall of to-be-forgotten trauma words than non-ASD participants (Moulds & Bryant, 2005). These findings suggest that people with ASD possess a cognitive style that avoids awareness of aversive or distressing information. This interpretation accords with findings that people with ASD use avoidant cognitive strategies to manage their trauma memories (Guthrie & Bryant, 2000; Warda & Bryant, 1998b). Avoidance of distressing information or memories may be associated with psychopathological responses because it may lead to impaired processing of trauma-related memories and affect. In terms of autobiographical memory, one study has found that ASD participants reported fewer specific positive memories than non-ASD participants, and this deficit contributed to subsequent PTSD severity (Harvey, Bryant, & Dang, 1998). This pattern may suggest that problems in retrieving positive memories about one's personal past may limit access to information that is useful in making adaptive appraisals about the trauma and its consequences (Ehlers & Clark, 2000).

BIOLOGICAL MECHANISMS OF ASD

Biological perspectives have focused on fear conditioning and progressive neural sensitization in the weeks after trauma as possible explanations of the genesis of PTSD (Kolb, 1987; Pitman, Shalev, & Orr, 2000). It is possible that sensitization occurs as a result of repetitive activation by trauma reminders, which elevate sensitivity of limbic networks (Post, Weiss, & Smith, 1995), and that as time progresses these responses become increasingly conditioned to trauma-related stimuli (LeDoux, Iwata, Cicchetti, & Reis, 1988). In support of these proposals, there is evidence that people who eventually develop PTSD display elevated resting heart rates in the initial week after trauma (Bryant, Harvey, Guthrie, & Moulds, 2000b; Shalev et al., 1998; see also Blanchard, Hickling, Gaslovski, & Veazey, 2002). There is also evidence that lower cortisol levels shortly after trauma predict subsequent PTSD (McFarlane, Atchison, & Yehuda, 1997; Delahanty, Raimonde, & Spoonster, 2000). Cortisol may act as an "anti-stress" hormone that restores equilibrium, and lower cortisol levels may reflect an incapacity to lower arousal following trauma (Yehuda, 1997). The importance of increased arousal in the acute phase is also indicated by the prevalence of panic attacks in people with ASD (Bryant & Panasetis, 2001; Nixon & Bryant, 2003). A promising finding emerged from a pilot study that attempted to prevent PTSD by administering propranolol (a beta-adrenergic blocker) within 6 hours of trauma exposure (Pitman et al., 2002); there is evidence that propanolol abolishes the epinephrine enhancement of conditioning (Cahill, Prins, Weber, & McGaugh, 1994). Although propanolol did not result in reduced PTSD relative to a placebo condition, patients receiving propanolol displayed less reactivity to trauma reminders 3 months later. A subsequent study has found that propanolol administered immediately after trauma does reduce PTSD severity 2 months later (Vaiva et al., 2003). This outcome suggests that propanolol administration shortly after trauma exposure may limit the fear conditioning that may contribute to subsequent PTSD development.

Measurement Tools for ASD

There are currently three structured measures specifically designed to assess for ASD. The first measure to be developed was the Stanford Acute Stress Reaction Questionnaire (SASRQ). The original version of the SASRQ (Cardeña, Classen, & Spiegel, 1991) was a self-report inventory that indexed dissociative (33 items), intrusive (11 items), somatic anxiety (17 items), hyperarousal (2 items), attention disturbance (3 items), and sleep disturbance (1 item) symptoms, and different versions of this measure have been employed by the authors across a range of studies (Cardeña & Spiegel, 1993; Classen, Koopman, Hales, & Spiegel, 1998; Freinkel et al., 1994; Koopman, Classen, & Spiegel, 1994). Each item asks respondents to indicate the frequency of each symptom on a 6-point Likert scale (0 = "not experienced"; 5 = "very often experienced") that may occur during and immediately following a trauma. The SASRQ possesses high internal consistency (Cronbachs alpha = .90 and .91 for dissociative and anxiety symptoms, respectively) and concurrent validity with scores on the IES (r = .52 − .69; Koopman et al., 1994). Different versions of the SASRQ have been employed in a number of studies conducted by the authors (Cardeña & Spiegel, 1989; Classen et al., 1998; Freinkel et al., 1994; Koopman et al., 1994). The current version of the SASRQ (Cardeña, Koopman, Classen, Waelde, & Spiegel, 2000) is a 30-item self-report inventory that encompasses each of the ASD symptoms. At this stage, the SASRQ has not been validated against independent clinician-diagnosed ASD diagnosis. Although SASRQ scores are predictive of subsequent posttraumatic stress symptomatology, there is limited data concerning SASRQ scores and subsequent PTSD diagnostic status.

The Acute Stress Disorder Interview (ASDI; Bryant, Harvey, Dang, & Sackville, 1998a) is a structured clinical interview that is based on DSM-IV criteria. The ASDI contains 19 dichotomously scored items that relate to the dissociative (cluster B, five items), reexperiencing (cluster C, four items), avoidance (cluster D, four items), and arousal (cluster E, six items) symptoms of ASD. Summing the affirmative responses to each symptom provides a total score indicative of acute stress severity (range, 1–19). The ASDI possesses good internal consistency ($r = .90$), test–retest reliability ($r = .88$), sensitivity (91%), and specificity (93%) relative to independent clinician diagnosis of ASD. The ASDI has also been used in prospective studies that have identified recently trauma-exposed people who subsequently develop PTSD (Bryant & Harvey, 1998; Harvey & Bryant, 1998, 1999, 2000).

The Acute Stress Disorder Scale (ASDS; Bryant, Moulds, & Guthrie, 2000a) is a self-report inventory that is based on the same items described in the ASDI. Each item on the ASDS is scored on a 5-point Likert scale that reflects degrees of severity. It was validated against the ASDI on 99 civilian trauma survivors assessed between 2 and 10 days posttrauma. Using a formula to identify ASD cases, the ASDS possessed good sensitivity (95%) and specificity (83%). Test–retest reliability was evaluated on 107 bushfire survivors 3 weeks posttrauma, with a re-administration interval of 2 to 7 days. Test–retest reliability of the ASDS scores was strong ($r = 0.94$). Predictive ability of the ASDS was investigated in 82 trauma survivors who completed the ASDS and were subsequently assessed for PTSD 6 months posttrauma. A cutoff score of 56 on the ASDS predicted 91% of those who developed PTSD and 93% of those who did not. The major limitation of the ASDS in predicting PTSD, however, was that one-third of people who scored above the cutoff did not develop PTSD.

It needs to be noted that these measures of ASD suffer from the same limitations of the ASD diagnosis. That is, requiring dissociation to be present will probably result in the oversight of many high-risk individuals, possibly preventing them from receiving treatment from which they could benefit. One way to increase the likelihood of accurately identifying people who will develop PTSD is to delay the assessment for several weeks after trauma exposure. It is very probable that the sooner a clinician diagnoses ASD after trauma exposure, the more likely he or she will confuse a psychopathological response with a transient stress reaction. There is some evidence from a study of civilians involved in the Gulf War that many people experience immediate posttraumatic stress reactions in the initial days after trauma exposure but that these reactions subsequently remit (Solomon, Laor, & McFarlane, 1996). One study found that whereas 77% of people who were diagnosed with ASD at 4 weeks posttrauma subsequently developed PTSD, only 32% of those diagnosed with ASD 1 week posttrauma subsequently met criteria for PTSD (Murray et al., 2002).

WHAT IS THE EVIDENCE FOR CBT'S EFFECTIVENESS?

Cognitive-behavioral therapy (CBT) typically comprises psychoeducation, anxiety management, stress inoculation, cognitive restructuring, imaginal and in vivo exposure, and relapse prevention. Although there is considerable evidence for the efficacy of CBT in reducing PTSD symptoms in people with chronic PTSD (for reviews, see Bryant & Friedman, 2001; Foa & Meadows, 1997; Foa, 2001; Harvey, Bryant, & Tarrier, 2002), there is a limited evidence base for early interventions using CBT. Apart from uncontrolled studies of early interventions that employed some CBT approaches (Brom, Kleber, & Hofman, 1993; Viney, Clark, Bunn, & Benjamin, 1985), the first attempts at controlled study of early intervention applied behavioral approaches. Kilpatrick and Veronen (1984) randomly allocated 15 recent rape victims to either repeated assessments, delayed assessment, or a brief behavioral intervention that comprised a 4- to 6-hour program that involved imaginal reliving of the trauma, education about psychological responses to trauma, cognitive restructuring, and anxiety management. The brief intervention was no more effective than the repeated assessments. This study was limited, however, by small sample sizes, the lack of rigorous application of exposure, and ambiguity about the degree of psychopathology experienced after the rape (Kilpatrick & Calhoun, 1988).

Foa and colleagues conducted a more rigorous study by providing brief CBT to victims of sexual and nonsexual assault shortly after the trauma (Foa, Hearst-Ikeda, & Perry, 1995). This study compared participants who received CBT (including exposure, anxiety management, *in vivo* exposure, and cognitive restructuring) to matched participants who received repeated assessments. Each participant received four treatment sessions and then received assessment by blind assessors at 2 months posttreatment and at 5-month follow-up. Whereas 10% of the CBT group met criteria for PTSD at 2 months, 70% of the control group met criteria; there were no differences between groups at 5 months, although the CBT group was less depressed. This study suggests that CBT may accelerate natural recovery from trauma. Inferences from this study were limited, however, by the lack of random assignment. In a subsequent study, Foa, Zoellner, and Feeny (2002) randomly allocated survivors of assault who met criteria for PTSD in the initial weeks after the assault to four weekly sessions of CBT, repeated assessment, or supportive counseling (SC). At posttreatment, patients in the CBT and repeated-assessment conditions showed comparable improvements. SC was associated with greater PTSD severity and greater general anxiety than the CBT group. At 9-month follow-up, approximately 30% of participants in each group met criteria for PTSD.

A potential limitation of these studies is that the inclusion of all recently distressed trauma survivors raises the possibility that treatment effects may overlap with natural recovery in the initial months after trauma exposure. In an attempt to overcome this problem, other studies have focused on people who meet criteria for ASD because of evidence that most people who do display ASD are at high risk for subsequent PTSD (Bryant, 2003). In an initial study of ASD participants, Bryant and colleagues randomly allocated motor vehicle accident or nonsexual assault survivors with ASD to either CBT or SC (Bryant, Harvey, Dang, Sackville, & Basten, 1998b). Both interventions consisted of five 1.5-hour weekly individual therapy sessions. CBT included education about posttraumatic reactions, relaxation training, cognitive restructuring, and imaginal and *in vivo* exposure to the traumatic event. The SC condition included trauma education and more general problem-solving skills training in the context of an unconditionally supportive relationship. At the 6-month follow-up, fewer participants in the CBT group (20%) met diagnostic criteria for PTSD, compared to SC control participants (67%). In a subsequent study that dismantled the components of CBT, 45 civilian trauma survivors with ASD were randomly allocated to five sessions of either (1) prolonged exposure, cognitive therapy, anxiety management; (2) prolonged exposure and cognitive therapy; or (3) SC (Bryant, Sackville, Dang, Moulds, & Guthrie, 1999). This study found that at the 6-month follow-up, PTSD was observed in approximately 20% of both active treatment groups compared to 67% of those receiving SC. A follow-up of participants who completed these two treatment studies indicated that the treatment gains of those who received CBT were maintained 4 years after treatment (Bryant, Moulds, & Nixon, 2003b).

Two recent studies by the same research group have supported the utility of CBT for people with ASD. One study randomly allocated civilian trauma survivors ($N = 89$) with ASD to either CBT, CBT associated with hypnosis, or SC (Bryant, Moulds, Guthrie, & Nixon, 2005). This study added hypnosis to CBT because some commentators have argued that hypnosis may breach dissociative symptoms that characterize ASD (Spiegel, 1996). To this end, the hypnosis component was provided immediately prior to imaginal exposure in an attempt to facilitate emotional processing of the trauma memories. In terms of treatment completers, more participants in the SC condition (57%) met PTSD criteria at 6-month follow-up than those in the CBT (21%) or CBT + hypnosis (22%) condition. Interestingly, participants in the CBT + hypnosis condition reported greater reduction of reexperiencing symptoms at posttreatment than those in the CBT condition. This finding suggests that hypnosis may facilitate treatment gains in ASD participants. Finally, a recent study replicated the original Bryant et al. (1998b) study with a sample of ASD participants ($N = 24$) who had sustained mild traumatic brain injury following motor vehicle accidents (Bryant et al., 2003a). This study investigated the efficacy of CBT in people who lost consciousness during the trauma as result of their injury. Consistent with the previous studies, fewer participants receiving CBT (8%) met criteria for PTSD at 6-month follow-up than those receiving SC (58%).

Gidron et al. (2001) provided a two-session CBT intervention that was intended to promote memory reconstruction in 17 survivors of accidents. This approach was based on the premise that facilitating people's organization of trauma memories would assist processing of these memories and thereby assist recovery. Using an entry criterion of a heart rate higher than 94 beats per minute at admission to the emergency room (see Bryant et al., 2000a; Shalev et al., 1998), participants in this study received a telephone-administered protocol 1–3 days after the accident. Patients who received this intervention had greater reductions in severity of PTSD symptoms 3–4 months after the trauma than did those who received two sessions of supportive listening over the telephone.

DELIVERING CBT SHORTLY AFTER TRAUMA

Prior to commencing therapy, it is imperative to make important decisions about treatment delivery. These decisions include (1) when should therapy begin?, (2) how long should therapy continue? (3) how often should therapy be provided?, and (4) to whom should therapy be delivered? In terms of the commencement of therapy, some commentators have proposed that treating the person with ASD should occur "as soon after the trauma as possible" (Spiegel & Classen, 1995, p. 1526). However, it may be better to delay active CBT for a week or several weeks after trauma exposure, if doing so would allow the individual to accrue more resources to allocate to therapy. Treating people several weeks after trauma (1) allows them additional time to muster the resources that they can allocate to therapy, (2) decreases the likelihood that presenting symptoms will prove to be transient reactions to the trauma, and (3) increases the opportunity to resolve the immediate problems associated with the traumatic event.

Duration of therapy should be determined by therapy response and factors occurring in the period following trauma. Although most published treatment studies have employed five or six therapy sessions of 1½–2 hours, additional sessions may be required if the individual displays some clinical gains from the therapy but has not achieved adequate recovery, or ongoing stresses are impeding recovery and the individual would benefit from additional work. Therapy typically occurs on a weekly basis, but this format may be modified for a number of reasons. Hospital patients who may be discharged or military personnel who will be deployed in the near future and cannot attend therapy may be given massed (i.e., perhaps daily) therapy sessions. Some individuals may display excessive avoidance that precludes effective therapy; these patients can also benefit from daily sessions to minimize the avoidance that may accumulate when a week separates each therapy session.

Perhaps the most important decision that needs to be made is whether an individual is suitable for CBT shortly after trauma. Although there is no uniform rule that precludes any individual from early intervention, there are several clinical factors that need to be considered carefully and that may lead to the clinical decision to delay active CBT for some individuals.

Excessive Avoidance

Although strong avoidance tendencies are present in nearly all cases of ASD, degree of avoidance in a proportion of individuals impedes any form of exposure-based therapy. For example, some patients may not attend therapy sessions, be late for sessions, refuse to comply with exposure homework, or perform exposure in a superficial manner. This level of avoidance can reduce therapy efficacy and can lead patients to believe that they are not responsive to CBT. In cases of extreme avoidance, the therapist should consider the functional significance of this behavior. Some individuals employ extreme avoidance in the acute phase as a means of warding off distress that they cannot tolerate. For instance, a patient who had a hand traumatically amputated in an industrial accident was not able to look at his hand during the initial interview. Even when the interviewer requested that he glance at his hand, he refused because of an inability to tolerate the resulting distress. It is often better not to use exposure-based therapies with these individuals because treatment in the acute phase may exacerbate, rather than alleviate, their distress.

Dissociation

The emotional detachment associated with dissociative responses can impede engagement with traumatic memories and thereby limit the utility of any therapy approach that requires emotional processing (Foa & Hearst-Ikeda, 1996). This problem can occur in ASD because of the prevalence of dissociation in this condition. Therapists should be sensitive to the presentation of marked dissociation because it may indicate a defense against overwhelming distress that the person may not be able to manage in the acute phase. Marked dissociation may include the absence of any apparent affect in a patient whom one would expect to be distressed, staring into space during discussion of the trauma, or persistent periods of thinking about other matters when asked to focus on the trauma. It is important to distinguish between distractibility associated with hyperarousal and dissociation. Many patients display poor attentional focus, but they can be directed back to their trauma narrative by simple requests. In contrast, dissociation tends to reflect a more pervasive and repetitive inability to focus on trauma memories. Breaching dissociative responses in the acute phase may be detrimental because it may reduce the individual's control over his or her distress. Therapists should be sensitive to the potentially protective role that dissociative and avoidant responses can play in the acute phase. Respecting this function of dissociation, therapists should consider patients' psychological resources and their capacity to tolerate their distress. Those individuals who display signs of psychological instability may fare better with supportive therapy, which would allow them to stabilize their acute reaction prior to more direct therapeutic intervention.

Anger

Anger is a very common response following a traumatic experience (Hyer et al., 1986; Riggs, Dancu, Gershuny, Greenberg, & Foa, 1992). It has been proposed that anger may serve to inhibit anxiety following a trauma, especially when effortful avoidance is unsuccessful (Riggs et al., 1995). Indeed, patients who display anger during the initial narrative tend not to respond positively to exposure therapy (Foa et al., 1995; Jaycox, Perry, Freshman, Stafford, & Foa, 1995). People who present with anger as the primary emotional response may benefit more from anger management strategies, including anxiety management and cognitive therapy techniques (Chemtob, Novaco, Hamada, & Gross, 1997).

Grief

Grief also is a very common reaction following a traumatic experience (Raphael & Martinek, 1997). Moreover, posttraumatic stress and grief can interact to compound the clinical presentation (Goenjian et al., 1995; Horowitz, Weiss, & Marmar, 1987). It is important to recognize that the bereavement process requires time, and it may not be appropriate to provide acutely grieving patients with exposure when they are coming to terms with their loss. One woman was referred to a PTSD unit after a road accident in which her young baby had died. She had been trapped in the car for several hours with her dead child lying on her lap. This scene represented the primary content of her intrusive memories. The referral document expressly requested exposure therapy to reduce this woman's intrusive images of her dead child lying in her lap. In the context of considerable grief and guilt issues that needed to be addressed, providing this woman with exposure therapy only weeks after the accident would most probably have been harmful. Therapists need to help people deal with their grief reactions and ensure that active interventions for ASD do not interfere with the natural grief process (see Fleming & Robinson, 2001).

Extreme Anxiety

Some individuals present with very extreme anxiety that often may reflect pretrauma anxiety states. Moreover, many people present with panic attacks following trauma (Nixon & Bryant, 2003). Employing exposure therapy with these individuals in the acute phase can compound their anxiety state and their posttraumatic difficulties. Instead, these individuals may require containment, support, and anxiety reduction strategies. Some individuals benefit from techniques that limit panic attacks, including interoceptive exposure and cognitive restructuring (Craske & Barlow, 1993). Many people in the acute phase also require assistance in learning how to tolerate distress and in developing skills in reducing their anxiety states (see Cloitre & Rosenberg, Chapter 13, this volume).

Catastrophic Beliefs

Individuals who present with strong ruminations or catastrophic appraisals of their experience and their capacity to cope may not benefit from exposure. One study found that exposure was not successful if the individual's narrative of the trauma was characterized by mental defeat or lack of mastery over the situation (Ehlers et al., 1998a). These individuals require careful cognitive restructuring, and exposure should be considered only when their tendency to ruminate has been modified.

Prior Trauma

It is common for people who have suffered unresolved traumatic experiences prior to the recent trauma to be distressed by memories of both the recent stressor and the earlier experience. A police officer who attended our PTSD unit denied any earlier traumatic experience but during exposure was very distressed by memories of childhood abuse that he had avoided for many years. Many people find it difficult to deal with developmental or previous traumatic experiences when they are in an emotionally fragile state because of the recent traumatic experience. Allowing the posttraumatic upheaval to settle before addressing longer-term traumatic memories can sometimes lead to a better outcome.

Comorbidity

Therapists need to be aware of comorbid (and often preexisting) disorders that may be exacerbated by the distress elicited by exposure. Some of the more problematic preexisting disorders include borderline personality disorder and people with psychotic histories. People with these problems can experience marked deterioration, including psychotic episodes, severe dissociative states, and self-destructive tendencies, when confronted with expo-

214 SPECIALIZED POPULATIONS AND DELIVERY

sure to traumatic memories. Caution is required; it is often wiser to offer support for containing their preexisting disorder than to resolve their traumatic experience in the acute phase. Managing the complexity of comorbid disorders often involves integration of other techniques (see Wagner & Linehan, Chapter 6, this volume),

Substance Abuse

Substance abuse is a common comorbidity following trauma (Kulka et al., 1990). Intake of abusing substances needs to be monitored carefully because it can limit the capacity of an individual to engage the anxiety response during exposure. Further, people who have a tendency toward substance abuse may increase their reliance on the substance as a means of coping with the distress associated with exposure. Moreover, reliance on substances in the acute phase may indicate a tendency to utilize avoidant coping mechanisms. If an individual presents with marked substance abuse in the acute phase, it is may be wiser to delay exposure-based therapy for some time. The problems arising from increased substance abuse may outweigh the benefits of exposure (see Naajavits, Chapter 10, this volume).

Depression and Suicide Risk

Individuals who are considered a suicide risk in the acute phase require support, containment, and possibly antidepressant medication or hospitalization. The risk of providing suicidal individuals with exposure is that it may enhance their attention toward the negative aspects of their experience. There is considerable evidence that depressed people have poor retrieval of specific positive memories (Williams, 1996), so depressed individuals may have difficulty reinterpreting their traumatic memories following exposure. In contrast, they may focus on pessimistic views of their trauma and engage in ruminative thoughts that can compound suicidal ideation. These possibilities indicate that depression and suicide should first be managed in seriously suicidal people; acute stress reactions can be addressed after these immediate problems are contained.

Ongoing Stressors

Many trauma survivors experience marked stressors in the initial period after trauma exposure. Severe pain, surgery, financial loss, criminal investigations, property loss, interpersonal breakdown, and media attention are some of the stressors that may make further demands on the acutely traumatized individual. Providing active therapy can represent an additional burden and compound the adjustment difficulties of some individuals in the context of ongoing stressors. Moreover, these individuals may not have sufficient resources to allocate to therapy if they have other excessive demands on them. For example, a burn patient who is attempting to cope with the severe pain of daily debridements and physiotherapy may require psychological support to assist him of her through these procedures. Attempting exposure may burden this patient with additional distress at a time when he or she requires all available energy for managing his or her medical condition.

It is important to note that there are important limitations to the current evidence for the effective use of CBT shortly after trauma exposure. First, although CBT does lead to significant reductions in recently traumatized people who complete treatment, a significant proportion of participants do drop out of treatment. For example, 20% of participants dropped out of both the Bryant et al. (1999) and Bryant et al. (2005) studies. That is, intent-to-treat analyses in these studies indicate modest benefits of CBT (Bryant et al., 1999, in press). This pattern clearly points to the need for interventions that are efficacious and manageable for more recently traumatized people. For example, providing nonexposure-based therapies (such as cognitive therapy) may be better tolerated by some patients. Alternately, teaching coping skills prior to exposure may help some patients cope with the exposure more effectively (Cloitre, Koenen, Cohen, Han, 2002). Second, most early intervention treatment studies for ASD have emerged from a handful of treatment centers, and there is a need for replication across sites to validate the generalizability of these findings. The available studies have also been conducted with survivors of assault or accident; we currently have no data pertaining to the utility of CBT approaches applied shortly after mass violence, disaster, or terrorism. Third, we have no evidence indicating that early provision of CBT is actually superior to later provision of CBT. There is evidence that CBT provided approximately 4 months posttrauma is beneficial (Ehlers et al., 2003; Öst, Paunovic, & Gillow, 2002). Moreover, there is overwhelming evidence of the efficacy of CBT for chronic PTSD (for reviews, see Foa & Meadows, 1997; Harvey et al., 2003). It has yet to be demonstrated that there are tangible benefits in providing CBT shortly after trauma exposure, apart from the obvious benefit of reducing distress sooner rather than later.

COMPONENTS OF CBT FOR ASD

Education

Therapy commences with education about stress reactions and the rationale for treatment, including a discussion of the specific treatment strategies. The aims of this education are to give the patient a framework in which they can understand their current symptoms, develop some mastery over their reactions, and acquire the foundations for participating in CBT. It is important to illustrate each point with examples from the individual's own experience. After explaining the rationale of treatment to the patient, it is useful to ask the patient to explain his or her understanding of the problematic response and why he or she thinks treatment may work. This exercise encourages the individual to process the information that has been provided and gives the therapist an opportunity to correct any misunderstandings that the patient may have.

Anxiety Management Skills

It can be useful to provide anxiety management strategies early in therapy because (1) they can give patients a degree of control over their distress, and (2) these techniques are relatively simple to use. Be aware that most patients experience considerable distress during the initial sessions because they are confronting and expressing upsetting memories. The utility of reducing arousal in the acute posttrauma phase is also indicated by evidence that acute arousal is associated with chronic PTSD (Shalev et al., 1998). Giving the patient some tools to assist mastery over the acute anxiety can provide both a sense of relief and a motivation to comply with more demanding therapy tasks. Anxiety management often involves progressive muscle relaxation (Öst, 1987) and breathing retraining, which aims to achieve 10 breaths a minute. Although these techniques are simple, therapists need to be aware that focusing on bodily sensation or on breathing can trigger reminders of the trauma. First, individuals who experienced panic, suffocation, or choking need to be approached with caution because muscle relaxation or breathing exercises can elicit flashbacks. Second, requesting recently traumatized people to close their eyes can be a threatening experience if they have concerns about losing control. Therefore, it may be better to conduct these exercises with eyes open.

Cognitive Therapy

Cognitive therapy is based on the notion that emotional dysfunction results from maladaptive or catastrophic interpretations of events (Beck, Rush, Shaw, & Emery, 1979). The relevance of cognitive therapy to ASD and PTSD is underscored by increasing evidence that catastrophic thoughts in the acute phase are predictive of subsequent PTSD (Ehlers et al., 1998b; Engelhard et al., 2002). Although it is beyond the scope of this chapter to provide an adequate outline of cognitive therapy (see Beck et al., 1979), it is important to note several points in relation to providing cognitive therapy to individuals with ASD.

First, it can be useful to provide cognitive therapy prior to employing exposure because it can be difficult to learn the cognitive therapy techniques if an individual is overly distressed by focusing on traumatic memories. Second, many beliefs that acutely traumatized patients report are based on recent and threatening experiences. Accordingly, their beliefs that they are not safe or that the world is inherently dangerous appear valid to them in the context of their recent trauma. Therapists need to emphasize to these individuals that their beliefs are understandable in the aftermath of their recent trauma, although they may be modified with consideration of other evidence. Third, it is important to recognize that cognitive therapy is not positive thinking. Whereas therapists should encourage individuals to consider alternative explanations in the light of all available evidence, there is a need to acknowledge that negative events can still persist following trauma. This approach is particularly important when treating people who are at high risk for ongoing trauma, including military personnel, police officers, firefighters, and paramedics. Fourth, clinicians should note that teaching cognitive therapy in the acute phase commences a learning process that will continue for months (hopefully) after therapy is complete. Therapists should not expect recently traumatized individuals to alter beliefs rapidly or easily, because the level of threat they may have experienced could be severe, and a period of time is often required for these individuals to learn through experience that their immediate beliefs are not evidence-based. Below is an example of cognitive therapy with a patient who has ASD.

THERAPIST: You mentioned that you feel that you can never feel safe again. How strongly do you feel this?

PATIENT: I know that for a fact. I will never feel safe again.

THERAPIST: OK. On a scale of 0–100, how sure are you of that?

PATIENT: Very sure. I'd say about 90.

THERAPIST: OK, now I wonder if you can tell me about other times in your life when you've felt strongly about something. What has happened to that feeling? Tell me about some of the worst things that have happened to you.

PATIENT: Well, about 4 years ago my mother died. That was pretty tough. We were close.

THERAPIST: How did you feel at the time?

PATIENT: Really bad. My life fell apart.

THERAPIST: At the time did you feel you would get over it?

PATIENT: Not at the beginning. It got better after a while.

THERAPIST: What other bad things have happened to you?

PATIENT: A friend of mime killed herself a few years ago. That was really bad.

THERAPIST: When you think back to these things, do you still feel as bad today about those losses as you did when they happened?

PATIENT: No. Things got better eventually.

THERAPIST: Have you *ever* had feelings about anything that have stayed as strong as they were initially?

PATIENT: Well, I guess if you put it that way, everything changes eventually.

THERAPIST: What about that feeling that you can't feel safe? Do you really feel that there is no place where you feel safe?

PATIENT: None.

THERAPIST: So you don't feel safe here right now?

PATIENT: No, that's different. I know you are not going to hurt me.

THERAPIST: So you do feel safe here? What about when you are with your wife at home?

PATIENT: No, I am safe there. Home is OK.

THERAPIST: OK. Now I want you to consider these points. You're saying that you feel safe here, and you fee safe at home. You are also saying that you realize that even strong feelings that you've had in the past usually change after a while. I want you to hold all those thoughts in your mind for a minute and then think again about how strongly you believe that you will never feel safe again. How strongly do you feel that on a scale of 0–100?

PATIENT: I guess it's only about 50.

THERAPIST: Why only 50?

PATIENT: When you point out that other stuff, I guess I'll probably feel better soon.

THERAPIST: The major point to note here is that when you let your mind accept all the evidence available, you can often come to a conclusion that is different from the one you often think of automatically. I don't expect you to really believe this right now. The real point is that the more you can think of all the evidence, the more you'll start to believe these more realistic conclusions. And they will probably help you feel a bit better. The belief that you will never feel safe leaves you feeling rather helpless about things. I think we need to start working on the evidence that you can feel better in the future, but it's probably a bit soon to expect yourself to be feeling great. Remember, it's only been a few weeks since you were assaulted.

In this excerpt the therapist does not insist that the patient alter his belief about his likelihood for change. The goal of the interaction is to (1) teach the patient the basic rationale of cognitive therapy, and (2) to assist him in recognizing that there is evidence that he can change how he feels—or that how he feels changes somehow. It may be premature to try to alter fundamental beliefs about feeling safe at this point. Instead, commencing cognitive therapy discussions about changes in feelings of safety is more likely to be successful and allow the patient to work within a cognitive therapy framework for some time before addressing more central issues.

Prolonged Exposure

Prolonged imaginal exposure requires the individual to vividly imagine the trauma for prolonged periods in a way that emphasizes all relevant details, including sensory cues and affective responses. To achieve this victimization, the patient is often asked to provide the narrative in the present tense, speak in the first person, and focus on the most distressing aspects. Prolonged exposure typically occurs for at least 50 minutes and is usually supplemented by daily homework exercises. Variants of imaginal exposure involve requiring patients to write down detailed descriptions of the experience repeatedly (Resick & Schnicke, 1993) and implementing exposure with the assistance of virtual reality paradigms produced via computer-generated imagery (Rothbaum, Hodges, Ready, Graap, & Alarcon, 2001). Most imaginal exposure treatments supplement this exercise with in vivo exposure that involves live graded exposure to the feared trauma-related stimuli. There is much debate concerning the change mechanisms operating in exposure; proposed mechanisms include habitation of anxiety, correction of the belief that avoidance is required to control anxiety, incorporation of corrective information, and self-mastery (Jaycox & Foa, 1996; Rothbaum & Mellman, 2001; Rothbaum & Schwartz, 2002).

In general, exposure for ASD utilizes the same exposure protocols as those described for chronic PTSD (see Riggs, Cahill, & Foa, Chapter 4, this volume; Foa & Rothbaum, 1997). The first stage in considering exposure is determining the patient's suitability for this procedure. As mentioned above in the context of assessment, caution should be exercised in providing exposure to any recently traumatized individual who displays signs of being at risk for an adverse reaction to the distress that will be elicited by exposure. When commencing exposure, some patients will skip over the most distressing aspects of the experience because they cannot tolerate the affective response. This self-editing can be permitted initially, but it is important that as therapy proceeds, these "hot spots" receive close attention. Once a patient demonstrates in therapy that he or she can tolerate the exposure, daily homework exercises should be initiated. It is also especially useful to integrate cognitive therapy immediately after each exposure exercise, because there is typically much cognitive material elicited during exposure that can be addressed in cognitive therapy.

In vivo exposure should be implemented in parallel with, or soon after, other treatment components. The initial step in in vivo exposure is to develop a hierarchy of feared or avoided situations. This procedure involves having the patient determine a graded series of situations that elicit varying degrees of anxiety. After the hierarchy is complete, the therapist should ask the patient to commence with the situation that is lowest on the hierarchy. It is advisable to start with a situation in which the patient can cope relatively easily to facilitate confidence in his or her ability and enhance compliance with more demanding items. It is useful to require the patient to remain in the situation until his or her distress has reduced by 50%. Once a situation is mastered, the therapist then requires the patient to undertake the next step on the hierarchy. In the acute phase, it is important to recognize that many avoidance behaviors are understandable and do not necessarily reflect maladaptive avoidance. For example, a man who was the victim of a home invasion was reluctant to return to his house several weeks posttrauma because his home was still stained with blood from the vicious attack. In a case such as this, it is reasonable to allow a degree of avoidance. Overall, it is useful to check that the person is engaging fully with the exposure to the feared stimulus and not engaging in safety behaviors that may minimize distress. For example, an assault victim may agree to remain in the shopping mall where the attack took place, but will carry a knife in his pocket as a means of protection. Such safety behaviors serve to minimize full exposure to the situation and should be removed from the exposure exercise.

SUMMARY

Treating ASD has significant benefits because it can limit posttraumatic stress reactions that can otherwise lead to a debilitating and long-term disorder. It should be noted, however, that early intervention should not be offered to all recent trauma survivors who are distressed. Available evidence suggests that treatment effects are comparable when we treat people in the initial month after trauma or several years later. Accordingly, clinicians should not assume that early intervention is an imperative. Indeed, in cases of mass violence or disaster, it is often impossible to allocate sufficient resources in the initial month to provide therapy to hundreds or thousands of trauma survivors. In these situations it is important to ensure that all high-risk people are identified and therapy provided within a reasonable period of time. Although our evidence for early intervention is growing, we require further research to develop better evidence-based approaches that can be utilized by a broader array of acutely traumatized people. In the context of terrorism, war, and natural disasters, developing strategies that can be delivered to many people who require it remains one of our highest priorities.

REFERENCES

American Psychiatric Association. (1994). *Diagnostic and statistical manual of mental disorders* (4th ed.). Washington, DC: Author.
Andrews, B., Brewin, C. R., Rose, S., & Kirk, M. (2000). Predicting PTSD in victims of

violent crime: The role of shame, anger and blame. *Journal of Abnormal Psychology, 109*, 69–73.

Beck, A. T., Rush, A. J., Shaw, B. F., & Emery, G. (1979). *Cognitive therapy of depression.* New York: Guilford Press.

Berah, E. F., Jones, H. J., & Valent, P. (1984). The experience of a mental health team involved in the early phase of a disaster. *Australian and New Zealand Journal of Psychiatry, 18*, 354–358.

Blanchard, E. B., Hickling, E. J., Barton, K. A., Taylor, A. E., Loos, W. R., & Jones Alexander, J. (1996). One-year prospective follow-up of motor vehicle accident victims. *Behaviour Research and Therapy, 34*, 775–786.

Blanchard, E. B., Hickling, E. J., Galovski, T., & Veazey, C. (2002). Emergency room vital signs and PTSD in a treatment seeking sample of motor vehicle accident survivors. *Journal of Traumatic Stress, 15*, 199–204.

Brewin, C. R., Andrews, B., Rose, S., & Kirk, M. (1999). Acute stress disorder and posttraumatic stress disorder in victims of violent crime. *American Journal of Psychiatry, 156*, 360–366.

Brom, D., Kleber, R. J., & Hofman, M. (1993). Victims of traffic accidents: Incidence and prevention of post-traumatic stress disorder. *Journal of Clinical Psychology, 49*, 131–140.

Bryant, R. A. (2000). Acute stress disorder. *PTSD Research Quarterly, 11*, 1–7.

Bryant, R. A. (2003). Early predictors of posttraumatic stress disorder. *Biological Psychiatry, 53*, 789–795.

Bryant, R. A., & Friedman, M. (2001). Medication and non-medication treatments of posttraumatic stress disorder. *Current Opinion in Psychiatry, 14*, 119–123.

Bryant, R. A., & Harvey, A. G. (1996). Initial post-traumatic stress responses following motor vehicle accidents. *Journal of Traumatic Stress, 9*, 223–234.

Bryant, R. A., & Harvey, A. G. (1997). Acute stress disorder: A critical review of diagnostic issues. *Clinical Psychology Review, 17*, 757–773.

Bryant, R. A., & Harvey, A. G. (1998). Relationship of acute stress disorder and posttraumatic stress disorder following mild traumatic brain injury. *American Journal of Psychiatry, 155*, 625–629.

Bryant, R. A., & Harvey, A. G. (2000). New DSM-IV diagnosis of acute stress disorder [Letter]. *American Journal of Psychiatry, 157*, 1889–1890.

Bryant, R. A., Harvey, A. G., Dang, S., & Sackville, T. (1998a). Assessing acute stress disorder: Psychometric properties of a structured clinical interview. *Psychological Assessment, 10*, 215–220.

Bryant, R. A., Harvey, A. G., Dang, S. T., Sackville, T., & Basten, C. (1998b). Treatment of acute stress disorder: A comparison of cognitive behavior therapy and supportive counseling. *Journal of Consulting and Clinical Psychology, 66*, 862–866.

Bryant, R. A., Harvey, A. G., Guthrie, R. M., & Moulds, M. (2000a). A prospective study of acute psychophysiological arousal, acute stress disorder, and posttraumatic stress disorder. *Journal of Abnormal Psychology, 109*, 341–344.

Bryant, R. A., Moulds, M., & Guthrie, R. M. (2000b). Acute Stress Disorder Scale: A self-report measure of acute stress disorder. *Psychological Assessment, 12*, 61–68.

Bryant, R. A., Moulds, M. L., Guthrie, R. M., & Nixon, R. D. V. (2003a). Treating acute stress disorder after mild brain injury. *American Journal of Psychiatry, 160*, 585–587.

Bryant, R. A., Moulds, M. L., Guthrie, R. M., & Nixon, R. D. V. (2005). The additive benefit of hypnotherapy and cognitive behavior therapy in treating acute stress disorder. *Journal of Consulting and Clinical Psychology, 73*(2), 334–340.

Bryant, R. A., Moulds, M. A., & Nixon, R. D. V. (2003b). Cognitive behaviour therapy of acute stress disorder: A four-year follow-up. *Behaviour Research and Therapy, 41*, 489–494.

Bryant, R. A., & Panasetis, P. (2001). Panic symptoms during trauma and acute stress disorder. *Behaviour Research and Therapy, 39*, 961–966

Bryant, R. A., Sackville, T., Dang, S. T., Moulds, M., & Guthrie, R. M. (1999). Treating acute stress disorder: An evaluation of cognitive behavior therapy and counseling techniques. *American Journal of Psychiatry, 156*, 1780–1786.

Butler, L. D. (2000). New DSM-IV diagnosis of acute stress disorder [Letter]. *American Journal of Psychiatry, 157*, 1889.

Butler, L., Duran, R. E. F., Jasiukaitis, P., Koopman, C., & Spiegel, D. (1996). Hypnotizability and traumatic experience: A diathesis–stress model of dissociative symptomatology. *American Journal of Psychiatry, 153*(Suppl. 7S), 42–63.

Cahill, L., Prins, B., Weber, M., & McGaugh, J. L. (1994). B-adrenergic activation and memory for emotional events. *Nature, 371*, 702–704.

Cardeña, E., Classen, C., & Spiegel, D. (1991). *Stanford acute stress reaction questionnaire.* Stanford, CA: Stanford University Medical School.

Cardeña, E., Koopman, C., Classen, C., Waelde, L. C., & Spiegel, D. (2000). Psychometric properties of the Stanford Acute Stress Reaction Questionnaire (SASRQ): A valid and reliable measure of acute stress. *Journal of Traumatic Stress, 13*, 719–734.

Cardeña, E., & Spiegel, D. (1993). Dissociative reactions to the San Francisco Bay Area earthquake of 1989. *American Journal of Psychiatry, 150*, 474–478.

Carlier, I. V. E., Lamberts, R. D., van Uchelen, A. J., & Gersons, B. P. R. (1998). Disaster related post-traumatic stress in police officers: A field study of the impact of debriefing. *Stress Medicine, 14*, 143–148.

Chemtob, C. M., Novaco, R. W., Hamada, R. S., & Gross, D. M. (1997). Anger regulation deficits in combat-related posttraumatic stress disorder. *Journal of Traumatic Stress, 10*, 17–36.

Classen, C., Koopman, C., Hales, R., & Spiegel, D. (1998). Acute stress disorder as a predictor of posttraumatic stress symptoms. *American Journal of Psychiatry, 155*, 620–624.

Cloitre, M., Koenen, K. C., Cohen, L. R., & Han, H. (2002). Skills training in affective and interpersonal regulation followed by exposure: A phase-based treatment for PTSD related to childhood abuse. *Journal of Consulting and Clinical Psychology, 70*, 1067–1074.

Craske, M. G., & Barlow, D. H. (1993). Panic disorder and agoraphobia. In D. H. Barlow (Ed.), *Clinical handbook of psychological disorders* (pp. 1–47). New York: Guilford Press.

Creamer, M. C., O'Donnell, M. L., & Pattison, P. (2004). The relationship between acute stress disorder and posttraumatic stress disorder in severely injured trauma survivors. *Behaviour Research and Therapy, 42*, 315–328.

Delahanty, D. L., Herberman, H. B., Craig, K. J., Hayward, M. C., Fullerton, C. S., Ursano, R. J., & Baum, A. (1997). Acute and chronic distress and posttraumatic stress disorder as a function of responsibility for serious motor vehicle accidents. *Journal of Consulting and Clinical Psychology, 65*, 560–567.

Delahanty, D. L., Raimonde, A. J., & Spoonster, E. (2000). Initial posttraumatic urinary cortisol levels predict subsequent PTSD symptoms in motor vehicle accident victims. *Biological Psychiatry, 48*, 940–947.

Difede, J., Ptacek, J. T., Roberts, J. G., Barocas, D., Rives, W., Apfeldorf, W. J., & Yurt, R. (2002). Acute stress disorder after burn injury: A predictor of posttraumatic stress disorder. *Psychosomatic Medicine, 64*, 826–834.

Ehlers, A., & Clark, D. (2000). A cognitive model of posttraumatic stress disorder. *Behaviour Research and Therapy, 38*, 319–345.

Ehlers, A., Clark, D. M., Hackmann, A., McManus, F., Fennell, M., Herbert, C., & Mayou, R. A. (2003). A randomized controlled trial of cognitive therapy, self-help, and repeated assessment as early interventions for PTSD. *Archives of General Psychiatry, 60*, 1024–1032.

Ehlers, A., Clark, D. M., Winton, E., Jaycox, L., Meadows, E., & Foa, E. B. (1998a). Predicting response to exposure treatment in PTSD: The role of mental defeat and alienation. *Journal of Traumatic Stress, 11*, 457–471.

Ehlers, A., Mayou, R. A., & Bryant, B. (1998b). Psychological predictors of chronic PTSD after motor vehicle accidents. *Journal of Abnormal Psychology, 107*, 508–519.

Engelhard, I. M., van den Hout, M. A., Arntz, A., & McNally, R. J. (2002). A longitudinal study of "intrusion-based reasoning" and posttraumatic stress disorder after exposure to a train disaster. *Behaviour Research and Therapy, 40*, 1415–1424.

Feinstein, A. (1989). Posttraumatic stress disorder: A descriptive study supporting DSM-III-R criteria. *American Journal of Psychiatry, 146*, 665–666.

Fleming, S., & Robinson, P. J. (2001). Grief and cognitive behavior therapy: the reconstruction of meaning. In M. S. Stroebe, R. O. Hansson, W. Stroebe, & H. A. W. Schut (Eds.), *Handbook of bereavement research: Consequences, coping, and care* (pp. 647–670). Washington, DC: American Psychological Association.

Foa, E. B., & Hearst-Ikeda, D. (1996). Emotional dissociation in response to trauma. In L. K. Michelson & W. J. Ray (Eds.), *Handbook of dissociation: Theoretical, empirical, and clinical perspectives* (pp. 207–222). New York: Plenum Press.

Foa, E. B., Hearst-Ikeda, D., & Perry, K. J. (1995). Evaluation of a brief cognitive behavioral program for the prevention of chronic PTSD in recent assault victims. *Journal of Consulting and Clinical Psychology, 63*, 948–955.

Foa, E. B., & Meadows, E. A. (1997). Psychosocial treatments for post-traumatic stress disorder: A critical review. *Annual Review of Psychology, 48*, 449–480.

Foa, E. B., & Rothbaum, B. O. (1997). *Treating the trauma of rape: Cognitive-behavioral therapy for PTSD.* New York: Guilford Press.

Foa, E. B., Zoellner, L. A., & Feeny, N. C. (2002). *An evaluation of three brief programs for facilitating recovery.* Manuscript submitted for publication.

Freinkel, A., Koopman, C., & Spiegel, D. (1994). Dissociative symptoms in media witnesses of an execution. *American Journal of Psychiatry, 151*, 1335–1339.

Galea, S., Vlahov, D., Resnick, H., Ahern, J., Ezra, S., Gold, J., Bucuvalas, M., & Kilpatrick, D. (2003). Trends of probable post-traumatic stress disorder in New York City after the September 11th terrorist attacks. *American Journal of Epidemiology, 158*, 514–524.

Galea, S., Resnick, H., Kilpatrick, D., Bucuvalas, M., Gold, J., & Vlahov, D. (2002). Psychological sequelae of the September 11 terrorist attacks in New York City. *New England Journal of Medicine, 346*, 982–987.

Gidron, Y., Gal, R., Freedman, S., Twiser, I., Lauden, A., Snir, Y., & Benjamin, J. (2001). Translating research findings to PTSD prevention: Results of a randomized-controlled pilot study. *Journal of Traumatic Stress, 14*, 773–780.

Goenjian, A., Pynoos, R. S., Steinberg, A. M., Najarian, L. M., Asarnow, J. R., Karayan, I., Ghurabi, M., & Fairbanks, L. A. (1995). Psychiatric co-morbidity in children after the 1988 earthquake in Armenia. *Journal of the American Academy of Child and Adolescent Psychiatry, 34*, 1174–1184.

Guthrie, R., & Bryant, R. A. (2000). Attempted thought suppression over extended periods in acute stress disorder. *Behaviour Research and Therapy, 38*, 899–907.

Harvey, A. G., & Bryant, R. A. (1998). Relationship of acute stress disorder and post-traumatic stress disorder following motor vehicle accidents. *Journal of Consulting and Clinical Psychology, 66*, 507–512.

Harvey, A. G., & Bryant, R. A. (1999). A two-year prospective evaluation of the relationship between acute stress disorder and posttraumatic stress disorder. *Journal of Consulting and Clinical Psychology, 67*, 985–988.

Harvey, A. G., & Bryant, R. A. (2000). A two-year prospective evaluation of the relationship between acute stress disorder and posttraumatic stress disorder following mild traumatic brain injury. *American Journal of Psychiatry, 157*, 626–628.

Harvey, A. G., & Bryant, R. A. (2002). Acute stress disorder: A synthesis and critique. *Psychological Bulletin, 128*, 892–906.

Harvey, A. G., Bryant, R. A., & Dang, S. (1998). Autobiographical memory in acute stress disorder. *Journal of Consulting and Clinical Psychology, 66*, 500–506.

Harvey, A. G., Bryant, R. A., & Tarrier, N. (2003). Cognitive behavior therapy of posttraumatic stress disorder. *Clinical Psychology Review, 23*, 501–522.

Hillman, R. G. (1981). The psychopathology of being held hostage. *American Journal of Psychiatry, 138*, 1193–1197.

Holeva, V., Tarrier, N., & Wells, A. (2001). Prevalence and predictors of acute stress disorder and PTSD following road traffic accidents: Thought control strategies and social support. *Behavior Therapy, 32*, 65–83.

Horowitz, M. J., Weiss, D. S., & Marmar, C. (1987). Diagnosis of posttraumatic stress disorder. *Journal of Nervous and Mental Disease, 175*, 267–268.

Hyer, L., O'Leary, W. C., Saucer, R. T., Blount, J., Harrison, W. R., & Boudewyns, P. A. (1986). Inpatient diagnosis of posttraumatic stress disorder. *Journal of Consulting and Clinical Psychology, 54*, 698-702.

Janet, P. (1907). *The major symptoms of hysteria.* New York: McMillan.

Jaycox, L. H., & Foa, E. B. (1996). Obstacles in implementing exposure therapy for PTSD: Case discussions and practical solutions. *Clinical Psychology and Psychotherapy, 3*, 176–184.

Jaycox, L. H., Perry, K., Freshman, M., Stafford, J., & Foa, E. B. (1995). Factors related to improvement in assault victims treated for PTSD. Paper presented at the annual meeting of the International Society of Traumatic Stress Studies, Boston, MA.

Kangas, M., Henry, J. L., & Bryant, R. A. (2005). A prospective study of autobiographical memory and posttraumatic stress disorder following cancer. *Journal of Consulting and Clinical Psychology, 73*(2) 293–299.

Keane, T. M., Kaufman, M. L., & Kimble, M. O. (2001). Peritraumatic dissociative symptoms, acute stress disorder, and the development of posttraumatic stress disorder: Causation, correlation or epiphenomena. In L. Sanchez-Planell & C. Diez-Quevedo (Eds.), *Dissociative states* (pp. 21–43). Barcelona, Spain: Springer-Verlag.

Kilpatrick, D. G., & Calhoun, K. S. (1988). Early behavioral treatment for rape trauma: Efficacy or artifact? *Behavior Therapy, 19*, 421–427.

Kilpatrick, D. G., & Veronen, L. J. (1984). Treatment of rape-related problems: Crisis intervention is not enough. In L. Cohen, W. Clairborn, & G. Specter (Eds.), *Crisis intervention* (2nd ed.). New York: Human Services Press.

Kolb, L. C. (1987). A neuropsychological hypothesis explaining post-traumatic stress disorder. *American Journal of Psychiatry, 144,* 989–995.

Koopman, C. (2000). New DSM-IV diagnosis of acute stress disorder [Letter]. *American Journal of Psychiatry, 157,* 1888.

Koopman, C., Classen, C., Cardeña, E., & Spiegel, D. (1995). When disaster strikes, acute stress disorder may follow. *Journal of Traumatic Stress, 8,* 29–46.

Koopman, C., Classen, C., & Spiegel, D. (1994). Predictors of posttraumatic stress symptoms among survivors of the Oakland/Berkeley, Calif., firestorm. *American Journal of Psychiatry, 151,* 888–894.

Kulka, R. A., Schlenger, W. E., Fairbank, J. A., Hough, R. L., Jordan, B. K., & Marmar, C. R. (1990). Trauma and the Vietnam War generation: Report of findings from the National Vietnam Veterans' Readjustment Study. New York: Brunner/Mazel.

LeDoux, J. E., Iwata, J., Cicchetti, P., & Reis, D. J. (1988). Different projections of the central amygdaloid nucleus mediate autonomic and behavioral correlates of conditioned fear. *Journal of Neuroscience, 8,* 2517–2529.

Marshall, R. D., Spitzer, R., & Liebowitz, M. R. (1999). Review and critique of the new DSM-IV diagnosis of acute stress disorder. *American Journal of Psychiatry, 156,* 1677–1685.

Marshall, R. D., Spitzer, R., & Liebowitz, M. R. (2000). New DSM-IV diagnosis of acute stress disorder. *American Journal of Psychiatry, 157,* 1890–1891.

McFarlane, A. C., Atchison, M., & Yehuda, R. (1997). The acute stress response following motor vehicle accidents and its relation to PTSD. In R. Yehuda & A. C. McFarlane (Eds.), *Psychobiology of posttraumatic stress disorder* (pp. 433–436). New York: New York Academy of Sciences.

McNally, R. J. (2003). *Remembering trauma.* Cambridge, MA: Belknap Press.

Mitchell, J. T., & Bray, G. (1990). *Emergency services stress.* Englewood Cliffs, NJ: Prentice-Hall.

Mitchell, J. T., & Everly, G. S., Jr. (2001). *Critical incident stress debriefing: An operations manual for CISD, defusing and other group crisis intervention services* (3rd ed.). Ellicott City, MD: Chevron.

Murray, J., Ehlers, A., & Mayou, R. A. (2002). Dissociation and post-traumatic stress disorder: Two prospective studies of road traffic accident survivors. *British Journal of Psychiatry, 180,* 363–368.

Moulds, M. L., & Bryant, R. A. (2002). Directed forgetting in acute stress disorder. *Journal of Abnormal Psychology, 111,* 175–179.

Moulds, M. L., & Bryant, R. A. (2005). An investigation of retrieval inhibition in acute stress disorder. *Journal of Traumatic Stress, 18*(3), 233–236.

Nemiah, J. C. (1989). Janet redivivus [Editorial]. *American Journal of Psychiatry, 146,* 1527–1529.

Nixon, R., & Bryant, R. A. (2003). Peritraumatic and persistent panic attacks in acute stress disorder. *Behaviour Research and Therapy, 41,* 1237–1242.

North, C. S., Smith, E. M., McCool, R. E., & Lightcap, P. E. (1989). Acute postdisaster coping and adjustment. *Journal of Traumatic Stress, 2,* 353–360.

Noyes, R., Hoenk, P. R., Kuperman, S., & Slymen, D. J. (1977). Depersonalization in accident victims and psychiatric patients. *Journal of Nervous and Mental Disease, 164,* 401–407.

Noyes, R., & Kletti, R. (1977). Depersonalization in response to life-threatening danger. *Comprehensive Psychiatry, 18,* 375–384.

Öst, L.-G. (1987). Applied relaxation: Description of a coping technique and review of controlled studies. *Behaviour Research and Therapy, 25,* 397–409.

Öst, L.-G., Paunovic, N., & Gillow, E.-M. (2002). *Cognitive-behavior therapy in the prevention of chronic PTSD in crime victims.* Manuscript submitted for publication.

Pitman, R. K., Sanders, K. M., Zusman, R. M., Healy, A. R., Cheema, F., Lasko, N. B., Cahill, L., & Orr, S. P. (2002). Pilot study of secondary prevention of posttraumatic stress disorder with propranolol. *Biological Psychiatry, 51,* 189–192.

Pitman, R. K., Shalev, A. Y., & Orr, S. P. (2000). Posttraumatic stress disorder: Emotion, conditioning and memory. In M. D. Corbetta & M. Gazzaniga (Eds.), *The new cognitive neurosciences* (2nd ed.). New York: Plenum Press.

Post, R. M., Weiss, S. R. B., & Smith, M. (1995). Sensitization and kindling: Implication for the evolving neural substrates of posttraumatic stress disorder. In M. J. Friedman, D. S. Charney, & A. Y. Deutch (Eds.), *Neurobiological and clinical consequences of stress: From normal adaptation to posttraumatic stress disorder.* Philadelphia: Lippincott-Raven.

Resick, P. A., & Schnicke, M. K. (1993). *Cognitive processing therapy for rape victims: A treatment manual.* London: Sage.

Riggs,, D. S., Dancu, C. V., Gershuny, B. S., Greenberg, D., & Foa, E. B. (1992). Anger and post-traumatic stress disorder in female crime victims. *Journal of Traumatic Stress, 5,* 613–625.

Riggs, D. S., Rothbaum, B. O., & Foa, E. B. (1995). A prospective examination of symptoms of posttraumatic stress disorder in victims of non-sexual assault. *Journal of Interpersonal Violence, 10,* 201–214.

Rothbaum, B. O., Foa, E. B., Riggs, D. S., Murdock, T., & Walsh, W. (1992). A prospective examination of post-traumatic stress disorder in rape victims. *Journal of Traumatic Stress, 5,* 455–475.

Rothbaum, B. O., Hodges, L. F., Ready, D., Graap, K., & Alarcon, R. D. (2001). Virtual reality exposure therapy for Vietnam veterans with posttraumatic stress disorder. *Journal of Clinical Psychiatry, 62,* 617–6 22.

Rothbaum, B. O., & Mellman, T. A. (2001). Dreams and exposure therapy for PTSD. *Journal of Traumatic Stress, 14,* 481–490.

Rothbaum, B. O., & Schwartz, A. C. (2002). Exposure therapy for posttraumatic stress disorder. *American Journal of Psychotherapy, 56,* 59–75.

Schnyder, U., Moergeli, H., Klaghofer, R., & Buddeberg, C. (2001). Incidence and prediction of posttraumatic stress disorder symptoms in severely injured accident victims. *American Journal of Psychiatry, 158,* 594–599.

Shalev, A. Y., Sahar, T., Freedman, S., Peri, T., Glick, N., Brandes, D., Orr, S. P., & Pitman, R. K. (1998). A prospective study of heart rate responses following trauma and the subsequent development of PTSD. *Archives of General Psychiatry, 55,* 553–559.

Simeon, D., & Guralnik, O. (2000). New DSM-IV diagnosis of acute stress disorder [Letter]. *American Journal of Psychiatry, 157,* 1888–1889.

Sloan, P. (1988). Post-traumatic stress in survivors of an airplane crash-landing: A clinical and exploratory research intervention. *Journal of Traumatic Stress, 1,* 211–229.

Smith, K., & Bryant, R. A. (2000). The generality of cognitive bias in acute stress disorder. *Behaviour Research and Therapy, 38,* 709–715.

Solomon, Z., Laor, N., & McFarlane, A. C. (1996). Acute posttraumatic reactions in soldiers and civilians. In B. A. van der Kolk, A. C. McFarlane, & L. Weisaeth (Eds.), *Traumatic stress: The effects of overwhelming experience on mind, body, and society* (pp. 102–114). New York: Guilford Press.

Spiegel, D. (1996). Dissociative disorders. In R. E. Hales & S. C. Yudofsky (Eds.), *Synopsis of psychiatry* (pp. 583–604). Washington, DC: American Psychiatric Press.

Spiegel, D., & Classen, C., (1995). Acute stress disorder. In G. O. Gabbard (Ed.), *Treatments of psychiatric disorders* (Vol. 2, pp. 1521–1535). Washington, DC: American Psychiatric Press.

Spiegel, D., Classen, C., & Cardeña, E. (2000). New DSM-IV diagnosis of acute stress disorder [Letter]. *American Journal of Psychiatry, 157*, 1890–1891.

Staab, J. P., Grieger, T. A., Fullerton, C. S., & Ursano, R. J. (1996). Acute stress disorder, subsequent posttraumatic stress disorder and depression after a series of typhoons. *Anxiety, 2*, 219–225.

Vaiva, G., Ducrocq, F., Jezequel, K., Averland, B., Lestavel, P., Brunet, A., & Marmar, C. R. (2003). Immediate treatment with propranolol decreases posttraumatic stress disorder two months after trauma. *Biological Psychiatry, 54*, 947–949.

van der Kolk, B. A., & van der Hart, O. (1989). Pierre Janet and the breakdown of adaptation in psychological data. *American Journal of Psychiatry, 146*, 1530–1540.

Viney, L. L., Clark, A. M., Bunn, T. A., & Benjamin, Y. N. (1985). Crisis intervention counseling: An evaluation of long- and short-term effects. *Journal of Consulting and Clinical Psychology, 32*, 29–39.

Warda, G., & Bryant, R. A. (1998a). Cognitive bias in acute stress disorder. *Behaviour Research and Therapy, 36*, 1177–1183.

Warda, G., & Bryant, R. A. (1998b). Thought control strategies in acute stress disorder. *Behaviour Research and Therapy, 36*, 1171–1175.

Williams, J. M. G. (1996). Depression and the specificity of autobiographical memory. In D. C. Rubin (Ed.), *Remembering our past: Studies in autobiographical memory* (pp. 244–267). Cambridge, UK: Cambridge University Press.

Yehuda, R. (1997). Sensitization of the hypothalamic–pituitary–adrenal axis in posttraumatic stress disorder. *Annals of the New York Academy Science, 821*, 57–75.

CHAPTER TEN

Seeking Safety

Therapy for Posttraumatic Stress Disorder and Substance Use Disorder

Lisa M. Najavits

"I just felt so ugly, hateful and evil. I hated myself. There was nothing good in me. I didn't know I was someone. I would always look down. But when I drank, it made me feel confident, secure and happy. It made me feel all the things I was not." (quoted in Stamm, 2002)

This client put into words what many live day to day: the use of substances to escape the emotional pain of trauma. Having suffered childhood physical and sexual abuse by multiple family members, the client began using substances at a young age. Despite attending self-help groups such as Alcoholics Anonymous (AA) and numerous treatment programs, she was unable to stop. Eventually she found a therapist who helped her explore the connection between her trauma and her substance use disorder (SUD). She views therapy as her foundation and has achieved 8 years of sobriety (Stamm, 2002).

There are many different client stories, types of trauma, substances, and treatment methods. However, research over the past decade has established the basic and important point that trauma and SUD frequently co-occur. For example, posttraumatic stress disorder (PTSD), the psychiatric disorder most directly related to trauma, is highly associated with SUD (for reviews, see Brady, 2001; Jacobsen, Southwick, & Kosten, 2001; Najavits, Weiss, & Shaw, 1997; Ouimette & Brown, 2002; Ruzek, Polusny, & Abueg, 1998; Triffleman, 1998). In community samples, men with PTSD have a 51.9% lifetime rate of alcohol use disorder, and 34.5% have drug use disorder; the respective rates for women are 27.9% and 26.9% (Kessler, Sonnega, Bromet, Hughes, & Nelson, 1995). In treatment settings, the rates are higher. For example, 33–59% of women in substance abuse treatment have current PTSD, and 55–99% report one or more lifetime traumas (Najavits et al., 1997). Among males the most common traumas associated with SUD are combat and crime victimization, whereas among females they are childhood physical and sexual abuse (Najavits et al., 1997). Large-scale traumatic disasters such as the 9/11 attacks, the Oklahoma City bombing, and Hurricane Hugo, are also associated with increased substance use (Clark, 2002; North et al., 1999). Substances are also used by trauma perpetrators, who may be under the influence at the time of assault or sedate the victim through use of a substance (Bureau of Justice, 1992). Various subgroups tend to have especially high rates of trauma and SUD, including women, veterans, the homeless, adolescents, prisoners, gays and lesbians, rescue workers such as firefighters and police, prostitutes, and victims of domestic violence (Davis & Wood, 1999; North et al., 2002; Smith, North, & Spitznagel, 1993; Substance Abuse and Mental Health Services Administration, 2001; Tarter & Kirisci, 1999; Teplin, Abram, & McClelland, 1996).

The clinical needs of this population are serious and urgent. A variety of studies indicates that those with the dual diagnosis of PTSD and SUD have worse outcomes than those with either disorder alone; higher rates of subsequent trauma; and greater impairment, including other Axis I and Axis II disorders, self-harm and suicidality, medical and legal problems, HIV risk, and lower work functioning (Brady, Killeen, Saladin, Dansky, & Becker, 1994; Grice, Brady, Dustan, Malcolm, & Kilpatrick, 1995; Hien, Nunes, Levin, & Fraser, 2000; Najavits et al., 1998a; Najavits et al., 1997; Najavits, Weiss, & Shaw, 1999b; Ouimette, Finney, & Moos, 1999). Abuse of substances itself is often construed as a reenactment of trauma. Substance use may represent harm to the body that symbolizes familiar traumatic experiences; living the role of the marginalized; or not caring about oneself after violation by others (Najavits, 2002d; Teusch, 2001). Notably, one of the major predictors of both trauma and SUD is a family history of these—the repeated generational cycles of this seemingly inexorable combination (Kendler, Davis, & Kessler, 1997; Yehuda, Schmeidler, Wainberg, Binder-Brynes, & Duvdevani, 1998).

Treatment of the dual diagnosis has historically been marked by a separation that only lately has begun to improve. A culture of "other" predominated in which many mental health clinicians believed that they could not adequately assess or treat SUD, and many SUD clinicians believed that they could not assess or treat PTSD (Najavits, 2002d; Najavits, Weiss, & Liese, 1996; Read, Bollinger, & Sharansky, 2002). There is now increasing awareness that a no-wrong-door approach is likely to be the most helpful (Clark, 2002). Regardless of how they enter treatment, clients need attention to both disorders. Split systems, wherein a client who uses substances is rejected from mental health treatment until abstinent, or the client with mental health problems is rejected from SUD treatment until stabilized, are believed less effective than concurrent or integrated treatment (Brady, 2001; Ouimette & Brown, 2002). Yet older messages abound, such as "Just get clean and sober first," "Go to Alcoholics Anonymous or I won't treat you,"

230 SPECIALIZED POPULATIONS AND DELIVERY

or "You're defocusing from your addiction if you talk about the past." Clinicians in a variety of settings may fail to assess routinely for trauma, PTSD, and SUD. Indeed, underdiagnosis or misdiagnosis of both PTSD and SUD are common (Davidson, 2001; Najavits, 2004b), and *most* SUD clients are neither assessed for PTSD nor given treatment for it (Brown, Stout, & Gannon-Rowley, 1998; Dansky, Roitzsch, Brady, & Saladin, 1997; Hyer, Leach, Boudewyns, & Davis, 1991; Najavits, Sullivan, Schmitz, Weiss, & Lee, 2004). Clients too tend to minimize both SUD and PTSD. Shame, guilt, denial, and lying are more common in these disorders than in many other psychiatric conditions. A client may say, "I drink alone so no one will see how much I'm using," or "I shouldn't feel bad about the trauma; I'm just being weak." In treatment, some clinicians may take too harsh a stance, such as threat of termination if the client relapses on substances. Newer approaches to SUD, including harm reduction (reinforcing any decrease in use rather than requiring full abstinence) and emphasis on choices and support (rather than confrontation) may be unfamiliar (Fletcher, 2001; Marlatt, Tucker, Donovan, & Vuchinich, 1997). Yet these modifications of standard treatment may be especially helpful for clients with dual diagnosis, in general, and those with PTSD, specifically, who often suffer from demoralization and hopelessness (Marlatt et al., 1997; Najavits, 2002d). The 12-step approach of AA, one of the mainstays of addiction recovery, has been helpful for many (Fletcher, 2001). However, for PTSD clients, abstinence may be more difficult, and such methods may not work as well (Ruzek et al., 1998; Solomon, Gerrity, & Muff, 1992). PTSD symptoms may worsen with abstinence, for example, leading the client back to a cycle of using substances to cope with overwhelming emotion (Brady et al., 1994; Kofoed, Friedman, & Peck, 1993).

A major clinical effort of the past several years has been the development of integrated therapies for PTSD and SUD. Working on both disorders at the same time from the start of treatment is now widely encouraged (Brady, 2001; Najavits et al., 1996; Ouimette & Brown, 2002). Clients too report a clear preference to include treatment of PTSD in SUD treatment (Brown et al., 1998; Najavits et al., 2004). Most of all, evidence thus far indicates that integrated approaches to PTSD and SUD result in positive outcomes in both domains as well as related areas. Contrary to older views, treating PTSD and SUD simultaneously appears to help clients with addiction recovery, rather than derailing them from attaining abstinence (Brady, Dansky, Back, Foa, & Caroll, 2001; Donovan, Padin-Rivera, & Kowaliw, 2001; Hien, Cohen, Litt, Miele, & Capstick, 2004; Najavits, Schmitz, Gotthardt, & Weiss, in press-a; Najavits, Weiss, Shaw, & Muenz, 1998b; Triffleman, 2000; Zlotnick, Najavits, & Rohsenow, 2003).

Treatment for trauma offers a depth to SUD treatment that many clients and clinicians find helpful. It honors what clients have lived through, encourages empathy and self-understanding, and may increase motivation for abstinence. It can be reassuring for clients to realize that they may have used substances to cope with overwhelming emotional pain, and to recognize that this pattern is common. Such understanding can move them beyond the revolving door of just more treatment, into different treatment. Rather than cycling back through standard treatment, the client can go down a new path. One client said, "I was relieved to find I had something with a name. I thought it was just me—I'm crazy. But I can deal with this now. Now I can put down the cocaine and work on what's behind it" (Najavits, 2002e, p. 81).

Integrated models that have been empirically studied (i.e., one or more published outcome trials) are Seeking Safety (Najavits, 2002d); Concurrent Treatment of PTSD and Cocaine Dependence (Back, Dansky, Carroll, Foa, & Brady, 2001; Brady et al., 2001); Substance Dependence PTSD Therapy, later relabeled Assisted Recovery from Trauma and Substances (ARTS, Triffleman, 2000; Triffleman, Carroll, & Kellogg, 1999); and Transcend (Donovan et al., 2001). Other models include the Addictions and Trauma Recovery Integrated Model (Miller & Guidry, 2001); Helping Women Recover (Covington, 1999; Covington, 2000); Trauma Adaptive Recovery Group Education and Therapy (Ford, Kasimer, MacDonald, & Savill, 2000); Trauma-Relevant Relapse Prevention Training (Abueg & Fairbank, 1991; Abueg et al., 1994); Treating Addicted Survivors of Trauma (Evans & Sullivan, 1995); Double Bind (Trotter, 1992); an unnamed group model (Meisler, 1999); and an inpatient model (Bollerud, 1990). The various models differ in their emphases. Some focus more on the present and others more on the past, some address both disorders throughout the therapy, whereas others attend more to one than the other at different times, some are fully manualized, with handouts and published materials, whereas others are briefer or not yet published. Models for PTSD alone or SUD alone also abound but are beyond the scope of this chapter.

DESCRIPTION OF SEEKING SAFETY

In this chapter the Seeking Safety model is described; it is the most studied treatment, thus far, for clients with PTSD and SUD (see the section, Empirical Results). It has also been implemented broadly with clients who do not necessarily meet diagnostic criteria for these disorders, such as those with trauma-related symptoms but not formal PTSD. The complete treatment manual is provided in book form (Najavits, 2002d), and the website *www.seekingsafety.org* provides materials that can be freely downloaded, including sample topics, a description of each empirical study, upcoming trainings, assessment tools, and journal articles (such as how to train clinicians in the model [Najavits, 2000] and implementation strategies [Najavits, 2004a]). Prior descriptions of the model are provided in book chapters and articles (Najavits, 2002b, 2002c; Najavits et al., 1996).

Overview

The title of the treatment, Seeking Safety, expresses a central idea: When a person has both active substance abuse and PTSD, the most urgent clinical need is to establish safety. "Safety" is an umbrella term that signifies various elements: safety from substances, safety from dangerous relationships (including domestic violence and drug-using friends), and safety from extreme symptoms, such as dissociation and self-harm. Many of these self-destructive behaviors reenact trauma—having been harmed through trauma, clients now harm themselves. "Seeking safety" refers to helping clients free themselves from such negative behaviors and, in so doing, to move toward freeing themselves from trauma at a deep emotional level.

Seeking Safety is an integrated treatment for SUD and trauma/PTSD that can be used from early recovery onward. It was designed to help explore the link between SUD and trauma/PTSD, but without delving into details about the past that may destabilize clients during early recovery. Its goal is a present-focused, empathic approach that helps clients "own" and name the trauma experience, validates the connection to substance use, provides psychoeducation, and offers specific "safe coping skills" to manage the often overwhelming impulses and emotions of this dual diagnosis. The model focuses equally on both disorders, at the same time, from the start of treatment, but in a way that is designed to be as safe, supportive, and containing as possible.

The treatment provides 25 topics to help clients attain safety. Topics are evenly divided among cognitive, behavioral, and interpersonal domains, with a clinician guide and extensive client handouts. Each topic addresses both trauma/PTSD and SUD.

The seven interpersonal topics are:

- Asking for Help
- Honesty
- Setting Boundaries in Relationships
- Healthy Relationships
- Community Resources
- Healing from Anger
- Getting Others to Support Your Recovery

The seven behavioral topics are:

- Detaching from Emotional Pain: Grounding
- Taking Good Care of Yourself
- Red and Green Flags
- Commitment
- Coping with Triggers
- Respecting Your Time
- Self-Nurturing

The seven cognitive topics are:

- PTSD: Taking Back Your Power
- Compassion
- When Substances Control You

- Recovery Thinking
- Integrating the Split Self
- Creating Meaning
- Discovery

The four combination topics are:

- Introduction to Treatment/Case Management
- Safety
- The Life Choices Game (review)
- Termination

See Table 10.1 for a brief description of all topics. The treatment manual provides a summary for each topic, a therapist orientation with background and clinical strategies for conducting the session, a quotation to read aloud at the start of each session to engage clients emotionally, client handouts, and examples of "tough cases" that the therapist can rehearse to prepare for the topic. Background chapters on the dual diagnosis and how to conduct the treatment are also provided.

The topics are written in simple language and designed to be emotionally compelling, with a respectful tone that honors clients' courage in fighting the disorders. The topics address new ways of coping and convey the idea that no matter what happens, clients can learn to cope in safe ways—without substance use or other destructive behavior. Special emphasis is placed on the clinician's role, such as countertransference and self-care, as this dual-diagnosis population is considered difficult to treat.

The treatment was developed to be broadly applicable in a wide variety of settings. It has been used for clients with formal diagnoses of both PTSD and SUD, those with one disorder but not the other, and those who do not meet diagnostic criteria (e.g., a trauma history but no PTSD, and/or a SUD history that is not current). For simplicity, the terms PTSD and SUD are used below, although clients do not have to meet formal criteria for these disorders. Topics can be conducted in any order, with the order selected by clients, clinicians, or both. Extensive handouts are available from which clients and clinicians can select those that are most relevant. Each topic is independent of the others and can be conducted as a single session or over multiple sessions, depending on the client's length of stay. Suggestions for how to select the order of topics are provided in the manual.

Session Structure

The session structure includes a check-in, a quotation (to emotionally engage clients), handouts, and a check-out (see Table 10.2). The structure is designed to model good use of time, appropriate containment, and achievement of goals. For clients with SUD and PTSD, who are often impulsive and

TABLE 10.1. Seeking Safety Topics

1. Introduction to Treatment/Case Management

   This topic covers (a) introduction to the treatment, (b) getting to know the client, and (c) assessment of case management needs.

2. Safety (*combination*)

   Safety is described as the first stage of healing from both PTSD and substance abuse, and the key focus of the treatment. A list of over 80 Safe Coping Skills is provided and clients explore what safety means to them.

3. PTSD: Taking Back Your Power (*cognitive*)

   Four handouts are offered: (a) What is PTSD?; (b) The Link between PTSD and Substance Abuse; (c) Using Compassion to Take Back Your Power; and (d) Long-Term PTSD Problems. The goal is to provide information as well as a compassionate understanding of the disorder.

4. Detaching from Emotional Pain: Grounding (*behavioral*)

   A powerful strategy, "grounding," is offered to help clients detach from emotional pain. Three types of grounding are presented (mental, physical, and soothing), with an experiential exercise to demonstrate the techniques. The goal is to shift attention toward the external world, away from negative feelings.

5. When Substances Control You (*cognitive*)

   Eight handouts are provided, which can be combined or used separately: (a) Do You Have a Substance Abuse Problem? (b) How Substance Abuse Prevents Healing from PTSD; (c) Choose a Way to Give Up Substances; (d) Climbing Mount Recovery, an imaginative exercise to prepare for giving up substances; (e) Mixed Feelings; (f) Self-Understanding of Substance Use; (g) Self-Help Groups; and (h) Substance Abuse and PTSD: Common Questions.

6. Asking for Help (*interpersonal*)

   Both PTSD and substance abuse lead to problems in asking for help. This topic encourages clients to become aware of their need for help and provides guidance on how to obtain it.

7. Taking Good Care of Yourself (*behavioral*)

   Clients explore how well they take care of themselves using a questionnaire that lists specific behaviors (e.g., "Do you get regular medical checkups?"). They are asked to take immediate action to improve at least one self-care problem.

8. Compassion (*cognitive*)

   This topic encourages the use of compassion when trying to overcome problems. Compassion is the opposite of "beating oneself up," a common tendency for people with PTSD and substance abuse. Clients are taught that only a loving stance toward the self produces lasting change.

Note. Each topic represents a *safe coping skill* relevant to both SUD and trauma/PTSD, and can be conducted over one or more sessions. After the first topic, the rest can be conducted in any order based on clinician and client preference. Domains are listed in parentheses (cognitive, behavioral, interpersonal, or a combination).

Adapted from (Najavits, 2002c). Copyright 2002 by the American Psychological Association Press. Reprinted by permission.

9. Red and Green Flags (behavioral)

Clients explore the up-and-down nature of recovery in both PTSD and substance abuse through discussion of "red and green flags" (signs of danger and safety). A Safety Plan is developed to identify what to do in situations of mild, moderate, and severe relapse danger.

10. Honesty (*interpersonal*)

Clients discuss the role of honesty in recovery and role-play specific situations. Related issues include: What is the cost of dishonesty? When is it safe to be honest? What if the other person does not accept honesty?

11. Recovery Thinking (*cognitive*)

Thoughts associated with PTSD and substance abuse are contrasted with healthier recovery thinking. Clients are guided to change their thinking using rethinking tools such as List Your Options, Create a New Story, Make a Decision, and Imagine. The power of rethinking is demonstrated through think-aloud exercises.

12. Integrating the Split Self (*cognitive*)

Splitting is identified as a major psychic defense in both PTSD and substance abuse. Clients are guided to notice splits (e.g., different sides of the self, ambivalence, denial) and to strive for integration as a means to overcome these.

13. Commitment (*behavioral*)

The concept of keeping promises, both to self and others, is explored. Clients are offered creative strategies for keeping commitments, as well as the opportunity to identify feelings that can get in the way.

14. Creating Meaning (*cognitive*)

Meaning systems are discussed with a focus on assumptions specific to PTSD and substance abuse, such as Deprivation Reasoning, Actions Speak Louder Than Words, and Time Warp. Meanings that are harmful versus healing in recovery are contrasted.

15. Community Resources (*interpersonal*)

A lengthy list of national nonprofit resources is offered to aid clients' recovery (including advocacy organizations, self-help, and newsletters). Also, guidelines are offered to help clients take a consumer approach in evaluating treatments.

16. Setting Boundaries in Relationships (*interpersonal*)

Boundary problems are described either in terms of too much closeness (difficulty saying no in relationships) or too much distance (difficulty saying yes in relationships). Ways to set healthy boundaries are explored, and domestic violence information is provided.

17. Discovery (*cognitive*)

Discovery is offered as a tool to reduce the cognitive rigidity common to PTSD and substance abuse (called "staying stuck"). Discovery is a way to stay open to experience and new knowledge, using strategies such as Ask Others, Try It and See, Predict, and Act As If. Suggestions for coping with negative feedback are provided.

cont.

TABLE 10.1. *cont.*

18. Getting Others to Support Your Recovery (*interpersonal*)

Clients are encouraged to identify which people in their lives are supportive, neutral, or destructive toward their recovery. Suggestions for eliciting support are provided, as is a letter that they can give to others to promote understanding of PTSD and substance abuse. A safe family member or friend can be invited to attend the session.

19. Coping with Triggers (*behavioral*)

Clients are encouraged to actively fight triggers of PTSD and substance abuse. A simple three-step model is offered: change *who* you are with, *what* you are doing, and *where* you are (similar to AA's "change people, places, and things").

20. Respecting Your Time (*behavioral*)

Time is explored as a major resource in recovery. Clients may have lost years to their disorders, but they can still make the future better than the past. They are asked to fill in schedule blanks to explore issues, such as the following: Do they use their time well? Is recovery their highest priority? Also addressed is how to balance structure versus spontaneity; work versus play; and time alone versus time in relationships.

21. Healthy Relationships (*interpersonal*)

Healthy and unhealthy relationship beliefs are contrasted. For example, the unhealthy belief, "Bad relationships are all I can get," is contrasted with the healthy belief, "Creating good relationships is a skill I can learn." Clients are guided to notice how PTSD and substance abuse can lead to unhealthy relationships.

22. Self-Nurturing (*behavioral*)

Safe self-nurturing is distinguished from unsafe self-nurturing (e.g., substances and other "cheap thrills"). Clients are asked to create a gift to the self by increasing safe self-nurturing and decreasing unsafe self-nurturing. Pleasure is explored as a complex issue in PTSD/substance abuse.

23. Healing from Anger (*interpersonal*)

Anger is explored as a valid feeling that is inevitable in recovery from PTSD and substance abuse. Anger can be used constructively (as a source of knowledge and healing) or destructively (when acted out against self or others). Guidelines for working with both types of anger are offered.

24. The Life Choices Game (*combination*)

As part of termination, clients are invited to play a game as a way to review the material covered in the treatment. Clients pull from a box slips of paper that list challenging life events (e.g., "You find out your partner is having an affair"). They respond with how they would cope, using game rules that focus on constructive coping.

25. Termination

Clients express their feelings about the ending of treatment, discuss what they liked and disliked about it, and finalize aftercare plans. An optional termination letter can be read aloud to clients to validate the work they have done.

overwhelmed, the predictable session structure helps them know what to expect. It offers, in its process, a mirror of the focus and careful planning that are needed for recovery from the disorders. Most of the session is devoted to the topic selected for the session (per Table 10.1), relating it to current and specific problems in clients' lives. Priority is on any unsafe behavior the client reported during the check-in. The tone of the treatment, when conducted well, feels like deep therapy rather than just psychoeducation or school. There is strong emphasis on rehearsal of the skills during sessions, using any of a number of methods (e.g., role play, experiential exercises, think-alouds, discussion, question–answer, replaying a scene of poor coping, and processing obstacles). There are no particular coping skills or topics clients must master; rather, they are offered a wide variety from which to choose. The goal is to "go where the action is"—to use the materials in a way that adapts to the client, the clinician, and the program.

TABLE 10.2. Session Format

1. Check-In

   The goal of the check-in is to find out how clients are doing (up to 5 minutes per patient). Clients report on five questions: Since the last session (a) How are you feeling? (b) What good coping have you done? (c) Any substance use or other unsafe behavior; (d) Did you complete your commitment? and (e) Community Resource update.

2. Quotation

   The quotation is a brief device to help emotionally engage clients in the session (up to 2 minutes). A client reads the quotation out loud. The clinician asks, "What is the main point of the quotation?" and links it to the topic of the session.

3. Relate the Topic to Clients' Lives

   The clinician and/or client select any of the 25 treatment topics (see Table 10.1) that feels most relevant. This is the heart of the session, with the goal of meaningfully connecting the topic to clients' experience (30–40 minutes). Clients look through the handout for a few minutes, which may be accompanied by the clinician summarizing key points (especially for clients who are cognitively impaired). Clients are asked what they most relate to in the material, and the rest of the time is devoted to addressing the topic in relation to specific and current examples from clients' lives. As each topic represents a safe coping skill, intensive rehearsal of the skill is strongly emphasized.

4. Check-Out

   The goal is to reinforce clients' progress and give the clinician feedback (a few minutes per client). Clients answer two questions: (a) Name one thing you got out of today's session (and any problems with the session); (b) What is your new commitment?; and (c) What community resource will you call?

Note. From Najavits (2002d). Copyright 2002 by The Guilford Press. Reprinted by permission.

At the end of each session clients are asked to select a commitment to try before the next session. Commitments are very much like cognitive-behavioral therapy (CBT) homework, but the language is changed to emphasize that clients are making a promise—to themselves, to the therapist, and, in group treatment, to the group—to promote their recovery by taking at least one action step forward. Commitments do not have to be written, because clinical experience with this population suggests that some clients do not like written assignments. Examples of commitments include "Ask your partner not to offer you any more cocaine," "Read a book on parenting," and "Write a supportive letter to the young side of you that feels scared." Ideas for commitments are offered at the end of each handout, but therapists are encouraged to customize them to best fit each client (see also Najavits, 2005).

The treatment is thus both highly structured yet also extremely flexible—characteristics that may be particularly important when working with severe populations. The multiple needs, impulsivity, and intense affect of such populations can lead to derailed sessions if the clinician does not impose clear structure. Yet the treatment is also highly flexible to allow clients' most important concerns to be kept primary, to allow adaptation to a variety of settings, to respect clinicians' clinical judgment, and to encourage clinicians to remain inspired and interested in the work. These considerations are believed to be paramount when working with a population such as this, where the risks of client dropout and clinician burnout are high (Najavits, 2001). Moreover, the model was designed to adapt to the managed care era, in which many clients have limited access to treatment. Thus the treatment can be extremely short-term (e.g., one or a few sessions, such as on a brief inpatient stay), or can be extended to long-term treatment. The therapy is also designed to be integrated with other treatments. Although it can be conducted as a stand-alone intervention, the severity of clients' needs usually suggests that they be in several treatments at the same time (e.g., 12-step groups, pharmacotherapy, individual therapy, group therapy). Thus, not only was the treatment designed to be used in conjunction with other treatments, but it also includes an intensive case management component to help engage clients in other treatments.

Seeking Safety has been conducted in a variety of formats, including group and individual; open and closed groups; sessions of varying lengths (50 minutes, 1 hour, 90 minutes, and 2 hours); sessions of varying pacing (weekly, twice weekly, and daily); singly and co-led; outpatient, inpatient, and residential; integrated with other treatments or as a stand-alone therapy; and single gender or mixed gender. Some programs have covered all 25 topics, others created two blocks of 12 sessions each, and others allowed clients to cycle through the entire treatment multiple times. In some programs particular topics were added to ongoing treatments (e.g., Healing from Anger was added to an existing anger management group), or only selected topics were covered. In general, however, it is recommended to first try conducting the treatment as planned, in terms of both the topics and the session format, before adapting it. Empirical studies of the treatment thus far, however, were conducted under constrained conditions to evaluate gains within the typical limits of managed care treatment. The treatments were time-limited (typically twice per week for 3 months), with one session per topic. A recent article (Brown et al., 2005) describes adaptations of Seeking Safety in three community programs, with a summary of satisfaction and feedback from both clients and clinicians.

The treatment was first described in an early paper (Najavits et al., 1996), although it evolved considerably after that: from a focus on women to both genders, from group modality to individual as well, and from outpatient to diverse settings. The therapy was developed over 10 years, beginning in the early 1990s, under grants from the National Institute on Drug Abuse. An iterative process was used, such that clinical experience with this dual-diagnosis population led to various versions of the manual over time, with the final version published in 2002. The treatment also drew on educational innovation and research (i.e., how to convey concepts in a way clients can understand). In the rest of this chapter, the treatment is described in more detail, and implementation and assessment considerations are offered.

KEY PRINCIPLES

Seeking Safety is based on five principles.[1]

Safety as the Priority of This First-Stage Treatment

The treatment fits what has been described as first-stage therapy for both PTSD and SUD. Experts within both fields have independently described an extremely similar first stage of treatment, termed "safety" or "stabilization," that prioritizes psychoeducation, coping skills, and reducing the most destructive symptoms (Herman, 1992; Kaufman & Reoux, 1988). Later stages, again quite similar for the two disorders, are conceptualized as "mourning" (facing one's past by exploring the impact of trauma and substance abuse) and "reconnection" (attaining a healthy engagement with the world through work and relationships), to use the language of Herman (Herman, 1992). The first stage, safety, is an enormous therapeutic task for some clients, and thus the Seeking Safety treatment addresses only that stage. Throughout the treatment, safety is addressed over and over, including the use of the topic Safety; a list of safe coping skills; a Safe Coping Sheet to explore recent unsafe incidents; a Safety Plan to identify stages of danger and how to address them; a Safety Contract; and a report of unsafe behaviors at each session's check-in. The concepts of safety and first-stage treat-

---

[1]This section is reprinted with minor edits from Najavits (2002c). Copyright 2002 by the American Psychological Association Press. Reprinted by permission.

ment are designed to protect the clinician as well as the client. By helping clients move toward safety, clinicians are protecting themselves from the sequelae of treatment that could move too fast without a solid foundation, resulting in vicarious traumatization, medicolegal liability, and/or dangerous transference dilemmas (Chu, 1988; Pearlman & Saakvitne, 1995). In particular, eliciting trauma memories too early in treatment when safety has not been established may have harmful consequences (Chu, 1988; Ruzek et al., 1998). Increased substance use and suicidality are of particular concern in this vulnerable dual-diagnosis population. Thus, seeking safety is, hopefully, both the client's and the clinician's goal.

Note that although clients do not delve into the past in the Seeking Safety model, the treatment can be combined with trauma-processing methods such as exposure therapy (Foa & Rothbaum, 1998), eye movement desensitization and reprocessing (Shapiro, 1995), and other models of trauma exploration. One pilot study on men, for example, combined Seeking Safety with a revised version of Exposure Therapy (Najavits et al., in press-a). At this stage, however, there has been little research on which SUD clients are best suited for trauma exploration and at what point in treatment. Indeed, within the mental health field, in general, it remains unclear whether all PTSD clients need to engage in trauma exposure therapy, whether some may benefit from both present- and past-focused PTSD treatment (and, if so, whether to combine the two treatments sequentially or concurrently), whether some may need just one or just the other type of treatment, and how to decide. Thus far, studies that directly compared present-focused versus past-focused PTSD approaches have found both to produce positive outcomes, without significant differences between them (e.g., Marks, Lovell, Noshirvani, Livanou, & Thrasher, 1998; Schnurr et al., 2003). In teaching clinicians about a present-focused treatment such as Seeking Safety, it is important for these issues to be raised. It is sometimes a surprise that treatment of PTSD does not necessarily have to involve exploration of trauma memories. Many assume that present-focused PTSD treatment is always a precursor to eventually doing the "real" treatment of trauma exposure. But more research is needed both in SUD and other samples to better understand when and under what conditions present- and past-focused PTSD methods are needed. See Coffey et al. (Coffey, Dansky, & Brady, 2002; Coffey, Schumacher, Brimo, & Brady, 2005) and Najavits et al. (Najavits et al., in press-a) for more on this issue.

Integrated Treatment of PTSD and Substance Abuse

Seeking Safety is designed to continually integrate attention to both disorders; that is, both are treated at the same time by the same clinician. This *integrated* model contrasts with a *sequential* model, in which the client is treated for one disorder, then the other; a *parallel* model, in which the client receives treatment for both disorders but by different treaters; or a *single* model, in which the client receives only one type of treatment (Weiss &

Najavits, 1997). An integrated model is consistently recommended as the treatment of choice for this dual diagnosis population (Abueg & Fairbank, 1991; Brady et al., 1994; Brown, Recupero, & Stout, 1995; Evans & Sullivan, 1995; Kofoed et al., 1993; Najavits et al., 1996; Ruzek et al., 1998). Furthermore, a survey of clients with this dual diagnosis found that clients also preferred simultaneous treatment of both disorders (Brown et al., 1998).

In practice, however, the two disorders are not usually treated simultaneously. Indeed, it is still the norm for clients to be told that they need to become abstinent from substances before working on PTSD—a mandate that does not work for many clients. In many settings clinical staff are reluctant to even assess for the other disorder; and clients' own shame and secrecy about trauma and substance abuse can further reinforce treatment splits (Brown et al., 1995). Integration is thus, ultimately, an intrapsychic goal for clients as well as a systems goal: to "own" both disorders, to recognize their interrelationship, and to fall prey less often to the vulnerability of each disorder triggering the other. Seeking Safety provides opportunities for clients to discover connections in their lives between the two disorders: in what order the disorders arose and why, how each affects healing from the other, and the origins of both disorders in other life problems (e.g., poverty). The clinician, too, is guided to use each disorder as leverage to help clients overcome the other disorder, because clients often have stronger motivation initially to work on one rather than the other. Finally, integration also occurs at the intervention level. Each safe coping skill in the treatment can be applied to both PTSD and substance abuse. For example, setting boundaries in relationships can apply to PTSD (e.g., leaving an abusive relationship) and to substance abuse (e.g., asking a friend to stop offering drugs). In sum, Seeking Safety was designed to attend equally strongly to both disorders. It was not originally a SUD treatment that later added a focus on PTSD, nor vice versa. Also, it directly targets improvements in both domains, although more empirical work is needed to evaluate whether, in fact, the treatment consistently has equal impact on both.

A Focus on Ideals

It is difficult to imagine two mental disorders that each individually, and especially in combination, lead to such demoralization and loss of ideals. This loss of ideals in PTSD has been written about, for example, in work on "shattered assumptions" (Janoff-Bulman, 1992) and the "search for meaning" (Frankl, 1963). Some research has found that trauma survivors who are able to create positive meanings from their suffering fare better than those who do not (Janoff-Bulman, 1997). There is also a loss of ideals in substance abuse—life narrows in focus, and, in its severe form, the person "hits bottom." It is notable that the primary treatment for substance abuse for most of this century, AA, is the only treatment for a mental disorder that has a heavily spiritual component. The AA goal of living a life of moral integrity is an antidote to the deterioration of ideals inherent in substance abuse.

Seeking Safety explicitly seeks to restore ideals that have been lost. The title of each topic is framed as a positive ideal, one that is the opposite of some pathological characteristic of PTSD and substance abuse. For example, the topic Honesty combats denial, lying, and the false self. Commitment is the opposite of irresponsibility and impulsivity. Taking Good Care of Yourself is a solution for bodily self-neglect. Throughout, the language of the treatment emphasizes values such as respect, care, integration, protection, and healing. By aiming for what can be, the hope is that clients can summon the motivation for the incredibly hard work of recovery from two difficult disorders.

Four Content Areas: Cognitive, Behavioral, Interpersonal, and Case Management

CBT is the basis for this treatment, because it so directly meets the needs of first-stage treatment through its high degree of structure, focus on problem solving in the present, educational emphasis, and time-limited framework. Moreover, in outcome studies CBT has been found to be one of the most promising approaches for the treatment of each of the disorders (PTSD and substance abuse) when treated separately (Najavits et al., 1996). The cognitive domain of Seeking Safety addresses beliefs and meanings associated with PTSD and SUD and explores how to rethink these in an adaptive way. The behavioral domain addresses how to take concrete actions in one's life, such as taking good care of one's body. The interpersonal domain is an area of special need because most PTSD arises from trauma inflicted by others (e.g., in contrast to natural disasters or accidents; Kessler et al., 1995). Whether the trauma involved childhood physical or sexual abuse, combat, or crime victimization, all have an interpersonal valence that may evoke distrust of others, confusion over what can be expected in relationships, and concern over reenactments of abusive power (Herman, 1992). Similarly, substance abuse is often associated with relationships. It is typically initiated in interaction with others and is frequently used to cope with interpersonal conflicts and anxiety in social situations (Marlatt & Gordon, 1985). The case management component arose because data in the first Seeking Safety pilot study showed that many clients were engaged in few treatment services (Najavits, Dierberger, & Weiss, 1999a). Most participants required significant assistance getting the care they needed, such as psychopharmacology, job counseling, and housing. Thus, case management (termed "community resources") is heavily emphasized, based on the idea that psychological interventions can work only if clients have an adequate treatment base.

Attention to Clinician Processes

Research shows that for substance abuse clients, in particular (and psychotherapy, in general), the effectiveness of treatment is determined as much or more by the clinician as by any particular theoretical orientation or client characteristics (Najavits, Crits-Christoph, & Dierberger, 2003; Najavits & Weiss, 1994). With dual-diagnosis clients, who are often considered difficult, severe, or extreme (Kofoed et al., 1993), providing effective therapy is a major challenge. Moreover, in conducting workshops for clinicians and listening to hundreds of therapy tapes using the model, it has become clear that some of the most frequent dilemmas that emerge are about process: for example, how to calm agitated clients and how to confront clients who have lied about substance abuse. Clinician processes emphasized in Seeking Safety include compassion for clients' experience, using the treatment's coping skills in one's own life (not asking the client to do things that one cannot do oneself), giving clients control whenever possible (because loss of control is inherent in trauma and substance abuse), modeling what it means to try hard by meeting the client more than halfway (e.g., heroically doing anything possible within professional bounds to help the client get better), "listening" to clients' behavior more than their words, learning to give both positive and negative feedback, and obtaining feedback from clients about their reactions to the treatment. The flip side of such positive clinician processes is negative countertransference, including harsh confrontation, sadism, inability to hold clients accountable because of misguided sympathy, becoming victim to clients' abusiveness; power struggles; and, in group treatment, allowing a client to be scapegoated. As Herman (1992) suggested, clinicians may unwittingly repeat the trauma roles of victim, perpetrator, or bystander. Attention is also directed to what I call the "paradox of countertransference" in PTSD and substance abuse; that is, each disorder appears to evoke opposite countertransference reactions that are difficult for clinicians to balance. PTSD tends to evoke identification with clients' vulnerability, which, if taken too far, may lead to excessive support at the expense of growth. Substance abuse tends to evoke anxiety about the client's substance use, which, if extreme, can become harsh judgment and control (e.g., "I won't treat you if you keep using"). The goal is thus for the clinician to integrate support and accountability, which are viewed as the two central processes in the treatment. Clinicians are encouraged to help clients seek explanations, but not excuses, for their unsafe behavior.

Training methods for the treatment (Najavits, 2000, 2004a) emphasize these various process issues as well as observation of he clinician in action (e.g., taped sessions) and intensive training experiences (e.g., watching videotapes of good vs. poor sessions; peer supervision, role plays, knowledge tests; identifying key themes; and think-aloud modeling). For every topic in the manual, "tough case" clinical scenarios are provided that also emphasize challenging statements clients may say. For example, when covering the topic Safety, the client may say, "I don't want to stay safe; I want to die." The clinician is encouraged to rehearse possible responses to such statements.

WHAT IS NOT PART OF THE TREATMENT

There are two main areas that this treatment explicitly omits, particularly when it is offered in group format: exploration of past trauma, and interpretive psychodynamic work.

Exploration of past trauma is, in and of itself, a major treatment intervention for PTSD. As noted above, it is conceptualized as the second stage of treatment, after the client has attained a foundation of safety (Herman, 1992; Kaufman & Reoux, 1988). A variety of PTSD treatment methods have as their central goal the evocation of traumatic memories as a means to process them. These include mourning (Herman, 1992), exposure therapy (e.g., Foa & Rothbaum, 1998), and eye movement desensitization and reprocessing (Shapiro, 1995). By directly processing trauma memories, they no longer hold such emotional power over the client.

Despite the known importance and efficacy of such treatments for PTSD (e.g., Marks et al., 1998), various experts have recommended the delay of such work for substance abusers until they have achieved a period of stable functioning and abstinence (Chu, 1988; Keane, 1995; Ruzek et al., 1998; Solomon et al., 1992). Until then, trauma processing may be too emotionally upsetting for clients who do not yet have adequate coping skills to control their impulses. Concerns repeatedly expressed in the literature are increased substance use, relapse (if already abstinent), or an increase in dangerous behaviors such as self-harm or suicidality (Keane, 1995; Ruzek et al., 1998; Solomon et al., 1992). Opening up the "Pandora's box" of trauma memories may destabilize clients when they are most in need of stabilization. Clients themselves may not feel ready for trauma processing early in SUD recovery; others may want to talk about the past but may underestimate the intense emotions and new disturbing memories.

Thus far, only a few studies of clients with PTSD and substance abuse have used exploration of past trauma as a key intervention. In one study (Brady et al., 2001) results indicated that the 39% of their sample who was able to complete at least 10 of the 16 sessions showed positive outcomes in PTSD symptoms and cocaine use (as well as other symptoms), which were maintained at the 6-month follow-up. However, most clients were noncompleters; and the researchers excluded clients with suicidal ideation, and thus likely selected a less impaired sample. In a study that combined Seeking Safety plus Exposure Therapy–Revised (Najavits et al., in press-a), positive outcomes were found in various domains, including psychiatric and substance abuse symptoms. However, a large number of modifications to standard exposure therapy was created, the treatment was conducted individually, and various "safety parameters" were put in place to maximize clients' ability to safely tolerate the work. For a description of the safety parameters and elaboration of how Seeking Safety was combined with exposure, see Najavits et al. (in press-a) and also Chapter 2 of the Seeking Safety manual (Najavits, 2002d). Finally, another study (Triffleman, Wong, Monnette, &

Bostrum, 2002) also reported positive outcomes for exposure therapy in opioid-dependent clients.

Thus, until further research explores the use of exposure techniques with this dual-diagnosis population, it is not included as part of Seeking Safety. Also, Seeking Safety was initially tested in a time-limited group format, which did not appear to be an appropriate context in which to conduct exposure methods for victims of repeated early trauma, who represent a large number of clients with this dual diagnosis (Najavits et al., 1997). Even the mention of trauma experiences has been found to trigger other clients, and in a short-term group treatment format, there may be insufficient ability to process the material fully. If a client brings up details of trauma during a Seeking Safety session, the clinician empathically validates the importance of such material but reminds the client that the treatment is present-focused and that description of trauma details may be overly upsetting for him or her (and to others, if it is a group therapy). The clinician gently refocuses the client on the present and how to cope with whatever is coming up. However, at any point in the treatment, clients can share in a brief phrase the type of trauma they experienced (such as child sexual abuse, rape, combat) if they choose to, which can help them feel understood and bond with others in a group without being overly destabilized.

Interpretive psychodynamic work is also specifically avoided in Seeking Safety. There is little, if any, transference-based exploration of the client's relationship with the clinician or, in group treatment, of members with each other. There is also no interpretation of intrapsychic motives or dynamic insights. Although these powerful interventions can be helpful in later stages of treatment, they are believed to be potentially too upsetting for clients at this stage. There is a lot of interaction and discussion in Seeking Safety, but the model primarily focuses on support, problem solving, and coping. The heavily confrontational style of some SUD group therapies is also avoided to maintain the safety of a trauma-focused treatment. Accountability, but not harsh confrontation, is emphasized.

CLIENT AND CLINICIAN SELECTION

In selecting clients, in general, the goal is to be as inclusive as possible, with a plan to monitor clients over time and evaluate whether the model appears helpful to them. As noted earlier, although most of the empirical studies on Seeking Safety were conducted on clients formally and currently diagnosed with both disorders, in clinical practice the range has been much broader. It has included clients with a history of trauma and/or SUD, clients with serious and persistent mental illness, clients with just one or the other disorder, and clients with other disorders (e.g., eating disorders). An important consideration is clients' own preference. Given the powerlessness inherent in both PTSD and SUD, empowerment is key. It appears best to describe the treatment and then give clients a choice in whether to participate. Letting them explore the treatment by attending a few sessions, without obligation to continue, is another helpful process. Thus far, there do not appear to be any particular readiness characteristics or contraindications that are easily identified. Because the treatment is designed for safety, coping, and stabilization, it is not likely to destabilize clients and thus has been implemented quite broadly. Similarly, clients do not need to attain stabilization before starting; Seeking Safety was designed for use from the beginning of treatment. Clients who have addictive or impulsive behavior in addition to substance abuse (e.g., binge eating, self-mutilation, gambling) are encouraged to apply the safe coping skills taught in Seeking Safety to those behaviors, while also participating in specialized treatment for such problems as part of the case management component. Clients are not discontinued from the treatment unless they evidence a direct threat to staff or other clients (e.g., assault, selling drugs). An open-door policy prevails; clients are welcome back at any time—a position advocated in early recovery (Herman, 1992).

The key criteria for selecting clinicians to conduct Seeking Safety are positive attitudes toward clients with PTSD and SUD, a willingness to use a treatment manual, a high degree of empathy, a willingness to cross-train (i.e., for mental health clinicians to learn about substance abuse, and vice versa), and a strong ability to hold clients accountable and work with aggression (Najavits, 2000). In early use of Seeking Safety, various professional characteristics were sought, such as a mental health degree and particular types of training (e.g., CBT, substance abuse). It became clear over time that far more important than any such credentials were the more subtle criteria mentioned above (Najavits, 2000). Clinicians who genuinely enjoy these clients, often perceiving the work as a mission or calling, bring a level of commitment that no degree, per se, can provide. Similarly, clinicians who are open to the value of a treatment manual, viewing it as a resource to help improve the quality of the work, can make the best use of the material. Because there are no strict criteria for selecting clinicians (such as degree or training), the treatment may be widely applicable. Many substance abuse programs, for example, do not have staff with advanced degrees or formal CBT training. Because the treatment focuses on stabilization rather than trauma processing, it is comparable to relapse prevention models and thus does not appear to exceed the training, licensure, or ethical limits of substance abuse counselors. However, they are guided to refer clients out for specialized professional mental health treatment if clients' problems exceed the parameters of their work (e.g., dissociative identity disorder). Per the manual, it is also important that if a clinician does not have any prior background in trauma work, PTSD, substance abuse, or CBT, some training and/or supervision in these areas should be sought.

Additional suggestions for selecting a Seeking Safety clinician are described in a protocol that can be downloaded from *www.seekingsafety.org*

(see Clinician Selection). Briefly, it suggests a try-out to determine whether the clinician might be a good match. The clinician conducts one or more audiotaped sessions using Seeking Safety with a real client, and the sessions are rated by the client as well as evaluated on the Seeking Safety adherence scale. Methods for training and implementation are described in the manual as well as related articles (Najavits, 2000, 2004). A study exploring clinicians' views on treating these clients with dual diagnoses may also be relevant (Najavits, 2002a).

EMPIRICAL RESULTS

Seeking Safety is the most studied treatment thus far for the dual-diagnosis of PTSD and SUD, with seven completed outcome trials: outpatient women, in a group modality (Najavits et al., 1998b); women in prison, in group modality (Zlotnick et al., 2003); women in a community mental health setting, in group format and combined with other manual-based treatments (Holdcraft & Comtois, 2002); low-income urban women, in individual format (Hien et al., 2004); adolescent girls, in individual format (Najavits, Gallop, & Weiss, 2005); men and women veterans, in group format (Cook, Walser, Kane, Ruzek, & Woody, in press); and outpatient men traumatized as children, in individual format (Najavits et al., in press-a). In all of the studies the clients were severe. That is, they had the disorders for many years and the majority of cases involved substance dependence. Most clients had a history of multiple traumas, often in childhood, and typically had additional co-occurring Axis I and/or Axis II disorders.

Participants in all seven studies of Seeking Safety evidenced positive outcomes. In the six studies that reported on substance use, improvements were found in that domain. The six studies that assessed PTSD and/or trauma-related symptoms found improvements in those areas. Improvements were also found in various other areas, including social adjustment, general psychiatric symptoms, suicidal plans and thoughts, problem solving, sense of meaning, depression, and quality of life. Treatment satisfaction and attendance were reported to be high. Four studies had follow-ups after treatment ended and found that some key gains were maintained (Hien et al., 2004; Najavits et al., 2005; Najavits et al., in press-a; Najavits et al., 1996; Zlotnick et al., 2003). Five studies were pilots, and two were randomized controlled trials (Hien et al., 2004; Najavits et al., 2005). In the study by Hien et al., both Seeking Safety and relapse prevention treatments showed positive effects with no significant difference between them, and both outperformed a nonrandomized treatment-as-usual control (unspecified and unlimited treatment in the community). In Najavits et al. (2005), Seeking Safety outperformed treatment-as-usual for adolescent outpatient girls. It can also be noted that two studies combined Seeking Safety with other manual-based therapies. The study of men (Najavits et al., in press-a) combined Seeking Safety with exposure therapy—revised (ETR), an adaptation for substance abuse clients of Foa and Rothbaum's exposure therapy for PTSD (Foa & Rothbaum, 1998). Clients were allowed to choose the number of sessions of each type and chose an average of 21 Seeking Safety sessions and 9 ETR sessions. The study of women in a community mental health center (Holdcraft & Comtois, 2002) combined Seeking Safety with Linehan's (1993) dialectical behavior therapy.

Future directions for empirical work on Seeking Safety include the need for more randomized controlled trials, more studies comparing the model to other manualized treatments (e.g., to PTSD treatment alone), exploration of mechanisms of action, evaluation of clinician selection and training, and further studies in community-based settings. A brief 12-session version is currently being evaluated in the National Institute on Drug Abuse Clinical Trials Network; Seeking Safety was also used by four sites in the Substance Abuse and Mental Health Services Administration study, Women, Co-Occurring Disorders and Violence (Cocozza et al., 2005).

ASSESSMENT

A recent book chapter describes, in detail, practical considerations in assessing SUD and PTSD (Najavits, 2004b). It includes a list of specific domains within each disorder to consider for assessment and provides websites from which free assessment measures for both disorders can be downloaded (see also *www.seekingsafety.org*, section Assessment, for links to key sites). Specific suggestions for assessment are provided, including the therapeutic benefit of clients' receiving information about each of their diagnoses; the importance of routinely assessing for both trauma and PTSD even in the context of clients' substance use or withdrawal; the use of brief screenings to address the resource limitations of many programs; the goal of collecting only minimal information on trauma early in treatment to avoid triggering the client; and the need to delay assessment if the client is intoxicated. Also discussed are issues of diagnostic overlap between the two disorders, misconceptions of SUD criteria, age-appropriate measures, secondary gain in PTSD and SUD, common misdiagnoses, memory issues, countertransference by assessors, and clinical versus research instruments.

Implementation[2]

Several key considerations in implementing the treatment are explored in this section. Additional implementation suggestions are provided elsewhere. These include (1) how to integrate trauma processing therapy with Seeking Safety (see Chapter 2 of the manual [Najavits, 2002d], and Najavits et al., in press-a); (2) emergency procedures (see Chapter 2 of the manual); (3) process and training issues (see Chapter 2 of the manual and related articles by Najavits, 2000, 2004a); and (4) a detailed description of the Seeking Safety format (see Chapter 2 of the manual). See also Brown et al. (2005) for examples of how community programs adapted Seeking Safety.

Diversity (Ethnicity, Race, Gender)

Before the manual was published, Seeking Safety was conducted with diverse clients, including two studies with diverse racial/ethnic samples (Hien et al., 2000; Zlotnick et al., 2003), women and men, and clients with various trauma histories (e.g., child abuse, crime victimization, combat). The examples and language in the book were written to reflect these experiences and to mention sexism, racism, poverty, and both female and male issues. Thus far, the treatment has obtained high client satisfaction ratings in these subgroups. However, clinicians working with particular populations may benefit from adding more examples from their lives, including cultural elements relevant to them, and addressing their particular context and burdens. In treating men, for example, exploring how certain traumas violate the masculine role may be helpful (e.g., themes of "weakness" and vulnerability). In treating Latinos, using the Spanish-language version of Seeking Safety (see *www.seekingsafety.org*, the section Seeking Safety) and providing cultural context may be useful (e.g., acculturation stress and concepts such as *familismo* and *marianismo*). In treating gay, lesbian, bisexual and transgendered clients, homophobia concerns may be central. If clients cannot read written materials or have very low intelligence, summarizing the material briefly or having other clients read small sections out loud in group may help.

Group Modality

Several issues are notable when conducting the treatment in a group format. First, the name of the group can make a difference. One program initially called their group "Trauma Group," and few clients wanted to attend. When they renamed it "Seeking Safety Group," the attendance improved considerably. If the group title includes the term "trauma" or "PTSD," clients may fear that they will be asked to describe their traumas or will have to listen to others do so, and may not feel ready for that step. If it has a more upbeat title, they may feel more reassured. Thus thr group might be called Safety Group, Seeking Safety, or Coping Skills, for example. Second, the number of group members should be planned carefully. Keeping in mind that the check-in allows up to 5 minutes per client (although it often goes more quickly) and that the average group is 1 hour in length, a group of five cli-

---

[2]This section is reprinted with minor edits from Najavits (2004a). Copyright by . Reprinted by permission.

ents is workable to allow up to 25 minutes of check-in. For longer sessions, such as 1.5 hours, more clients can be added. However, adaptability is important here too. One residential program, for example, decided to conduct very large groups with 30 clients and to make the treatment psychoeducational rather than therapy-oriented (thus leaving out the check-in and check-out), because clients already participated in small groups where they received more personal attention. Third, because Seeking Safety focuses on trauma, the tone of the group may be different from typical substance abuse groups. In the latter, confrontation may be accepted (e.g., a client may tell another that he or she is "in denial" or "being too self-pitying"). In the Seeking Safety model such statements would be seen as detracting from the emotional safety of the group. The clinician is asked to train clients to focus on their own recovery work and to interact primarily in supportive and problem-solving ways rather than confrontational ways. Fourth, single-gender groups are the most common way of implementing the treatment, because trauma is often sexual or physical in nature, and clients are likely to feel more comfortable with others of the same gender. However, Seeking Safety has been implemented with mixed-gender groups as well, but only when none of the clients had a major history as a perpetrator (which could be too triggering), and only when clients agreed to join a mixed-gender group. The clinicians, too, have typically been the same gender as the group, although it could be argued that having a group leader of the opposite gender can create positive new experiences that may be healing for trauma survivors (Chu, personal communication). Finally, as noted earlier, the treatment has shown positive outcomes both in open and closed group formats, and when both singly-led and co-led. If clients miss a session, they are offered the handouts, if desired, as a way to keep up with the group. If clients plan to join an open group once it has begun, it is suggested that they review the topic "PTSD: Taking Back Your Power" prior to attending their first session, to learn about trauma and PTSD.

Typical Difficulties

One of the most common difficulties is talking too much or lecturing clients. In keeping with the goal of deep-level learning, an 80/20 rule is suggested; that is, clients talk 80% of the session, and clinicians 20%. This ratio preserves the feeling that the session is more like therapy than school, and it promotes success by having the clinician listen closely enough to clients to help solve their problems in a realistic way. When the clinician does not listen sufficiently, interventions tend to be less effective and more simplistic. Clinicians are encouraged to use the treatment's coping skills in their own lives, to give them a personal understanding of how the skills may (or may not) work.

A second major difficulty is not following the structure of the treatment. Although Seeking Safety is highly adaptable and flexible, it nonetheless asks clinicians to follow a structured format. This format was based on empirical testing conducted over many years with diverse populations. Even the wording of check-in questions, for example, was tested in different versions to identify ones that worked best. Thus clinicians are asked to start by using the structure as planned, only adapting it if clients provide negative feedback about it. In the projects that have used Seeking Safety thus far, clients have reported liking the structure and they learned it quickly with minimal instruction. Clinicians, however, particularly those who are not used to using a treatment manual, have needed more time and effort to adjust to it.

Finally, a third issue is staying "real." Because the treatment emphasizes validation, support, and empathy for clients' difficult trauma histories, clinicians sometimes overemphasize these processes at the expense of constructive feedback and setting limits. For example, when a client does a role play, clinicians sometimes offer only praise, rather than giving feedback on both strengths and weaknesses. Yet growth-oriented feedback is essential for clients to improve. Another example is owning anger, both seeing it in clients and in oneself. In the topic "Healing from Anger," it is suggested that clients' anger is inevitable in recovery from PTSD and substance abuse, and that it is a common countertransference reaction in clinicians as well. Yet in an attempt to be sympathetic, clinicians sometimes ignore or repress anger to a degree that is unhelpful. For example, a client may continually reject every suggestion offered, but the clinician keeps offering additional ideas to placate the client. It would be more helpful to process the dynamic of anger that typically underlies this help-rejecting client stance.

CONCLUSIONS AND RECOMMENDATIONS

Integrated therapies for dual diagnosis have become prominent in the past decade to help clients better overcome SUD and co-occurring mental disorders. A variety of integrated therapies has emerged for SUD and trauma/ PTSD, with positive outcomes evidenced thus far in empirical trials. Seeking Safety is the most studied therapy to date for this particular dual diagnosis. It is described in detail in this chapter, including assessment and implementation considerations.

Despite advances in this area of work, there is a tremendous need for more research. Few randomized controlled therapy trials have been conducted, and no trials comparing integrated models versus other models have been published (e.g., sequential or parallel treatment). Studies of mechanisms of treatment have not yet occurred. Innovative methods for training clinicians to work with such clients who have severe and complex conditions also need research. Clinically, there remains significant concern that assessment and treatment of PTSD in SUD settings is not widespread, and similarly, in mental health settings both PTSD and SUD may not be adequately addressed. Rigorous and large-scale studies are relatively rare, as are studies of long-term outcomes (1 year or more). Given the often chronic course of both PTSD and SUD through the lifespan (e.g., Port, 2001), more research and clinical help may be necessary than are reflected in the largely short-term outcome studies conducted thus far. If, how, and when to use trauma-processing models in SUD clients is a particular question in the literature, and more studies on this issue are needed. More generally, how best to combine treatments for this dual diagnosis has rarely been studied. Hopefully over time, further insights from both the clinical and research domains can help improve services for a population that is greatly in need.

ACKNOWLEDGMENTS

Preparation of this chapter was supported in part by grants K02DA00400 and R43DA018437 from the National Institute on Drug Abuse. Parts of this chapter were adapted from Najavits (2002c, 2004a). Copyright by The Guilford Press and the American Psychological Association Press. Adapted by permission.

REFERENCES

Abueg, F. R., & Fairbank, J. A. (1991). Behavioral treatment of the PTSD-substance abuser: A multidimensional stage model. In P. Saigh (Ed.), *Posttraumatic stress disorder: A behavioral approach to assessment and treatment* (pp. 111–146). New York: Pergamon Press.

Abueg, F. R., Lang, A. J., Drescher, K. D., Ruzek, J. I., Aboudarham, J. F., & Sullivan, N. (1994). *Enhanced relapse prevention training for posttraumatic stress disorder and alcoholism: A treatment manual.* Menlo Park, CA: National Center for PTSD.

Back, S., Dansky, B., Carroll, K., Foa, E., & Brady, K. (2001). Exposure therapy in the treatment of PTSD among cocaine-dependent individuals: Description of procedures. *Journal of Substance Abuse Treatment, 21*, 35–45.

Bollerud, K. (1990). A model for the treatment of trauma-related syndromes among chemically dependent inpatient women. *Journal of Substance Abuse Treatment, 7*, 83–87.

Brady, K. T. (2001). Comorbid posttraumatic stress disorder and substance use disorders. *Psychiatric Annals, 31*, 313–319.

Brady, K. T., Dansky, B., Back, S., Foa, E., & Caroll, K. (2001). Exposure therapy in the treatment of PTSD among cocaine-dependent individuals: Preliminary findings. *Journal of Substance Abuse Treatment, 21*, 47–54.

Brady, K. T., Killeen, T., Saladin, M. E., Dansky, B. S., & Becker, S. (1994). Comorbid substance abuse and posttraumatic stress disorder: Characteristics of women in treatment. *American Journal on Addictions, 3*, 160–164.

Brown, P. J., Recupero, P. R., & Stout, R. (1995). PTSD substance abuse comorbidity and treatment utilization. *Addictive Behaviors, 20*(2), 251–254.

Brown, P. J., Stout, R. L., & Gannon-Rowley, J. (1998). Substance use disorders–PTSD comorbidity: Patients' perceptions of symptom interplay and treatment issues. *Journal of Substance Abuse Treatment, 14*, 1–4.

Brown, V. B., Najavits, L. M., Cadiz, S., Finkelstein, N., Heckman, J., Gatz, M., et al. (2005). *Implementing an evidence-based practice: Seeking Safety.* Manuscript under review.

Bureau of Justice. (1992). *Criminal victimization in the U.S. 1992.* Washington, DC: Author.

Chu, J. A. (1988). Ten traps for therapists in the treatment of trauma survivors. *Dissociation: Progress in the Dissociative Disorders, 1,* 24–32.

Clark, H. W. (2002, January). *Meeting overview.* Paper presented at the Trauma and Substance Abuse Treatment Meeting, Bethesda, MD.

Cocozza, J. J., Jackson, E., Hennigan, K., Morrissey, J. P., Reed, B. G., Fallot, R., & Banks, S. (2005). Outcomes for women with co-occurring disorders and trauma: Program-level effects. *Journal of Substance Abuse Treatment, 28*(2), 109–119.

Coffey, S. F., Dansky, B. S., & Brady, K. T. (2002). Exposure-based, trauma-focused therapy for comorbid posttraumatic stress disorder–substance use disorder. In P. Ouimette & P. J. Brown (Eds.), *Trauma and substance abuse: Causes, consequences, and treatment of comorbid disorders* (pp. 209–226). Washington, DC: American Psychological Association.

Coffey, S. F., Schumacher, J. A., Brimo, M. L., & Brady, K. T. (2005). Exposure therapy for substance abusers with PTSD: Translating research to practice. *Behavior Modification, 29*(1),10–38.

Cook, J. M., Walser, R. D., Kane, V., Ruzek, J. I., & Woody, G. (in press). Dissemination and feasibility of a cognitive-behavioral treatment for substance use disorders and posttraumatic stress disorder in the Veterans Administration. *Journal of Psychoactive Drugs.*

Covington, S. S. (1999). *A woman's journal: Helping women recover. Special edition for use in the criminal justice system.* San Francisco: Jossey-Bass.

Covington, S. S. (2000). Helping women recover: A comprehensive integrated treatment model. *Alcoholism Treatment Quarterly, 18*(3), 99–111.

Dansky, B. S., Roitzsch, J. C., Brady, K. T., & Saladin, M. E. (1997). Posttraumatic stress disorder and substance abuse: Use of research in a clinical setting. *Journal of Traumatic Stress, 10,* 141–148.

Davidson, J. R. T. (2001). Recognition and treatment of posttraumatic stress disorder. *Journal of the American Medical Association, 286,* 584–588.

Davis, T. M., & Wood, P. S. (1999). Substance abuse and sexual trauma in a female veteran population. *Journal of Substance Abuse Treatment, 16,* 123–127.

Donovan, B., Padin-Rivera, E., & Kowaliw, S. (2001). Transcend: Initial outcomes from a posttraumatic stress disorder/substance abuse treatment study. *Journal of Traumatic Stress, 14,* 757–772.

Evans, K., & Sullivan, J. M. (1995). *Treating addicted survivors of trauma.* New York: Guilford Press.

Fletcher, A. (2001). *Sober for good: New solutions for drinking problems–advice from those who have succeeded.* Boston: Houghton Mifflin.

Foa, E. B., & Rothbaum, B. O. (1998). *Treating the trauma of rape: Cognitive-behavioral therapy for PTSD.* New York: Guilford Press.

Ford, J., Kasimer, N., MacDonald, M., & Savill, G. (2000). *Trauma adaptive recovery group education and therapy (TARGET): Participant guidebook and leader manual.* Unpublished manuscript, University of Connecticut Health Center, Farmington, CT.

Frankl, V. E. (1963). *Man's search for meaning.* New York: Pocket Books.

Grice, D. E., Brady, K. T., Dustan, L. R., Malcolm, R., & Kilpatrick, D. G. (1995). Sexual and physical assault history and posttraumatic stress disorder in substance-dependent individuals. *American Journal on Addictions, 4*(4), 297–305.

Herman, J. L. (1992). *Trauma and recovery.* New York: Basic Books.

Hien, D. A., Cohen, L., Litt, L., Miele, G., & Capstick, C. (2004). Promising empirically supported treatments for women with comorbid PTSD and substance use disorders. *American Journal of Psychiatry, 161,* 1426–1432.

Hien, D. A., Nunes, E., Levin, F. R., & Fraser, D. (2000). Posttraumatic stress disorder and short-term outcome in early methadone maintenance treatment. *Journal of Substance Abuse Treatment, 19,* 31–37.

Holdcraft, L. C., & Comtois, K. A. (2002). Description of and preliminary data from a women's dual diagnosis community mental health program. *Canadian Journal of Community Mental Health, 21,* 91–109.

Hyer, L., Leach, P., Boudewyns, P. A., & Davis, H. (1991). Hidden PTSD in substance abuse inpatients among Vietnam veterans. *Journal of Substance Abuse Treatment, 8,* 213–219.

Jacobsen, L. K., Southwick, S. M., & Kosten, T. R. (2001). Substance use disorders in patients with posttraumatic stress disorder: A review of the literature. *American Journal of Psychiatry, 158,* 1184–1190.

Janoff-Bulman, R. (1992). *Shattered assumptions: Towards a new psychology of trauma.* New York: Free Press.

Janoff-Bulman, R. (1997). The impact of trauma on meaning: From meaningless world to meaningful life. In M. J. Power & C. R. Brewin (Eds.), *The transformation of meaning in psychological therapies: Integrating theory and practice* (pp. 91–106). Chichester, UK: Wiley.

Kaufman, E., & Reoux, J. (1988). Guidelines for the successful psychotherapy of substance abusers. *American Journal of Drug and Alcohol Abuse, 14,* 199–209.

Keane, T. M. (1995). The role of exposure therapy in the psychological treatment of PTSD. *Clinical Quarterly (National Center for Posttraumatic Stress Disorder), 5*(1), 3–6.

Kendler, K. S., Davis, C. G., & Kessler, R. C. (1997). The familial aggregation of common psychiatric and substance use disorders in the National Comorbidity Survey: A family history study. *British Journal of Psychiatry, 170,* 541–548.

Kessler, R. C., Sonnega, A., Bromet, E., Hughes, M., & Nelson, C. B. (1995). Posttraumatic stress disorder in the national comorbidity survey. *Archives of General Psychiatry, 52,* 1048–1060.

Kofoed, L., Friedman, M. J., & Peck, R. (1993). Alcoholism and drug abuse in inpatients with PTSD. *Psychiatric Quarterly, 64,* 151–171.

Linehan, M. M. (1993). *Skills training for treating borderline personality disorder.* New York: Guilford Press.

Marks, I., Lovell, K., Noshirvani, H., Livanou, M., & Thrasher, S. (1998). Treatment of posttraumatic stress disorder by exposure and/or cognitive restructuring: A controlled study. *Archives of General Psychiatry, 55,* 317–325.

Marlatt, G., & Gordon, J. (1985). *Relapse prevention: Maintenance strategies in the treatment of addictive behaviors.* New York: Guilford Press.

Marlatt, G., Tucker, J., Donovan, D., & Vuchinich, R. (1997). Help-seeking by substance abusers: The role of harm reduction and behavioral-economic approaches to facilitate treatment entry and retention. In L. Onken, J. Blaine & J. Boren (Eds.), *Beyond the therapeutic alliance: Keeping the drug-dependent individ-*

ual in treatment (pp. 44–84). Rockville, MD: U.S. Department of Health and Human Services.

Meisler, A. W. (1999). Group treatment of PTSD and comorbid alcohol abuse. In B. H. Young & D. D. Blake (Eds.), *Group treatments for post-traumatic stress disorder* (pp. 117–136). Philadelphia: Brunner/Mazel.

Miller, D., & Guidry, L. (2001). *Addictions and trauma recovery.* New York: Norton.

Najavits, L. M. (2000). Training clinicians in the Seeking Safety treatment for post-traumatic stress disorder and substance abuse. *Alcoholism Treatment Quarterly, 18,* 83–98.

Najavits, L. M. (2001). Early career award paper: Helping difficult patients. *Psychotherapy Research, 11,* 131–152.

Najavits, L. M. (2002a). Clinicians' views on treating posttraumatic stress disorder and substance use disorder. *Journal on Substance Abuse Treatment, 22,* 79–85.

Najavits, L. M. (2002b). Seeking Safety therapy for trauma and substance abuse. *Corrections Today, 64,* 136–140.

Najavits, L. M. (2002c). Seeking Safety: A new psychotherapy for posttraumatic stress disorder and substance use disorder. In P. Ouimette & P. J. Brown (Eds.), *Trauma and substance abuse: Causes, consequences, and treatment of comorbid disorders* (pp. 147–170). Washington, DC: American Psychological Association.

Najavits, L. M. (2002d). *Seeking Safety: A treatment manual for PTSD and substance abuse.* New York: Guilford Press.

Najavits, L. M. (2002e). *A woman's addiction workbook.* Oakland, CA: New Harbinger.

Najavits, L. M. (2004a). Treatment for posttraumtic stress disorder and substance abuse: Clinical guidelines for implementing the Seeking Safety therapy. *Alcoholism Treatment Quarterly, 22,* 43–62.

Najavits, L. M. (2004b). Assessment of trauma, PTSD, and substance use disorder: A practical guide. In J. P. Wilson & T. M. Keane (Eds.), *Assessing psychological trauma and PTSD* (2nd ed., pp. 466–491). New York: Guilford Press.

Najavits, L. M. (2005). Homework in cognitive-behavioral therapy for substance use disorders: A clinical guide. In N. Kazantzis, F. P. Deane, K. R. Ronan, & L. L'Abate (Eds.), *Using homework assignments in cognitive-behavior therapy.* Brunner-Routledge.

Najavits, L. M., Crits-Christoph, P., & Dierberger, A. E. (2003). Clinicians' impact on the quality of substance use disorder treatment. In M. Galanter (Ed.), *Research on alcoholism treatment* (Vol. 35, pp. 55–68). New York: Plenum Press.

Najavits, L. M., Dierberger, A. E., & Weiss, R. D. (1999a, November). *PTSD/substance abuse patients: Treatment utilization and satisfaction.* Poster presented at the annual meeting of the International Society for Traumatic Stress Studies, Miami, FL.

Najavits, L. M., Gallop, R. J., & Weiss, R. D. (2005). Seeking Safety therapy for adolescent girls with PTSD and substance use disorder: A randomized controlled trial. Manuscript under review.

Najavits, L. M., Gastfriend, D. R., Barber, J. P., Reif, S., Muenz, L. R., Blaine, J., et al. (1998). Cocaine dependence with and without posttraumatic stress disorder among subjects in the NIDA Collaborative Cocaine Treatment Study. *American Journal of Psychiatry, 155,* 214–219.

Najavits, L. M., Schmitz, M., Gotthardt, S., & Weiss, R. D. (in press). Seeking Safety plus exposure therapy—revised: An outcome study in men with PTSD and substance dependence. *Journal of Psychoactive Drugs.*

Najavits, L. M., Sullivan, T. P., Schmitz, M., Weiss, R. D., & Lee, C. S. N. (2004). Treatment utilization of women with PTSD and substance dependence. *American Journal on Addictions, 13*, 215–224.

Najavits, L. M., & Weiss, R. D. (1994). Variations in therapist effectiveness in the treatment of patients with substance use disorders: An empirical review. *Addiction, 89*, 679–688.

Najavits, L. M., Weiss, R. D., & Liese, B. S. (1996). Group cognitive-behavioral therapy for women with PTSD and substance use disorder. *Journal of Substance Abuse Treatment, 13*, 13–22.

Najavits, L. M., Weiss, R. D., & Shaw, S. R. (1997). The link between substance abuse and posttraumatic stress disorder in women: A research review. *American Journal on Addictions, 6*, 273–283.

Najavits, L. M., Weiss, R. D., & Shaw, S. R. (1999b). A clinical profile of women with PTSD and substance dependence. *Psychology of Addictive Behaviors, 13*, 98–104.

Najavits, L. M., Weiss, R. D., Shaw, S. R., & Muenz, L. R. (1998b). "Seeking Safety": Outcome of a new cognitive-behavioral psychotherapy for women with posttraumatic stress disorder and substance dependence. *Journal of Traumatic Stress, 11*, 437–456.

North, C. S., Nixon, S. J., Shariat, S., Mallonee, S., McMillen, J. C., Spitznagel, E. L., et al. (1999). Psychiatric disorders among survivors of the Oklahoma City bombing. *Journal of the American Medical Association, 282*, 755–762.

North, C. S., Tivis, L., McMillen, J. C., Pfefferbaum, B., Spitznagel, E. L., Cox, J., et al. (2002). Psychiatric disorders in rescue workers after the Oklahoma City bombing. *American Journal of Psychiatry, 159*, 857–859.

Ouimette, P., & Brown, P. J. (2002). *Trauma and substance abuse: Causes, consequences, and treatment of comorbid disorders*. Washington, DC: American Psychological Association.

Ouimette, P. C., Finney, J. W., & Moos, R. H. (1999). Two-year posttreatment functioning and coping of substance abuse patients with posttraumatic stress disorder. *Psychology of Addictive Behaviors, 13*, 105–114.

Pearlman, L. A., & Saakvitne, K. W. (1995). *Trauma and the therapist: Countertransference and vicarious traumatization in psychotherapy with incest survivors*. New York: Norton.

Port, C. L. (2001). New research on the course of PTSD. *American Journal of Psychiatry, 158*, 1474–1479.

Read, J. P., Bollinger, A. R., & Sharansky, E. (2002). Assessment of comorbid substance use disorder and posttraumatic stress disorder. In P. Ouimette & P. J. Brown (Eds.), *Trauma and substance abuse: Causes, consequences, and treatment of comorbid disorders* (pp. 111–125). Washington, DC: American Psychological Association.

Ruzek, J. I., Polusny, M. A., & Abueg, F. R. (1998). Assessment and treatment of concurrent posttraumatic stress disorder and substance abuse. In V. M. Follette, J. I. Ruzek, & F. R. Abueg (Eds.), *Cognitive-behavioral therapies for trauma* (pp. 226–255). New York: Guilford Press.

Schnurr, P. P., Friedman, M. J., Foy, D. W., Shea, M. T., Hsieh, F. Y., Lavori, P. W., et al. (2003). Randomized trial of trauma-focused group therapy for posttraumatic stress disorder: Results from a Department of Veterans Affairs cooperative study. *Archives of General Psychiatry, 60*, 481–490.

Shapiro, F. (1995). *Eye movement desensitization and reprocessing: Basic principles, protocols, and procedures*. New York: Guilford Press.

Smith, E. M., North, C. S., & Spitznagel, E. L. (1993). Alcohol, drugs, and psychiatric comorbidity among homeless women: An epidemiologic study. *Journal of Clinical Psychiatry, 54*(3), 82–87.

Solomon, S. D., Gerrity, E. T., & Muff, A. M. (1992). Efficacy of treatments for posttraumatic stress disorder. *Journal of the American Medical Association, 268,* 633–638.

Stamm, M. K. (2002). *Posttraumatic stress disorder and substance abuse: Perspectives of women in recovery.* Unpublished dissertation, Massachusetts School of Professional Psychology, Boston, MA.

Substance Abuse and Mental Health Services Administration. (2001). *A provider's introduction to substance abuse treatment for lesbian, gay, bisexual, and transgender individuals.* Rockville, MD: U.S. Department of Health and Human Services.

Tarter, R. E., & Kirisci, L. (1999). Psychological evaluation of alcohol and drug abuse in youth and adults. In P. J. Ott & R. E. Tarter (Eds.), *Sourcebook on substance abuse: Etiology, epidemiology, assessment, and treatment* (pp. 212–226). Needham Heights, MA: Allyn & Bacon.

Teplin, L. A., Abram, K. M., & McClelland, G. M. (1996). Prevalence of psychiatric disorders among incarcerated women. I: Pretrial detainees. *Archives of General Psychiatry, 53,* 505–512.

Teusch, R. (2001). Substance abuse as a symptom of childhood sexual abuse. *Psychiatric-Services, 52,* 1530–1532.

Triffleman, E. (1998). An overview of trauma exposure, posttraumatic stress disorder, and addictions. In H. R. Kranzler & B. J. Rounsaville (Eds.), *Dual diagnosis and treatment: Substance abuse and comorbid medical and psychiatric disorders* (pp. 263–316). New York: Dekker.

Triffleman, E. (2000). Gender differences in a controlled pilot study of psychosocial treatments in substance dependent patients with post-traumatic stress disorder: Design considerations and outcomes. *Alcoholism Treatment Quarterly, 18*(3), 113–126.

Triffleman, E., Carroll, K., & Kellogg, S. (1999). Substance dependence posttraumatic stress disorder therapy: An integrated cognitive-behavioral approach. *Journal of Substance Abuse Treatment, 17,* 3–14.

Triffleman, E., Wong, P., Monnette, C., & Bostrum, A. (2002). *A pilot trial of treatments for PTSD–substance use disorders among the opioid addicted.* Paper presented at the International Society for Traumatic Stress Studies, Baltimore, MD.

Trotter, C. (1992). *Double bind.* Minneapolis: Hazelden Press.

Weiss, R. D., & Najavits, L. M. (1997). Overview of treatment modalities for dual diagnosis patients: Pharmacotherapy, psychotherapy, and twelve-step programs. In H. R. Kranzler & B. J. Rounsaville (Eds.), *Dual diagnosis: Substance abuse and comorbid medical and psychiatric disorders* (pp. 87–105). New York: Dekker.

Yehuda, R., Schmeidler, J., Wainberg, M., Binder-Brynes, K., & Duvdevani, T. (1998). Vulnerability to posttraumatic stress disorder in adult offspring of Holocaust survivors. *American Journal of Psychiatry, 155,* 1163–1171.

Zlotnick, C., Najavits, L. M., & Rohsenow, D. J. (2003). A cognitive-behavioral treatment for incarcerated women with substance use disorder and posttraumatic stress disorder: Findings from a pilot study. *Journal of Substance Abuse Treatment, 25,* 99–105.

CHAPTER ELEVEN

Cognitive Therapy
for Trauma-Related Guilt and Shame

Edward S. Kubany
Tyler C. Ralston

There is considerable evidence that cognitions play an important role in the maintenance or chronicity of posttraumatic stress (e.g., Brewin, Dalgleish, & Joseph, 1996; Ehlers & Clark, 2000; Foa, Ehlers, Clark, Tolin, & Orsillo, 1999; Kubany et al., 1996; Kubany & Watson, 2002, 2003a). This research has emphasized survivors' phenomenology, much of which involves guilt and shame (see Kubany, 1998, for a brief review).

Research reviewed elsewhere shows that trauma-related guilt is a common problem for survivors of many different kinds of traumatic events—including survivors of combat, physical and sexual abuse, technological disasters, and surviving family members of victims of accidents, suicide, homicide, and sudden illness (Kubany et al., 1995; Kubany & Manke, 1995). Our own research documents that trauma-related guilt is pervasive both within and across survivor groups (Kubany et al., 1996, 2000). In a mixed sample of treatment- and non-treatment-seeking Vietnam veterans, nearly two-thirds (65%) reported experiencing at least moderate guilt, and almost one-third (32%) reported guilt in the considerable-to-extreme range (Kubany et al., 1996). Among 168 women participating in support groups for battered women, almost half (49%) reported moderate or greater guilt related to their abuse (Kubany et al., 1996). Only six of these women had no abuse-related guilt. Among 212 physically and/or sexually abused women with diagnoses of posttraumatic stress disorder (PTSD) (based on structured interviews), 75% reported moderate or greater abuse-related guilt (Kubany, 2000).

Guilt is positively and significantly related to the severity of PTSD. In three separate samples of Vietnam combat veterans, combat-related guilt was correlated between .67 and .81 with combat-related PTSD (Kubany, Abueg,

Kilauano, Manke, & Kaplan, 1997; Kubany et al., 1995, 1996). In a sample of 50 women in support groups for battered women, an index of partner-abuse-related guilt was correlated .51 with PTSD (Kubany et al., 1995). Similarly, in a sample of 68 women in support groups for battered women, the Global Guilt and Guilt Cognitions scales of the Trauma-Related Guilt Inventory (TRGI) were both correlated .55 with partner-abuse-related PTSD (Kubany et al., 1996).

In our conceptualization of chronic PTSD, guilt-associated beliefs and guilt-associated language repertoires contribute significantly to the persistence or chronicity of trauma-related distress and depression (Kubany & Watson, 2002, 2003a). An important reason why memories of trauma may not lose their capacity to evoke emotional pain over time may be due to higher order language conditioning (Kubany & Watson, 2002)—whereby guilt-associated appraisals that have acquired the ability to evoke negative affect (e.g., "I never should have . . . I could have prevented it")—function as conditioned language stimuli in pairings with images or thoughts of the trauma (Staats, 1972, 1996). Such appraisals may also control or lead to shame-related statements, such as, "There's something wrong with me . . . so stupid . . . I'm a bad mother." If habitually paired with recollections of trauma, such affect-evoking appraisals may repeatedly recondition memories of the trauma with distress. Affect-evoking cognitions of guilt may also function as a form of self-punishment that contributes to depression (e.g., Pitman et al., 1991), and tendencies to suppress or avoid trauma-related memories that evoke guilt may interfere, due to insufficient exposure duration, with the process of spontaneous recovery or natural extinction (Rohrbaugh, Riccio, & Arthur, 1972).

A GUIDING CONCEPTUALIZATION OF GUILT

We have conceptualized and obtained empirical support for guilt as a multidimensional construct comprised of negative affect and four guilt-related beliefs or cognitions: (1) perceived responsibility, (2) perceived insufficient justification for actions taken, (3) perceived violation of values, and (4) perceived foreseeability and preventability of negative outcomes (which are often distorted by hindsight bias; Fischhoff, 1975; Kubany & Watson, 2003a). In a two-factor analysis of the TRGI, all negative affect items loaded on a Distress factor, and all cognitive items loaded on a Cognitions factor (Kubany et al., 1996). Guilt is defined phenomenologically as *an unpleasant feeling accompanied by a belief (or beliefs) that one should have thought, felt, or acted differently* (Kubany & Watson, 2003a). This definition has guided our theoretical work on guilt (e.g., Kubany & Watson, 2003b; Kubany et al., 1995), our guilt assessment research (e.g., Kubany et al., 1996), and our development of a cognitive therapy model, which is the topic of this chapter.

Shame and Its Relationship with Guilt

Many trauma survivors experience both guilt and shame (e.g., Dutton, 1992; Hogland & Nicholas, 1995; Lisak, 1994). Guilt and shame tend to be yoked in trauma, because when survivors implicate themselves as playing a significant role in a tragic, irreparable outcome, they are also prone to conclude that the outcome reflects on their entire self, personality, or character (Kubany & Watson, 2003b). For example, one woman concluded that she was "evil" and a "monster" because she believed there were things she "could have done" to prevent her mother's death from cancer (Lindsay-Hartz et al., 1995, p. 277). As another example, Kubany and Watson (2005) cite a survivor of acquaintance rape who concluded that there was "something wrong with me" for not preventing the assault, in light of the fact that she, herself, was a sex abuse counselor and "should have seen the signs." Thus, guilt and shame often seem to go together in the experience of trauma survivors because distress and guilt cognitions of high magnitude would often lead to shame cognitions and shame.

It is important, though, to differentiate shame from guilt, precisely because shame is an emotional experience so closely associated with guilt and elicited by the same kinds of events or situations as guilt (Harder, 1995; Johnson et al., 1987; Tangney & Fischer, 1995). Perhaps the essential distinction between guilt and shame is that guilt involves depreciation of specific actions or behaviors, whereas shame involves depreciation of the entire self (Barrett, 1995; Ferguson & Stegge, 1995; Harder, 1995; Lewis, 1971; Tangney, 1998). In line with this distinction, shame can be defined *as an unpleasant feeling plus a negative evaluation of one's entire self, personality, intelligence, or character* (e.g., "I feel inadequate"; Kubany & Watson, 2003b; cf. Foa et al.'s [1999] construct of "negative cognition about the self"). Shame is associated with a negative evaluation about one's entire self, whereas guilt is associated with a negative evaluation of one's specific actions in specific situations.

ERRONEOUS THINKING AMONG TRAUMA SURVIVORS

Because many trauma survivors exaggerate or distort the importance of their roles in traumatic events, they experience guilt and shame that have little or no rational basis (see Kubany & Manke, 1995). Kubany and Manke (1995) observed that trauma survivors tend to draw four kinds of faulty conclusions concerning their roles in the trauma, each of which involves distortion of a cognitive component of guilt. First, many survivors believe, in retrospect, that trauma-related outcomes were foreseeable, hence preventable; that is, they may believe falsely that they "knew" what was going to happen before it was possible to know, or that they dismissed or overlooked clues that "signaled" what was going to occur (*foreseeability and preventability distortion*). Second, many survivors accept an inordinate share of responsibility for causing the trauma or related negative outcomes (*responsibility distortion*). Third, many survivors believe that their trauma-related actions were less justified than would be concluded on the basis of an objective analysis of the facts (*justification distortion*). Fourth, many survivors believe they violated personal or moral convictions, even though their intentions and actions were consistent with their convictions (*wrongdoing distortion*).

OVERVIEW OF COGNITIVE THERAPY FOR TRAUMA-RELATED GUILT

The goal of cognitive therapy for trauma-related guilt (CT-TRG) is to help clients achieve an objective and accurate appraisal of their roles in trauma. CT-TRG focuses on correcting thinking errors that can lead trauma survivors to draw faulty conclusions about the importance of the roles they played in traumatic events. We have identified 18 such thinking errors, which are shown in Table 11.1 (Kubany, McCaig, & Laconsay, 2004b).

There are three phases in CT-TRG: (1) assessment, (2) guilt incident debriefings, and (3) CT proper, which involves separate, semistructured procedures for correcting thinking errors that lead to faulty conclusions associated with guilt. The main procedures used in CT-TRG are briefly discussed below. These procedures are described and illustrated in greater detail elsewhere (Kubany, 1997, 1998; Kubany & Manke, 1995), and clinicians who are interested in using CT-TRG are encouraged to examine these other sources.

Guilt Assessment

Assessment is an integral part of the CT-TRG model. We use a structured interview and specially designed questionnaires (1) to identify idiosyncratic sources of trauma-related guilt, (2) to assess clients' faulty thinking patterns, and (3) to evaluate treatment efficacy.

Structured Guilt Assessment Interview

We use a structured interview to identify important issues across five domains of guilt (Kubany & Manke, 1995). This interview (which also includes follow-up probes) consists of five core questions about the trauma that ask whether respondents feel guilty about (1) anything they did, (2) anything they *did not do*, (3) feelings they had, (4) feelings they *did not have*, and (5) *thoughts or beliefs* they had. For example, clients may be asked, "Do you feel guilty about anything you did related to the trauma? . . . Tell me about that."

TABLE 11.1. Thinking Errors That Lead to Faulty Conclusions and Trauma-Related Guilt

Thinking error that contributes to faulty conclusions about knowledge possessed before outcome was known (regarding the *foreseeability and preventability* of negative outcomes)

    HB   Hindsight-biased thinking

Thinking errors that contribute to faulty conclusions about *justification* or goodness of reasons for acting as one did

    J#1:   Weighing the merits of actions taken against idealized actions that did not exist

    J#2:   Weighing the merits of actions taken against options that only came to mind later

    J#3:   Focusing only on "good" things that might have happened had an alternative action been taken

    J#4:   Tendency to overlook "benefits" associated with actions taken

    J#5:   Failure to compare available options in terms of their perceived probabilities of success before outcomes were known

    J#6:   Failure to realize that (a) acting on speculative hunches rarely pays off, and (b) occurrence of a low-probability event is not evidence that one should have "bet" on this outcome before it occurred

    J#7:   Failure to recognize that different decision-making "rules" apply when time is precious than in situations that allow extended contemplation of options

    J#8:   Failure to recognize that in heightened states of negative arousal, one's ability to think clearly and make logical decisions is impaired

Thinking errors that contribute to faulty conclusions about degree of *responsibility* for causing negative outcomes

    R#1:   Hindsight-biased thinking

    R#2:   Obliviousness to totality of forces that cause traumatic events

    R#3:   Equating a belief that one could have done something to prevent the traumatic event with a belief that one caused the event

    R#4:   Confusion between responsibility as accountability (e.g., "my job") and responsibility as having the power to cause or control outcomes

    R#5:   Existential beliefs about accountability and the need to accept the consequences of one's actions—which fail to take into account the causal power of situational forces

Thinking errors that contribute to faulty conclusions about *wrongdoing* or violation of values

    W#1:   Tendency to conclude wrongdoing on the basis of outcome rather than on the basis of one's intentions before the outcome was known

    W#2:   Failure to realize that strong emotional reactions are not under voluntary control (i.e., not a matter of choice or willpower)

    W#3:   The tendency to "inflate" the seriousness of a minor moral violation—from "misdemeanor" to "felony" status—when the minor violation leads unforeseeably to a traumatic outcome

cont.

W#4:   Failure to recognize that when all available options have negative
        outcomes, the least bad option is a sound and moral choice

Thinking error that contributes to all of the faulty conclusions

ALL: Belief that an emotional reaction to an idea provides evidence for the
        idea's validity—also called *emotional reasoning*

Attitudes About Guilt Survey

The Attitudes About Guilt Survey (AAGS) is a brief questionnaire that is
used to assess the presence and magnitude of guilt components with regard
to highly specific guilt issues (Kubany et al., 1995; Kubany & Manke, 1995;
Kubany et al., 2004b). The AAGS, which is reproduced at the end of this
chapter in Appendix 11.1, assesses the magnitudes of four guilt-related
beliefs and the magnitudes of distress and guilt related to specified guilt
issues. Clients are asked to fill out a separate AAGS for each guilt issue targeted for intervention, and before each guilt issue is analyzed, they are asked
to explain their responses to the guilt-cognition items (items 1–4). In addition to its value for initial assessment, the AAGS can be readministered as
therapy proceeds to assess progress, lack of progress, or "slippage" (i.e.,
reversion to faulty logic that seemed to have been corrected) and the need
for additional work.

Trauma-Related Guilt Inventory

The TRGI (Kubany et al., 1996; Western Psychological Services, 2004) was
constructed to assess guilt and cognitive and emotional aspects of guilt associated with specified traumatic events (e.g., combat, physical or sexual
abuse). The TRGI includes three scales and three subscales. The scales
include a Global Guilt Scale, a Distress Scale, and a Guilt Cognitions Scale,
which includes items that comprise the three subscales—Hindsight-Bias/
Responsibility, Wrongdoing, and Lack of Justification. The TRGI is meant to
be used as a molar measure of trauma-related guilt (e.g., combat-related
guilt, incest-related guilt) rather than as a measure of more specific guilt
issues occurring within the context of the trauma (e.g., guilt about having
been afraid or trading places with someone who got killed). The TRGI,
which assesses 22 specific trauma-related beliefs, may have considerable utility as a treatment-outcome measure in CT-TRG and other cognitive-behavioral interventions aimed at modifying trauma survivors' beliefs about their
role in trauma.

Guilt Incident Debriefings

Prior to CT proper (with *each* targeted guilt issue), a guilt incident debriefing
is conducted. Clients are asked to give a detailed description of what hap-

pened during and immediately preceding the event in question (e.g., "Tell me in three-dimensional living color what happened, leading up the exact day and time when you think you should have left your abusive boyfriend"). Clients are asked, "What did you see, hear, feel, and smell? Who did what, who said what, what thoughts were going through your mind?" We have found that detailed retelling of exactly what happened—as opposed to superficial retelling—is more likely to facilitate tearful grieving, and is also more likely to yield useful assessment information about distortions in logic (see Kubany, 1998, pp. 150–151). After clients have described what happened, they are asked, "What was the worst part of what happened?" "What were your feelings during the worst part?" and "What were your thoughts during the worst part?"

CT Proper

After the initial guilt incident debriefing, the therapist discusses the meaning of guilt, its conceptualization as a multidimensional construct, and its various components. Clients are then given an overview of CT-TRG procedures and goals. They are told that they will be involved in an "intellectual analysis," the goal of which is "to achieve an accurate and objective appraisal of your role in the trauma."

The process of correcting thinking errors associated with faulty conclusions is conducted in the context of four semistructured procedures. These four procedures were designed to teach clients to distinguish what they knew then (i.e., at the time of the trauma) from what they know now and as a means to analyze and reappraise perceptions of justification, responsibility, and wrongdoing—in light of knowledge possessed when the trauma occurred.

The CT component of CT-TRG is a "successive approximations" approach in which guilt issues are addressed one at a time. With each issue, guilt is broken into its component parts, which are also treated one at a time—in isolation from the other components. The therapist and client actively engage in assessing the client's beliefs and considering alternative explanations. Much of this process is characterized by a Socratic line of inquiry, during which clients are asked many questions that challenge their logic and noncritical thinking.

Correcting Faulty Beliefs about Outcome Foreseeability and Preventability (Hindsight Bias)

Because of a common thinking error called "hindsight bias," trauma survivors commonly believe that unforeseeable traumatic outcomes were foreseeable and preventable. Hindsight bias is the human tendency to allow knowledge of an event's outcome to bias recollection of knowledge possessed before the outcome was known (Fischhoff, 1975; Hawkins & Hastie, 1990).

The first step in correcting faulty beliefs about outcome foreseeability and preventability is to identify what clients falsely believe they "knew" before outcomes were known, which would have enabled them to prevent or avoid the trauma-related outcome. The second step is to help clients realize that it is *impossible* for knowledge obtained after making a decision to guide the earlier decision-making process. Clients are then taught about hindsight bias and told anecdotes about trauma survivors who engaged in hindsight-biased thinking. Clients are helped to realize that if they had known *in advance* what outcome was going occur, they would not have acted as they did, and that an outcome which is not foreseeable is not preventable.

Justification Analysis: Were the Reasons for the Actions Taken Good Ones?

The "most justified" course of action in a situation is the best course of action among those that were actually considered at the time. A person's justification for acting as he or she did cannot be weighed against ideal or fantasy choices that never existed, or against options that only came to mind *later*. When all contemplated courses of action have adverse consequences, the course of action with the least negative consequences is the best course of action—and completely justified.

In the justification analysis, clients are asked to describe their reasons for acting as they did. Then they are asked what other courses of action they considered but ruled out and to describe what they thought *at the time* would have happened, had these courses been selected. Finally, clients are asked which choice—of options actually considered—was the most justified choice (knowing only what they knew and believed then); when this line of thinking is pursued, the course of action that was taken is almost always selected as *completely justified*.

Causal Responsibility Analysis

Almost all events have multiple contributing causes. In the responsibility analysis, we identify a list of contributing causes outside of self, and we assign a percentage of causation to each. Then we reappraise the client's share of responsibility in light of the total percentage of contributing causes.

Wrongdoing Analysis

Clients learn that a value judgment of wrongdoing is usually assigned when someone intentionally or deliberately causes foreseeable harm. Clients are asked whether they knew a negative outcome (which is the source of guilt) was going to occur when they acted as they did and whether they wanted the negative outcome to occur. The answers to these questions are almost always *no*, to which the therapist might then say that a judgment of wrongdoing does not apply. When clients experience guilt that stems from situations in which all courses of action had negative consequences, they are helped to realize that the least bad choice is a sound and moral choice.

CT-TRG as a Treatment for Shame as Well as Guilt

CT-TRG is considered to be a treatment for shame as well as guilt because the procedures that impact guilt-related beliefs and guilt also impact shame-related beliefs and shame. That is, guilt-related beliefs (e.g., "I blame myself") often contribute directly to shame-related beliefs ("I was stupid"; see Kubany & Watson, 2003b), and when guilt-related beliefs are corrected (e.g., "It wasn't my fault"), the reason for a shame-related negative evaluation ceases to exist. When irrational guilt cognitions are corrected, shame almost always dissipates without any direct intervention. We give one example to illustrate.

CT-TRG was the sole intervention employed in treating a Vietnam veteran who was troubled by multiple sources of combat-related guilt (Kubany, 1997). The veteran's scores on a guilt index—averaged for six targeted guilt issues—went from 5.8 (on a scale of 0–6) before therapy to 1.5 after therapy, gains that were maintained for almost 2 years. Even though the intervention focused exclusively on the veteran's *guilt-related* beliefs about his role in Vietnam trauma, his perceptions of the degree to which he considered himself to be a bad person for what he had done changed from "a very bad person" (*mean* = 2.83 on a 5-point scale from 0 to 4) to "not a bad person" (*mean* = 0) after therapy.

Later in this chapter we describe two case studies that illustrate CT-TRG, primarily the procedures for correcting faulty beliefs about foreseeability and preventability. Correcting foreseeability/preventability beliefs often represent a formidable challenge for therapists new to CT-TRG, especially when clients persist in maintaining that they "knew" in advance what was going to happen and could have prevented the trauma-related outcomes.

MODIFYING GUILT- AND SHAME-RELATED SELF-TALK

Guilt- and shame-related beliefs can have a devastating effect on a person's mood or state of mind when these beliefs are manifested in conscious thoughts and speech (e.g., "I never should have done that! I am so stupid"). In the early stages of therapy, many clients are extremely self-critical and repeatedly drag themselves down by the way they talk to themselves in their public and private speech.

Using procedures that complement CT-TRG, we teach clients to break negative self-talk habits. Early in therapy, we may draw clients' attention to negative self-talk immediately after it occurs in the session. We may say, "There are certain words and phrases that if you never use again, you will be a happier person. Are you aware of what you just said?" Clients learn that awareness precedes change, and if they are not aware of the negative things that they say to themselves, they are out of control and cannot regulate how they feel.

Considerable research has shown that self-monitoring can aid in modifying a variety of habits, including ruminative thinking (e.g., Korotitsch & Nelson-Gray, 1999; Frederiksen, 1975). Clients are given an ongoing homework assignment to monitor three categories of maladaptive self-talk (thoughts and speech). These three categories are (1) the word "should," the phrases "should have" and "could have," and "why" questions; (2) global, shame-related put-downs of self (e.g., "I'm stupid . . . I'm a coward"); and (3) saying "I feel . . . " in sentences that end with words that are not emotions (e.g., "I *feel* obligated . . . stuck . . . overwhelmed . . . responsible . . . unsafe"). Clients are taught to keep track of these words and phrases during all waking hours for the remainder of therapy, using a Self-Monitoring Recording Form, shown in Figure 11.1. On the form, days are broken into 4-hour blocks, and clients are instructed to record (in code, with numbers 1, 2, or 3) *only the first occurrence* of each type of statement *in the interval in which it is observed* to occur (e.g., between 4 P.M. and 8 P.M.). If a type of statement does not occur in an interval, nothing is recorded. The total number of observations (for each type of statement) for each day is the total number out of six daily 4-hour time intervals in which the statement was observed to occur. Requiring individuals to document only the first occurrence of a behavior in each observation interval is easier and elicits greater compliance than procedures that require clients to record *every* occurrence of a behavior being monitored.

The therapist emphasizes that heightened awareness of mental activity is a necessary precursor to breaking any self-talk habit, and conscientious performance of the self-talk monitoring homework is a means toward that end. Clients are instructed to carry the self-monitoring form with them at all times and to record instances of negative self-talk as soon as they occur. They may be told:

"Waiting until later defeats the purpose of the exercise. It may be inconvenient or mildly punishing to write it down at the time. But that's the idea. Mild punishment will help break the negative self-talk habit."

Clients learn that the first goal of the self-monitoring homework is to increase their awareness of their mental life, and that awareness precedes change. Clients may learn:

"After a while you will start catching yourself when you start to think or say these words, and this may interrupt a chain of negative self-talk, which in the past may have had a life of its own—of which you may not even have been aware."

Person Observed: _____ Dates: From _____ To _____

Phrases of Concern:	1 =	"should . . . I should have . . . I could have . . . Why . . . ?"
	2 =	Self put-downs of your entire personality or character (e.g., "I'm stupid . . . I'm inadequate . . . I'm a wimp . . . There's something wrong with me")
	3 =	"I *feel* . . ." statements ending with words that are not emotions (e.g., "I *feel* obligated . . . responsible . . . overwhelmed . . . sorry for")

Dates	Mon.	Tues.	Wed.	Thurs.	Fri.	Sat.	Sun.
8 am – 12 pm							
12 pm – 4 pm							
4 pm - 8 pm							
8 pm – 12 am							
12 am – 8 am							

Monday Phrases:	1: _____ 2: _____ 3: _____
Tuesday Phrases:	1: _____ 2: _____ 3: _____
Wednesday Phrases:	1: _____ 2: _____ 3: _____
Thursday Phrases:	1: _____ 2: _____ 3: _____
Friday Phrases:	1: _____ 2: _____ 3: _____
Saturday Phrases:	1: _____ 2: _____ 3: _____
Sunday Phrases:	1: _____ 2: _____ 3: _____

FIGURE 11.1. Self-Monitoring Recording Form.

If clients express pessimism about being able to modify the way that they talk to themselves, we ask them if they ever played sports. If they did, and if they had a bad habit, such as a slice in golf or a faulty serve in tennis, we ask them if they would be able to break the habit if they had a good coach and practiced diligently. Clients usually agree that they could break such a habit, and then we may say, "Changing the way that you talk to yourself is exactly the same thing. It simply involves breaking a bad habit."

We ask clients if they would want to go to a therapist who treated them with disrespect—someone who called them *stupid* and said that they could have and should have prevented trauma-related negative outcomes. Of course, clients say they would not want to go to such a therapist, and then we may say:

> "If I'm treating you with respect, and you're treating yourself with disrespect, we're canceling each other out. We need to be working together, "on the same side of the ball." And you need to start giving yourself the same respect you want to get—and deserve to get—from others."

EMPIRICAL OUTCOMES OF CT-TRG

CT-TRG is a central feature of cognitive trauma therapy (CTT), a highly psychoeducational intervention for the treatment of PTSD, depression, and guilt. The efficacy of CTT has been evaluated in two treatment-outcome studies with samples of PTSD-suffering battered women (Kubany et al., 2003, 2004). In both studies, CT-TRG (which was conducted in the larger context of CTT) resulted in quite significant reductions in guilt, as assessed by the TRGI. The studies also found that these reductions in guilt were associated with significant reductions in PTSD and depression and quite significant increases in self-esteem. For example, in the first treatment-outcome study (Kubany et al., 2003), 30 of 32 women who completed CTT (94%) were PTSD negative at the end of treatment, and 29 of these women (88%) had scores on the Beck Depression Inventory (BDI) of 10 or less—showing an absence of depression.

There is also some case-study-based evidence for the efficacy of CT-TRG. For example, as described in Kubany (1997), I (EK) conducted CT-TRG in a single 7-hour session with a Vietnam combat veteran suffering from multiple sources of Vietnam-related guilt. After therapy, the veteran reported dramatic reductions in guilt, which were accompanied by the aforementioned reductions in PTSD and depression and increases in self-esteem.

In the studies of CT-TRG efficacy conducted thus far, we have not been able to evaluate what precisely about CT-TRG is causing these reductions in PTSD and depression symptomatology, but we believe the CT-TRG is clearly having causal effects. Definitive studies have yet to be conducted.

SPECIAL ISSUES IN CT-TRG

Client Resistance

Occasionally, clients resist or are skeptical of therapists' overtures to treat their guilt, perhaps because they think they "deserve" to feel guilty; or because only someone cold and callous wouldn't feel guilty about what they did; or because mentally "tricking" oneself into reducing guilt might be thought of as avoiding taking responsibility for what happened, thus a "cop-out"; or because it might be thought of as dishonoring those who didn't survive or who who suffered more than they did (Kubany & Manke, 1995, pp. 56–57). For example, in the case of a man who accidentally shot and killed a close friend—described later in this chapter—it was inconceivable to this man at the beginning of therapy that he could be taught to experience less guilt—because he believed he "deserved" to feel guilty.

Thus, at the beginning of therapy, we do not make direct attempts to get clients to endorse or "buy into" our model of guilt therapy, which generally assumes that survivors tend to experience guilt that has little or no rational basis. Early on, we might tell clients about the high prevalence of trauma-related guilt and findings that trauma survivors tend to distort or exaggerate the importance of their roles in trauma (see Kubany & Manke, 1995). We also share anecdotes of survivors who experienced guilt, which had absolutely no rational basis, and may tell clients, "You probably don't believe me now, but I am going to show you that your guilt is just as irrational as the guilt of the people in the stories I just told you." As the psychoeducation in CT-TRG proceeds, clients learn about the thinking errors that lead to guilt (e.g., hindsight-biased thinking) and how these thinking errors may apply to them. Typically, "resistance" that clients have had dissolves as they see and begin to understand how the thinking errors apply to them too.

Educational Level of Clients

Some readers may wonder whether CT-TRG works as well with clients who are less educated or less verbal as it does with more highly educated clients. CT-TRG appears to work equally well regardless of clients' educational level. For example, in the two-treatment outcome studies of CTT mentioned earlier, approximately half of the 162 enrolled women had no more than a high school education, some, less than that; yet, almost 90% of the women who completed treatment no longer had PTSD at the end of the therapy, and almost all reported substantial reductions in guilt.

Principles taught to clients in CT-TRG are easy to grasp and understand because they are relatively simple and straightforward, and are presented in plain language. The emphasis on using survivor anecdotes to illustrate principles in CT-TRG helps less well-educated clients comprehend the principles. With more well-educated clients, knowledge of the principles tends to remind them of their own anecdotes.

Didactic Nature of CT-TRG

CT-TRG tends to have an educational quality, because it involves the transmission of large amounts of information. Therapists who are more comfortable with passive therapy approaches, such as listening or being reflective, than with the kind of active teaching CT-TRG entails may find some difficulty getting used to imparting large amounts of information and playing a role that is more didactic or education-oriented.

Applications of CT-TRG to Those Who Have Perpetrated Suffering

Some readers may be interested in knowing whether CT-TRG is applicable for socially deviant individuals who have intentionally committed acts of violence, such as physical or sexual abuse. Such individuals, often referred to as *perpetrators*, include murderers, rapists, child molesters, and individuals who abuse or batter their wives and girlfriends. Many such individuals are psychopaths—with diagnoses of antisocial personality disorder—who exhibit pervasive empathy deficits, and who may rarely or never experience guilt. As characterized in the DSM-IV, they "frequently lack empathy and tend to be callous, cynical, and contemptuous of the feelings, rights, and sufferings of others" (American Psychiatric Association, 1994, p. 647). Since distress is a component of guilt, and without distress there can be no guilt, CT-TRG would not be expected to work with perpetrators/psychopathic individuals of this type who do not experience distress or unpleasant feelings when they think about what happened and what they did.

However, there are many people who would be considered perpetrators in a sense who do experience genuine guilt about their previous aggressive or antisocial actions. Included in this group are many combat veterans who engaged in deliberate brutality or used excessive force in the war zone (e.g., "atrocities") but who feel bad when they think about what happened. They may even be tormented by guilt. CT-TRG is definitely applicable for such individuals; however, for CT-TRG to be effective, it is crucial for the individuals to be able to accurately recall how they felt at the time, and what they knew and believed when they engaged in the brutality or used the excessive force. An example of such a case is a Vietnam War combat veteran I (EK) treated, described in Kubany (1997). He experienced severe guilt over having mutilated enemy dead and taking a body part as a war souvenir. He said, "What bothers me so much is . . . that I took a knife and cut off a human ear and wore it on a bracelet around my wrist as a war souvenir. At the time I was proud of it" (p. 235). This veteran was helped to realize that many American troops in Vietnam were impaired in their capacity to experience compassion, empathetic distress, and guilt because they had become numbed by the trauma of war. In combination with a certain degree of a social consensus that extreme or brutal behavior might be excusable or necessary, the lowering of empathy in response to human suffering certainly raised the probability that extreme or brutal behavior would occur. Similarly, many Americans in Vietnam came to hold the belief about life, death, and human nature that it "don't mean nothing"—that life (and death) is of little value or importance. One can see how extreme or inhumane behavior may be perceived as justifiable, once one comes to believe that life has little or no value. In addition, research on cue-controlled aggression has shown that aggressive cues in the environment can "release" impulsive aggressive behavior in individuals who are negatively aroused (e.g., Berkowitz & LePage, 1967; Kubany, Bauer, Richard, & Muraoka, 1995). Circumstances of horror and rage over the gruesome deaths of fellow Americans triggered impulsively hostile behavior, which in retrospect would be considered brutal or overly aggressive.

TWO CASE STUDIES

Man Who Accidentally Shot a Friend When He Was 12 Years Old

When Peter was 12 years old, he and one of his closest friends, Tom, were planning to play basketball. When Tom called that morning, Peter suggested that, before they go to play basketball, Tom come to his house briefly to shoot at birds with a 22-gauge rifle his uncle had loaned to his father. Peter's father had been using the gun to teach Peter about gun safety. No one else was home that day, and Peter knew he was only supposed to use the gun under his father's supervision; however, he was confident in his ability to use the gun safely.

When Tom came over, they crawled out of an upstairs window onto the roof to shoot at birds in the trees. They waited for about 10 minutes but there were no birds, so they crawled back into the house. Peter emptied out the bullets and was about to put the gun away. Then they saw a bird land in a nearby tree, and Peter decided to give it one more chance. Peter put one bullet back in the chamber, but by the time he turned around, the bird was gone. So he took the bullet out. He had the gun over his shoulder when all of a sudden the gun went off inexplicably. When Peter turned, he saw Tom slumped down in the corner of the room, with blood trickling down his face. Tom never regained consciousness and 2 days later he died.

As Peter discovered later, the gun was defective and a bullet remained lodged in the chamber after the rifle was presumably emptied. Unfortunately, this fact provided little consolation to Peter. Although many years had passed since the incident, Peter was still tormented by guilt. In fact, his responses on the AAGS reflected extreme distress, extreme guilt, and extreme guilt cognitions. For example, Peter indicated on the AAGS that he "absolutely should have known better" than to play with the gun, was "not justified in any way," was "completely responsible" for the death of his friend ("100%"), and was "extremely wrong" to have used the gun. Peter was also deeply ashamed about the shooting accident—so much so that it influenced his choice of friends. For years, Peter had associated with a very unsavory circle of friends—high school dropouts and heavy users of alcohol and drugs.

Peter thought that he "didn't deserve" to have friends "with class"—those who were well-educated, sophisticated, and successful.

Foreseeability and Preventability Analysis

Here we will provide highlights of the CT-TRG foreseeability and preventability analysis conducted with Peter. This analysis was critical in getting Peter to realize that he had played only a minimal role in the death of his friend. We present the analysis as dialogue between Peter and his therapist.

THERAPIST: What should you have known better?

PETER: I should have known better than to play with a firearm. I'm not the first person that that happened to. Happens all the time in the news. I should have known, if you play with guns, somebody is bound to get hurt, or worse.

THERAPIST: And what should you have done differently?

PETER: Made a better decision. I knew it was stupid and reckless; but I did it anyway, even though part of me was telling me it's not the right thing to do. Too easy to screw up—way too easy.

THERAPIST: And exactly what is it you should have done differently?

PETER: I shouldn't have played with the gun, period, without my dad there.

THERAPIST: Exactly what should you have done then?

PETER: When Tom called me to go play basketball, I should have gone.

THERAPIST: You shouldn't have suggested he come over?

PETER: Right. Because . . . the thought just occurred to me that morning—it's not as if I planned for him to come over. It was just a secondary thought. An impulse. We knew we were going to the basketball court the night before, so he was just calling me to say, "Let's go," and I said, "Hey, before we go . . . "

THERAPIST: When did you first realize or learn that you weren't supposed to say, "Hey, before we go, why don't you come over here?"?

PETER: I knew it even before I said anything—that it was wrong when the idea [for Tom to come over] occurred to me.

THERAPIST: We were talking about what negative outcomes were foreseeable. Did you know that Tom was going to die when you invited him over?

PETER: No.

THERAPIST: OK. So that outcome wasn't foreseeable.

PETER: No, not his death . . . I guess.

THERAPIST: What you did know is that you were breaking a rule.

PETER: Yeah.

THERAPIST: Mischief. A misdemeanor. So that was foreseeable. That's what you knew.

PETER: I had to have known the potential was there because we weren't playing with a basketball; we were playing with a weapon.

THERAPIST: Well . . . When did it first occur to you that inviting him over had the potential to cause his death?

PETER: Not until I saw blood dripping down into his ear.

THERAPIST: That's exactly right . . . Do you see what's happening here? What you are doing is remembering yourself knowing something—when you talked to Tom on the telephone—that you didn't learn until you saw blood dripping down his face. You can't use knowledge acquired after making a decision to help you make that earlier decision. You can't use information you acquire on Wednesday to help you with a decision you had to make 2 days earlier on Monday. You can't use knowledge that the stock market went up 500 points today to help you with an investment decision you made 2 days ago. Did you ever see the TV program *Early Edition*?

PETER: Yes.

THERAPIST: The star of the show gets tomorrow's newspaper today. And because he knows what's going to happen tomorrow, tomorrow is preventable. And that's the story line. He spends all day today preventing some bad thing that is going to occur tomorrow, because tomorrow is foreseeable. It's like having a crystal ball. But we don't have crystal balls to guide us. Still, we think we do when we engage in hindsight bias. Read the paragraph in your workbook in the middle of the page.

PETER: "Hindsight bias occurs when knowledge of an event's outcome (e.g., 'who won') distorts or biases a person's memory of what (s)he knew before the outcome was known. Hindsight biased thinking is similar to 'Monday morning quarterbacking' and is implied by statements such as 'I should have known better . . . I should have done something differently . . . I saw it coming . . . I knew what was going to happen (before outcomes were known)' and 'I could have prevented it.' As applied to trauma, many survivors falsely believe that the events were foreseeable—hence preventable."

THERAPIST: It's like having a crystal ball. It's remembering yourself as being smarter than you were capable of being, as if you knew something you did not find out until later. It's something that trauma survivors do, but everyone has a tendency to do it; and it has been demonstrated over and over again in studies with college students and other populations.

There was even a big review article published about hindsight bias [Hawkins & Hastie, 1990].

Peter's therapist then illustrated the concept by telling Peter about the type of study that is conducted to demonstrate hindsight bias.

THERAPIST: Imagine you're taking a class in psychology, and everyone in the class volunteers to participate in a research project for extra credit. Your professor then divides the class into three groups and says, "Your task is to predict who is going to win the big game tomorrow. I am going to give you lots of information about the two teams—for example, their win–loss records—and you are to use this information to help you make your predictions. But I'm not going to let you watch the game. Instead, I am going to put you up in three hotel rooms." On the day after the game, the professor goes into the first room and says, "The red team won. Oops! I wasn't supposed to tell you that. Disregard what I just said. Just tell me who you think won, based on the information I gave you in class." Then he goes into the second room and says, "The black team won. Oops! I wasn't supposed to tell you, so disregard this information. Tell me who won based on the information I gave you." In the third room the professor simply asks who won without giving the group any information about the game's outcome. What do you think the predictions were of the three different groups?

PETER: The first group would probably choose the red team. The second group would probably choose the black team, and the third would probably be split down the middle.

THERAPIST: Right. That's what most people say. And that's not too surprising. But what is surprising is what the students say when they are asked, "Did you know my telling you the outcome biased your recollection of who won?" They are unaware that the outcome knowledge affected their recollection of their preoutcome knowledge and may even deny it. If good things happen, there is no problem and the individual can take credit for his or her retrospective wisdom. But if bad things happen, and you're recalling bad things as foreseeable and preventable, then it's trouble, and you know exactly where that goes.

PETER: Yeah.

To further illustrate how hindsight bias works, Peter's therapist described anecdotes of trauma survivors who engaged in hindsight biased-thinking. In one story he told Peter about three women who had the same guilt issue related to being molested when they were between the ages of 4 and 7 years old by someone who was older but who did not scare them—two father figures, and an older cousin.

THERAPIST: When asked, "What is it you should have known better?", the women all claimed they should have known better than to permit molestation (e.g., "I should have known that a daughter isn't supposed to have sex with her father"). When asked what she should have done differently, each woman said, "I should have said 'no' and not let him do that." When asked when they first learned or realized they were supposed to say "no," one of the girls laughed nervously and said, "Much later." One of the other women became confused by this question and started to cry. When asked again, the woman replied that it did not occur to her that she was supposed to say "no" until 4 years later, in sex education class.

Peter's therapist concluded his discussion of foreseeability and preventability with an anecdote about President Harry Truman that illustrates the kind of clear thinking that can inoculate a person from falling into the trap of hindsight-biased thinking in regard to *any* potential guilt issue.

THERAPIST: President Truman was asked by a reporter about 3 years after the end of World War II whether he had made the right decision in ordering the atomic bomb to be dropped on two Japanese cities. If President Truman had been a "should have/could have" kind of guy, do you think he might experience some guilt?

PETER: Yeah.

THERAPIST: But he seemed to be doing fine, and his clear thinking was reflected in the way he answered the reporter's question. President Truman purportedly said something to the effect that, "Knowing in 1945 what I know today, maybe I would have, and maybe I wouldn't have ordered the bomb to be dropped. But I would have to give that a lot of additional thought. However, knowing today only what I knew in 1945, I would do exactly what I did back then." President Truman could separate what he knew from what he subsequently learned, and he did not allow subsequent knowledge to filter back into his memory of what he knew before he ordered the bombs to be dropped.

I would suggest that there is no possible way you could have known Tom was going to die. Otherwise, you wouldn't have invited Tom to come to your house. If you knew with certainty, or even thought that there was a remote chance he might die, would you have taken that kind of chance with a close friend's life?

PETER: No way.

THERAPIST: No way. No way. You didn't know what was going to happen. Otherwise, you wouldn't have done what you did.

To reassess Peter's beliefs about the foreseeability and preventability of Tom's death, his therapist asked him to reanswer item #1 on the AAGS.

THERAPIST: What's the correct answer, the answer that reality would dictate?

PETER: Reality dictates "a" ("There is no possible way I could have known better"). But I still believe I should have known better.

THERAPIST: Let's not confuse bad feelings, the sadness, the grieving—with guilt. By saying "I should have known better," you're saying that you were obligated to know something you didn't know.

PETER: I didn't know that Tom was going to die, but I had to know there was a potential . . .

THERAPIST: You had to know? You can only know something if you knew it. If you believed it was going to be dangerous to play with that gun—that you were putting Tom's life at risk—would you have played with the gun?

PETER: No, I wouldn't have.

THERAPIST: Then you can't say, "I should have. . . . " We have to analyze the facts. You can only be obligated to do something that you know how to do. You can have an obligation to prevent something only if you know it is going to happen. That was the obligation of the star in the TV series *Early Edition*, which I told you about earlier. We're going to come at this from several different directions. Next time, we are going to analyze your beliefs about justification, and responsibility, and wrongdoing. But before we end our discussion today, I want to mention one more point about hindsight bias, and why it is so harmful. Hindsight bias not only goes straight to guilt; it also contributes to distortions in the other three guilt-related beliefs. For example, if you think you could have prevented Tom's death, it's just a few small steps to, "Therefore, to some extent, I caused his death." This is a thinking error because to say, "I could have prevented something" is not the same thing as "I caused it." As one battered woman realized when she said, "You're right. I didn't pull his fist into my face."

With respect to wrongdoing, the faulty logic is that wrongdoing is often concluded on the basis of a tragic outcome—even though it was unforeseeable. An example that comes to mind is the case of a man whose 16-year-old daughter died from alcohol poisoning after he put her to bed. This man said, "For the rest of my life, I'm going to have to live with the fact that I *murdered* my daughter." That's condemning himself to an unforgivable sin when, in fact, he was just being a loving and caring father who put his intoxicated daughter to bed instead of scolding her. When do you think he found out he should have walked his daughter around until she sobered up a little? Not until after she was dead, at the very earliest, maybe not until after the autopsy.

What are some of the things that you learned today?

PETER: We talked about hindsight bias, which I apparently have a lot of.

THERAPIST: You are not alone.

PETER: Basically, that I thought I could have prevented something that I didn't know was going to happen.

THERAPIST: All your answers [on the AAGS] are going to change—based on an analysis of the facts, not based on some kind of subliminal hidden persuasion.

PETER: It's not like I never thought about this. I didn't know what the outcome was going to be, and I didn't know the rifle was defective, and Tom didn't have to say "yes" and come over. But like the woman you told me about who had a stranglehold on guilt, and it took you three sessions to help her get rid of it—I feel like I have a stranglehold. I've thought about it a lot, and logically . . .

THERAPIST: We can't do it all at once.

PETER: When you tell me stories of other people, I can immediately see their thinking errors—there's no way they could have foreseen what happened. I can understand feeling bad, but not that bad. But when it's my story, I feel so incredibly bad.

THERAPIST: It goes back to emotional reasoning. The horrible feeling leads to the conclusion that you could have prevented the accident. By the way, you have been engaging in another common thinking error: the tendency to "inflate" the seriousness of a minor moral violation—from "misdemeanor" to "felony" status—when the minor violation leads unforeseeably to a traumatic outcome. When someone knew they were breaking a rule, but they didn't know a tragedy was going to occur, they often consider themselves to have violated a huge value—because of the tragedy. A woman, as a teen, played hooky from school to go to the beach with a much older boyfriend. And he raped her. She said, "I knew I shouldn't have played hooky. I wouldn't have been raped if I hadn't played hooky." If that relationship had worked out and she had married that guy, do you think that day when she played hooky would have had any significance in her life whatsoever? If nothing bad had happened and she had a great time at the beach, do you think she would feel any guilt about playing hooky that day?

PETER: Now that story is a lot closer to my story.

THERAPIST: Yeah. Gives you something to think about. I've got other stories like that too.

Two more sessions were needed to complete the analysis of Peter's guilt about the shooting accident. Peter's view of himself changed greatly, as is illustrated by his response to the following statements that he was asked to write at the start and then again at the end of therapy: "I am an *innocent* survivor and am likable and lovable. I also *deserve* to be happy!!" At the start of therapy, Peter wrote: "I have a hard time believing this." Before his last therapy session, Peter wrote, "This is the first time since I was a boy that I have believed these statements."

Woman with Guilt and Shame about Not Disclosing Childhood Sexual Abuse

Mary, who was in her mid-30s, had a longstanding history of drug abuse and had been in two relationships with boyfriends who were abusive. She had had almost 2 years of "sobriety" when she volunteered to receive cognitive trauma therapy (CTT).

Mary was tormented by guilt. First we analyzed her guilt about not breaking off her relationship with an abusive boyfriend sooner. Even though she achieved considerable relief in resolving this issue, the reduction in guilt did not generalize or transfer to her guilt about not disclosing the molestation by her uncle, which occurred the first time when Mary was 7 or 8 years old. This incident occurred when her father, uncle, and other relatives were drinking on the back porch. She was running by when her uncle took her aside, away from the others, and made her sit on his lap. Then he started to touch her inappropriately. Mary said:

> "I was surprised. It was like, 'Wow! Why is he doing this?' And all the while, in the back of my mind, I was thinking, 'You know, I know this isn't right, and maybe I should say something to somebody.' But then I was thinking, 'Oh, maybe it would be my fault.' "

Foreseeability and Preventability Analysis

Like many trauma survivors, Mary believed that negative outcomes that occurred after her molestation—in Mary's case, long after her molestation—were foreseeable and preventable when she was a young girl. Following are portions of the foreseeability and preventability analysis conducted with Mary.

THERAPIST: What is it that you should have known better?

MARY: I should have known better than to let my uncle fool around with me, as far as sex is concerned.

THERAPIST: What were some of the negative outcomes that could have been prevented had you disclosed the abuse?

MARY: I could have prevented 5 years of molestation and all the guilt and shame that came with it. . . . Looking back, I should have told my mother the first time it happened. And then there was the time when my sister came home, and my uncle and I were in the house, and I wanted to tell her. I wanted to tell her, but when I looked at him, all pathetic-looking, I said, "Screw it. Just ride it out." I wanted to say something, but this had gone on for so long. I got myself into this, and hopefully I can get myself out of it, not realizing that today I feel partly responsible for what happened. I know he had a big part of it, but I feel, I also had a part because I let it go on."

THERAPIST: You looked at him, and he looked pathetic? . . . What were your feelings when your sister came in?

MARY: Uh, scared. I felt like I didn't belong. I was different. I was less than. . . . If anybody knew, they wouldn't like me. I must be bad. Who else is as low as this? . . . If you murder somebody you can go to jail, you know. What are they going to do with me now?

THERAPIST: Worse than stealing. You put it in the same sentence as murder!

MARY: (*Laughs.*)

THERAPIST: Who is the victim here?

MARY: Uh . . . me.

THERAPIST: And what is it you should have done differently?

MARY: I should have said something the first time it happened.

THERAPIST: Well, when did you first realize or learn that you were supposed to tell your mother that he was molesting you?

MARY: I knew *then*! I knew the first time it occurred. I knew every time it came up.

At this point, Mary's therapist shifted the focus from what Mary *knew*, to what she *didn't know* back then—the outcomes that were unforeseeable when she chose to "ride it out" and keep the molestation a secret.

THERAPIST: Many things were completely unforeseeable when you decided to keep the abuse to yourself. Was it foreseeable that it was going to go on for 5 years when you kept it to yourself?

MARY: No.

THERAPIST: Was it even foreseeable that it was going to happen a second time when you chose not to tell your mother after the first time?

MARY: No. I didn't think he would molest me again.

THERAPIST: Was it foreseeable that your opinion of yourself was going to go as low as it could go?

MARY: No.

THERAPIST: If you had known that it was going to lead to your dropping out of school and getting into drugs when he did it the first time, would you have kept it to yourself?

MARY: No, I wouldn't have. No.

THERAPIST: If you had known that each time you didn't tell your mother, after that first time, that it was going to make you look even guiltier and more implicated, would you have kept it to yourself after the first time?

MARY: No. I would have told her.

THERAPIST: All right. Now, I want you to re-answer this question on the Attitudes About Guilt Survey again: "To what extent do you think that you should have known better and could have prevented or avoided the outcome?"

MARY: The answer is "a": "There is no possible way I could have known better." There's no possible way I could have known all those things were going to happen.

THERAPIST: Before we move on, let's take a look at how false beliefs about foreseeability and preventability not only contribute directly to guilt but also contribute to faulty beliefs about responsibility. If you believe that you "could have prevented" a negative outcome, can you see how easily it would be to then conclude that, to some extent, you caused the outcome?

MARY: I understand.

Justification Analysis

The most justified course of action in any situation is the best course of action among the courses of action actually considered at the time. A person's justification for acting as he or she did cannot be weighed against ideal or fantasy choices which never existed or against options that only came to mind *later*. When all contemplated courses of action have adverse consequences, the course of action with the least negative consequences is the best course of action, and it is completely justified.

THERAPIST: What were your reasons for not telling your mom?

MARY: I thought she wouldn't believe me—and then she would tell everyone, and then there would be a big blowout with the family, and then the finger would be pointed toward me.

THERAPIST: So here we have a situation in which all courses of action have some negative consequences. There are no unequivocally good choices. When we have a situation in which all courses of action have negative consequences, the best course of action is the one with the least bad consequences—the least negative fallout. Why did you rule out telling your mother?

MARY: By keeping it to myself, I thought that the whole incident would blow over, and we would just forget about it.

THERAPIST: You made the least bad choice. Do you agree?

MARY: I do now.

Responsibility Analysis

Almost all events have multiple contributing causes. In the responsibility analysis, we identify a list of contributing causes outside of self, and we assign a percentage of causation to each. Then we reappraise the client's share of responsibility in light of the total percentage of contributing causes.

THERAPIST: You indicated that you were 60% responsible for keeping it to yourself. What people, factors, forces—outside of yourself—contributed to your keeping the molestation to yourself? I'll help you get started. There were a lot of fears.

MARY: Fears?

THERAPIST: Fear of you being blamed?

MARY: Yeah.

THERAPIST: And fear of being rejected?

MARY: Yeah.

THERAPIST: And your fear that everything would explode and your belief that the family would go into turmoil. And your belief that other people would not only blame you; they would think you were a bad person.

MARY: Hmm.

THERAPIST: You were taught to believe that if something bad happened, it's your fault.

MARY: I always got blamed if something went wrong.

THERAPIST: And you already had a low opinion of yourself.

MARY: I wanted to play sports—baseball, track—but my mother wouldn't let me. She wanted me to be a ballerina. I felt like I wasn't getting attention from my mother because I didn't dance.

THERAPIST: The withdrawal of attention of your mother . . . all right, here you are. You're a little child who's told to go out and play, and nobody's protecting you or watching after you to be sure no harm comes to you. How much—from 0% to 100%—did your fear of being blamed contribute to your not telling?

MARY: I would say 100%. I was really scared.

THERAPIST: How about your fear that the family would be thrown into turmoil?

MARY: 100%.

THERAPIST: And what about your learning experiences that caused you to have such low self-esteem?

MARY: I would say that would be 100% too.

THERAPIST: And what about your mother's disapproval of you and withdrawal of all that attention for not being interested in ballet?

MARY: 100%.

THERAPIST: We could go on, but let's add this up. All outside sources of causation add up to—let's see—400%. But it all has to fit into 100%, including the 60% that you said belonged to you. An event cannot be more than 100% caused. How responsible were you for not telling?

MARY: Not any.

THERAPIST: Let's say there was a lion outside this room. Do you think that lion would have anything to do with your decision to stay in here?

MARY: Oh, yeah.

THERAPIST: The lion would be the source of the fear that would keep you in here. You were like a little twig in a 150-mile-per-hour hurricane wind who thinks she's responsible for all the destruction on the ground. You were like the beautiful oak tree in that storm who thinks she murdered all her leaves.

MARY: Yeah.

Wrongdoing Analysis

Clients learn that a person is ordinarily judged to have committed a wrongful act if he or she deliberately causes harm or damage that was foreseeable—for example, intentionally stealing something of value belonging to someone else. In analyzing Mary's degree of wrongdoing, it became immediately clear that she had had good intentions, and that the terrible consequences of her actions were unforeseeable.

THERAPIST: You indicated that what you did was "extremely wrong." Did you want to cause harm to yourself?

MARY: No way.

THERAPIST: Was all the harm that ensued foreseeable?

MARY: No.

THERAPIST: OK. What is the answer to the wrongdoing item on the Attitudes About Guilt Survey?

MARY: "A." "What I did was not wrong in any way."

THERAPIST: Not in any way. You were in a cornered situation—you were trapped. "Terrible things are going to happen if I do this. Terrible things are going to happen if I don't do this! But which terrible things will I choose?" Somehow, you were fantasizing an ideal choice that would keep everyone happy and stop the abuse. Did that option exist?

MARY: No, it didn't.

THERAPIST: It was a fantasy. You were comparing what you did against fantasy choices. What are some of the things you learned today?

MARY: I learned that I can use what I learned with every guilt issue I have ever had.

THERAPIST: That's right.

MARY: And I think I am going to be OK. I *am* OK.

Commentary and Conclusions

To correct hindsight-biased thinking, it is critical to identify negative outcomes that were unforeseeable. Recalling unforeseeable outcomes as foreseeable reflects hindsight-biased thinking, and if outcomes were not foreseeable, they were not preventable. Mary's therapist established that many important outcomes were not foreseeable when Mary "chose" to keep the molestation a secret after it first happened. Mary did not know that her uncle was going to molest her again, that the abuse was going to continue for 5 years, and that it was going to result in her dropping out of school and engaging in years of drug addiction. In addition, she did not know that, when she was molested on subsequent occasions, it was going to make her appear more implicated and responsible because she didn't tell her mother after the first time. Mary "knew" that the molestation was "wrong" and that she was "supposed" to tell her mother when it first occurred, but she *did not know* any of the long-term negative sequelae associated with not telling her mother.

In Peter's case, he did not know the gun was defective when he and Tom tried to shoot at birds. When he decided to use the gun without his parents around, he did not know that his friend would die. To say that Peter "should have known" the risk involved does not alter the fact that he did not know the risk. It never occurred to Peter—indeed, it was unthinkable—that Tom would be shot and die when they used the gun that morning.

Both Peter and Mary engaged in the thinking error of elevating a relatively minor transgression to "felony status" when the minor transgression was followed by a tragic but unforeseeable outcome. Peter knew that he was breaking a family gun-safety rule when he invited Tom to shoot at birds. He considered this transgression to be a grievous violation of values *after* Tom was shot and died. In Mary's case, not telling her mother about the molestation violated a "supposed to" rule. Mary viewed this violation as reflecting a serious character flaw *after* she became aware of the unforeseeable long-term negative effects of the abuse.

The "bottom line" to the successful resolution of guilt is the development of a full recognition of *what one knew and believed* at the time of the event. When Mary came to appreciate what she knew and believed as an 8-year-old girl—that disclosing the abuse to her mother would be fraught with negative consequences, whereas if she just kept quiet, the matter would "blow over" and go away—her actions *at that time* made complete sense. When Peter realized how naïve he was as a 13-year-old boy who believed that he and his close friend were impervious to serious harm—the actions of "that boy" who was Peter seemed reasonable, after all. This conclusion came into clear perspective when Peter was visited by two young nephews who were about the same age as Peter was when the shooting incident had occurred. Peter observed how naïve and carefree his nephews were. He realized that he was not capable, as a 13-year-old boy, of knowing or even imagining beforehand the horrible outcome of that fateful day.

In closing, our continuing work with trauma survivors has reinforced our belief that how we think is an important determinant of how we feel, and that how trauma survivors view their role in trauma-related events has a major effect on their recovery from posttraumatic stress. We believe that widespread availability of CT-TRG may enable therapists to help trauma survivors achieve a peace of mind about their role in trauma to a degree that was previously believed unattainable.

REFERENCES

American Psychiatric Association. (1994). *Diagnostic and statistical manual of mental disorders* (4th ed.). Washington, DC: Author.

Barrett, K. C. (1995). A functionalist approach to shame and guilt. In J. P. Tangney & K. W. Fischer (Eds.), *Self-conscious emotions: The psychology of shame, guilt, embarrassment, and pride* (pp. 25–63). New York: Guilford Press.

Berkowitz, L., & Le Page. (1967). Weapons as aggression-eliciting stimuli. *Journal of Personality and Social Psychology, 7*, 202–207.

Brewin, C. R., Dalgleish, T., & Joseph, S. (1996). A dual representation theory of posttraumatic stress disorder. *Psychological Review, 103,* 670–686.

Dutton, M. A. (1992). *Empowering and healing the battered woman: A model for assessment and intervention: A model for assessment and intervention.* New York: Springer.

Ehlers, A., & Clark, D. M. (2000). A cognitive model of posttraumatic stress disorder. *Behaviour Research and Therapy, 38,* 319–345.

Ferguson, T. J., & Stegge, H. (1995). Emotional states and traits in children: The case of guilt and shame. In J. P. Tangney & K. W. Fischer (Eds.), *Self-conscious emo-*

tions: The psychology of shame, guilt, embarrassment, and pride (pp. 174–197). New York: Guilford Press.

Fischhoff, B. (1975). Hindsight does not equal foresight: The effect of outcome knowledge on judgment under uncertainty. *Journal of Experimental Psychology: Human Perception and Performance, 1,* 288–299.

Foa, E. B., Ehlers, A., Clark, D. M., Tolin, D. F., & Orsillo, S. M. (1999). The Posttraumatic Cognitions Inventory (PTCI): Development and validation. *Psychological Assessment, 11,* 303–314.

Frederiksen, L. W. (1975). Treatment of ruminative thinking by self-monitoring. *Journal of Behavior Therapy and Experimental Psychiatry, 6,* 258–259.

Harder, D. W. (1995). Shame and guilt assessment, and relationships of shame- and guilt-proneness to psychopathology. In 1. P. Tangney & K. W. Fischer (Eds.), *Self-conscious emotions: The psychology of shame, guilt, embarrassment, and pride* (pp. 368–392). New York: Guilford Press.

Hawkins, S. A., & Hastie, R. (1990). Hindsight: Biased judgments of past events after outcomes are known. *Psychological Bulletin, 107,* 311–327.

Hogland, C. L., & Nicholas, K. B. (1995). Shame, guilt, and anger in college students exposed to abusive family environments. *Journal of Family Violence, 10,* 141–157.

Johnson, R. C., Danko, G. P., Yau-Huang, H., Park, Y. J., Johnson, S. B., & Nagoshi, C. (1987). Guilt, shame, and adjustment in three cultures. *Personality and Individual Differences, 8,* 357–364.

Korotitsch, W. J., & Nelson-Gray, R. O. (1999). An overview of self-monitoring research in assessment and treatment. *Psychological Assessment, 11,* 415–425.

Kubany, E. S. (1997). Application of cognitive therapy for trauma-related guilt (CT-TRG) with a Vietnam veteran troubled by multiple sources of guilt. *Cognitive and Behavioral Practice, 3,* 213–244.

Kubany, E. S. (1998). Cognitive therapy for trauma related guilt. In V. Follette, J. Ruzek, & F. Abueg, (Eds.), *Cognitive behavioral therapies for trauma* (pp. 124–161). New York: Guilford Press.

Kubany, E. S. (2000, November). *Cross validation of the Trauma-Related Guilt Inventory.* Poster presented at the 16th annual meeting of the International Society for Traumatic Stress Studies, San Antonio, TX.

Kubany, E. S., Abueg, F. R., Brennan, J. M., Owens, J. A, Kaplan, A., & Watson S. (1995). Initial examination of a multidimensional model of trauma-related guilt: Applications to combat veterans and battered women. *Journal of Psychopathology and Behavioral Assessment, 17,* 353–376.

Kubany, E. S., Abueg, F. R., Kilauano, W., Manke, F. P., & Kaplan, A. (1997). Development and validation of the Sources of Trauma-Related Guilt Survey—War-Zone Version. *Journal of Traumatic Stress, 10,* 235–258.

Kubany, E. S., Bauer, G. B., Richard, D. C., & Muraoka, M. Y. (1995). Impact of labeled anger and blame in intimate relationships. *Journal of Social and Clinical Psychology, 14,* 53–63.

Kubany, E. S., Haynes, S. N., Abueg, F. R., Manke, F. P., Brennan, J. M., & Stahura, C. (1996). Development and validation of the Trauma-Related Guilt Inventory (TRGI). *Psychological Assessment, 8,* 428–444.

Kubany, E. S., Hill, E. E., & Owens, J. A. (2003). Cognitive trauma therapy for battered women with PTSD: Preliminary findings. *Journal of Traumatic Stress, 16,* 81–91.

Kubany, E. S., Hill, E. E., Owens, J. A, Iannce-Spencer, C., McCaig, M. A., Tremayne,

K., & Williams, P. (2004a). Cognitive trauma therapy for battered women with PTSD (CTT-BW). *Journal of Consulting and Clinical Psychology, 72*(1), 3–18.

Kubany, E. S., & Manke, F. P. (1995). Cognitive therapy for trauma-related guilt (CT-TRG): Conceptual bases and treatment outlines. *Cognitive and Behavioral Practice 2,* 23–61.

Kubany, E. S., McCaig, M. A., & Laconsay, J. R. (2004b). *Healing the trauma of domestic violence: A workbook for women.* Oakland, CA: New Harbinger.

Kubany, E. S., & Watson, S. B. (2002). Cognitive trauma therapy for formerly battered women with PTSD (CTT-BW): Conceptual bases and treatment outlines. *Cognitive and Behavioral Practice, 9,* 111–127.

Kubany, E. S., & Watson, S. B. (2003a). *A fear-loss model of chronic PTSD that emphasizes the role of irrational beliefs and evaluative language.* Manuscript in preparation.

Kubany, E. S., & Watson, S. B. (2003b). Guilt: Elaboration of a testable multidimensional model. *Psychological Record, 53,* 51–90.

Kubany, E. S., & Watson, S. B. (2005). *Multiple tests of a multidimensional model of guilt: An analogue investigation.* Manuscript submitted for publication.

Lewis, H. B. (1971). *Shame and guilt in neurosis.* New York: International Universities Press.

Lindsay-Hartz, J., de Rivera, J., & Mascolo, M. A. (1995). Differentiating guilt and shame and their effects on motivation. In J. P. Tangney & K. W. Fischer (Eds.), *Self-conscious emotions: The psychology of shame, guilt, embarrassment, and pride* (pp. 274–300). New Yark: Guilford Press.

Lisak, D. (1994). The psychological impact of sexual abuse: Content analysis of interviews with male survivors. *Journal of Traumatic Stress, 7,* 525–548.

Pitman, R. K., Altman, B., Greenwald, E., Longpre, R. E., Macklin, M. L., Poire, R. E., & Steketee, G. S. (1991). Psychiatric complications during flooding therapy for posttraumatic stress disorder. *Journal of Clinical Psychiatry, 52,* 17–20.

Rohrbaugh, M., Riccio, D. C., & Arthur, A. (1972). Paradoxical enhancement of conditioned suppression. *Behaviour Research and Therapy, 10,* 125–130.

Staats, A. W. (1972). Language behavior therapy: A derivative of social behaviorism. *Behavior Therapy, 3,* 165–192.

Staats, A. W. (1996). *Behavior and personality: Psychological behaviorism.* New York: Springer.

Tangney, J. P. (1998). How does guilt differ from shame? In J. Bybee (Ed.), *Guild and children* (pp. 1–18). New York: Academic Press.

Tangney, J. P., & Fischer, K. W. (Eds.). (1995). *Self-conscious emotions: The psychology of shame, guilt, embarrassment, and pride.* New York: Guilford Press.

Western Psychological Services. (2004). *Trauma assessment inventories: The Trauma-Related Guilt Inventory (TRGI).* Beverly Hills, CA: Author.

APPENDIX: Attitudes About Guilt Survey (AAGS)

Individuals who have experienced traumatic events often experience guilt which is related to these events. They may feel guilty about something they did (or did not do), about beliefs or thoughts that they had (that they now believe to be untrue), or about having had certain feelings (or lack of feelings). The purpose of this questionnaire is evaluate how you feel about ONE (and only one) guilt issue.

Please take a moment to think about your experience. Briefly describe what happened:

_____

_____

I should have / shouldn't have (*circle one*): _____

_____

_____

In answering each of the following questions, please circle <u>ONE</u> answer that best describes your view of what happened.

1. **To what extent do you think that you should have known better and could have prevented or avoided the outcome?**
   a. There is no possible way that I could have known better.
   b. I believe slightly that I should have known better.
   c. I believe moderately that I should have known better.
   d. For the most part I believe that I should have known better.
   e. I absolutely should have known better.

2. **How justified was what you did? (i.e., How good were your reasons for what you did?)**
   a. What I did was completely justified (excellent reasons).
   b. What I did was mostly justified.
   c. What I did was moderately justified.
   d. What I did was slightly justified.
   e. What I did was not justified in any way (very poor reasons).

3. **How personally responsible were you for causing what happened?**
   a. I was in no way responsible for causing what happened.
   b. I was slightly responsible for causing what happened.
   c. I was moderately responsible for causing what happened.
   d. I was largely responsible for causing what happened.
   e. I was completely responsible for causing what happened.

   Your percentage of responsibility _____ percent

---

4. **Did you do something wrong? (i.e., Did you violate personal standards of right and wrong by what you did?)**
   a. What I did was not wrong in any way.
   b. What I did was slightly wrong.
   c. What I did was moderately wrong
   d. What I did was very wrong.
   e. What I did was extremely wrong.

5. **How distressed do you feel when you think about what happened?**
   a. I feel no distress when I think about what happened.
   b. I feel slightly distressed when I think about what happened.
   c. I feel moderately distressed when I think about what happened.
   d. I feel very distressed when I think about what happened.
   e. I feel extremely distressed when I think about what happened.

6. **Circle the answer which indicates <u>how often</u> you experience guilt that relates to what happened.**
   Never   Seldom   Occasionally   Often   Always

7. **Circle the answer which indicates the <u>intensity or severity</u> of guilt that you typically experience about what happened.**
   None   Slight   Moderate   Considerable   Extreme

CHAPTER TWELVE

Treatment of Complicated Grief

Integrating Cognitive-Behavioral Methods with Other Treatment Approaches

Katherine Shear
Ellen Frank

WHAT IS COMPLICATED GRIEF?

Bereavement and grief are universal experiences. Many features of acute grief resemble symptoms of major depression. Consequently, there is a long history of linking grief and depression in psychiatric thinking. Bereavement triggers an episode of major depression in about 20% of individuals who lose a loved one. However, not all grief-related problems meet criteria for major depressive disorder. There is a rich clinical literature describing pathological grief reactions, under various designations, including abnormal grief, unresolved grief, and complicated grief (CG). However, the absence of a reliable method of identifying the condition and/or for evaluating its severity has obstructed the development and testing of treatments. This problem was addressed when Prigerson et al. developed a simple 19-item questionnaire that reliably identifies bereaved individuals who have persistent, intense grief and poor long-term outcomes (Prigerson et al., 1995a, 1995b). The condition so described, called either "complicated grief" or "traumatic grief," is a chronic debilitating condition characterized by symptoms of separation distress, traumatic distress, sadness and other dysphoric affects, and social withdrawal. Armed with a reliable and valid assessment instrument, we embarked on a project to find an efficacious treatment for this condition.

CG involves such as involves symptoms that are similar to those of post-traumatic stress disorder (PTSD), intrusive thoughts and images and avoidance behaviors. Additionally, the presence of separation distress differentiates CG from major depression and PTSD, as well as other existing DSM-IV diagnoses. Unique to this grief-based syndrome, separation distress is characterized by intense yearning and longing, a tendency to engage in reveries about the deceased, and the desire to remain close to, or seek proximity to, items belonging to the deceased. Thus, given that CG includes symptoms not targeted by other approaches, and given disappointing results in most intervention studies, we concluded that we needed to develop a targeted approach.

A significant portion of the literature related to abnormal grief consists of clinical reports and conjectures. Although clinical observations can be very valuable, little emphasis is placed on the ability to systematically replicate findings, and little attention is paid to standardizing terminology. As a result, terms such as "bereavement," "grief," and "mourning" are used inconsistently and sometimes interchangeably. In this chapter we follow suggestions of Stroebe (1997) in defining "bereavement" as the state of having lost someone close. We use the term "grief" to designate the response to bereavement that generally consists of a distressing state of unease, with yearning and longing for the person who died, preoccupation with thoughts and images of the deceased, pangs of sadness, especially upon contact with reminders of the deceased, and transient social withdrawal. Consistent with existing data, we view natural grief as varying in intensity and characteristics, depending upon the circumstances of the death, the nature of the relationship to the deceased, and the life context of the bereaved person. We further consider grief to be an enduring reaction to loss that is initially preoccupying and later recedes in importance, as it becomes integrated as a "background" state. Notwithstanding variability in early manifestations, most bereaved individuals eventually experience a diminution in grief intensity and reengage in a satisfying life without the deceased. For an unfortunate minority, grief remains the primary focus and becomes a chronic condition, associated with high levels of distress and serious functional impairment. Accumulating evidence suggests that the state of the bereaved at 6 months after the loss predicts the long-term outcome.

Until the past few decades, ideas about grief were dominated by psychoanalytic thinking that included several basic assumptions. Effective grief was considered to require a period of emotionally intense "grief work" that progressed to resolution. If grief work was not done, a delayed grief reaction could be expected. If grief work was not effective, the bereaved individual would experience unresolved, incomplete, or pathological grief. There was a belief that one could not "move on" until the attachment to the deceased was relinquished, a process often referred to as "letting go." The origin of a pathological grief reaction was considered to reside in an ambivalent relationship to the deceased. Data were not available when these ideas were formulated. Now that empirical evidence is accumulating, many of the findings challenge these basic assumptions.

Evidence indicates that intense negative emotion in early bereavement is associated with a higher rather than a lower likelihood of persistent grief intensity (Bonanno, Keltner, Holen, & Horowitz, 1995), and the corollary, the experience of positive emotions early in bereavement predicts better outcome (Bonanno & Keltner, 1997). Studies of the trajectory of grief over as long as 5 years have failed to document the occurrence of delayed grief (Bonanno & Field, 2001). This finding suggests that a substantial number of mourners experience a relatively brief period of dysphoric emotions and that these individuals generally have a benign course. Thus there is little evidence for the need for "grief work" in order to come to terms with the death of a loved one.

Other data challenge the idea that detachment from the deceased (i.e., "letting go") is the optimal outcome (Field, Nichols, Holen, & Horowitz, 1999; Reisman, 2001; Russac, Steighner, & Canto, 2001). Instead, the relationship to the loved one is often a permanent, ongoing one, in which the deceased person continues to influence the life and the thinking of the bereaved. The relationship being characterized by an ambivalent, avoidant attachment style is associated with a better, not a worse, grief outcome (Bonanno, Notarius, Gunzerath, Keltner, & Horowitz, 1998), whereas closer, more satisfying relationships often produce more grief. The syndrome of complicated grief, therefore, is more likely to happen when there has been a very positive relationship to the deceased, rather than a troubled or ambivalent relationship (Prigerson et al. 1997b; van Doorn, Kasl, Beery, Jacobs, & Prigerson, 1998). These findings have important implications for understanding risk and for designing a treatment approach for CG.

The field has been slow to specify criteria for abnormal grief reactions, in spite of the fact that pathological grief is well described in the clinical literature (Bowlby, 1973; Lindemann, 1944; Parkes, 1998; Raphael & Martinek, 1997). Additionally, lack of consensus regarding the best name for a pathological grief reaction is a problem in both the clinical and research literature. In this chapter, we utilize the term "Complicated Grief" to refer to the syndrome described by Horowitz (Horowitz et al., 1997) and Prigerson (Prigerson et al. 1999). Analogous to the situation that existed for a trauma-related syndrome a few decades ago, clinical descriptions abound, but diagnostic criteria have not been agreed upon. This means that CG is not widely recognized and no proven efficacious treatment yet exists for this condition. As several authors have noted (Middleton & Raphael, 1987; Sireling, Cohen, & Marks, 1988), the absence of criteria is an important obstacle to the development and testing of efficacious treatment. There is a growing movement to redress this problem.

The ability to identify reliably those bereaved individuals with clinically significant grief-related symptoms was made possible by the creation of the Inventory of Complicated Grief (ICG; Prigerson et al., 1995b). A score exceeding 25 on the ICG 6 months after a loss predicts poor mental and physical outcomes at 18 months (Prigerson et al., 1997a). Diagnostic criteria for a clinically significant grief syndrome of complicated grief were proposed by Horowitz et al. (1997) and later by Prigerson et al. (1999). Prigerson et al. designated the syndrome "complicated grief" because of the similarity of symptoms to PTSD. Symptoms on the ICG, listed in Table 12.1, include an inability to accept the death, intense yearning and longing for the deceased, bitterness and anger about the death, intrusive images of the dying person, avoidance of reminders of the loss, and a general inability to function effectively.

WHAT IS CG TREATMENT?

CGT treatment (CGT) is a 16-session psychotherapy model that is delivered in three phases consisting of a beginning, middle, and termination (see Figure 12.1). In the beginning phase the therapist provides an introduction to the treatment model, in which grief is understood to be a natural inborn, biopsychosocial pathway to adjustment to a painful loss. Characteristic features of grief are reflections of separation distress and traumatic distress, manifested in various ways that can be influenced by cultural practice. The trajectory of natural grief is to move from an engrossing primary state in which grief exerts a psychological and emotional preeminence to an integrat-

TABLE 12.1. Items Rated on the Inventory of Complicated Grief

1. I think about this person so much that it's hard for me to do the things I normally do.
2. Memories of the person who died upset me.
3. I feel I cannot accept the death of the person who died.
4. I feel myself longing for the person who died.
5. I feel drawn to places and things associated with the person who died.
6. I can't help feeling angry about his/her death.
7. I feel disbelief over what happened.
8. I feel stunned or dazed over what happened.
9. Ever since he/she died it is hard for me to trust people.
10. Ever since he/she died I feel like I have lost the ability to care about other people or I feel distant from people I care about.
11. I have pain in the same area of my body or have some of the same symptoms as the person who died.
12. I go out of my way to avoid reminders of the person who died.
13. I feel that life is empty without the person who died.
14. I hear the voice of the person who died speak to me.
15. I see the person who died stand before me.
16. I feel that it is unfair that I should live when this person died.
17. I feel bitter over this person's death.
18. I feel envious of others who have not lost someone close.
19. I feel lonely a great deal of the time ever since he/she died.

Beginning Phase	Introduction and rapport building History of relationship, loss, and grief Introduction to the treatment model and procedures Introduction to personal goals work	
Middle Phase	LOSS FOCUS Grief monitoring Imaginal revisiting Cognitive work Situational revisiting Memories work Imaginal conversation with the deceased	RESTORATION FOCUS Goals work Situational revisiting Interpersonal work
Termination phase	Discussion of treatment progress Plans for reinforcing and continuing progress Feelings about termination of treatment	

FIGURE 12.1. Overview of the structure of CGT.

ed state of subdued background grief, that continues to evolve and change. The process by which this transition is achieved has been usefully described as the "dual process model" of coping (Stroebe & Schut, 2000). Bereaved individuals are seen as entering an oscillating state of loss-focused and restoration-focused coping. Such oscillation is seen as the optimal way for treatment to proceed in CGT. The goal of CGT is to help a person create a state of integrated grief.

Integrated grief is a part of the life of the bereaved individual. Many people experience a sense of disbelief in the immediate aftermath of the death of someone to whom they were very close. Even if the death is expected, loss of a loved one can be an intense experience for the bereaved family and friends. Often there is a period (variable in length) of intense emotions, primarily sadness, and sometimes guilt, anger and/or fear. Thoughts and images of the deceased typically flood the mind of those left behind. For most people, there is a period of turning inward, away from the hustle and bustle of everyday life. Many cultures support this period of withdrawal, which may provide an optimal context from which progression of grief can occur. In most people this progression happens naturally, eventuating in a muted, integrated form of grief. There is some indication that movement out of a primary grief state is facilitated by meaning-making experiences or activities and by positive emotions (optimism, compassion, acceptance, and forgiveness).

Once achieved, integrated grief can be a positive force in a person's life, providing a meaningful lifelong link to an important relationship. Rather than promoting detachment from the deceased, integrated grief is accompanied by a reconfigured relationship to the loved one. Grief contains within it personal implications of the death of the loved one for the bereaved individual, and these typically change over time. As an example of this, a leading author in the field, Robert Neimeyer (a prominent thanatology researcher and editor of the journal *Death Studies*), wrote the following:

> Many of the subsequent emotional, relational and occupational choices made by my mother, my brother, my little sister, and me can be read as responses to my father's fateful decision [to commit suicide], although their meaning continues to be clarified, ambiguated, and reformulated across the years. (2001, p. xi)

CG is a maladaptive grief reaction that can be conceptualized as a state of being "stuck" in primary grief. Rather than taking its place in the background, integrated into the life of the bereaved person, CG remains "center stage." Instead of providing a link to a positive, nurturing relationship, this form of grief is focused on reminders of a terrible loss. Consequently, the person experiencing CG continually feels as if the death happened very recently, even though many months or even years have passed since its actual occurrence. CG interferes with the natural ability to feel a positive connection to the deceased, because attention is focused on the magnitude and pain of the loss. People experiencing CG typically feel estranged from others and unable to feel satisfaction or interest in daily activities.

CGT is conceptualized as an intervention that seeks to remove impediments to the progression of primary grief and facilitate integration of loss-related thoughts and feelings into the mental and emotional life of the bereaved. Impediments include dysphoric emotions and problematic attitudes or beliefs about the death. CGT targets blocked positive as well as negative emotions and seeks to relieve guilt about positive as well as negative emotions. For the person with CG, the event of the death was a psychological trauma that has led to a PTSD-like reaction. Thus techniques to relieve traumatic distress are a key augmentation component of CGT. Difficulty feeling a positive connection to the deceased and yearning and longing for the lost relationship are forms of separation distress. Several components of CGT target this problem. In addition, given that positive emotions of optimism, compassion, acceptance, and forgiveness contribute to a favorable outcome in natural grief, we seek to develop and enhance these. As noted above, reports in the literature support the idea that a deficiency of positive emotions is associated with prolonged, intense grief (Bonanno, 2001; Lindstrom, 2002), as is an excess of negative emotions. CGT identifies putative sources of enhanced negative emotions and diminished positive ones as treatment targets.

The CGT model considers that adjustment to a loss requires a vision of the world that includes a potential for gratification even without the physical presence of the deceased. However, we do not consider psychological detachment as the goal of successful grief. Instead, the CGT therapist works to facilitate integration of the relationship to the deceased into current and future life, while encouraging development of satisfying personal goals and relationships. The therapist helps the patient reestablish interests and relationships, taking the position that the relationship to the deceased is ongoing in memory, and that memory is not a static entity but rather a living, dynamic process. As eloquently described by Buechner (1991) and Neimeyer (2001), a person we love continues to live with us, even after he or she dies, and to influence our lives forever. Thus the emphasis in CGT is on helping the bereaved person to live fully again, "accompanied" by the deceased person alive in memory.

A novel component of CGT entails a focus on long-term personal goals and discussion of ways to achieve them. This segment is a component of the restoration-focus strategy in CGT. Motivation to go on living can be a problem for individuals with CG. We have documented suicidal ideation in more than half of the individuals with CG whom we have treated, and nearly a third have either made a suicide attempt or engaged in indirect self-destructive behavior. In addition, a kind of reluctance to give up grieving is often seen in CG. The person with CG often fears that grief is all that is left of the relationship to the deceased and if he or she has less grief, then he or she risks losing the deceased forever. Survivor guilt about still being alive and free to enjoy the world may also be present. There may be reticence to develop a close relationship because of fear of being hurt again by its loss. Some people are convinced that no one can understand them, or they feel resentment because they experience others as pushing them to relinquish guilty or angry or sad feelings before they are ready. Still others are very afraid or ashamed of their own emotions. Thus we have learned that it is a good idea to address ambivalence about changing right from the beginning. To do this, we draw upon motivational enhancement strategies.

The primary motivational enhancement strategy we use is that of personal goals work. CGT uses a modified motivational interviewing approach to elicit, discuss, and monitor progress of personal goals, beyond grief. The therapist helps the patient consider things that he or she would like to be doing if he or she were no longer grieving. This exercise conveys to the patient that the therapist (1) believes it is possible for this person to feel less pain from grief, (2) finds less painful grief perfectly acceptable, even desirable, and (3) considers the life of the bereaved person to be important, completely apart from his or her grief and loss. The procedure used encourages patients to identify their own life goals. Sometimes it is surprising how ready patients are to do this. Other times, several sessions are required before goals are elicited. Once identified, the therapist invites patients to identify specific ways they would know if a given goal were accomplished, how committed they are to their goal, what stands in their way (other than grief), and who can help them achieve their goal. Goals work is introduced early in the treatment, usually at the second session. Thereafter, the therapist monitors progress toward goals and discusses strategies and achievements with patients. In implementing this component we were surprised to find that many people with CG do harbor such goals. Even in early sessions, an individual's affect becomes noticeably more positive as he or she focuses full attention on the discussion of personal goals and dreams.

CGT includes a structured procedure for revisiting the death and surrounding events, using a procedure similar to that developed by Foa and colleagues (Foa, 1995) for the treatment of PTSD following rape and other types of trauma. This technique was initially based upon research documenting anxiety reduction during prolonged exposure to fear cues. It is clear how this procedure can be useful in PTSD; it is somewhat less clear in complicated grief, because grief comprises a more complex emotional reaction in which fear is not predominant. However, many people struggling with grief are very frightened of talking about the death. The imaginal revisiting exercise helps ameliorate this fear. Moreover, Foa has found that prolonged exposure is a powerful way to facilitate the evolution of new ways of thinking about the trauma. We have observed this improvement as well in grief treatments. Most striking is the way in which this exercise seems to enhance the patient's nonjudgmental acceptance of the death. By using Foa's technique of tape recording and relistening to the story, the patient sees clearly how the story evolves and often notices aspects of his or her own story that he or she has not attended to previously. For example, some patients come to the realization that there were many very supportive people present at the time of the death. Others notice how helpful they really were in comforting or taking care of the deceased. Still others find that they are reassured about how little the person they loved suffered at the time of the death. Thus a key procedure in CGT is modified use of the procedure that Foa and her colleagues referred to as "prolonged exposure." For grief treatment we call this procedure "revisiting." We chose this name deliberately, as described below.

The revisiting procedure entails asking the patient to tell and retell the story of the death, eventually focusing on the most painful moments. The therapist gradually encourages disclosure of all emotionally relevant details. For bereaved individuals, the initial exercises of imaginal revisiting are often very frightening as well as intensely painful, but with repetition we have found that the fear diminishes noticeably and this diminishment reduces the pain of other emotions as well. Later revisiting exercises can then focus on the most intensely emotional thoughts and memories. Accompanying reduction in emotional intensity achieved through successful revisiting, a more satisfactory narrative of the death usually emerges. There is also a decrease in the sense of confusion and disbelief. The process of repeated revisiting facilitates acceptance of the death and clarification of problematic expectations and beliefs underlying associated emotions. The death becomes "thinkable" and looms less large on the landscape of the overall relationship to the deceased.

There are several reasons why we chose the term "revisiting" for this procedure. We wanted to change the terminology because we found that the idea of reliving the death is very frightening to most bereaved people. Moreover, we believe the exercise is not accurately described as "reliving" or "reexperiencing" because it really entails repeatedly activating ("revisiting") a memory. The goal is to work on solving a problem related to the death. Often in solving problems it is helpful to think about the problem, leave it for a while, and then revisit it. In this sense we are revisiting the problem of the death in CGT. "Visitation" is also a term we use when referring to a time to honor the person who died and a time to comfort the bereaved. Revisiting is meant to provide another opportunity to honor the dead and to be comforted, now by the therapist.

During revisiting exercises, specific beliefs that trigger guilt, anger, shame, and fear emerge and are reevaluated. Beliefs such as "I will fall apart," "I will start to cry and never stop," or "I will be shunned and ostracized when I confront the strong emotions of my grief" are proved erroneous when these feared outcomes do not occur. The belief that negative feelings will continue at unbearably high levels, unabated and intolerable, unless the patient avoids talking about the death, is also proven wrong. The overall experience of being able to face painful emotions helps to correct these fears and to reduce denigration of self as weak or "wimpy." Thus imaginal revisiting of the loved one's death is a highly effective and useful technique.

Also important is an extensive debriefing period following each revisiting exercise, during which the therapist guides the patient in techniques to reduce emotional distress and refocus on the present. Unlike interpersonal psychotherapy (IPT), in which the therapist is instructed to simply listen when the patient is experiencing very intense emotion, in CGT the therapist is instructed to work with the patient on active techniques to reduce the emotion. The CGT therapist is interested in helping the patient see that he or she has the control to think about the death and also to set it aside. For example, the patient is asked to imagine that the story he or she has told is on a video cassette, and that he or she is rewinding the cassette and putting it away. The therapist then guides the patient in refocusing attention elsewhere. The conversation moves to the topic of plans for the rest of the day or the week, and to a discussion of other people in the patient's life. The therapist explains that part of the effectiveness of revisiting as a problem-solving strategy is to leave the problem for a while. In addition, because the person has been willing to undergo tremendous pain in order to revisit the death in the spirit of honoring the deceased, it is important to acknowledge this effort and make plans to take proper care of him- or herself.

Another component of CGT is situational revisiting exercises. This intervention bears some resemblance to the *in vivo* exposure technique used in PTSD and other anxiety disorder treatments. Situational revisiting focuses on identifying and confronting situations and people that have been actively avoided, neglected, or shunned since the death. Often avoidance behaviors in bereavement are subtle and not immediately recognized. Still, they can contribute substantially to impairment and to the sense of incompetence and isolation. Avoidance can also interfere with resolution of emotions. Major treatment goals are to reduce intensity of grief-related emotions and to decrease isolation. Thus, the therapist uses situational revisiting to help the bereaved person identify interesting activities and again form satisfying relationships, including reestablishing relationships that have been neglected. However, it is important to be aware that shunning situations that evoke painful emotions is common and can be adaptive. Oscillation between avoidance and confrontation is often very helpful in coming to terms with an unthinkable reality and/or solving a difficult problem. To be effective, however, this oscillation requires a delicate balance, because the relief that ensues from turning away from the evocative situation can serve to reinforce avoidance, particularly if repeated confrontation does not result in lessening of emotion or movement toward problem solving. In this situation the reinforcing relief gradually renders avoidance an ingrained habit.

For individuals with CG, avoidance of activities and places can interfere considerably with adaptive adjustment to the loss and can lead to negative consequences such as a self-concept of incompetence and/or a view of the world as hostile. Avoidance also interferes with the task of resolving the emotional pain in order to find comfort in memories of the deceased. At the same time, avoidance can be helpful in allowing people to focus attention on their current lives and begin to derive life-sustaining pleasure and satisfaction despite the absence of the loved one. Therefore, the therapist needs to find a workable balance between fostering needed contact with evocative stimuli and focusing elsewhere. CGT incorporates exercises focused specifically on revisiting activities, places, and people that the patient has eschewed. Revisiting focuses primarily on situations that the patient would like to do but finds too painful. This exercise helps to reinstate the normal oscillatory process, and the therapist intervenes to facilitate the consequent reduction in affect and problem-solving increase in effectiveness. Revisiting ,in and of itself, can enhance feelings of competence, especially for places patients want to be free to visit, activities they wish to engage in, and people they want to see. Situational revisiting that focuses on enjoyable activities can be a powerful antidote to thoughts of never again being able to experience joy or satisfaction without the loved one.

It is worth noting that many individuals with CG have a problem with preoccupation with the deceased. At first blush, preoccupation with the deceased may seem to be the antithesis of avoidance. However, in reality this is not the case. Preoccupation often this takes the form of lengthy, dreamy reveries that focus on idealized moments in the relationship with the deceased. Such behaviors actually resemble avoidance in that they temporarily protect the bereaved person from feelings of loss, and they also prevent the person from engaging in satisfying activities and forming new relationships.

CGT seeks to enhance patients' ability to access positive, comforting memories of the deceased. It is helpful to be at ease with negative memories as well. For individuals with CG, intrusive memories or images of the death are usually dominant, to the exclusion of a wider access to long-term memories. Sometimes good memories become easily available once grief intensity is reduced through imaginal and *in vivo* revisiting exercises. However, specific work on memories is also done in CGT. The CGT therapist uses a set of simple forms to facilitate accessibility of memories. Administered over a 5- to 6-week period, beginning after two imaginal revisiting sessions, these forms focus initially on positive, comforting memories. Later, the patient is invited to review "least favorite" memories and things that were annoying about the person who died. Some patients tell us these memory forms were the most helpful component of the treatment. Of note, we have found that memory forms are difficult to use before several sessions of the imaginal revisiting exercises have been completed. The positive memories evoke too much sadness if used early.

Imaginal conversation is a technique used in the second half of CGT. The exercise is structured in a manner similar to imaginal revisiting. However, instead of reporting the memory of events related to the death, we invite patients to imagine that they are with the deceased after the death. If they were present at a natural illness-related death, the conversation is held immediately after the person died. Very often, distressed, bereaved patients comment that they very much wish they could have had one last conversation with the deceased. Usually they have questions they would like answered and/or things they wanted to say but did not have the opportunity to express. We have found that such questions can be answered very effectively in an imaginal conversation with the deceased.

The therapist is instructed to invite patients to talk with the deceased. Patients are instructed to close their eyes and imagine they are with the deceased after the death, telling the loved one anything they wish, including asking any questions. Then patients are instructed to imagine (pretend) that the deceased can actually hear them and respond. Then patients are invited to take the role of the person who died, and to answer.

This exercise helps bereaved individuals feel a sense of connection with the deceased—which, in turn, provides experiential evidence for the idea that a strong sense of the loved one is internalized. In successfully undertaking this exercise, patients report that it seems much clearer to them how the loved one still resides within them. Patients frequently report that having this "conversation" is very powerful—that it makes them feel a sense of deep attachment to the person who died.

This exercise further facilitates a connection with the loving side of the deceased because the questions are usually ones that cause the bereaved person pain, and the responses are invariably comforting. For example, "Did you feel I abandoned you because I was not there when you died?" The response might be, "Of course, not. I never doubted for a minute that you love me very much and that you would have been there if you could have." Although this may be the response the patient most wants to hear, it is also very convincing that the loved one would have, in fact, responded in this way. The relationship to the deceased for CG patients is virtually always a very positive and loving one. Even when there were difficulties in the relationship, the strength of its constructive, loving side is clear. Recall that CGT seeks to enhance this positive connection rather than encourage disengagement. The imaginal conversation serves this purpose very well. This technique has proven to be extremely powerful when administered at the right time in the treatment.

IPT: THE MATRIX FOR CGT

Our initial treatment approach was standard IPT, a proven efficacious treatment for depression that includes abnormal grief as a possible problem area. Complicated grief resembles major depression in symptoms of dysphoric affect, guilty ruminations, suicidality, and social withdrawal so it seemed reasonable that IPT would be an efficacious treatment. Surprisingly, though, we found that standard IPT did not appear to sufficiently reduce CG symptoms in many patients. Consistent with this observation, CG appears to be only minimally responsive to antidepressant medication. Lack of efficacy of standard treatments for depression fit with a growing body of data indicating that CG is a separate condition, distinct from major depression (Prentice & Brown, 1989; Prigerson, Frank, et al., 1995). One difference in CG is the presence of symptoms resembling PTSD (Jacobs, Mazure, & Prigerson, 2000). CGT thus includes techniques to target the separation and traumatic distress symptoms related primarily to the loss-oriented coping process. For the restoration-orientation phase, IPT plays a significant role.

In several large studies IPT has been shown to be an excellent treatment for major depressive disorder (MDD; DiMascio et al., 1979; Frank, 1991; Frank et al., 2000; Prusoff, Weissman, Klerman, & Rounsaville, 1980; Weissman et al. 1979). IPT was devised by Dr. Gerald Klerman and his colleagues during the 1970s. It is a practical, innovative approach that is relatively easy for most practicing therapists to learn. IPT fosters a strong therapeutic alliance, and dropout rates are generally low. The review provided here is derived from Klerman, Weissman, Rounsaville, and Chevron (1984, 1996) and Weissman, Markowitz, and Klerman (2000). The interested reader is referred to these seminal texts for a more detailed explication of IPT.

The original version of IPT rests on a foundation of social–relational research that was available in the early 1970s. This literature includes the work of sociologists, anthropologists, and the interpersonal school of psychotherapy. Particularly influential were observations that marital discord was a frequent harbinger of depression onset (Paykel et al., 1969). Researchers further observed that "exit events" that included various kinds of losses were also observed in depressed individuals more often than controls (Paykel et al., 1969). These findings led to the idea that IPT might target interpersonal conflict and/or significant losses. The importance of supportive relationships was repeatedly confirmed. Studies in the 1970s defined and emphasized the importance of strong social relationships in protecting against neurosis (Overholser & Adams, 1997; Pearlin & Johnson, 1977). Investigators discovered that although they reported spending time with others, individuals with neurosis, especially depression, also reported that this time was often unpleasant (Henderson, 1991, 1977). This work reaffirmed the logic of a treatment that would improve existing relationships. Brown and Harris's work extended these observations to include the importance of an intimate confidant (Brown, Harris, & Copeland, 1977). Other studies elucidated interpersonal communication problems in depressed individuals that could contribute to disruption of social relationships (Bloom, Asher, & White, 1978; Ilfeld, 1977; Pearlin & Lieberman, 1977). From this body of empirical data, the developers of IPT concluded that depressed patients were suffering from interpersonal problems that might be amenable to intervention. To this end, they devised a novel and highly innovative interpersonal treatment approach.

The treatment was developed specifically to target the episodic occurrence of major depression, which was seen as arising from three interacting domains: (1) symptoms of depression, thought to have both biological and psychological underpinnings; (2) social and interpersonal relations that have both trait- and state-like features; and (3) pathogenic personality traits. IPT targets symptoms and interpersonal functioning. Personality traits are not a focus of the treatment, but therapists are encouraged to be cognizant of existing personality problems. IPT is typically provided in approximately 16 sessions. The initial first through third sessions, called the initial phase, focus on assessment and presentation of the treatment model. The middle phase of approximately 10 sessions focuses on the chosen problem area(s). The final phase of one to three sessions focuses on termination of the treatment. Goals are outlined for each of these phases, and strategies and techniques are provided. Unlike most cognitive-behavioral treatments, the IPT manual (Weissmann, Markowitz, & Klerman, 2000) does not prescribe specific interventions in a detailed manner. Instead, treatment objectives are outlined and suggestions for ways to meet these objectives are provided. Goals of the initial phase of IPT are common to all four of the problem areas and include (1) dealing with the depression, (2) relating the onset of depression to the patient's interpersonal context, (3) identifying a problem area, and (4) explaining IPT concepts and developing a contract for treatment.

The therapist first addresses the depressive episode by reviewing the symptoms, naming the syndrome, and giving patients the "sick role." This procedure helps patients to see their symptoms in a somewhat detached, nonblaming way, similar to how people might see themselves when diagnosed with diabetes or pneumonia. In this way, the model of depression in IPT is similar to that used in medication treatments. Depression is considered to be the product of malfunctioning brain mechanisms that is not related to personal or moral weakness and need not be intrinsic to the person's sense of self. The therapist helps patients to see that self-blame and low self-esteem are symptoms of the depression. Naming symptoms in this manner can be a powerful intervention in itself. Furthermore, such a practice supports a discussion of the possible use of medication—also a charge to the therapist in the initial phase of IPT. Cognitive-behavioral therapy (CBT) practitioners also name symptoms and provide a nonblaming way to think about the symptoms.

Next, the IPT therapist conducts an in-depth review of the patient's interpersonal relationships, attending especially to any changes or problems related to the onset of depression. Links between depression and the patient's interpersonal functioning are examined by discussing important current and past relationships, including the nature of the interactions, mutual expectations of the patient and important others, aspects of relationships that are satisfying and unsatisfying, and changes the patient would like to make in his or her important relationships. From this thorough discussion of current and past relationships, the therapist and patient identify one of the four IPT problem areas on which they will focus their work. These include grief, interpersonal role dispute, role transition, and interpersonal deficits. The final task of the initial phase is to explain IPT concepts and develop a contract for treatment. The remainder of our discussion focuses on the problem area of grief. We highlight instances in the IPT manual (Weissmann et al., 2000) that needed revision because they did not fit with existing data about CG.

The basis for the IPT focus on grief is the assumption that bereavement-related depression is a result of inadequate grieving. Depression that results from inadequate grieving can occur immediately following a loss or at a later time, when the patient is reminded of the loss. According to the IPT manual, evidence suggestive of "pathological mourning" includes multiple losses, inadequate grief in the bereavement period, avoidance behavior in relation to the death, symptoms around a significant date, fear of the illness that caused the death, history of preserving the environment as it was at the time of the death, and absence of social supports during the bereavement period. Patients with grief as a problem are expected to evidence low self-esteem and to idealize the deceased.

Goals of grief-focused IPT are twofold: (1) to facilitate dealing with the loss, and (2) to help the patient reestablish relationships to substitute for what was lost. In conducting the treatment, regardless of the focus, the IPT therapist reviews depressive symptoms and relates symptom onset to the problem area. For a grief-focused treatment, the problem area is the death of a loved one. Other strategies used in grief-focused IPT include reconstructing the relationship with the deceased, discussing events at the time of the death, exploring feelings, and considering possible ways of becoming involved with others. The therapist is instructed to assume that there was an insufficient social network to provide support at the time of the death, to act as a substitute for the deficient support, and to gently encourage the identification of negative emotions related to the deceased. Using Horowitz's (1976) model of reaction to stress, the IPT manual identifies seven typical stress reactions, encouraging the therapist to be alert to these. The seven problematic responses include (1) fear of repetition of the event, (2) shame at helplessness to prevent the death, (3) rage at the person who died, (4) guilt about aggressive impulses or fantasies, (5) survivor guilt, (6) fear of identification or merger with the deceased, and (7) sadness about the loss. The therapist is further instructed to anticipate these types of emotional responses by inquiring about them before the patient mentions them.

The IPT therapist works to reconstruct the relationship to the deceased, suggesting strategies such as reviewing old pictures or reminiscing with friends and family who knew the deceased. An important idea is that ambivalent feelings toward the deceased are assumed to underlie the development of depression. Patients are thought to idealize the deceased. Thus a special emphasis is placed on negative feelings toward the deceased. The therapist is warned to elicit such feelings very gently, and to reassure the patient that positive and comforting feelings will follow the exploration of negative ones. Providing this reassurance also averts the possibility that negative feelings toward the deceased would be transferred to the therapist, causing the patient to discontinue treatment. Thus the goal to develop a more balanced awareness in the patient of his or her positive and negative feelings toward the deceased is focused mostly on the long-ignored negative feelings.

Catharsis is considered important in IPT work with grief. "Catharsis" generally refers to the therapeutic effect of emotional release or expression. The idea is that once released, the affective intensity diminishes. The therapist is instructed to encourage the patient to contact and express painful emotions of grief and then, when they surface, to respond with attentive listening. A pitfall for the therapist to avoid is the impulse to intervene in an attempt to help the patient with this affect; intervening could convey the message that the patient's feelings are dangerous or intolerable. Through catharsis, the patient is expected to lose a (presumed) investment in maintaining abnormal grief. After release has been accomplished, the IPT therapist is instructed to actively help the patient develop new relationships to "fill the 'empty space' left by the lost loved one" (Weissmann et al., 2000, p. 67). The technique of revisiting, similar to imaginal exposure for PTSD, also includes evocation of intense emotion. However, the experience is tape recorded and the patient is asked to listen to the tape. The effectiveness of this technique is thought to stem from the opportunity to observe self and rethink the experience, rather than simply to release pent-up emotion.

Weissman et al. (2000) acknowledge that bereavement-related depression is different from complicated grief. They further note that use of IPT with complicated grief has not been studied. Around the time of the IPT manual's publication in 2000, our group reported that only a small reduction in grief symptoms occurs in bereaved depressed patients treated with IPT (Reynolds et al., 1999). We have now replicated this finding of minimal improvement in a larger group of individuals who participated in a randomized controlled trial comparing IPT to CGT (Shear et al., 2005, NIMH Grant No. MH 60783). The IPT approach is a useful one, in that it focuses the therapist's attention on the dual goals of successful grief: addressing feelings about the loss and reengaging in satisfying life. However, it is clear that the strategies described in the published manuals require modification and enhancement in order to effectively treat CG.

Some modification is needed in order to be consistent with data about the course of grief, the relationship context in which CG occurs, and the impediments to making progress in a natural grief process. CG is a condition in which an intense, primary grief reaction persists. This point is important because there is no evidence of *insufficient* negative emotions, as is assumed in the delayed or distorted grief model. Instead, CG symptoms are better explained as unresolved traumatic and separation distress. CGT targets these problems. The IPT focus on grief does not provide a clear description of the syndrome of CG because the focus is on depression. Although there is some overlap in symptoms, it is not clear that CG is a distinct disorder. There is a need to provide a clear definition of this syndrome for the purpose of patient psychoeducation and therapist clarity.

An important aspect of the distinction is that CG patients rarely idealize the deceased. Instead, they describe a relationship that was very close and identity-defining. In part for this reason, the therapeutic goal in CG is not to assist patients to "emancipate themselves from a crippling attachment to the dead person, thus becoming free to cultivate new interests" (Weissmann et al., 2000, p. 64). Instead, the therapist seeks to help the patient gain a transformed relationship to the deceased that can be comfortably integrated into ongoing life without the lost loved one. A corollary of this idea is that as CGT therapists work to help patients reengage in life, they do not see this reengagement as filling a gap but as pursuing meaningful personal goals that have been set aside because of traumatic and separation distress.

IPT therapists typically work with patients to enrich their current and future interpersonal life. Important people are identified and personal goals are often discussed. However, in grief-focused IPT the therapist is told that this work is best done after the pathological "crippling" attachment to the deceased has been relinquished. By contrast, the CGT therapist frames this work as one of two simultaneous tracks that characterize successful grief. Rather than encouraging the patient to relinquish a crippling attachment, the CGT therapist helps the patient to solidify a more comforting, ongoing "relationship" to the deceased, taking the position that this relationship remains a living, changing one, even though it has a different quality because the loved one has died. Finding a satisfying way to live without the person who died is considered an important aid to the transformation in the relationship, rather than a way to "fill the gap" left by the deceased. Thus the CGT therapist begins work on personal goals at the beginning of the treatment

In working with loss, the therapeutic focus in CGT is on increasing the range of accessible memories and reducing the pain associated with these memories. Rather than focusing on suppressed or denied rage at the person who died, guilt about aggressive impulses or fantasies, or other evidence of underlying ambivalence, the therapist encourages a comfortable, realistic view of the deceased. Instead of placing a special emphasis on negative feelings toward the deceased, the emphasis is on the ability to take comfort in positive feelings. The impediment to effective grief is seen as the presence of too much negative emotion and too little positive, whereas in IPT it is the opposite—the negative emotion is seen as trauma related in an important way. Thus, whereas catharsis is considered important in IPT work with grief, emotional processing—a cognitive process—is considered essential to resolution in CGT. As noted, the IPT therapist is instructed to encourage the expression of painful emotions of grief and then, when they surface, to respond with listening. The role of the CGT therapist is more active; he or she encourages active cognitive work on the part of the patient. In our experience, most patients need assistance in making needed cognitive changes to reduce problematic emotions. Most require tools with which to manage high levels of affect, and the therapist provides these as a part of the work with the intensely painful emotions related to the death. Thus CGT differs from IPT with regard to its (1) underlying model of grief, which is presented to the patient, (2) structuring of the therapist's stance toward the patient, and (3) decisions about when and how to provide support.

INTEGRATING CBT AND IPT IN CGT

Because IPT already has a grief focus with goals that are consistent with treating CG, and our group has extensive experience using IPT effectively, we decided to base our targeted CGT in an IPT framework. Goals for treating CG were similar to IPT grief-focus goals, and we included the core three-phase IPT method as an organizing framework. We integrated CBT strategies for treatment of PTSD as well as cognitive strategies for dealing with separation distress into this framework. We found that these additional complicated grief-specific components could be easily blended in an IPT grief-focused treatment that is time-limited and present-oriented.

Both CBT and IPT are short-term, focused treatments that are present-oriented and practical. Both are very different from psychodynamic psychotherapy. Neither attempts to ameliorate psychological symptoms through addressing intrapsychic problems, such as conflict or defense, nor is an attempt made to interpret transference. IPT differs from CBT in placing interpersonal relationships at the center of the therapeutic work, and in eschewing formal structure (e.g., systematic homework) as a means to uncover distorted thoughts. Whereas it is usual for the IPT therapist to provide suggestions that the patient try new behaviors or pay attention to feelings between sessions, the CBT therapist assigns "homework." Nevertheless, as documented in a recent report (Ablon & Jones, 2002), striking similarities exist between IPT and CBT when the nature of the interaction between the patient and therapist is the focus of comparison. As Ablon and Jones (2002) point out:

> In both treatments, the therapist assumes an authoritative role and coaches patients to think or conduct themselves differently and encourages them to test out these new ways of thinking and behavior in everyday life. . . . Taken together, the results of our two studies suggest that what was shared between the two forms of therapy in the NIMH Treatment of Depression Collaborative Research Program was more salient and defining of the treatments than what was different. (p. 781)

This similarity in therapist behavior supports the feasibility of a merged intervention. We have successfully integrated behavioral and cognitive techniques in two other IPT projects, one targeting bipolar disorder (Frank, Swartz, & Kupfer, 2000) and one that addresses comorbid panic and depression (Cyranowski et al., 2004). Thus, in developing CGT, we began with standard grief-focused IPT and developed some CBT-informed modifications, drawing especially upon Foa's approach to PTSD (Jaycox, Zoellner, & Foa, 2002; Zoellner, Fitzgibbons, & Foa, 2001).

The CGT therapist does utilize IPT facilitative, supportive, cognitive, and behavioral techniques. These core IPT therapeutic techniques, as outlined in the Weissman et al. (2000) manual, include nondirective exploration, encouragement and acceptance of affect, helping the patient generate suppressed and/or avoided affect, and clarification and communication analysis. Directive behavioral change techniques are also outlined and include education, advice and suggestions, modeling and direct help. Into this matrix CGT inserts techniques drawn from CBT for PTSD. Daily symptom monitoring is encouraged. The CGT revisiting procedures are modified versions of prolonged imaginal and *in vivo* exposure techniques. Two cognitive therapy techniques that are used are (1) "memories forms," in which the client is asked to recall specific types of memories of the deceased, and (2) for the client to have an imaginal conversation with the deceased. A segment on personal goals is adapted from motivational interviewing.

The use of these CBT-informed techniques entails more structured plans for continuing therapeutic activities between sessions. The CGT therapist uses a less rigorous approach than CBT, but a more structured one than IPT. The CGT therapist offers a simple monitoring form to track the ups and downs of the patient's grief, and asks the patient to complete this form daily. Taped revisiting and imaginal conversation exercises are sent home with the encouragement to listen to them. Memories forms are provided to guide the patient's reminiscences during a part of the treatment. Weekly plans are discussed with the patient at the end of each session, and these plans are recorded and given to the patient to serve as reminders of the discussion. CGT utilizes assessment forms to examine the kinds of beliefs about grief the person might harbor and to begin to identify what is being avoided. These are completed prior to some sessions, in the waiting room. A midtreatment assessment of progress is conducted. These procedures are easily integrated because they are similar to the weekly depression ratings often used in IPT In general, IPT therapists are encouraged to track symptoms systematically and to use assessment tools to do so. In the section that follows we describe the five key augmentation strategies used in CGT, explaining their rationale and providing a general description of procedures.

CASE EXAMPLE

Angela was a 45-year-old married woman who entered treatment 4 years after her mother died at the end of a 2-year bout with an aggressive form of cancer. Angela knew her mother was very ill, but felt convinced that the doctors would find a cure somehow. She reacted to the news of her mother's death with hysterical screaming and crying. Attempts made by the nurses to soothe her were met with angry rebuffs. She said she just couldn't believe that her mother really had died. She cried almost continually over the ensuing period, including the visitation, and was unable to participate in preparations for the funeral. Her younger sisters took over and organized these events, as well as the selection of a casket and decisions about the burial. She found respite only by falling into an exhausted dreamless sleep, assisted by hypnotic medication prescribed by her concerned physician. She sobbed throughout the funeral service.

Angela was inconsolable for weeks after her mother's death. She alternated between periods of intense emotion and a kind of dulled emptiness when she felt numb. She experienced a strange sense of alienation from her family and friends, almost like she was living in a dream. She forgot to eat and hardly left the house. She got almost no physical exercise and engaged in only minimal social interaction. She looked forward to the night when she could go to bed, and assisted by the pills from her doctor, escape from the nightmarish reality of her days.

During the first few months after her mother's death, Angela's friends and family were warm and comforting and did their best to help take care of her and her family. They made needed school pick-up and transportation arrangements for her two children, ages 7 and 12. Her sisters and best friend either arranged to cook dinner or made sure that they provided food that could be stored in the freezer and easily heated. At least one of them called Angela on a daily basis and expressed her sympathy, while also gently trying to distract her from the pain of the loss. After about 6 months of this, the three women started to become impatient. They talked among themselves about how tiresome this was getting and shared the observation that Angela still seemed to be in the frame of mind that emerged in the early days after her mother's death. They became concerned that their sympathy and support were impeding her progress and decided together that they would need to take a different tack.

Maria, Angela's closest friend, called her to tell Angela that she and her sisters felt that it was time to move on. She gently urged Angela to push herself to do more and reminded her that her children and husband needed her. She said that the three women would no longer arrange for after-school management of the children and would stop providing dinners. She said that she would call later in the week to see how things were going, and she invited Angela to go shopping with her. Angela heard all this as though it were being said across a deep chasm. She felt several pangs of guilt as Maria talked, and started wondering what was wrong with her. She agreed with everything Maria said and accepted the invitation to go shopping. However, she felt dead inside and wondered how she was going to manage. In recalling this period, she reported that she "went on auto-pilot." She began to take care of things that were necessary, as her sisters and friends hoped she would do. However, her sense of estrangement from them increased as she realized they had no understanding of how she was feeling. Moreover, because they were her closest companions with whom she had always shared everything, she now decided that she was "damaged goods" to feel so estranged.

She told herself that she could have prevented her mother's death if she had only taken her to a different doctor. At the same time, she also felt that she was wrong to be so devastated by the death. She thought that her sisters and friend were right. She should be over it by now. She began to wonder if others would be better off without her and stopped using her asthma medication. She occasionally ran a red light when driving—something very uncharacteristic for her. Although she was seriously angry with God, she had always been a religious person and she feared that taking her own life might mean that she would never see her mother again.

Angela had returned to her work as an assistant store manager at a local pharmacy after just a week of bereavement leave. Her job hours allowed her to be home by 3:30 to meet her children when they arrived home from school. After her mother died, her boss was sympathetic but refused to allow more time off. Angela went through the motions at work, but found herself escaping to the ladies room to cry several times a day. She made mistakes at work, though she was usually a careful employee. Her boss was understanding at first, but after several months of persistent, obvious reduction in her job quality, had given her a verbal warning. This occurred around the same time that Maria was telling her that she should "move on."

Angela's was a close-knit family. Her parents had lived two blocks away (her father was still there) and two of her four sisters lived in the neighborhood as well. Her oldest brother had married a woman that the sisters did not like, and he lived in another part of town. Angela was the oldest of the five children and was especially close to her mother. She saw her mother almost every day and talked to her on the telephone at least daily. She secretly felt that she was her mother's favorite, and this feeling of specialness meant everything to her. A quiet, conscientious person, Angela had been plagued for most of her life with mild but persistent feelings of insecurity. These feelings evaporated when she was with her mother. She felt the glow of her mother's admiration and valued her advice and counsel. Angela rarely made a decision without first discussing it with her mother. Once, about 10 years before her mother's death, her parents had rented a cabin for 2 weeks over the summer. Angela recalled that she had felt lost during that time without her mother and thereafter persuaded her husband and her parents that it would be more fun to take vacations together.

Angela presented for treatment of CG after her daughter, now 16, was caught drinking with her friends and taken to a local police station. Angela was devastated. She decided that she had ruined her daughter's life, and the daughter was on the road to being an alcoholic or even a drug addict. She said she knew that she could not raise her children without her mother. When she began telling her sister that she would be better off dead, her sister brought her for psychiatric treatment.

On admission to the clinic, Angela told the clinician that she had not been the same since her mother had died. She described persistent, intense yearning and longing for her mother and a feeling of disbelief about her death. She reported frequently having the feeling that she would round a corner and her mother would be there. When she was alone, she would often daydream about the times she had shared with her mother, and hours would pass before she realized that she had not accomplished something she had set out to do. At the same time, she often had recurrent intrusive images of her mother's face just before she died. Her mother had lost considerable weight in the final months of her illness, and her wasted, exhausted body and tired eyes would appear as a frightful image in Angela's mind.

Angela refused to go anywhere that she had regularly gone with her mother, or anyplace where they had shared a particularly special time. However, she also did not want to do anything new, because she felt that taking steps in a new direction would distance her from her mother. Thus her activities were markedly constricted, and she engaged in only those pursuits that were necessary to care for her family. Additionally, she was plagued with self-doubt about her relationship with her mother, especially the period of her mother's illness. Angela was preoccupied with thoughts about how she might have taken better care of her mother and/or made her death easier. Sometimes, when she focused on the fact that her mother had died, she experienced a panicky feeling and thought she was going crazy.

Angela felt reassured when she was told by the therapist that her experiences were typical of the syndrome of CG. The therapist explained the concept of primary and integrated grief and suggested that Angela had gotten stuck, through no fault of her own, in primary grief. Because most people experience the progress of grief differently from this, it was understandable that her family and friends did not understand. One of the things the therapist suggested was that Angela invite one of her sisters or her friend Maria to come to a session, so that she could hear our view of the situation and (hopefully) become an ally in the treatment. Angela reluctantly agreed to this idea. The therapist told Angela that he could provide a treatment approach that has been successful with this problem, and that, with some work, it would be very possible for her to feel a good deal better. She was relieved to hear this view.

Angela learned how to recognize her feelings of grief and to rate her grief intensity on a scale of 0–10. She began keeping a grief diary and noticing when her feelings were highest and lowest. The therapist explained that both are important because getting the grief process moving entails both engaging with the higher levels of emotions and also learning how to set the grief aside. The situations associated with lower levels of grief during the week would begin to provide clues about what she could do that would make it easier to set her grief aside for a time. At the same time, the cues for higher intensity grief would help in deciding how to work best with the painful emotions.

In the second session the therapist encouraged Angela to think about her personal goals. He asked the question, "If you were feeling much better and your grief was not so preoccupying, what do you think you would like to be doing with your life?" Angela thought for a minute and said she would like to be more engaged with her children and her husband and take better care of them. The therapist accepted this statement and then encouraged her to think of something she would also like for herself. At this point Angela smiled broadly for the first time since he had met her. She said that she had an "old dream" of becoming a physician's assistant. She shyly told the therapist that she had been a pretty good student in high school and also had done pretty well in community college. She had dreamed of being a nurse or a physician's assistant because she found herself very attracted to medicine. However, when she met her husband-to-be after her second year of college and they decided to get married, her mother encouraged her to quit school and get a job so that they could save up to buy a house. At that point, Angela got her job at the pharmacy. She said she had been thinking a lot lately about going back to school, but she wasn't sure if her mother would approve. Her mom always thought a woman's place was in the home, and her younger child was still 11 years old. Still, she had gone as far as looking on the Internet to see if there were any physician assistant programs in the area. It turned out that her own community college offered such a program. She had begun daydreaming guiltily about what it would be like to go there again. She asked the therapist if he thought this was wrong.

The therapist reassured her that he definitely did not think it was wrong, and in fact, told her it was very interesting to him to see how much her mood brightened when she talked about this topic. She said that it made her happy to think that she could possibly get more education that would help her to do something very useful in the world. She said she had always felt it would be important to make a contribution to the community, but her mother did not agree, so she felt uncertain about her own feelings in this area. She longed for a feeling of independence that she could not seem to get in her family. However, since her mother's death, she had been feeling guilty about these wishes, even sometimes thinking that her disagreement with her mother about this issue had so troubled her mother that it had somehow caused her illness. Angela knew this line of thinking was irrational, but still she had this thought and it troubled her.

The therapist told her that he was quite certain that this wish on Angela's part did not cause her mother's illness, and he also said that he thought it would be very important to pursue her desire to enlarge this area of her life. He asked her what she would need to do in order to know that she was moving forward on this possibility. He also asked her to consider who could help her with her goal and what might stand in the way of her achieving it. The therapist explained that dealing with the loss of a very important person can really only proceed naturally if the bereaved person deals with the emotional side of the loss—the sadness and the guilt and anxiety, and even with anger about the death—at the same time he or she is rebuilding own life. He said that if you try to do one of these coping tasks without the other, it tends to hold both back. Imagine two little toy trains tied together with a string, he said. If you shoot one of them forward, it will go for a while but then the other one will stop it and pull it back a little. So to move them forward, you need to push them both at once. Angela smiled. She said it made sense.

The ensuing session included imaginal revisiting and situational revisiting exercises. Angela agreed to participate in the revisiting exercise but expressed concerns that it might be very upsetting and that she honestly didn't see how it would help her. The therapist explained that in telling and retelling this story, and in listening to herself do this, she would likely come to see some of the most troubling elements in a new way. He assured her that he would help her as she moved through this process.

Angela then closed her eyes and told the story of her mother's death. She was alone with her mother, sitting with her in the hospital, and her mother was very weak and tired. She had not eaten for several days and spent most of her time sleeping. The sisters were taking turns being at her bedside. Usually there were two of them, but at this time Angela happened to be alone. She walked out of the room to use the bathroom and when she returned, she noticed that her mother did not seem to be breathing. She shook her mother's arm, and her mother opened her eyes and looked at Angela. "I'll never forget that look," Angela said. "It was like she was angry with me. It was like she was saying, 'How did you let this happen? Why didn't you help me?'" Then she said her mother smiled and opened her hand "like she wanted me to hold it. I took her hand and she gently squeezed. She whispered, 'I love you, Angela.' And then she took a strange-sounding deep breath and looked distant. She didn't breathe again for about a minute, and it really scared me. I was going to run for the nurse when she did that again. This time she closed her eyes and didn't breathe again. I kept waiting for another breath, and then it suddenly occurred to me that she was gone. I started to scream at her, 'Breathe!! Breathe, Mom! You can't go away! You can't leave me!' I don't know what else I said because I started to cry hysterically, and a nurse rushed into the room and took my arm. She tried to calm me down, but she just made me mad. She seemed to be saying that my mother was at peace, but I did not want to hear it. After a while my sisters came and then the rest of the family. Everyone was crying. We were all hysterical. Honestly, I don't remember much about what happened after that. The next thing I remember was being at my parents' home with my father and all of the family and lots of friends and other people around. Our family doctor came over to talk to me, and he gave me a sedative. Eventually I fell asleep."

Telling this story took about 10 minutes, and the therapist provided periodic encouragement and asked for subjective units of distress (SUDs) levels every 2–3 minutes. Angela started the story at a 70, on a scale of 1–100, and quickly increased to a 100. She stayed at a 100 for most of the story. She began crying soon after starting to tell this story and was sobbing by the end. This exercise was tape recorded. After Angela said she fell asleep, the therapist asked her to open her eyes and again asked her SUDs level. She said it was 80. The therapist asked what this experience was like for her. Angela said that it seemed very real, and that she had not told anyone this part of the story. She reported feeling very guilty about the part when she almost went to get the nurse, but then her mother breathed again so she didn't. Angela said she should have gone to get the nurse—that maybe her mother would still be alive if she had done that. The therapist asked her if she really thought that was true. She said "yes and no." Part of her, she said, knew that her mother had a terminal illness. The doctors told her that there was no more they could do to cure the cancer, but somehow she still felt that this was not true and that if she had taken better care of her mother, she would have lived.

Angela was crying again, saying, "I really didn't want her to die." The therapist said that he understood this and that he knew it had been very difficult for her to lose her mother. He then said that she had done an outstanding job with this exercise and that he wanted her to do another brief exercise in order to set this story aside. He suggested that she close her eyes and imagine that the story she just told was on a videotape. He suggested she rewind the tape and put it away. He asked her to describe this process, which she did, and the therapist then asked her SUDs level. She said it was 40. She opened her eyes, and the therapist asked if she were willing to listen to the tape during the week. She said she would try. He then asked how she planned to spend the rest of the day.

The remainder of the session was spent (1) discussing how she would take care of herself and reward herself for this hard work, (2) planning situational revisiting exercises, (3) planning when she would listen to the tape, and (4) discussing where she stood on her progress toward finding a way to enter the physician's assistant program or something similar. At the end of the session her SUDs level was a 20.

Angela listened to the imaginal revisiting exercise four times during the week. She found it too hard to do this every day, as suggested by the therapist, but she did learn that by the end of the week her SUDs had come down to 70–80 for most of the tape. When she described her mother's eyes, the SUDs went to 100 and stayed there until she reported being at home with her family. This story was repeated during the subsequent four sessions, and more details were filled in. During the fourth of these, the therapist focused on the last part, where the SUDs were still high. They repeated this part of the story three times sequentially in the seventh session.

Angela noticed several things as she repeatedly told the story. First, she commented on how well the sisters had worked together during their mother's illness and how supportive they had been of each other. She said she had forgotten all about that. As she came to this realization, she decided to go out with her sisters and discuss this period with them. Their lunch together went very well, and Angela reported that she felt very close to them again, for the first time since her mother had died. During the "hot spot" repetition of the scene regarding her mother's "angry" look, Angela began to consider the possibility that the look she recalled might have been one of confusion upon being awakened. She began to think that her mother was disoriented and did not recognize her at first. Then, when she realized Angela was with her, she smiled and took her hand and said she loved her. Angela began to cry with relief. She said that she was sure this was what happened and was amazed at her own distortion of this over all these months.

As Angela worked on the imaginal and situational revisiting exercises, she also began to complete memory forms. Over therapy weeks 5–9 she listed (1) things she liked about her mother, (2) more things she liked about her mother, (3) her favorite things about her mother, (4) things she didn't like so well, and (5) things she liked and didn't like. During this time, the therapist asked her to bring in pictures of her mother and to talk about her and her relationship with her mother, telling stories related to the pictures.

By the eighth session the SUDs levels in the imaginal revisiting story had come down to 50–60 throughout the story, and a revisiting story of the funeral produced SUDs levels of 50–70. At the ninth session the therapist suggested that Angela might want to have an imaginal conversation with her mother. He described this procedure as one in which Angela would again close her eyes and imagine herself at the bedside of her mother. However, this time it would be after her mother had died. She could imagine that everyone else had left the room and she had a few minutes alone with her mother, who had now died. The therapist invited Angela to imagine that she could actually talk with her mother at this time and suggested she tell her mother anything she would like and/or ask her any questions that she would like to have answered. After Angela spoke to her mother, the therapist would ask her to imagine that she was her mother and to respond. This "conversation" could go back and forth several times. Angela agreed to do this exercise.

During the imaginal conversation, Angela first told her mother how much she loved her and missed her. Her mother "responded" by saying that she loved Angela very much too. Angela then asked her mother if she thought that she could have done more to make her comfortable or prevent her death. Her mother then "said" that it was a great comfort to her that Angela was with her when she died. She said that she knew she had frightened Angela and she was sorry about that. However, she was ready to go. She said that the last few months of her life had been very painful. She knew her family would miss her, so she tried very hard to hang on, but it was exhausting. No one could have prevented her death. She said it was a great relief to let go and that she was at peace. She added that she very much wanted her daughter to be at peace too. She said that death is a natural thing and that she knew her daughter could accept that. She "told" Angela that God was looking after her and that her spirit would always be with her family on earth. Angela ended this conversation feeling greatly relieved. She said it was hard to do this exercise, but it also made her feel closer to her mother than she had since her mother had died.

In the 10th session the therapist conducted a brief review of their progress to date. Both agreed that it was very dramatic. Angela was feeling much better. Her relationships with her friends and family had improved dramatically. She had stopped having intrusive images of her mother dying and she was able to really have fun with her 11-year-old son. She was still avoiding the hospital where her mother had died, and she still had three large boxes of her mother's clothes and possessions that she had not opened since she and her sisters had packed them in the weeks after the death. She wanted to give some of the things away, and she wanted to decide what to keep. In addition, she had not yet gone back to the restaurant that her family's favorite place to eat with their mother. She had decided that she wanted to try taking a course in the physician's assistant curriculum during the next semester, and the school had agreed that she could do that. She thought that embarking seriously on this route would require some changes in her relationship with her husband and children, and she was unsure how to negotiate these changes. The therapist suggested that in the remaining sessions they focus on continuing the situational revisiting exercises, the work on goals, and this new work on role transition. In addition, he suggested that Angela have another imaginal conversation with her mother to "discuss" her plans to go to school. Angela was agreeable to this suggestion.

Over the course of the next five sessions Angela worked with the therapist, using IPT techniques to elucidate and discuss her feelings about the planned transition to studying and then work as a physician's assistant. She became aware of feeling anxiety about her ability to succeed, guilt about her wish to do so, and sadness that her mother was not there to share this new plan with her. She and the therapist discussed her guilt about doing something that would affect the lives her husband and children, especially given her fear that her mother would not approve. She began to talk first with her husband and later with her children about her plans and was able to be assertive in the face of their doubts and reluctance. In the end her family agreed to do what was needed to support her. During this period she realized that her husband had his own insecurities, and the therapist helped her provide support for him as they progressed in this work. Angela held another "conversation" with her mother, in which she told her mother of her feelings about becoming a physician's assistant and her mother responded supportively. In the course of this work, the families went to dinner at the previously avoided restaurant, and she and her sisters went through her mother's belongings and disposed of them in ways to which they all agreed.

The final sessions of the treatment focused on termination. The therapist asked Angela to think about what had helped her and what she thought had changed through the treatment. Angela said the revisiting exercises were clearly the turning point for her. Additionally, she said that talking about her wish to work in medicine and then taking steps toward achieving this goal were very important. She said that, quite honestly, she felt like a different person from when she began the treatment, and really a different person than she had been even before her mother had died. The therapist encouraged her to plan activities she would continue when therapy ended. They discussed her feelings, including her fears and happiness, about ending the sessions.

CONCLUSIONS

CGT is an IPT-based psychotherapy that targets the specific occurrence of a dysfunctional primary grief reaction. Underlying the CGT model is the idea that grief itself can go awry, and that this is different from the onset or worsening of a DSM-IV disorder that might be triggered by the stress of a loss. Grief is a problem primarily because of the strength of the lost attachment relationship and the perceived internal psychological ramifications of its loss. Thus, whereas IPT is a highly effective treatment for mood disorders, its model of grief does not fit our conception of CG, nor does it necessarily describe the process of natural grief as elucidated by empirical data. IPT strategies focus on the hypothesized therapeutic value of cathartic expression of negative emotion, articulation of ambivalent attitudes toward the deceased, and encouragement to loosen the attachment, which is considered to be "crippling" and essentially pathological. CGT focuses on the need to address simultaneously the loss and restoration of functioning. Dealing with the loss entails reducing the traumatic and separation distress related to the death. Decreasing separation distress is achieved through improving patients' ability to reconfigure their mental models of the deceased in such a way as to enhance a sense of connection to the person who died. Ameliorating traumatic distress is achieved through cognitive change in the experience of the death. Restoration coping is targeted with work on personal goals and improving satisfaction in ongoing relationships and daily activities.

To construct CGT, we modified IPT and added CBT-based enhancements. These include (1) revisiting of the time of the death, (2) revisiting activities, people, and objects that the patient is avoiding, (3) directed work with memories, and (4) an imaginal conversation with the deceased. CBT is procedurally compatible with IPT. Memories work, imaginal revisiting, and engagement with avoided objects are similar to stated procedures in the standard IPT manual, though specifics of the techniques are somewhat different in CGT. IPT instructs therapists to discuss the relationship to the person who died and the events prior to, during, and after the death, and encourages the patient to look through belongings or pictures of the deceased. The use of imaginal conversation and the development of personal goals are not mentioned in the standard manual, but are also very consistent with the procedures used in standard grief-focused IPT. Pilot work with CGT showed it to be very promising, with large reductions in scores on the ICG. A follow-up randomized controlled trial ($N = 95$) has just been completed, and initial analyses show greater improvement with CGT than IPT, with the same percentage of treatment dropouts (26%) in each treatment.

ACKNOWLEDGMENTS

This work was supported by National Institute of Mental Health Grant Nos. MH-60783, 30915, and 52247.

REFERENCES

Ablon, J. S., & Jones, E. E. (2002). Validity of controlled clinical trials of psychotherapy: Findings from the NIMH treatment of depression collaborative research program. *American Journal of Psychiatry 159*(5), 775–783.

Bloom, B. L., Asher, S. J., & White, S. W. (1978). Marital disruption as a stressor: A review and analysis. *Psychological Bulletin, 85,* 867–894.

Bonanno, G. A. (2001). Grief and emotion: A social-functional perspective. In M. S. Stroebe, R. O. Hansson, W. Stroebe, & H. Schut (Eds.), *Handbook of bereavement research: Consequences, coping and care* Washington, DC: American Psychological Association.

Bonanno, G. A., & Field, N. P. (2001). Examining the delayed grief hypothesis across 5 years of bereavement. *American Behavioral Scientist, 44*(5), 798–816.

Bonanno, G. A., & Keltner, D. (1997). Facial expressions of emotion and the course of conjugal bereavement. *Journal of Abnormal Psychology 106*(1), 126–137.

Bonanno, G. A., Keltner, D., Holen, A., & Horowitz, M. J. (1995). When avoiding unpleasant emotions might not be such a bad thing: Verbal-autonomic response dissociation and midlife conjugal bereavement. *Journal of Personality and Social Psychology 69*(5), 975–989.

Bonanno, G. A., Notarius, C. I., Gunzerath, L., Keltner, D., & Horowitz, M. J. (1998). Interpersonal ambivalence, perceived relationship adjustment, and conjugal loss. *Journal of Consulting and Clinical Psychology 66*(6), 1012–1022.

Bowlby, J. (1973). *Attachment and loss. Vol. II: Separation, anxiety and anger.* London: Hogarth Press.

Brown, G. W., Harris, T., & Copeland, J. R. (1977). Depression and loss. *British Journal of Psychiatry, 130*, 1–18.

Buechner, F. (1991). *The sacred journey: A memoria of early days.* San Francisco: Harper Books.

Cyranowski, J. M., Frank, E., Shear, M. K., Swartz, H. A., Fagiolini, A., Scott, J., & Kupfer, D. J. (2004). Interpersonal psychotherapy for depression with panic spectrum symptoms (IPT-PS): A pilot study. *Depression and Anxiety, 21*(3), 140–142.

DiMascio, A., Weissman, M. M. Prusoff, B. A., Neu, C., Zwilling, M., & Klerman, G. L. (1979). Differential symptom reduction by drugs and psychotherapy in acute depression. *Archive of General Psychiatry, 36*, 1450–1456.

Field, N. P., Nichols, C., Holen, A., & Horowitz, M. J. (1999). The relation of continuing attachment to adjustment in conjugal bereavement. *Journal of Consulting and Clinical Psychology, 67*(2), 212–218.

Foa, E. B. (1995). *Post Traumatic Stress Diagnostic Scale Manual.* Minneapolis: National Computer Systems.

Frank, E. (1991). Interpersonal psychotherapy as a maintenance treatment for patients with recurrent depression. *Psychotherapy, 28*(2), 259–266.

Frank, E., Grochocinski, V. J., Spanier, C. A., Buysse, D. J., Cherry, C. R., Houck, P. R., et al. (2000a). Interpersonal psychotherapy and antidepressant medication: Evaluation of a sequential treatment strategy in women with recurrent major depression. *Journal of Clinical Psychiatry, 61*(1), 51–57.

Frank, E., Swartz, H. A., & Kupfer, D. J. (2000). Interpersonal and social rhythm therapy: Managing the chaos of bipolar disorder. *Biological Psychiatry, 48*, 593–604.

Henderson, A. S. (1991). Social support and depression. In H. Veiel & U. Baumann (Eds.), *The meaning and measurement of social support.* Washington, DC: Hemisphere.

Henderson, S. (1977). The social network, support and neurosis: The function of attachment in adult life. *British Journal of Psychiatry, 131*, 185–191.

Horowitz, M. J. (1976). *Stress response syndromes.* New York: Aronson.

Horowitz, M. J., Siegel, B., Holen, A., Bonanno, G. A., Milbrath, C., & Stinson, C. H. (1997). Diagnostic criteria for complicated grief disorder. *American Journal of Psychiatry, 154*(7), 904–910.

Ilfeld, F. W. (1977). Current social stressors and symptoms of depression. *American Journal of Psychiatry, 119,* 243–252.

Jacobs, S. C., Mazure, C., & Prigerson, H. G. (2000). Diagnostic criteria for traumatic grief. *Death Studies, 24,* 185–199.

Jaycox, L. H., Zoellner, L., & Foa, E. B. (2002). Cognitive-behavior therapy for PTSD in rape survivors. *Journal of Clinical Psychology, 58*(8), 891–906.

Klerman, G. L., Weissman, M. M., Rounsaville, B. J., & Chevron, E. S. (1984). *Interpersonal psychotherapy of depression.* New York: Basic Books.

Klerman, G. L., Weissman, M. M., Rounsaville, B. J., & Chevron, E. S. (1996). Interpersonal psychotherapy for depression. In E. J. Groves (Ed.), *Essential papers on short-term dynamic therapy.* New York: New York University Press.

Lindemann, E. (1944). Symptomatology and management of acute grief. *American Journal of Psychiatry, 101,* 141–148.

Lindstrom, T. C. (2002). "It ain't necessarily so" . . . Challenging mainstream thinking about bereavement. *Family and Community Health, 25*(1), 11–21.

Middleton, W., & Raphael, B. (1987). Bereavement: State of the art and state of the science. *Psychiatric Clinics of North America, 10*(3), 329–343.

Neimeyer, R. A. (2001). *Meaning reconstruction and the experience of loss.* Washington, DC: American Psychological Association.

Overholser, J. C., & Adams, D. M. (1997). Stressful life events and social support in depressed psychiatric inpatients. In T. W. Miller (Ed.), *Clinical disorders and stressful life events..* Madison, CT: International Universities Press.

Parkes, C. M. (1998). Bereavement in adult life. [Review] [9 refs]. *BMJ* 316, no. 7134:856-859.

Paykel, E. S., Myers, J. K., Dienelt, M. N., Klerman, G. L., Lindenthal, J. J., & Pepper, M. P. (1969). Life events and depression: A controlled study. *Archive of General Psychiatry, 21*(6), 753–760.

Pearlin, L. I., & Johnson, J. S. (1977). Marital status, life-strains and depression. *American Sociological Review, 42*(5), 704–715.

Pearlin, L. I., & Lieberman, M. A. (1977). Social sources of emotional distress. In R. Simmons (Ed.), *Research in community and mental health.* Greenwich, CT: JAI Press.

Prentice, A., & Brown, R. (1989). Fetal tachyarrhythmia and maternal antidepressant treatment. *British Medical Journal, 298*(6667), 190.

Prigerson, H. G., Bierhals, A. J., Kasl, S. V., Reynolds, C. F., Shear, M. K., Day, N., et al. (1997a). Complicated grief as a risk factor for mental and physical morbidity. *American Journal of Psychiatry, 154*(5), 616–623.

Prigerson, H. G., Frank, E., Kasl, S. V., Reynolds, C. F., Anderson, B., Zubenko, G. S., et al. (1995a). Complicated grief and bereavement-related depression as distinct disorders: Preliminary empirical validation in elderly bereaved spouses. *American Journal of Psychiatry, 152*(1), 22–30.

Prigerson, H. G., Maciejewski, P. K., Reynolds, C. F., Bierhals, A. J., Newsom, J. T., Fasiczka, A., et al. (1995b). Inventory of Complicated Grief: A scale to measure maladaptive symptoms of loss. *Psychiatry Research, 59*(1-2), 65–79.

Prigerson, H. G., Shear, M. K., Beirhals, A. J., Pilkonis, P. A., Wolfson, L., Hall, M., et al. (1997b). Case histories of traumatic grief. *Omega: Journal of Death and Dying, 35*(1), 9–24.

Prigerson, H. G., Shear, M. K., Jacobs, S. C., Reynolds, C. F., Maciejewski, P. K.,

Rosenheck, R., et al. (1999). Consensus criteria for traumatic grief: A rationale and preliminary empirical test. *British Journal of Psychiatry*, *174*, 67–73.

Prusoff, B., Weissman, M. M., Klerman, G. L., & Rounsaville, B. J.(1980). Research diagnostic criteria subtypes of depression: Their role as predictors of differential response to psychotherapy and drug treatment. *Archives of General Psychiatry*, *37*, 796–803.

Raphael, B., & Martinek, N. (1997). Assessing traumatic bereavement and posttraumatic stress disorder. In J. P. Wilson & T. M. Keane (Eds.), *Assessing psychological trauma and PTSD*. New York: Guilford Press.

Reisman, A. S. (2001). Death of a spouse: Illusory basic assumptions and continuations of bonds. *Death Studies*, *25*(5), 445–460.

Reynolds, C. F., Miller, M. D., Pasternak, R. E., Frank, E., Perel, J. M., Cornes, C., et al. (1999). Treatment of bereavement-related major depressive episodes in later life: A randomized, double-blind, placebo-controlled study of acute and continuation treatment with nortriptyline and interpersonal psychotherapy. *American Journal of Psychiatry*, *156*(2), 202–208.

Russac, R. J., Steighner, N. S., & Canto, A. I. (2001). Grief work versus continuing bonds: A call for paradigm integration or replacement? *Death Studies*, *26*, 463–478.

Shear, K. Frank, E., Houck, P., Reynolds, C. F. (2005). Treatment of complicated grief: A randomized controlled trial. *Journal of the American Medical Association*, *293*(21), 2601–2608.

Sireling, L., Cohen, D., & Marks, I. (1988). Guided mourning for morbid grief: A controlled replication. *Behavior Therapy*, *19*(2), 121–132.

Stroebe, M. S., & Schut, H. (1999). The dual-process model of coping with bereavement: Rationale and description. *Death Studies*, *23*, 197–224.

Stroebe, M. S. (1997). Bereavement research and theory: Retrospective and prospective. In *Handbook of bereavement: Theory, research, and intervention*.

van Doorn, C., Kasl, S., Beery, L. C., Jacobs, S. C., & Prigerson, H. G. (1998). The influence of marital quality and attachment styles on complicated grief and depressive symptoms. *The Journal of Nervous and Mental Disease*, *186*(9), 566–573.

Viederman, M. (1995). Grief: Normal and pathological variants [Editorial]. *American Journal of Psychiatry*, *152*(1), 1–4.

Weissman, M. M., Markowitz, J. C., & Klerman, G. L. (2000). *Comprehensive guide to interpersonal psychotherapy*. New York: Basic Books.

Weissman, M. M., Prusoff, B. A., DiMascio, A., Neu, C., Goklaney, M., & Klerman, G. L. (1979). The efficacy of drugs and psychotherapy in the treatment of acute depressive episodes. *American Journal of Psychiatry*, *136*, 555–558.

Zoellner, L. A., Fitzgibbons, L. A., & Foa, E. B. (2001). Cognitive-behavioral approaches to PTSD. In J. P. Wilson & M. J. Friedman (Eds.), *Treating psychological trauma and PTSD*. New York: Guilford Press.

CHAPTER THIRTEEN

Sexual Revictimization

Risk Factors and Prevention

Marylene Cloitre
Anna Rosenberg

Sexual assault is one of the most frequent types of trauma associated with the development of posttraumatic stress disorder (PTSD; Norris, 1992) and is a highly prevalent event, with one out of every eight women experiencing a sexual assault some time in her life (National Victim Center and Crime Victims Research and Treatment Center, 1992). Of note however, sexual assault in adulthood is not evenly distributed across the female population. Rather, certain subgroups of women are more at risk than others. One of the most robust risk factors for sexual assault is a history of childhood abuse. Among clinical samples, women who have experienced childhood sexual abuse are 2.3–3.7 times more likely to experience a sexual assault in adulthood than those without an abuse history (Cloitre, Tardiff, Marzuk, Leon, & Potera, 1996). In community samples, risk is also heightened. For example, college women with a history of childhood sexual abuse are 1.4–2.1 times more likely to experience adult sexual assault than their nonabused counterparts (Roodman & Clum, 2001). A review of epidemiological data collected on the prevalence and types of sexual assault and abuse in a community sample has revealed that among women reporting a history of sexual assault, the majority (59%) reported having been assaulted in both childhood and adulthood, with much smaller numbers reporting only one or the other form of assault (Wyatt, Guthrie, & Notgrass, 1992).

These data indicate that retraumatized women make up the largest subgroup of sexually assaulted women. Given this fact, sexual assault research should prioritize identifying the psychological characteristics of women with a history of childhood sexual abuse that put them at risk for adult sexual assault. It is also important to begin developing prevention programs for at-risk women and adolescent girls that target and reduce these risk factors.

This chapter reviews the available data on the potential intrapersonal and interpersonal assault risk factors among women with a history of childhood abuse. It also presents a developing model of retraumatization and an intervention designed to reduce risk for repeated sexual assaults.

CHARACTERISTICS OF CHILDHOOD VICTIMIZATION

Victimization during childhood varies dramatically in its content, context, and consequences. Specific aspects of childhood abuse increase the risk of revictimization. Women who experience other types of abuse in childhood in addition to sexual abuse are at greater risk for adult victimization. In addition, severity of the abuse and the relationship to the perpetrator also influence the likelihood of future interpersonal violence.

Co-occurrence of Child Sexual and Physical Abuse

Physical abuse frequently co-occurs with sexual abuse and is an independent and additional contributor to adult revictimization. It has sometimes been found to have even greater predictive weight than sexual abuse, depending on the severity and complexity of the adult trauma. Merrill and colleagues (1999) found that childhood sexual abuse was a stronger determinant than physical abuse in predicting adult rape. In contrast, a similar study found that both sexual and physical abuse independently contributed to adult sexual revictimization, but physical abuse was a stronger predictor (Arata & Lindman, 2002). In addition, Schaaf and McCane (1998) found that women with the highest rate of adult sexual and/or physical victimization reported experiencing both child physical and sexual abuse. Women with childhood physical abuse only had the second highest rates of adult victimization, followed by women with only child sexual abuse. The results suggest that physical abuse is a stronger predictor of adult victimization when defined to include a wide range of outcomes (i.e., rape, domestic violence, sexual and physical assault), and there is some ambiguity in regard to the relative role of childhood sexual versus physical abuse when the outcome is limited to adult rape.

Cumulative Effects of Childhood Maltreatment

Apart from child sexual and physical abuse, other forms of childhood maltreatment increase the risk of adult victimization. A dose–response effect exists such that experiencing more types of victimization in childhood results in a stronger likelihood of adult victimization (Sanders & Moore, 1999; Irwin, 1999; Clemmons, DiLillo, Martinez, DeGue, & Jeffcott, 2003). A study of college women found that those who experienced date rape in adolescence/young adulthood had greater total childhood traumatic experiences than women who had not been raped (Sanders & Moore, 1999). Childhood traumatic experiences were measured by combining the three subscales of the Child Abuse and Trauma Scale: Negative Home Environment/Neglect, Punishment, and Child Sexual Abuse. When women were compared on individual subscales, the difference between the raped and nonraped groups remained on the Negative Home Environment/Neglect subscale but was not apparent on the Child Sexual Abuse and Punishment subscales. In a community sample of 155 Australian women, individual types of childhood maltreatment were not predictive of adult physical and/or sexual assault, although the total number of traumatic experiences was related to adult assault (Irwin, 1999). Similarly, in a sample of Latina undergraduates, Clemmons et al. found no differences in level of trauma symptomatology between women who experienced a single form of child maltreatment and those who experienced no maltreatment; however, those who experienced two or more types of maltreatment (29% of the sample) had greater symptomatology than those with a single type of maltreatment or none at all. Types of maltreatments included sexual abuse, physical abuse, emotional abuse, and witnessing violence. The authors also noted, however, that the number of types of maltreatment was positively related to severity of maltreatment. In summary, traumatic events typically do not occur in isolation during childhood. When researchers assess for only a specific type of abuse, they risk drawing inadequate conclusions about which kinds of abuse are driving the consequences.

Severity of Childhood Sexual Abuse and Type of Perpetrator

Severity of abuse has a great impact on future interpersonal violence (Ferguson, Horwood, & Lynskey, 1997; Kessler & Bieschke, 1999; Irwin, 1999; Clemmons et al., 2003). In a meta-analysis of 19 empirical studies Roodman and Clum (2001) found that defining child sexual abuse as involving physical contact yielded a greater effect size for predicting revictimization than a broader definition of childhood abuse. These findings also indicate the importance of providing a precise definition of childhood sexual abuse, suggesting that variation in measurement contributes to the noted variation in sexual abuse prevalence rates and revictimization rates. Studies with carefully operationalized definitions of sexual abuse have produced more coherent relationships with revictimization. For example, a study of 520 New Zealand 18-year-olds showed a linear increase in odds of revictimization with increasing severity of childhood sexual abuse (Ferguson et al., 1997). Odds of rape/attempted rape were 11:1 for those whose childhood sexual abuse involved intercourse, as compared to the nonabused group, whereas they were 2:1 for those who had experienced noncontact childhood sexual abuse.

In addition, there are some data indicating that the relationship of the perpetrator to the victim plays an important role. Kessler and Bieschke (1999) found that women who were abused incestuously had higher odds of revictimization than those abused by a nonfamily member adult or peer. Furthermore, women abused by a peer were more likely to experience revictimization than those abused by a nonfamily member adult.

THEORETICAL ORIENTATION:
A SOCIAL–DEVELOPMENTAL PERSPECTIVE

Whether an assault occurred in childhood or adulthood matters because the impact of interpersonal violence first occurring in childhood may be qualitatively different from that occurring in adulthood. The preponderance of data indicates that women who were sexually abused in childhood experience more severe and more diverse negative effects than women who were victimized only in adulthood (Follette, Polusny, Bechtle, & Naugle, 1996; Messman-Moore & Long, 2000). Furthermore, it has been suggested that understanding the sequelae of childhood sexual violence in terms of a PTSD model alone underestimates the range of deleterious consequences, which have been found to include significant problems in the emotional and social–developmental and domains of functioning.

Contemporary developmental theorists posit that abuse that takes place in childhood profoundly interferes with developmental tasks of that period, among which are included the critical development of affect regulation and interpersonal relatedness. There is substantial research in the developmental and community psychology literature indicating that childhood abuse has a negative impact on the acquisition of appropriate emotion regulation and interpersonal skills (e.g., Cicchetti & White, 1990; Shields & Cicchetti, 1998), a prerequisite to effective functioning in later life. For instance, early maltreatment, including both sexual and physical abuse, is associated with high levels of negativity and anger in toddlers and lack of self-control in preschoolers (Erickson, Egeland, & Pianta, 1989). Hostility and difficulty with peers (bullying or experiencing victimization) are seen in older children with histories of abuse (e.g., Hennessy, Rabideau, Cicchetti, & Cummings, 1994; Howes & Eldredge, 1985; Shields, Ryan, & Cicchetti, 1994). Sexual abuse, in particular, is associated with a variety of symptoms in childhood, including oppositional behaviors, sexualized behaviors, anxiety, and depression (Kendall-Tackett, Williams, & Finkelhor, 1993).

The disruption of affect regulation and interpersonal relatedness skills is hypothesized to create risk for subsequent assault in various ways. Below are descriptions of developmental processes associated with affect regulation and interpersonal relatedness, how these processes may be disrupted as a result of abuse, and the way in which these disruptions may create risk for future assaults.

AFFECT REGULATION

The capacity to regulate internal states and behavioral responses to external stressors is a skill facilitated by caretakers. For example, children's excitement about, and/or fear of, the new and unknown is moderated by the provision of parental soothing and guidance concerning appropriate approach and avoidance behaviors. In general, effective caretakers engage in behaviors that modulate the child's physiological state, providing a balance between reassurance and stimulation (Bowlby, 1984; van der Kolk, 1987). Under these circumstances, children learn how to take care of themselves effectively and, alternatively, how to get help when they are distressed (van der Kolk, 1996).

Sexual abuse can interfere with affect regulation development in two ways. First, the abuse itself directly contributes to affect regulation problems because it promotes chronic arousal. Second, the family environments of children who experience abuse provide little learning opportunity to develop affect regulation skills. Caregivers in such families often have affect regulation and impulse control problems themselves, such as mood disorders, domestic violence, and substance abuse problems (Shearer, Peters, Quaytman, & Ogden, 1990; Kellogg & Hoffman, 1997).

Risk Factors Related to Affect Dysregulation

Evidence is accumulating that certain problems associated with affect regulation, such as alexithymia and dissociation, are risk factors for sexual assault (Cloitre, Scarvalone, & Difede, 1997). In addition, there is anecdotal evidence that affect dysregulation, defined as a state of alternating experiences of emotional flooding and numbing, may also be a contributing risk factor. Lastly, use of alcohol and drugs, often reported as coping mechanisms intended to blunt painful or overwhelming affect, has been repeatedly demonstrated as a risk factor for sexual assault.

Alexithymia

"Alexithymia" refers to difficulties in identifying and labeling feeling states. This difficulty may have its source in chronic hyperarousal experiences in which the intensity of arousal may make it difficult to discriminate among feelings such as anger, fear, and anxiety. It is also possible that problems in appropriately labeling feelings are the result of poor or inaccurate instruction from caretakers, who themselves have limited abilities in this regard, or who are motivated to mislabel a child's emotional states to normalize or deny abuse. Differentiation among feeling states is a skill that develops in childhood, and recent data suggest that childhood abuse may subvert this skill (Cicchetti & White, 1990). One study found that women whose first sexual assault occurred in childhood were more likely to be alexithymic than women who had been assaulted for the first time in adulthood, even when other additional traumatic events in adulthood, such as domestic violence, were taken into account (Cloitre et al., 1997).

Alexithymia may especially be associated with acquaintance assaults. Difficulty identifying and labeling feeling states results in a diminished emotional vocabulary and an affectively out-of-sync self-presentation, which may lead others to more easily minimize or actively disregard an alexithymic individual's "no." Perhaps equally important, such individuals may be less able to accurately read others' emotional cues (e.g., to distinguish anger that is appropriate vs. dangerous), thus diminishing their capacity to respond effectively in interpersonally threatening situations.

Dissociation

Dissociation has also been suggested as a risk factor for subsequent assault among individuals with childhood abuse. Although there has been some controversy about the definition of dissociation, it is typically understood as an experience in which the individual is cognitively and emotionally removed from the current circumstance and has reduced or no available memory of it. The high level of dissociation among retraumatized women may make them frequently unaware of their environment and insensitive to potential risks. In addition, being in a dissociative state may make them look confused or distracted, marking them as "easy targets" to sexual and other predators. Lastly, poor recall of experiences and events occurring during a dissociative state may make an assaulted woman less likely to reach out for help and/or to be believed, thus decreasing the chances of employing any psychological, social, or legal intervention that can reduce risk for future events.

Cross-sectional studies have found that dissociation is higher among revictimized women than women victimized once (Cloitre et al., 1997; Wilson, Calhoun, & Bernat, 1999). In the study described earlier, women with both adult and childhood sexual assaults were found to report more frequent dissociative experiences than women who had been assaulted for the first time in adulthood and those who had never been assaulted (Cloitre et al., 1997). In a retrospective study of 51 childhood sexual abuse survivors, Field et al. (2001) reported that those revictimized in the 6 months prior to assessment had more somatic and psychological symptoms, including dissociation, than those who had not been revictimized during that period. These cross-sectional and retrospective study designs, however, cannot determine whether dissociation is a risk for revictimization, a consequence of it, or both.

Prospective and mediational studies suggest that recent revictimization is associated with dissociation (Sandberg, Matorin, & Lynn, 1999; Irwin, 1999; Kessler & Bieschke, 1999). The only prospective study of revictimization, which had a 10-week time frame, found dissociation to be associated with childhood sexual abuse, and even more strongly with childhood abuse and adult victimization combined. It was not, however, associated with revictimization during the 10-week period. The study provides evidence for dissociation as a consequence of victimization that develops in a cumulative fashion over multiple traumatic events. However, because the time period for the study was relatively short, and the number of women who experienced victimization during that period were few, further testing is necessary to determine whether or not dissociation is a risk for future revictimization as well as a consequence of it.

Further research might also explore whether other characteristics associated with dissociation, such as poor problem-solving strategies, may affect risk for revictimization. One study found that women with a history of child or adolescent sexual abuse were more likely to use disengagement coping methods to deal with an adult sexual assault than women without such a history (Gibson & Leitenberg, 2001). Disengagement coping was also associated with more general distress ($r = .27$, $p = .007$) and more PTSD symptoms ($r = .50$, $p < .001$).

Emotional Flooding and Numbing

Emotional flooding and numbing have been anecdotally reported as potential risk factors for assault. A "flood" of fearful feelings, or the absence of such feelings in the face of threat triggers can derail appropriate fight-or-flight responses. Women who have been repeatedly assaulted report overreaction to low-level threats and, alternatively, a lack of reaction or appropriate response to an event or trigger that indicates risk of assault. High-level triggers such as trespassing of physical boundaries (e.g., being touched at work, being approached on the street) or the presence of a weapon may not generate a fear response strong enough or early enough to initiate protective action.

Risk Recognition

Because affect regulation problems may lead an individual to high-risk situations and may hinder proper response in these situations, recent studies have attempted to assess the relationship between a history of repeated trauma and the capacity for accurate, subjective experiences of threat. For example, Meadows and colleagues (Meadows, Jaycox, Webb, & Foa, 1996) evaluated single-event rape narratives and found that victims with higher numbers of sexual assaults identified fewer danger cues, suggesting a relationship between poor risk recognition and a history of multiple assaults. A client at our clinic remarked that her feelings of fear alternated so wildly that she could never trust them to function as a guide for action. She said she had been physically abused so often as a child that her "danger sensor was smashed."

Several studies have used an audiotaped vignette of a date rape scenario that progresses from verbal appeals to coercion (Marx & Gross, 1995) to examine when female subjects thought the man had gone "too far" (which they indicated by pressing a button). In a study by Wilson et al. (1999) women who had been revictimized waited significantly longer, until a more coercive section of the tape, to press the button, as compared to nonvictimized women and to women victimized once in adolescence/adulthood, suggesting that revictimized women recognized threat only at more coercive circumstances. A relationship was not found between decision latency (i.e., the length of time to recognize the risk of the situation) and trauma symptoms for the entire sample. However, for the revictimized women decision latency was negatively related to (MPSS-SR; Modified PTSD Symptom Scale–Self-Report; Resick, Falsetti, Resnick, & Kilpatrick, 1991) scores, suggesting that revictimized women who waited until higher risk segments of the tape reported less PTSD symptoms than the revictimized women who pressed the button at an earlier point in the tape. Further examination of subscales showed that women with higher decision latency had lower reported arousal, whereas they did not differ on reexperiencing or avoidance scores.

In a later prospective study using the same tape scenario, Marx, Calhoun, Wilson, and Meyerson (2001) found a difference in decision latency between victimized college women (victimization age < 14) who reported being raped between the time of assessment and at 2 months follow-up and those who had not been raped during this time. However, when a broader definition of sexual victimization was used, ranging from any unwanted sexual contact to rape, no difference was found in decision latency between women who had experienced some form of sexual revictimization during this time and those who had not.

Lastly, in a variation of the risk recognition paradigm described above, participants watched a videotaped dating situation that highlighted the risk of sexual assault and then wrote down anything that would make them uncomfortable in the same situation (Breitenbecher, 1999). Perception of threat cues was unrelated to both prior sexual abuse and revictimization at a 5 month follow-up. The open response and broad definition of victimization, which included any type of unwanted sexual contact, may explain the discrepancy between these two studies.

Alcohol and Drug Use

Alcohol and drug use are well-known risk factors for sexual assault, especially among adolescents (Gidycz, Hanson, & Layman, 1995; Koss & Dinero, 1989; Greene, Navarro, & Gidycz, 1995; Muelenhard & Linton, 1987). In addition, drug and alcohol abuse are highly prevalent among individuals with childhood sexual abuse (Browne & Finkelhor, 1986; Polusny & Follette, 1995). Recent data suggest that alcohol consumption is a risk factor for sexual assault as well as a consequence of childhood abuse. However, it seems that although alcohol consumption is a consequence of childhood sexual abuse, it becomes an independent and additional risk factor for later assault. In a study of navy recruits, Merrill et al. (1999) found that childhood sexual abuse, alcohol problems, and number of sexual partners were distinct and independent predictors of adult rape. Similarly, Messman-Moore and Long (2002) found that childhood sexual abuse, alcohol-related diagnoses, and substance-related diagnoses each predicted rape and coerced intercourse. However, no significant interaction was found between child sexual abuse and either diagnostic status in predicting rape or coerced intercourse.

INTERPERSONAL AND SELF-APPRAISAL

A developmentally sensitive assessment of potential risk factors among childhood abuse survivors cannot overlook the temporal context in which the abuse occurs. During this time a child is organizing views of the self and templates or schemas for relating to others. Bowlby (1969) and others have suggested that there is a biologically wired-in propensity for maintaining closeness to the available caretaker. This biological imperative has its basis in the enormous dependency of the young on the caretaker for basic survival-relevant activity, such as provision of safety and sustenance. One way in which this attachment is organized and maintained is through the development of interpersonal schemas that provide information to the child about the conditions and circumstances under which relatedness occurs, so that the child may utilize this information to facilitate attachment to the caretaker and thus maximize survival. Typically, simple behaviors such as proximity and vocal calls elicit protection from caretakers, and caretakers, in turn, receive intrinsic satisfaction from the provision of protection and safety to their offspring.

Interpersonal Schemas Associated with Childhood Abuse

The interpersonal schema for attachment that emerges in an abusive caretaking setting deviates from the format proposed above. For example, in a physically assaultive home, proximity, a condition for care, may also elicit physical assault. Thus *care* and *physical assault* become paired. In sexually abusive homes, proximity may elicit sexual activity. Such contingency experiences might lead to templates of interpersonal relatedness that, whatever their particulars, suggest that to be interpersonally engaged means to be abused, and that abuse is a way to be connected.

Because these schemas are assumed to be the templates for future behaviors, and because they are automatically activated, it is easy to see how negative patterns set down in childhood can guide the adult toward repeating activities that are maladaptive in adulthood. For example, a young woman from an abusive family who has developed the understanding that interpersonal relatedness is contingent on sexual behavior is more likely to accept sexual activity as a way of emotionally connecting to others, whether or not she is interested in sex. Women from abusive homes are relatively unlikely to recognize the negative aspects of exchanging sex for human connection, because the pattern was established and accepted in early key relationships.

Interpersonal schema theory is valuable because it provides a non-victim-blaming way to understand repeated abusive relationships and assaults experienced by childhood abuse victims. The theory suggests that there is a predisposition to form attitudes and actions based on past experience and that the interpersonal belief system that emerges from these experiences has its origins in efforts to adapt effectively to the given environment for satisfaction of relational and survival needs. For those whose lives have been comprised of positive experiences and loving interpersonal relationships, the automatic activation of interpersonal schemas does them no harm and, in fact, probably enhances the probability of positive relationships (e.g., "Having my needs recognized/recognizing those of others is a way to attach"). In contrast, those whose lives have been comprised of trauma and negative relationships are at risk for continued or repeated negative relationships, a form of "self-fulfilling prophecy." Clinicians should note that such individuals carry a burden from their childhood experiences: namely, ways of thinking about themselves and others that are automatic and maladaptive. The challenge for client and therapist is to identify and change the automatic schemas in order to protect the individual from the negative consequences of inadvertently repeating his or her own history.

A recent study suggested that the tendency to "repeat" one's history via automatic application of interpersonal schemas is a behavior that is typical of both abused and nonabused individuals; the difference is found in the contents and consequences of the schemas. In a recent study based in the circumplex model of interpersonal functioning, we assessed the interpersonal schemas of several groups of women with differing trauma histories (Cloitre, Cohen, & Scarvalone, 2002a). The interpersonal beliefs of the revictimized women (incest survivors with adult sexual assault experiences) were strongly negative and reflected the expectation for others to respond to them in cold and controlling ways, for all the "others" they were asked to consider (i.e., mother, father, or friend) and across a variety of situations (e.g., competitive, cooperative). In contrast, never-assaulted women generally expected responses of warmth and low control (i.e., respect for autonomy) from the various people and circumstances they were asked to imagine. Thus both groups showed relatively "rigid" interpersonal expectations that differed only in valence (positive vs. negative) but not in range or flexibility. Notably, incest survivors who had not been assaulted in adulthood differed from both of these groups. Whereas women in this group held somewhat negative interpersonal beliefs, they showed more variable expectations of others, depending on the person and situation. Thus the non-revictimized women showed a greater range of interpersonal expectations, which suggests the presence of greater flexibility in their approach to interpersonal events.

Although the data are cross-sectional and causal inferences must be made with caution, we surmise that the characteristic of relatively high interpersonal flexibility among the subgroup of incest survivors may make them less at risk for abusive relationships or assaults, because they may be sensitive to opportunities for more positive relating and/or reworking of negative circumstances. Research is under way to identify the experiential factors that may contribute to interpersonal flexibility, such as the presence of role models outside of the abusive family system (e.g., teachers, strong peer friendships, aunts or uncles), positive therapy experiences, or the good fortune of having developed and sustained healthy intimate relationships in early adulthood.

Self-Appraisal: Shame

From a biosocial perspective, shame may result from physical and sexual assaults through the experience of submission and defeat. Andrews, Brown, Rose, and Kirk (2000) assessed individuals 1 month after they had experienced a violent crime, and again 6 months after initial assessment. The researchers found that feelings of shame at initial assessment were predictive of PTSD symptoms at time 1 and PTSD development at time 2. Of the respondents reporting high shame, the most common reason for feeling shame was that they had not taken effective action to prevent the victimization or trauma. This type of appraisal may also occur in children in abusive homes, despite their relative dependency and limited cognitive, physical, and social resources. One study noted that women with moderate or severe levels of child sexual abuse had significant levels of internalized shame (Playter, 1990). In addition to risk for PTSD, there is some evidence that shame is associated with risk for revictimization. In a large retrospective study of 548 college women, Kessler and Bieschke (1999) determined that shame mediated the relationship between childhood sexual abuse and adult victimization. Results also indicated that childhood sexual abuse survivors with higher levels of shame were more likely to be revictimized than both nonabused women and abused women with lower levels of internalized shame.

Shame appears to represent a sense of failure via experiences of defeat or submission. Beliefs that one is not competent to defend or protect oneself or others may create risk for successful revictimization via a self-fulfilling prophecy: "Given that I failed to protect myself then, I can't protect myself or don't deserve to protect myself now." Some data indicate that women who suffer from shame tend to become socially isolated and thus more vulnerable to future assaults (Kessler & Bieschke, 1999). It may be that a woman with high shame appraisal in a high-risk situation may quickly feel defeated or undeserving of escape and thus incapable of responding appropriately. Prospective studies are necessary to learn more about shame as a mediator between childhood sexual abuse and adult victimization.

PTSD AS A RISK FACTOR FOR RETRAUMATIZATION

Several epidemiological studies have found that after an individual has experienced one high-magnitude stressor, he or she is at risk for experiencing additional traumatic events over the lifespan (Breslau, Davis, Andreski, & Peterson, 1991; Kilpatrick, Saunders, Veronen, Best, & Von, 1987). Of even greater significance is the report that, at least among rape victims, the presence of PTSD, in and of itself, contributes to risk for repeated traumatization (National Victim Center and Crime Victims Research and Treatment Center, 1992). Given these findings, it becomes critical to determine whether individuals abused as children have PTSD related to the childhood abuse and/or assault.

There has been less than a complete consensus concerning the existence of a diagnostic category that adequately captures the range of symptoms associated with a history of childhood abuse. However, the accumulation of data indicates that PTSD is a salient, if not core, component of the complex of symptoms related to childhood sexual abuse (CSA). Accumulating evidence indicates that PTSD is a central and significantly debilitating outcome of childhood abuse. The DSM-IV field trials for PTSD identified the prevalence of CSA-related PTSD as 68% in a combined community and clinical sample (Roth, Newman, Pelcovitz, van der Kolk, & Mandel, 1997). A study assessing a clinical sample of 47 women with CSA found that 69% had PTSD (Rowan, Foy, Rodriquez, & Ryan, 1994). In another clinical study of 26 women with a history of CSA, 73% were diagnosed with PTSD (O'Neill & Gupta, 1991). In our own clinical sample of 98 women with CSA, Structured Clinical Interview for DSM-III-R (SCID-III-R) assessments revealed that 73% had DSM-III-R PTSD and that PTSD was the most prevalent Axis I disorder.

In a prospective study Sandberg et al. (1999) found that posttraumatic symptomatology moderated the relationship between child/adolescent sexual abuse and adult sexual abuse. Previous sexual victimization became more strongly associated with subsequent sexual victimization when posttraumatic symptomatology was taken into account. A limitation to the study was the length of the design, 10 weeks. Thirty percent (n = 98) of the sample had been sexually victimized during childhood and/or adolescence, and 8% (n = 27) had been victimized over the 10-week period. However, the study did not specify the number of women revictimized. The investigators did not find a mediating effect for posttraumatic symptomatology between childhood/adolescent sexual abuse and revictimization during said period.

Given that PTSD has been identified as a risk factor for additional sexual assaults among rape victims, it is possible that PTSD associated with CSA may be associated with even greater risk for subsequent assault than PTSD related to adulthood rape. This is because individuals who have PTSD deriving from childhood abuse are at risk for a greater portion of their lifespan, and the risk includes a period of life (childhood/adolescence) in which coping strategies for responding effectively to risk may be underdeveloped.

REVICTIMIZATION IN DIVERSE POPULATIONS

Much of the data on revictimization have focused on white and female samples. Evidence suggests that there is little difference across different ethnic groups of females. In addition, we consider the risk of revictimization among men, who are typically researched only in terms of their risk as perpetrators of violence rather than as victims of it.

Minority Samples

Prevalence rates of CSA are uniformly high across ethnicities. In a study of 1,093 women, Merrill et al. (1999) found similar rates across Hispanic (14%), black (13%) and white (19%) women in the sample. In addition, predictors of adult rape did not differ significantly between Hispanic, black, and white women. Similarly, Wyatt (1985) reported no differences in CSA prevalence rates between black and white women. A decade later, however, she assessed 18- to 36-year-old black and white women, comparable to the first sample (Wyatt, Burns Loeb, Solis, Vargas Carmona, & Romero, 1999). This time the difference in prevalence of sexual abuse was marginally significant: 29% of black compared to 39% of white women reported CSA, the result of increased reporting of abuse among white women as compared to the earlier sample. This difference may be due to either actual increased rates of abuse in white families or cultural differences in changes across time in labeling, defining, or willingness to report CSA, or some combination of both.

In contrast with childhood abuse, rates of reported revictimization appear to vary significantly by ethnicity. A study of 243 community college females found rates of revicimization higher for black women than white women (Urquiza & Goodlin-Jones, 1994). Among women reporting CSA, rates of later sexual assault (i.e., rape) were 44% of white women, 62% of black women, 40% of Hispanic women, and 25% of Asian American women. It seems that although prevalence rates of CSA do not vary significantly, revictimization rates might. Identifying the reasons for this disparity would potentially provide further insight into the relationship between childhood abuse and revictimization.

Male Samples

Sexual abuse occurs among boys about one-third as often as among girls. Community sample studies have found rates of sexual abuse among boys to range from 2.5 to 17%, depending on the definition of sexual abuse (Urquiza & Keating, 1990). A recent study of 17,337 adult health plan members found a prevalence of CSA to be 25% for women and 16% for men, using a contact definition for sexual abuse (Dong, Anda, Dube, Giles, & Felitti, 2003). A study of 7,850 male navy recruits found prevalence rates of 11–12% for CSA (Merrill, Thomsen, Gold, & Milner, 2001). A similar sample of female navy recruits found prevalence rates of 39% for CSA (Merrill et al., 1999). These data are consistent with the overall 1:3 sex ratio for CSA. In contrast, however, it should be noted that boys experience physical abuse more frequently than girls, particularly during the younger years (ages 1–11; National Center on Child Abuse and Neglect [NCCAN], 1994, 1995; Raiha & Soma, 1997).

Community studies have determined that one of the more disturbing consequences of childhood sexual and physical abuse in boys is increased risk of violent behavior in adulthood (see Finkelhor & Dziuba-Leatherman, 1994; Malinosky-Rummell & Hansen, 1993; Widom, 1989, for reviews). These studies have led to the general notion that, among men, "violence breeds violence." However, the evidence supporting this relationship is relatively weak and hampered by methodological limitations, such as failure to include appropriate comparison groups and disregard of confounding factors of childhood abuse, such as poverty and low educational attainment.

A large study that included a control group and attention to demographic variables (Merrill et al., 2001) found that men who had experienced only childhood physical abuse or only CSA were about twice as likely to commit rape than nonabused men, whereas men who had experienced both types of abuse were four to six times more likely to commit rape than nonabused men. However, like other research (e.g., Widom, 1989), this study limited the examination of consequences of childhood abuse among men to adult aggressive behaviors and did not investigate the potential relationship between a history of childhood abuse and an increased risk for adult victimization.

One study examined risk for both victimization and perpetration in a large sample of male psychiatric patients (Cloitre, Tardiff, Marzuk, Leon, & Potera, 2001). Prevalence rates of childhood abuse were 20% for physical abuse only, 7% sexual abuse only, and 10% both. This study investigated the relationship between childhood abuse and three violent adult outcomes: becoming (1) a perpetrator of interpersonal violence, (2) a victim of interpersonal violence, and (3) both perpetrator and victim of adult interpersonal violence. Controlling for diagnostic and demographic variables, men abused as children were two and a half times as likely as nonabused men to be victims of interpersonal violence and five times as likely to be both victims and perpetrators in adulthood. No relationship was found between childhood abuse and the perpetrator-only group. These data suggest that the relationship between childhood abuse and adulthood violence among men is more complex than was originally considered. The most common consequence of childhood abuse, at least among psychiatrically impaired men, is becoming both a victim and a perpetrator. Cloitre et al. reanalyzed the data to parallel previous studies, defining the adult outcome variable as perpetration of violence regardless of victimization status. They obtained results consistent with the other studies: Men who had been abused as children were nearly twice as likely to be perpetrators of violence in adulthood. These data demonstrate that neglect to examine male adult revictimization may generate results that provide only a partial picture and underestimate the impact of childhood abuse. These data have implications for the development of intervention and prevention programs for men with adulthood violence, focusing on the identification of past abuse and the relationship between acts of violence as perpetrator and as victim.

IMPLICATIONS FOR A TREATMENT MODEL

The model from which the treatment intervention described here is derived assumes that there are three categories of psychological risk factors for revictimization: (1) problems in affect regulation, (2) problems in interpersonal relatedness and self-appraisal, and (3) PTSD symptoms. The model also identifies two related sources of these problems. One derives from the abuse itself and its direct psychological sequelae, such as disrupted thresholds for arousal and posttraumatic stress symptoms. The other is the familial or caretaking situation, which is frequently limited or highly maladaptive in providing a learning environment for the development of basic affect regulation skills, adaptive beliefs about self and others, and associated interpersonal behaviors. This assessment suggests that the reduction of risk for future assault will require a two-component intervention: one focused on skills training related to the development of affect regulation and adaptive interpersonal beliefs and abilities, and the second on the amelioration of the direct psychological sequelae of trauma, such as PTSD.

Prevention programs to reduce risk of sexual assault have proven successful for women who did not have sexual assault histories, but not for women with histories of revictimization (Breitenbecher & Gidycz, 1998; Hanson & Gidycz, 1993). The most intensive prevention program designed to date, developed specifically for sexual abuse survivors to prevent revictimization, has shown success (Marx et al., 2001). The protocol combined the psychoeducational program developed by Hanson and Gidycz (1993) with a modified relapse prevention approach, including identification of high-risk situations, problem solving, coping skills training, assertiveness training, and development of communication skills. The intervention consisted of two 2-hour group sessions of 5–10 participants, held at a maximum of 2 days a part. Sixty-six undergraduate women with a history of sexual victimization (defined as any unwanted sexual contact) from the age of 14 were randomly assigned to either an intervention or a control group. Rates of overall revictimization during the 2 months prior to follow-up did not differ between the control group and the intervention group. However, a significant difference was found between the two groups for experiencing completed rape: 30% (20) of control group participants versus 12% (8) of intervention group participants reported being raped during the 2-month follow-up period ($X^2 = 2.45$, $p = .05$, one-tailed). These types of programs are useful because they take a prevention approach to a young and highly at-risk population and cast a wide net in a nonstigmatizing environment. The following model serves a clinical population in which many have experienced multiple traumas and have developed PTSD. Both models share a common assumption about the need for interventions that enhance or rehabilitate interpersonal and coping skills to protect the individual and reduce the risk of continued victimization.

A PROPOSED TREATMENT MODEL: SKILLS TRAINING IN AFFECT AND INTERPERSONAL REGULATION/ MODIFIED PROLONGED EXPOSURE

The treatment model recommended for retraumatized women is a two-phase model in which the first phase of treatment focuses on skills training in affect and interpersonal regulation (STAIR). Training includes skills development in (1) identifying and labeling feeling states (especially feelings of threat), (2) tolerating distress and modulating negative affect, and (3) identifying abuse-related interpersonal schemas that initiate and shape negative interpersonal situations and developing alternative, more adaptive schemas, (4) developing an expanded interpersonal behavioral repertoire, and (5) practicing and testing it in the "real world." Cognitive-behavioral techniques used to meet these goals include monitoring and rating feeling states, use of positive imagery and self-statements, identifying and challenging maladaptive cognitions, and role plays that emphasize context-sensitive and flexible interpersonal responses. Treatment is organized into eight sessions, although the treatment can be lengthened depending on the client's needs.

The second phase of treatment is an eight-session modified prolonged exposure (MPE) treatment adapted from Foa's treatment for rape-related PTSD (Foa, Rothbaum, Riggs, & Murdock, 1991). The goal of this phase is to help the patient engage in exposure to the trauma memory in order to resolve posttraumatic stress symptoms such as fearfulness, nightmares, and irritability.

In the two-module approach, the STAIR phase takes place first. STAIR provides the client and therapist with a stabilization phase in which the therapeutic relationship can develop, and in which the client can acquire and practice skills that are intended to improve functioning in day-to-day life and, accordingly, that provide a sense of success and competence. Furthermore, skills training precedes exposure so that the increased ability to regulate feeling states obtained from phase 1 can be utilized to enhance the effectiveness of the PTSD-related exposure work of phase 2. However, the modules can be used separately. In particular, the STAIR module can be used alone as a skills training/prevention program for individuals at risk for assault who do not suffer from significant PTSD symptoms. Table 13.1 summarizes the sessions included in STAIR and MPE intervention approaches.

TABLE 13.1. Summary of STAIR/MPE Sessions

Session	Focus and content
STAIR	
Session 1	*Introduction to treatment:* Psychoeducation on effects of childhood abuse on three problem domains: emotion regulation, interpersonal functioning, and PTSD symptoms; treatment overview and goals; psychoeducation and practice of focused breathing
Session 2	*Identification and labeling of feelings:* Psychoeducation on impact of childhood abuse on experiencing emotions; introduction and practice of self-monitoring of feelings, triggers, intensity, and coping/reaction
Session 3	*Emotion regulation:* Psychoeducation on connection between feelings, thoughts, and behaviors; identification of strengths and weaknesses in emotion regulation skill (cognitive, behavioral, social network domains); practicing new coping skills
Session 4	*Distress tolerance:* Psychoeducation on acceptance of feelings/distress tolerance; assessment of pros and cons of tolerating distress; identification and practice of pleasurable activities
Session 5	*Distinguishing between past trauma schemas and current goals:* Psychoeducation on interpersonal schemas related to childhood traumatic events as self-fulfilling prophecies; distinguishing between trauma-related schemas and "here-and-now" interpersonal goals; identification of schemas in a current problematic situation
Session 6	*Alternative interpersonal schemas:* Psychoeducation on role playing; identification of relevant interpersonal situations and enactment via role plays; generation of alternative schemas
Session 7	*Assertivenesss and control schemas:* Psychoeducation on assertiveness; discussion of alternative schemas and behavioral responses; implementation of role plays requiring assertiveness; generation of alternative schemas
Session 8	*Flexibility in schema application:* Psychoeducation on flexibility in interpersonal relationships; implementation of role plays requiring flexibility; generation of alternative schemas; discussion of transition from phase 1 to phase 2 of treatment
MPE	
Session 9	*Introduction to imaginal exposure:* Psychoeducation on rationale and technique; development of a narrative; creation of trauma memory hierarchy
Session 10	*Imaginal exposure to first memory:* Implementation of prolonged imaginal exposure; postexposure implementation of stabilization exercise; identification and labeling of feelings narratives identification of schemas embedded in narrative; contrast of trauma schemas with current developing schemas
Sessions 11–15	*Continued work on imaginal exposure:* Working through memory hierarchy with probes, clarifications, and greater evocative details; continuation of feeling and schema analysis of narrative
Session 16	*Wrapping up:* Identification of progress, risk for relapse, relapse prevention strategies

ASSESSMENT

There is growing evidence that the psychological effects of trauma are cumulative (Follette et al., 1996; Nishith, Mechanic, & Resick, 1997). Thus it is important to obtain a thorough history of trauma across the lifespan, ranging from childhood physical, sexual, and emotional abuse to adult events, including exposures to natural or human-made disasters.

Assessment of PTSD can be accomplished effectively by using the Clinician Administered PTSD Scale (CAPS), which includes separate frequency and intensity scales for PTSD symptoms and items that assess social and occupational functioning (Blake et al., 1995). In addition, the Structured Clinical Interview for DSM-IV (SCID; Spitzer, Williams, Gibbon, & First, 1994) is useful in assessing the entire range of Axis I and Axis II disorders. Of special diagnostic interest in this population is the presence of complex PTSD, which can be assessed using the Structured Interview for Disorders of Extreme Stress (SIDES; Pelcovitz et al., 1997). This clinician-administered instrument systematically assesses typical problems in affect regulation, somatization, dissociation, and problems in meaning systems concerning self and the world.

A comprehensive history of physical health status should be obtained because women with multiple traumas tend to have a relatively large number of health problems, some of which (e.g., sexually transmitted diseases) may impact psychological and interpersonal issues that emerge during treatment. Self-report questionnaires, which may not be typical in general treatment settings but are useful for assessment of trauma-related problems and symptoms and can be used by both client and therapist during the course of treatment, include assessment of alexithymia (Toronto Alexithymia Scale; Taylor, Bagby, Ryan, Parker, & Doody, 1988), anger expression (State–Trait Anger Expression Inventory; Spielberger, 1988), Negative Mood Regulation (Catanzaro & Mearns, 1990), and dissociative experiences (Dissociative Experiences Scale; Bernstein & Putnam, 1986). Last, use of self-report measures that evaluate social support (e.g., Social Adjustment Scale; Weissman & Bothell, 1976), interpersonal skills (e.g., Inventory of Interpersonal Problems; Horowitz, Rosenberg, Baer, Ureno, & Villasenor, 1988) and coping skills (e.g., Coping Orientation to Problems Experienced; Scheier & Carver, 1985) will help identify strengths and characteristic responses to stressors—all of which will help shape treatment goals and activities.

A complete evaluation of a multiply traumatized woman is a lengthy and emotionally draining experience for the client. The client may be providing information about her history that she has never revealed and aspects of her functioning about which she is embarrassed. Although this self-revelation can be painful, it is often a relief for the client to be given a coherent understanding of her symptom picture and to engage in a collaborative and supportive effort in organizing a plan for treatment.

GUIDELINES FOR SELECTION

Any individual who has experienced CSA and additional assaults in childhood or adulthood may be considered for this treatment. Assessment of role functioning, dissociation, alexithymia, interpersonal schemas, and posttraumatic stress symptomatology will help determine where the emphases in treatment should be placed. There are certain problems for which this treatment is not ideally suited and which require referral to alternative programs. These include substance dependence, moderate to severe self-mutilation, high risk for suicide, and presence of a dissociative disorder. We have been successful in treating individuals with substance abuse, mild self-mutilation, and chronic suicidal ideation. The judgment remains with the clinician to determine the degree of coping skills available to the patient to manage states of high distress as well as the degree of his or her motivation to learn new skills. Individuals in domestic violence situations or battering relationships also need direct and immediate help from programs developed specifically for these problems. Last, it should be noted that women who have chronic mental illnesses, such as schizophrenia or schizoaffective disorder, are among the group of women most at risk for retraumatization (Cloitre et al., 1996). Often, these women have expressed concerns that traditional cognitive-behavioral programs are not geared toward them: They do not understand the material, nor do they share the same perspective. There are programs currently being developed for people with chronic mentally illness with these issues in mind, and referral such a program would be ideal (Jonikas & Cook, 1994).

CLINICAL APPLICATION

The following case describes the situation of a multiply traumatized woman whose most significant symptom was avoidance of cognitive, emotional, and behavioral difficulties associated with her many traumas. Underlying her avoidant style in all of these domains was a sense of helplessness–hopelessness regarding her recovery and, more particularly, her ability to protect herself from future traumas. As treatment progressed, it became clear that she viewed herself as having one source of strength from which she derived great pride, and that was her ability to withstand the abuse of others. The client not only believed that she was "fated" for a life of trauma, but also she embraced it as a guiding principle in her life. This perspective had multiple functions: It provided (1) a source of personal identity and stability in an otherwise chaotic life, (2) a sense of control and mastery over herself and others, and (3) a sense of meaning and purposefulness for herself. Her core interpersonal schema was "If I am abused, then I am worthwhile," and her self-appraisal involved pride about, rather than shame in, her experiences of "defeat and submission." In her self-appraisal, wrought of desperation, she reversed the typical beliefs about consequences of chronic abuse to psychologically buoy herself up: In submission, she had found her strength.

The treatment focused on (1) identifying and counteracting her trauma-related emotional, cognitive, and behavioral avoidance activities; (2) identifying existing coping skills, which would provide evidence that she was not as helpless–hopeless as she felt herself to be; (3) providing motivation for her to "give up" her identity as a victim by identifying alternative interpersonal schemas and behaviors that would support connection to others and the development of healthy, nonabusive relationships; and (4) further motivating "letting go" of her identify as victim via realistic appraisals of success and competence in day-to-day life rather than only in traumatic circumstances.

Once these tasks were set in motion, the emotional processing of the trauma via prolonged exposure to the trauma memories was initiated and successfully completed.

Case Description

Ms. F came for evaluation of PTSD under the recommendation of her psychopharmacologist, whom she had been seeing for treatment of moderate to severe depression. Ms. F, 48 years old, spoke in a soft voice with a faint Hungarian accent and revealed herself to be a gentle and well-educated individual. Approximately 1 year earlier, Ms. F had been raped by an intruder into her fiancé's apartment while he was away. Her recollection of the rape and the accompanying violent physical assault was vivid, although she had no memory of the several hours after the rape, which she had spent in a local emergency room. Following the rape, she had not been able to shake a growing conviction that the world was a dangerous place and that she was constitutionally unable to protect herself.

She had quit her job as a manager of a small art gallery because the presence of men alone in the store with her made her feel vulnerable and elicited frightening images of being attacked, raped, and even tortured. She began feeling highly anxious and avoided situations that reminded her of the rape and in which she felt she might be attacked, particularly elevators, taxis, and empty streets. She retreated to the comfort and safety of her apartment but in the process lost connection with some of her friends, who, over the year, lost sympathy with her situation. She had also broken off her engagement because she believed her fiancé blamed her for the rape and had lost desire for her. She maintained her income by translating art history books, but her concentration had deteriorated to the point that she was unable to translate more than a paragraph a day. She had begun sleeping a lot to escape her preoccupation with her fears and from exhaustion derived from the anxiety symptoms she experienced when she did venture out. Her sleep was fitful and punctuated with nightmares of violence.

Upon questioning, Ms. F revealed a history of having been emotionally and physically abused by her mother throughout her childhood. Also, she was born in Hungary at the outset of World War II, and thus spent the first 5 years of her life exposed to "bombs, fire, deaths, and hysterical adults." At ages 5–8, she was sexually abused by a neighborhood man. The abuse ended when her family relocated. In her late teens she came to the United States and began a successful career as a model, followed by graduate training and employment as an art historian, which she enjoyed very much. She had had a few long-term and passionate romances but had left those relationships when discord or conflict developed and had never married or had children. She had experienced a rape previous to the rape for which she had come into treatment. The man had been a stranger who had assaulted her in the vestibule of her home. He was eventually identified as a serial rapist in the neighborhood and was convicted of rape and imprisoned. She had also experienced a mugging and a significant accident in which she broke her arm and leg, and for which she required extensive physical rehabilitation.

The second and most recent rape seemed to have crystallized trauma-based beliefs about herself and the world that had otherwise lain dormant. She viewed the world as a dangerous place, believed that there was something about herself that attracted violence, and was convinced that she was entirely responsible for the traumas and problems she had experienced, from the rapes to the failed relationships. She felt fated to a life of accumulated traumas and expected that she would die a horrible, violent death. She had never been in individual psychotherapy. Shortly after the second rape, she had entered a rape survivor group but had become extremely upset listening to the experiences of other rape victims and had left the group after the second session.

Treatment Overview: The Therapeutic Alliance

Regardless of the form of intervention applied in the treatment of the multiply traumatized woman, there is one unifying aspect of treatment, and that is the therapist–client alliance. Because clients with a history of childhood abuse may have negative responses to perceived authority figures, a first and perhaps continuing challenge throughout the treatment is managing issues of power, control, and trust in the treatment process. The therapist must be aware that the client has little reason to expect good to come from those in positions of authority and that he or she is likely to react negatively to strongly didactic approaches to treatment. It is easy for client and therapist to "lock horns" on issues that threaten the client's sense of safety, such as changing comfortable but maladaptive behaviors. The therapist can step out of power struggles by simply presenting the alternatives to the client and letting the client select the treatment activity for him- or herself. Usually, the ultimate choice is between continuing in patterns of behavior that the client has already decided to reject and taking risks in doing new and frightening things. The client will need to decide for him- or herself what he or she wishes to do.

Early in the treatment the therapist and client should identify goals and the means by which they will be achieved. The therapy thereby becomes a partnership in which the client and therapist identify problems, the therapist proposes interventions, and both therapist and client tailor the interventions as needed to the specific situation. In the case of Ms. F, it seemed wiser to encourage her take a strong lead in the treatment and use her keen intelligence to work through some of the conflicting issues for herself and take responsibility for solving the problems at hand. For example, although Ms. F's avoidance behaviors made her feel somewhat safe, she realized they never made her feel free or happy. It was her choice to decide between feeling "safe" in the short run versus "free" in the long run. This process provided a more thorough analysis of the pros and cons of a choice point in treatment than the therapist might otherwise have obtained. It also instilled a sense of responsibility and mastery in the client and increased motivation for follow-through on behavioral plans.

Phase 1: Skills Training in Affective and Interpersonal Regulation

Affective Regulation

Skills training in affective regulation involves (1) enhancing emotional awareness and (2) developing greater ability in modulating negative feelings and tolerating distress. In the first sessions clients are introduced to the activity of self-monitoring of feelings of distress, including identifying triggering situations and the intensity and frequency of the distress. Clients are also taught how to label and identify different feeling states (e.g., happy, sad, mad). Although this exercise appears quite simple, it can be a revolutionary experience for individuals who, from early life, have avoided or have never been guided in differentiating and labeling their own feeling states. Often these exercises provide validation of feelings that were previously ignored or unrecognized. Such exercises can also produce experiences of self-expansion in clients: a "filling out" of their emotional self that is validated by the therapist's interest in the client reports, thoughts, and concerns.

Clients are also quickly introduced to self-soothing and affect-regulation activities, so that as feelings emerge they have some ability to moderate or control them. These coping strategies include deep breathing, utilization of time-outs (which can vary from 3 minutes to a weekend), and cognitive exercises such as thought stopping, shifting of attention, and positive imagery and self-statements. In addition, the concept of identifying and countering maladaptive cognitions is introduced in the context of inquiring about clients' fears around experiencing and expressing their feelings. Frequent beliefs that emerge are "I'll get out of control," "I'll hit someone," and "I'll become my abuser." Elaborating on and countering these beliefs helps clients engage more readily and confidently in emotional experiencing. New coping techniques are introduced every session with demonstration and practice and followed by "between-session" daily practice of each skill. Each session also includes review of the between-session work and additional practice focused on trouble spots.

In the fourth session, after clients have begun to develop some affect regulation skills, they or are introduced to the concept of allowing and accepting the experience of distress. Significant psychoeducation takes place on this point, because many find the concept of accepting pain somewhat counterintuitive. However, the goal is for clients to understand that some distress in life is unavoidable. This truism is particularly relevant for clients who will ultimately need to confront and assimilate the pain of their trauma histories. Other psychoeducational aspects of distress tolerance include the notions that distress is a part of the process of changing oneself, that in order to experience positive feelings, one must allow for negative feelings, and that the inability to accept unavoidable distress leads to increased pain and suffering.

Client and therapist review situations that the client finds distressing and review the pros and cons of tolerating each situation. For example, Ms. F and her therapist reviewed the distress Ms. F experienced with even the smallest of physical intimacies with her boyfriend. Being embraced by him made her feel nauseous and disgusted. Her sole desire in these moments was to jump out of the embrace. Client and therapist reviewed reasons why she might want to tolerate this experience, which included her desire to connect with someone who seemed to understand her history and genuinely liked her, and, more generally, to be able to have positive reactions to touch and physical contact.

Client and therapist should, in addition, identify and practice coping techniques to assist in distress tolerance. These can include titrating the duration of the experience, deep-breathing exercises, self-statements such as "I can bear this for a little while," or temporarily leaving the upsetting situation and finding a soothing alternative activity (e.g., resting, taking a walk, washing hands and face).

Interventions for Affective Regulation Treatment Obstacles

The program described thus far is composed of relatively standard cognitive-behavioral techniques. The demonstration and practice of these techniques will pose little difficulty for the therapist. More challenging is coping with clients' desires to avoid feelings and their lack of confidence and sense of mastery in the process. These difficulties are often bound up with clients' history of abuse and their family–social learning experiences. The therapist will need to find ways to maintain clients' motivation and to introduce coping skills in ways that have value and meaning to individuals with chronic and early life trauma. Listed below are four interventions for coping with avoidance and sense-of-mastery problems.

1. *Provide a historical frame for avoidant behaviors.* Retraumatized individuals may believe that by using avoidance strategies they are behaving in ways that will protect them physically and emotionally. This belief may stem from the fact that the coping strategies they use, such as emotional numbing, denial, and acceptance of abuse, were actually adaptive under the circumstances of inescapable and chronic abuse. Because such strategies have worked in the past, their current application may give clients some sense of mastery, whereas the application of new strategies may engender anxiety. In addition, these avoidant strategies may be deeply entrenched because their use may extend as far back as childhood, and clients may believe that they are the best and only coping strategies available to them.

One way to reduce anxiety and rigidity about coping strategies is to first point out the effectiveness of clients' coping strategies as they applied to past situations. Clients have, after all, managed to survive through a series of traumas or escape from a chronically traumatizing environment. Pointing out clients' basic success establishes the fact that they have the capacity and resources to cope with difficult situations. With this reassurance in mind, they may be better able to begin contemplating both the frightening and wonderful view that they are no longer in the chronically abusive situation and that they need to change their coping strategies to adapt to a changed or changing life context.

2. *Provide psychoeducation about the negative consequences of avoidance.* Clients with trauma histories who avoid their feelings also often avoid thinking about their avoidance. It is useful to draw out explicitly the burdens of avoidance—a consideration to which clients may have given little focused attention. It is useful to review the fact that although avoidance appears to give a person control in the short run (e.g., immediate reduction in symptoms), he or she is really out of control with regard to long-term goals. For example, Ms. F avoided many situations—cars, elevators, downtown areas, and certain park areas. Although this activity provided her with immediate relief from her anxiety, her life began faltering, especially her search for a job, because there were so many places to which she would not travel for interviews. Furthermore, avoidance limited her life experience, including pleasurable activities and feelings. Despite the fact that avoidance seemed to provide Ms. F with brief emotional respites, she experienced almost chronic anxiety and fear, with little room for other feelings. She had few experiences with which to counter the powerful images and feelings that were associated with her catastrophic predictions of what would happen if she ventured out. Her form of emotional experiencing—a rather exhausting blend of fear, anxiety, and depression—became her uniform. For many individuals abused as children, avoiding feelings and engaging in a limited set of prescribed behaviors were among the few coping strategies available in their chronically abusive homes. Therapist and client need to review ways in which these behaviors ultimately create a prison in adulthood.

3. *Assess coping skills.* In order to help clients leave behind familiar but

maladaptive coping strategies, it is extremely useful to identify coping skills that are currently effective and others that, with some adaptation, can be put to good use. Client and therapist should systematically review the coping strategies the client currently uses to deal with difficult feelings and situations. The Negative Mood Regulation self-report instrument (Cantanzaro & Mearns, 1990) is one measure that can be used to assess baseline coping skills. This measure rates how strongly a client believes him- or herself capable of engaging in a particular coping strategy (e.g., "Telling myself it will pass will help calm me down").

Sometimes clients cannot report any coping strategies that they view positively. Often, however, the client does have some good coping skills—they are simply not discernible from within a negative or abusive life context. The therapist can help the client "translate" skills used in negative life circumstances for healthier purposes. For example, a recovered heroin addict was reminded that she had always been able to "hustle" enough money together to satisfy her addiction. She did, in fact, have a very good "sales person" personality and was very likable. Her therapist was able to help her view these behaviors as skills that could aid her in finding satisfactory employment in a people-oriented setting. Successful transition of behaviors from one life circumstance to another can provide a sense of continuity in self-identity and speed the process of skills enhancement. In the case of Ms. F, it was noted that she was well able to identify and monitor the mood of a potentially threatening person. This was an activity she had practiced extensively in childhood in order to manage and subdue her mother's irritability and reduce the risk of getting a beating. This interpersonal sensitivity was identified as a skill ready for "translation" to current circumstances. Her ability to detect the pleasure–displeasure of others was keen. The reorganization of this skill required disconnecting her monitoring skills from the automatic behavior of acquiescing to the source of threat. Client and therapist were able to identify a few alternative behaviors that would better protect her from danger.

4. *Give recognition to realistic fears and risks of relapse.* Standard cognitive-behavioral interventions, such as identifying and correcting faulty thinking patterns (e.g., exaggerating the probabilities of a negative emotional event), are a valuable component in reducing avoidance. The countering of maladaptive beliefs, however, must be framed realistically in the context of a life history of abuse. For example, Ms. F identified the following: "There is something vulnerable about me. My anxiety might attract someone to harm me. I've been assaulted before. That means I am likely to be assaulted again." Ms. F's thinking had some basis in facts. Her history did indicate increased risk for future assaults. She might have been correct that her anxiety was one of several cues that indicated that she was an "easy target" to potential perpetrators. Nevertheless, as treatment progressed, she learned to accept accurate and effective alternative thoughts, including "I am not as easy a target as I was a few months ago" and "I am in better control of my anxiety." These

types of statements should be reinforced with evidence. For example, Ms. F's treatment work led to improvement in her ability to assess more versus less dangerous situations. A decrease in hypervigilance led to a better sense of reality and better apportioning of her attention to actual threats.

Interpersonal Schemas and Interpersonal Skills Training

The second part of the treatment flows directly from the skills training in affect regulation, which serves as a foundation for the development of more adaptive interpersonal behaviors. One "transition session" is devoted to a discussion about the tendency for individuals with affect regulation problems to engage in excessively confrontational and/or avoidant behaviors when dealing with interpersonal conflict (see Linehan, 1993). In addition, clients are invited to consider ways in which the feelings they experience in some settings have little to do with the interpersonal demands and goals of the situation and more to do with the presence of emotional triggers associated with their abuse. The client is asked to describe various relationship difficulties. The goal for the client and therapist is to extract the core interpersonal schema from these situations. Typical core schemas include "If I express feelings, then I will be punished" or "If I ask for my needs to be met, I will be abandoned." Stripped down to caricature, the schemas often express the relationship between self and other in black-and-white terms, particularly in regard to themes of power and control: someone is a victim (powerless and with no control), and the other is a perpetrator (with unmitigated power and control).

Identification of interpersonal schemas is the foundation for all other intervention efforts. Identification of the core schema provides a guide for the analysis of future or ongoing interpersonal situations, with rapid detection of the key difficulties followed by corrective intervention. The identification of the core schema also provides a (foil?) with which to contrast alternative schemas (e.g., "Some of my friends welcome me to express my feelings"). The new schema is treated as a hypothesis that is tested in the "real world," with the use of appropriate interpersonal skills that are developing or being reinforced in the treatment. Furthermore, the notion of the interpersonal schema is the conceptual bridge between the phase 1 skills and phase 2 exposure components of the treatment. During phase 1, established schemas are identified, and new, more adaptive schemas are formulated and tested. During phase 2, the client is asked, after every new exposure, to identify the interpersonal schemas within the trauma narrative. The goal is to contrast the "old" schema with the "new" one and, by doing so, facilitate an awareness of the passage of time and the occurence of change since the non-distant trauma. Placing distance between the past and present allows the client to consider that the old schema, once justified and perhaps necessary, is now obsolete. The schemas emerging from more recent experience ideally take on more relevance and influence. These ideas are reinforced during phase 2 exposure exercises.

Self-Appraisal and Shame

The notion of interpersonal schema has its basis in attachment theory and accordingly assumes that sense of self develops inextricably in the context of relationship to others. Self-definition is shaped and informed by the content and character of interpersonal experiences. For this reason, work on self-appraisals follows work on interpersonal schemas. Identification of self-appraisals often emerges from, or is highly consistent with, identified interpersonal schemas. Clients' schemas and negative beliefs about self are often derived from experiences with, and feedback from, abusive caretakers. Clients frequently assume that they were treated badly because they were bad. Ms. F, for example, believed that she was bad for letting herself be abused as a child. This belief was maintained because of the distorted, unrealistic expectations she currently held concerning her own autonomy and mastery as a child. In addition, Ms. F's belief in "self as bad" stemmed from being told that she was bad by her mother and other family members. This label organized her experience: It created consistency between what was happening to her (how she was treated) and who she was.

Ms. F's feelings of shame alternated between the belief that she "let the abuse happen to her" (experiences of submission and defeat) and that she must have deserved the abuse (experience of self as bad). Sometimes these beliefs were toxically combined: She felt shamed that she let the abuse happen. In considering the possibility that she had not deserved the abuse (i.e., she was not a "bad child"), she then became bad for letting the abuse happen. In her adulthood Ms. F tired of the burden of such shame but could not extend her repertoire of behaviors beyond those defined by a victim role. This limitation resulted in her reorganization of a core schema to support the belief that victim behaviors were reasons to be proud. Ms. F desperately wanted to think well of herself. She simply could not imagine behaviors and ways of relating to others that did not include victimization. Ms. F concluded that "my only strength is in understanding and accepting people whose inner turmoil leads them to be abusive." More problematic was the firm belief that she could not create relationships based in schemas other than variants of the victim–abuser dyad. She was convinced that "if I try to be with others who don't abuse me, they don't want me or don't accept me."

Various interventions were implemented to help change these beliefs. We first addressed her belief that she was bad because she had "let the abuse happen." Review of the dependence of children on adults for basic survival needs, as well as their relatively underdeveloped resources in cognitive and emotional domains, was helpful in revising this distorted perspective. Of greatest impact, however, was engaging in "homework" to watch neighborhood children approximately the same age as she was (between 5 and 8 years) when she was abused. Watching them play and interact with adults provided very concrete and realistic information about the significant levels of dependency and trust children exhibit toward adults. Next we addressed the belief that she deserved the abuse because she was a bad person. This belief was challenged in a straightforward way by asking Ms. F to assess the quality and soundness of her mother's judgment, whom she had described in ways that suggested her mother's functioning was globally impaired. We also searched for alternative sources of information: What bad things had she done lately? Had she ever done anything good? Positive responses in this area provided a small but accumulating foundation of "evidence" for the creation of positive self-regard, which was reinforced by the therapist. These more positive views of herself were explored and tested frequently in well-considered interpersonal exchanges in the "real world," as described below.

Obstacles in Identifying and Changing Interpersonal Schemas and Self-Appraisal

Those abused as children often "protect" or avoid designating any blame to their perpetrators, even into adulthood. This behavior is often related to the fact that the perpetrator of the assault was a caretaker and expected to provide love, concern for, and protection of the child. Recognition of the caretaker's failure in this regard often engenders a great sense of loss and betrayal. In the language of interpersonal schema theory, the survivor of childhood abuse is confronted with the fact that the ordinary contingencies for obtaining protection from a care-figure, which are considered a biological given or "birthright," did not occur for him or her. This realization leads to more and sometimes new negative feelings of anger, hurt, and confusion.

Still, identifying and exploring the responsibility of the care-figure for the abuse is an important component of the treatment. The survivor's assumption of blame often functions to protect the past and current relationship with the abusive caretaker. However, it also keeps intact a maladaptive schema. This, in turn, places the client at risk for using such a schema in the development of future relationships. For example, if the victim does not recognize that it was wrong for his or her caretaker to provide care contingent upon sexual favors, then he or she is at risk for finding this contingency acceptable in future relationships. The person will have reasons "at the ready" for finding such behavior acceptable (e.g., "He [or she] can't help himself [herself]").

Interpersonal Skills Training

Problems with assertiveness and conflict resolution are often related to poor skills in these areas. The client has extensive experience interacting with abusive care-figures. Thus it is likely that the client's behavioral repertoire is heavily based on internalized interpersonal schemas related to victim–abuser roles. The victim role tends to present the self as unquestioning, undeserving, fearful, and groveling. The abuser role tends to present the self as bullying, inconsiderate of the needs of others, and operating from ultimatums. Neither of these roles is an appropriate or effective starting point for successful assertive behavior or conflict resolution. Client and therapist can role-play specific scenarios to provide "practice" experiences in doing things differently. Such scenarios may include interviewing for a job, asking for a raise, or expressing preferences for what to do on a Friday night out with a friend. The goal is to identify the client's goals and feelings and practice how they can be expressed in words and actions. Often the therapist can help the client find the right language, explore with the client the feelings he or she experienced in the role play (e.g., feeling scared, strange, or "fake"), and identify and challenge the activation of maladaptive cognitions during the role play (e.g., "I don't deserve a raise").

Ms. F, for example, really did not want to go to a party given by a friend because he had been bullying her. Client and therapist role-played a phone conversation with this friend, in which the client stated she would not be attending the party. The client role-played herself and the therapist role-played the bullying friend. The client's initial role play immediately placed her in a position in which she was overly apologetic, defensive, and whining in tone. The therapist reversed this role play, explaining to the friend in a sensitive but unapologetic manner that she would not be able to attend the party but would want to meet with the friend at another time when they could spend some private time together. The client oriented herself to this language and tone and practiced in an effective way. The role play was also useful because it facilitated identification and processing of Ms. F's conflicting beliefs about herself (e.g., "I am being selfish; although he is a bully, he really needs me" vs. "I have a right to be treated well by my friend and should be able to talk with him about this").

Obstacles in Interpersonal Skills Training

1. *Staying focused on the here-and-now goal.* Often the client's feelings from the past contradict (or oppose) and overwhelm current interpersonal goals. The client with an abuse history is typically easily distressed or angered by interpersonal conflict. Through general coaching and role play, the client can learn how to allow interpersonal situations to be guided by the goals of the interaction (e.g., obtaining a preferred vacation time from boss) rather than an emerging feeling state (e.g., anger at boss for exploiting and overworking client). Frequently, intensive work is required in this area, and skills training in affect regulation is critical to moving forward. Clients need to learn how to use self-soothing skills and appropriate cognitive reframing skills in order to maintain focus on, and achieve, an interpersonal goal.

2. *Creating context sensitivity and flexibility in interpersonal roles and reactions.* Clients with an abuse history often have difficulty trusting their judgments and evaluating the appropriate level of assertiveness in a situation. Because they tend to have limited and rigid schemas, they may assess a situation in such a way that results in their taking on a stance that is either too passive (the victim role) or too controlling (the abuser role), and in which the particulars of the situation are not well addressed. It is useful for the client and therapist to review situations in which the client may have been either too controlling or too assertive and identify ways to modify his or her behavior. This review highlights the importance of context: Who, what, and where determine the appropriate action and reaction. Next the client is asked to engage in multiple role plays involving particular types of interpersonal conflict in which the therapist plays a different significant other each time (e.g., client's boss, spouse, child, mother). These role plays provide material for discussion of the fact that different assumptions, attitudes, language, and behavior occur with different people, even when the goals are quite similar. The role plays are also intended to (a) contribute to the construction of a variety of new interpersonal schemas, especially as they relate to person- and situation-specific differences, and (b) provide clients with an opportunity to enhance their self-experience (i.e., understand themselves as persons who can be flexible in behaviors and attitudes).

3. *Pacing behavioral change and risk of relapse.* The skills training module includes a substantial amount of role playing involving difficult interpersonal situations. This training is intended to help clients create or expand a behavioral repertoire that will support them in avoiding high-risk situations and foster the development of successful interactions and relationships. However, many therapists note that individuals with repeated traumas have difficulty entering and staying in nonabusive relationships and that progress in treatment is often followed by relapse into abusive relationships and behaviors. One reason for this difficulty is the large number of behavioral and cognitive changes required by individuals as they move out of abuse schemas and begin identifying and experimenting with healthier interpersonal behaviors. These changes entail a reorganization of their sense of self, and in this reorganizational period, clients are in an emotionally fragile state. Unexpected stressors that occur when clients enter a new relationship or job situation may overwhelm them. They may literally not know what to say, do, or feel in these new situations. Some clients report losing sight of what they want and who they think they are. In this state, it is easy for clients to fall back into abusive relationships and behaviors, not because they feel good, but because they are familiar, predictable, and controllable, all of which brings relief from what is nothing less than an existential crisis.

In order to reduce the anxiety associated with the transition to healthier functioning, the therapist and client should slowly titrate and carefully target specific changes in behaviors and lifestyle. It is important for the client to experiment with new situations and new people, but this experimentation should be done in a way that maximizes success in these ventures: Task demands should match the client's abilities and readiness. Lastly, relapses are likely to occur. The therapist and client should think ahead about when and under what types of situations relapses are most likely to occur and have a relapse response plan ready.

Phase 2: Emotional Processing of Trauma Memories

Once the eight sessions of skills training are completed, the client moves directly to the second phase of treatment: the processing of the trauma memories. Although a therapist may wish to add a few more skills training sessions for clients who seem to need further training, and despite clients' trepidation about being "ready" for the work, it is best to move on to the memory-processing phase. Delay in moving to the second phase of treatment reinforces avoidance behaviors as well as clients' generally unfounded belief that they are not capable of mastering their affect-laden memories. Skills may not seem completely solidified, and that is to be expected. Review and practice of skills are included in every session of the processing phase. Clients' difficulties in processing their memories can be titrated by the depth and detail of the memories. It is expected that the narrative work will involve increased elaboration more negatively valenced material across time.

We have adapted Foa's prolonged exposure treatment for rape-related PTSD (Foa et al., 1991) for use with women who have a history of childhood abuse. This exposure treatment complements the skills training work of phase 1 with very little redundancy in tasks. It should be noted, however, that current data indicate that at least two forms of treatment for rape-related PTSD (Foa et al., 1991; Resick & Schnicke, 1992) are of equal effectiveness in the resolution of the PTSD diagnosis (Resick, Nishith, & Astin, 1996). It remains to be seen whether one form of treatment is more effective than the other in the resolution of PTSD symptoms experienced by women with chronic trauma histories.

Phase 2 of the treatment begins with the development of a hierarchy of abuse-related trauma memories ranked by the level of distress they induce. The sessions involve 45 minutes of imaginal exposure work, followed by practice of coping skills, including refining those used in association with the exposure completed during the session. The therapist begins imaginal exposure using the most distressing sexual-abuse memory the client feels is tolerable. The client describes the episode of abuse in the present tense, including visual and somatosensory detail. The goal is to elicit a significant level of distress and to sustain the exposure for the allotted time or until reported distress level declines. The therapist makes encouraging and directive remarks during this effort (e.g., "You are doing fine, stay with the image"). A tape is made of the narrative, and the client is encouraged to listen to the tape at least once a day. As the client habituates to the initial memory, she is asked to describe the events in greater detail and to focus more on her emotional response to the image. As the habituation process continues, additional memories are incorporated into the exposure exercises, and new exposures are constructed. The therapist and client may also include exercises that focus on fostering habituation to emotional "hot spots" in the client's memory.

The second narrative clearly includes not only greater details of the client's subjective experience but also an array of feelings, including fear, shame, anger, and aggression. These feelings, especially fear and anger, were emotions that Ms. F feared would overwhelm her (via a panic attack, crying jag, sense of disintegration, or assaulting someone) if she were to get close to them. Repeated exposure to these emotions in the sessions was followed by discussions of how it felt to experience them and the skills she had acquired with which to moderate them. The realization that she could handle these feelings significantly improved her day-to-day functioning by allowing her to engage in activities and situations that had the potential to elicit such feelings. She traveled more and she was less frightened of confronting situations that might involve interpersonal discord.

Modification of Prolonged Exposure: Identification of Interpersonal Schemas in the Trauma Narrative

After every exposure is completed, the client is asked to identify the interpersonal schemas embedded in the narrative. Often these are variants of the schemas with which they came into treatment: for example, "I am not able to take care of myself" or "If I don't ask for anything, I will not be hurt." Identifying the origins of the client's established schema as rooted in the childhood abuse trauma is often validating for him or her, providing a context and reason for beliefs that have been criticized by adulthood acquaintances. This exercise often demonstrates the logic or adaptive value of the schema under circumstances of chronic abuse. However, the client is also asked to compare the schema within the trauma narrative with the new schema, for which experiential evidence has accumulated during phase 1. This comparison helps organize and relate the schemas from the past with those of the present into a narrative of changing self. During skills training, "old" and "new" schemas can often be viewed as conflicting principles of action. During phase 2, the schemas can be understood from a historical perspective, as coexisting in the context of different life experiences in a developing life narrative.

Completion of Prolonged Exposure: Obstacles and Interventions

Typical obstacles encountered in processing trauma memories are avoidance of narrative work (e.g., not doing out-of-session narrative activity) and the absence of emotional engagement during trauma-processing activity. The introduction of the STAIR component of treatment is intended to ameliorate these difficulties. Skills training helps the client to be more emotionally engaged and aware during the processing work and to have greater ability to tolerate the distress associated with trauma processing.

During the actual processing work, the therapist should provide encouragement and validation of the client's skill and ability in processing the trauma. The goal of this treatment component is to reduce PTSD symptoms. Perhaps equally important is the sense of personal mastery and control the client will gain through successful processing of the trauma. The traumatic memory and associated feelings are likely to have dominated the emotional life of the client with PTSD. The review and controlled experiencing of these memories reverses this relationship: The individual takes ownership of the traumatic memory, rather than the memory driving the life decisions of the individual.

Termination and Follow-Up Care

Termination of treatment can be difficult because it is often clear to both therapist and client that more work could be done. However, significant gains often have been made in PTSD symptoms, depression, and role functioning. The final session is devoted to reviewing the client's experience with the treatment and identifying progress and future goals, including referrals appropriate to those goals. In addition, the client should be encouraged to call the therapist, as needed. Such situations may include experiences in which there are new stressors exacerbating symptoms or when the client is presented with a "choice point" or life decision. These phone calls can be viewed as "booster" sessions that reinforce established skills, guide the application of established skills to new circumstances, or provide support for tough decisions and emotional transitions. The client's awareness of the availability of continued care is reassuring and is likely to keep him or her from panicking into a relapse of maladaptive behaviors (e.g., substance abuse). Often a single session can prevent derailment into a spiral of decreased functioning and the need for reentering an extended therapy. The availability of follow-up care also sends the message that both therapist and client are aware that the recovery from trauma is a journey that will not be completed when therapy ends but continues for an unspecified time.

Ms. F wrote a summary of her progress a couple of weeks after her treatment ended, identifying where changes had been made and where she thought work remained to be done. She remained in contact with our clinic as she set about keeping her home, providing employment for herself, and making new relationships.

"Before I came to treatment, the violent incidences of my life were very present in mind, body, and soul. Those incidences are now a less integral part of who I am. I hope it stays that way. I still feel 'danger everywhere,' but it is less intense. I feel safer. Emotions are steadier. The fears of fear feelings have vanished! It is a tremendous relief.

"It is wonderful to have new guidelines for relationships. I've learned how to protect myself in knowing how to assess others' trustworthiness, their negative judgments of me, and their reactions to my requests. These guidelines give me a sense of control and help me feel less vulnerable. Unfortunately, I can hold these standards to new people but cannot yet apply them to my [past abusers].

"I still have self-doubt on all fronts and criticize myself excessively. I have thought about my past relationships and found, to my great surprise, that I was not entirely responsible for their failure. I am relieved to know that it is a human responsibility not to hurt someone, and that everyone is accountable for their actions. I have learned that I am more than other people's reactions to me.

"The ever-intrusive thought of meeting death by violence has moved farther to the background, being replaced by hope for the future. There actually appear thoughts of the possibility of nice things happening—a mere glimpse but a revelation nonetheless.

"I realize that I will have to continue to work on all this, so that my fears continue to diminish. Unfortunately, I have a problem trusting myself with accomplishing anything. Maybe this is the next thing I need to work on."

EFFICACY OF STAIR/MPE

The two-phase STAIR/MPE treatment has been evaluated in a randomized control trial (Cloitre, Koenen, Cohen, & Han, 2002b). Compared to a waiting-list control group, women who completed the treatment showed significant decreases in PTSD symptoms, affect regulation problems, and interpersonal problems. At the end of treatment, 75% of the sample no longer maintained the diagnosis of PTSD. Affect regulation skills were significantly improved, as were affect-related problems of alexithymia, dissociation, and anger expression. Interpersonal problems were significantly reduced in all areas measured, including assertiveness, control, and trust. In addition, reports of perceived social support and functional status in home, work and social domains were also improved. These gains were all maintained at both 3- and 9-month follow-up. Indeed, PTSD symptoms and interpersonal problems continued to show further and significant resolution. Clients' continued improvement after the end of treatment may result from their continued practice of interpersonal and affect regulation skills, allowing for the strengthening of skills and the accumulation of a positive experiential base by which to observe their effectiveness and value. The data suggest that the treatment is effective in resolving many of the hypothesized risk factors for revictimization. The impact of this treatment on rates of revictimization will require a larger sample and longer follow-up periods. Observation data, however, are encouraging. Of the 22 women who completed treatment, 12% experienced some form of revictimization (rape, attempted rape, domestic violence, or physical abuse) during the 9 months following treatment, as compared to a rate of 25% before treatment for the same sample and approximately same duration.

FUTURE DIRECTIONS

This chapter proposed several risk factors for revictimization. A careful review of the data, however, indicate that only two factors, PTSD and substance abuse, have significant empirical support from well-designed, large-sample, prospective studies. Many of the other proposed risk factors have some support, but conclusions are limited by small sample sizes, selective samples (i.e., college students), retrospective reporting, and the potential presence of unidentified and confounding risk factors. The public and personal cost of revictimizaton is significant and indicates the importance of undertaking large, prospective studies in which multiple risk factors can be tracked over time, with careful attention to the potential specificity of risk–outcome relationships. In addition, interventions should be developed in tandem with risk-factor identification, which may vary by population. Treatment programs such as STAIR/MPE serve women who are significantly impaired: They have full PTSD, and the majority has already experienced repeated victimizations beyond the childhood abuse. Lastly, and most importantly, intervention and prevention programming is needed for larger community-based populations, such as college and high school students, whom we can hope to characterize as predominantly carrying the risk, rather than the burdensome reality, of revictimization.

REFERENCES

Andrews, B., Brewin, C. R., Rose, S., & Kirk, M. (2000). Predicting PTSD symptoms in victims of violent crime: The role of shame, anger, and childhood abuse. *Journal of Abnormal Psychology, 109*(1), 69–73.

Arata, C. M. (2002). Child sexual abuse and sexual revictimization. *Clinical Psychology: Science and Practice, 9*(2), 135–164.

Arata, C. M., & Lindman, L. (2002). Marriage, child abuse, and sexual revictimization. *Journal of Interpersonal Violence, 17*(9), 953–971.

Bernstein, E. M., & Putnam, F. (1986). Development, reliability and validity of a dissociation scale. *Journal of Nervous and Mental Disease, 174,* 727–735.

Blake, D. D., Weather, F. W., Nagy, L. M., Kaloupek, D. G., Gusman, F. D., Charney, D. S., & Keane, T. M. (1995). The development of a clinician-administered PTSD scale. *Journal of Traumatic Stress, 8,* 75–90.

Bowlby, J. (1969). *Attachment and loss* (Vol. 1). New York: Basic Books.

Bowlby, J. (1984). Violence in the family as a disorder of the attachment and caregiving systems. *American Journal of Psychoanalysis, 44,* 9–27.

Breitenbecher, K. H. (1999). The association between the perception of threat in a dating situation and sexual victimization. *Violence and Victims, 14*(2), 135–146.

Breitenbecher, K. H., & Gidycz, C. A. (1998). An empirical evaluation of a program designed to reduce the risk of multiple sexual victimization. *Journal of Interpersonal Violence, 13,* 472–488.

Breslau, N., Davis, G. C., Andreski, P., & Peterson, E. (1991). Traumatic events and posttraumatic stress disorder in an urban population of young adults. *Archives of General Psychiatry, 48,* 216–222.

Briere, J. N. (1992). *Child abuse trauma: Theory and treatment of the lasting effects.* Newbury Park, CA: Sage.

Browne, A., & Finkelhor, D. (1986). Impact of child sexual abuse: A review of the research. *Psychological Bulletin, 99,* 66–77.

Cantanzaro, S. J., & Mearns, J. (1990). Measuring generalized expectancies for negative mood regulation: Initial scale development and implications. *Journal of Personality Assessment, 54,* 546–563.

Cicchetti, D., & White, J. (1990). Emotion and developmental psychopathology. In N. Stein, B. Leventhal, & T. Trebasso (Eds.), *Psychological and biological approaches to emotion* (pp. 359–382). Hillsdale, NJ: Erlbaum.

Clemmons, J. C., DiLillo, D., Martinez, I. G., DeGue, S., & Jeffcott, M. (2003). Co-occurring forms of child maltreatment and adult adjustment reported by Latina college students. *Child Abuse and Neglect, 27,* 751–767.

Cloitre, M., Cohen, L. R., & Scarvalone, P. (2002a). Understanding revictimization among childhood sexual abuse survivors: An interpersonal schema approach. *Journal of Cognitive Psychotherapy: An International Quarterly, 16,* 91–111.

Cloitre, M., Koenen, K. C., Cohen, L. R., & Han, H. (2002b). Skills training in affective and interpersonal regulation followed by exposure: A phase-based treatment for PTSD related to childhood abuse. *Journal of Consulting and Clinical Psychology, 70,* 1067–1074.

Cloitre, M., Scarvalone, P., & Difede, J. (1997). Post-traumatic stress disorder, self and interpersonal dysfunction among sexually revictimized women. *Journal of Traumatic Stress, 10,* 435–450.

Cloitre, M., Tardiff, K., Marzuk, P. M., Leon, A. C., & Potera, L. (1996). Childhood abuse and subsequent sexual assault among female inpatients. *Journal of Traumatic Stress, 9,* 473–482.

Cloitre, M., Tardiff, K., Marzuk, P. M., Leon, A. C., & Potera, L. (2001). Consequences of childhood abuse among male psychiatric inpatients: Dual roles as victims and perpetrators. *Journal of Traumatic Stress, 14,* 47–61.

Dietrich, A. M. (2003). *Posttraumatic stress disorder and associated features as predictors of revictimization and perpetration with samples of adults abused during childhood.* Unpublished doctoral dissertation, University of British Columbia, Vancouver, Canada.

Dong, M., Anda, R. F., Dube, S. R., Giles, W. H., & Filetti, V. J. (2003). The relationship of exposure to childhood sexual abuse to other forms of abuse, neglect, and household dysfunction during childhood. *Child Abuse and Neglect, 27,* 625–639.

Elliott, D. M., & Briere, J. (1992). Sexual abuse trauma among professional women: Validating the Trauma Symptom Checklist-40. *Child Abuse and Neglect, 16,* 391–398.

Erickson, M. F., Egeland, B., & Pianta, R. (1989). The effects of maltreatment on the development of young children. In D. Cicchetti & V. Carlson (Eds.), *Child maltreatment: Theory and research on the causes and consequences of child abuse and neglect* (pp. 674–684). Minneapolis: University of Minnesota Press.

Ferguson, D. M., Horwood, L. J., & Lynskey, M. T. (1997). Childhood sexual abuse, adolescent sexual behaviors, and sexual revictimization. *Child Abuse and Neglect, 21,* 789–803.

Field, N. P., Classen, C., Butler, L. D., Koopman, C., Zarcone, J., & Spiegel, D. (2001). Revictimization and information processing in women survivors of childhood sexual abuse. *Journal of Anxiety Disorders, 15,* 459–469.

Finkelhor, D. (1990). Early and long-term effects of child sexual abuse: An update. *Professional Psychology: Research and Practice, 21,* 325–330.

Finkelhor, D., & Dziuba-Leatherman, J. (1994). Victimization of children. *American Psychologist, 3,* 173–183.

Foa, E. B., Rothbaum, B. O., Riggs, D. S., & Murdock, T. B. (1991). Treatment of posttraumatic stress disorder in rape victims: A comparison between cognitive-behavioral procedures and counseling. *Journal of Consulting and Clinical Psychology, 60,* 715–723.

Follette, V. M., Polusny, M. A., Bechtle, A. E., & Naugle, A. E. (1996). Cumulative trauma: The impact of child sexual abuse, adult sexual assault, and spouse abuse. *Journal of Traumatic Stress, 9*(1), 25–35.

Gibson, L. E., & Leitenberg, H. (2001). The impact of child sexual abuse and stigma on methods of coping with sexual assault among undergraduate women. *Child Abuse and Neglect, 25,* 1343–1361.

Gidycz, C. A., Hanson, K., & Layman, M. J. (1995). A prospective analyses of the relationship among sexual assault experiences: An extension of prior findings. *Psychology of Women Quarterly, 19,* 5–29.

Gilbert, P., & McGuire, M. (1998). Shame, status and social roles: The psychobiological continuum from monkey to human. In P. Gilbert & B. Andrews (Eds.), *Shame: Interpersonal behavior, psychopathology and culture* (pp. 99–125). New York: Oxford University Press.

Greene, D. M., & Navarro, R. L. (1998). Situation-specific assertiveness in the epidemiology of sexual victimization among university women. *Psychology of Women Quarterly, 22,* 589–604.

Greene, D. M., Navarro, R. L., & Gidycz, C. A. (1995). *Secondary prevention of sexual victimization based on a prospective study of protective and risk factors.* Poster presented at the meeting of the Association for Advancement of Behavior Therapy, Washington, DC.

Hanson, K. R., & Gidycz, C. A. (1993). Evaluation of a sexual assault prevention program. *Journal of Consulting and Clinical Psychology, 6,* 1046–1052.

Hennessy, K. D., Rabideau, G. J., Cicchetti, D., & Cummings, E. M. (1994). Responses of physically abused and nonabused children to different forms of interadult anger. *Child Development, 63*(3), 815–828.

Herman, J. L. (1992). *Trauma and recovery.* New York: Basic Books.

Himelein, M. J. (1995). Risk factors for sexual victimization in dating: A longitudinal study of college women. *Psychology of Women Quarterly, 19,* 31–48.

Horowitz, L. M., Rosenberg, S. E., Baer, B. A., Ureno, G., & Villasenor, V. S. (1988). Inventory of Interpersonal Problems: Psychometric properties and clinical applications. *Journal of Consulting and Clinical Psychology, 56,* 885–892.

Howes, C., & Eldredge, R. (1985). Responses of abused, neglected, and non-maltreated children to the behaviors of their peers. *Journal of Applied Developmental Psychology, 6*(2–3), 261–270.

Irwin, H. J. (1999). Violent and nonviolent revictimization of women abused in childhood. *Journal of Interpersonal Violence, 14*(10), 1095–1110.

Jonikas, J. A., & Cook, J. A. (1994). *Safe, secure and street smart: Empowering women with mental illness to achieve greater independence in the community.* Chicago: Thresholds Research and Training Center.

Kellogg, N. D., & Hoffman, T. J. (1997). Child sexual revictimization by multiple perpetrators. *Child Abuse and Neglect, 21*, 953–964.

Kendall-Tackett, K. A., Williams, L. M., & Finkelhor, D. (1993). Impact of sexual abuse on children: A review and synthesis of recent empirical studies. *Psychological Bulletin, 113*(1), 164–180.

Kessler, B. L., & Bieschke, K. J. (1999). A retrospective analysis of shame, dissociation, and adult victimization in survivors of childhood sexual abuse. *Journal of Counseling Psychology, 46*(3), 335–341.

Kessler, R. C., Molnar, B. E., Feurer, I. D., & Applebaum, M. (2001). Patterns and mental health predictors of domestic violence in the United States: Results from the National Comorbidity Survey. *International Journal of Law and Psychiatry, 24*, 498–508.

Kilpatrick, D. G., Saunders, B. E., Veronen, L. J., Best, C. L., & Von, J. M. (1987). Criminal victimization: Lifetime prevalence, reporting to police, and psychological impact. *Crime and Delinquency, 33*, 479–489.

Koss, M. P., & Dinero, T. E. (1989). Discriminant analysis of risk factors for sexual victimization among a national sample of college women. *Journal of Consulting and Clinical Psychology, 57*, 242–250.

Linehan, M. M. (1993). *Cognitive-behavioral treatment of borderline personality disorder.* New York: Guilford Press.

Lisak, D., Hopper, J., & Song, P. (1996). Factors in the cycle of violence: Gender rigidity and emotional constriction. *Journal of Traumatic Stress, 9*, 721–743.

Malinosky-Rummell, R., & Hansen, D. J. (1993). Long-term consequences of childhood physical abuse. *Psychological Bulletin, 114*(1), 68–79.

Marx, B. P., Calhoun, K. S., Wilson, A. E., & Meyerson, L. A. (2001). Sexual revictimization prevention: An outcome evaluation. *Journal of Consulting and Clinical Psychology, 69*(1), 25–32.

Marx, B. P., & Gross, A. M. (1995). Date rape: An analysis of two contextual variables. *Behavior Modification, 19*, 451–463.

Mayall, A., & Gold, S. R. (1995). Definitional issues and mediating variables in the sexual revictimization of women sexually abused as children. *Journal of Interpersonal Violence, 10*(1), 26–42.

Meadows, E., Jaycox, L. H., Webb, S., & Foa, E. B. (1996). Risk recognition in narratives of rape experiences. In S. M. Orsillo & L. Roemer (Chairs), *The use of narrative methodologies to explore cognitive and emotional dimensions among women with post-traumatic stress disorder.* Symposium conducted at the meeting of the Association for Advancement of Behavior Therapy, New York, NY.

Merrill, L. L., Newell, C. E., Thomsen, C. J., Gold, S. R., Milner, J. S., Koss, M. P., et al. (1999). Childhood abuse and sexual revictimization in a female navy recruit sample. *Journal of Traumatic Stress, 12*(2), 211–225.

Merrill, L. L., Thomsen, C. J., Gold, S. R., & Milner, J. S. (2001). Childhood abuse and premilitary sexual assault in male navy recruits. *Journal of Consulting and Clinical Psychology, 69*(2), 252–261.

Messman-Moore, T. L., & Long, P. J. (2000). The revictimization of child sexual abuse survivors: An examination of the adjustment of college women with child sexual abuse, adult sexual assault, and adult physical abuse. *Child Maltreatment, 5*(1), 18–27.

Messman-Moore, T. L., & Long, P. J. (2002). Alcohol and substance use disorders as predictors of child to adult sexual revictimization in a sample of community women. *Violence and Victims, 17*(3), 319–340.

Messman-Moore, T. L., & Long, P. J. (2003). The role of childhood sexual abuse sequelae in the sexual revictimization of women: An empirical review and theoretical reformulation. *Clinical Psychology Review, 23*, 537–571.

Metcalfe, M., Oppenheimer, R., Dignon, A., & Palmer, R. L. (1990). Childhood sexual experiences reported by male psychiatric patients. *Psychological Medicine, 20*(4), 925–929.

Muelenhard, C. L., & Linton, M. A. (1987). Date rape and sexual aggression in dating situations: Incidence and risk factors. *Journal of Consulting and Clinical Psychology, 34*, 186–196.

National Center on Child Abuse and Neglect. (1994). *Child maltreatment 1992: Reports from the states to the National Center on Child Abuse and Neglect.* Washington, DC: U.S. Government Printing Office.

National Center on Child Abuse and Neglect. (1995). *Child maltreatment 1993: Reports from the states to the National Center on Child Abuse and Neglect.* Washington, DC: U.S. Government Printing Office.

National Victim Center and Crime Victims Research and Treatment Center. (1992). *Rape in America: A report to the nation.* Arlington, VA: Author.

Nishith, P., Mechanic, M., & Resick, P. (1997). Childhood sexual and physical abuse as predictors of adult sexual and physical revictimization in a sample of female crime victims. In M. Cloitre (Chair), *Sexual revictimization of women: Risk factors and prevention strategies.* Symposium conducted at the meeting of the Association for Advancement of Behavior Therapy, Miami, FL.

Norris, F. H. (1992). Epidemiology of trauma: Frequency and impact of different potentially traumatic events on different demographic groups. *Journal of Consulting and Clinical Psychology, 60*, 409–418.

O'Neill, K., & Gupta, K. (1991). Post-traumatic stress disorder in women who were victims of childhood sexual abuse. *Irish Journal of Psychological Medicine, 8*, 1224–1227.

Pelcovitz, D., van der Kolk, B., Roth, S., Mandel, F., Kaplan, S., & Resick, P. (1997). Development of a criteria set and a structured interview for disorders of extreme stress (SIDES). *Journal of Traumatic Stress, 10*(1), 3–16.

Playter, J. (1990). *The effect of childhood sexual abuse on internalized shame in adult women in treatment for chemical dependency.* Unpublished masters thesis, University of Wisconsin, Stout.

Polusny, M. A., & Follette, V. M. (1995). Long term correlates of child sexual abuse: Theory and review of the empirical literature. *Applied and Preventive Psychology: Current Scientific Perspectives, 4*, 143–166.

Raiha, N. K., & Soma, D. (1997). Victims of child abuse and neglect in the U.S. Army. *Child Abuse and Neglect, 21*, 759–768.

Resick, P. A., Falsetti, S. A., Resnick, H. S., & Kilpatrick, D. G. (1991). *The Modified*

PTSD Symptom Scale–Self Report. St. Louis, MO: University of Missouri and Charleston, SC: Crime Victims Treatment and Research Center, Medical University of South Carolina.

Resick, P. A., Nishith, P., & Astin, M. C. (1996, November). Results of an outcome study comparing cognitive processing therapy and prolonged exposure. In P. Resick (Chair), *Treating sexual assault/sexual abuse pathology: Recent findings*. Symposium conducted at the meeting of the Association for Advancement of Behavior Therapy, New York.

Resick, P. A., & Schnicke, M. K. (1992). Cognitive processing therapy for sexual assault victims. *Journal of Consulting and Clinical Psychology, 60,* 748–756.

Roodman, A. A., & Clum, G. A. (2001). Revictimization rates and method variance: A meta-analysis. *Clinical Psychology Review, 21*(2), 183–204.

Roth, S., Newman, E., Pelcovitz, D., van der Kolk, B., & Mandel, F. (1997). Complex PTSD in victims exposed to sexual and physical abuse: Results from the DSM-IV field trial for posttraumatic stress disorder. *Journal of Traumatic Stress, 10,* 539–555.

Rowan, A. B., Foy, D. W., Rodriquez, N., & Ryan, S. (1994). Posttraumatic stress disorder in a clinical sample of adults sexually abused as children. *Child Abuse and Neglect, 182,* 145–150.

Safran, J. D. (1990). Towards a refinement of cognitive therapy interpersonal theory: I. Theory. *Clinical Psychology, 56,* 5–8.

Sandberg, D. A., Matorin, A. I., & Lynn, S. J. (1999). Dissociation, posttraumatic symptomatology, and sexual revictimization: A prospective examination of mediator and moderator effects. *Journal of Traumatic Stress, 12,* 127–138.

Sanders, B., & Moore, D. L. (1999). Childhood maltreatment and date rape. *Journal of Interpersonal Violence, 14*(2), 115–124.

Schaaf, K. K., & McCanne, T. R. (1998). Relationship of childhood sexual, physical, and combined sexual and physical abuse to adult victimization and posttraumatic stress disorder. *Child Abuse and Neglect, 22*(11), 1119–1133.

Scheier, M. F., & Carver, C. S. (1985). Optimism, coping, and health: Assessment and implications of generalized outcome expectancies. *Health Psychology, 4*(3), 219–247.

Shearer, S. L., Peters, C. P., Quaytman, M. S., & Ogden, R. L. (1990). Frequency and correlates of childhood sexual and physical female borderline inpatients. *American Journal of Psychiatry, 147,* 214–216.

Shields, A. M., & Cicchetti, D. (1998). Reactive aggression among maltreated children: The contributions of attention and emotion dysregulation. *Journal of Clinical Child Psychology, 27,* 381–395.

Shields, A. M., Ryan, R. M., & Cicchetti, D. (1994). The development of emotional and behavioral self-regulation and social competence among maltreatment school age children. *Developmental Psychopathology, 6,* 57–75.

Spielberger, C. D. (1988). Manual for the state–trait anger expression inventory. In M. Hersen & A. S. Bellack (Eds.), *Dictionary of behavioral assessment techniques* (pp. 446–448). New York: Pergamon Press.

Spitzer, R. L., Williams, J. B., Gibbon, M., & First, M. B. (1994). *Clinical Interview for DSM-IV–Patient Edition.* New York: New York State Psychiatric Institute, Biometrics Research Department.

Taylor, G. J., Bagby, R. M., Ryan, D. P., Parker, J. D. A., & Doody, D. P. (1988). Criterion validity of the Toronto Alexithymia Scale. *Psychosomatic Medicine, 50,* 500–509.

Urquiza, A. J., & Goodlin-Jones, B. L. (1994). Child sexual abuse and adult revictimization with women of color. *Violence and Victims, 6,* 223–232.

Urquiza, A. J., & Keating, L. (1990). The prevalence of sexual victimization of males. In M. Hunter (Ed.), *The sexually abused male: Prevalence, impact and treatment* (Vol. 1, pp. 89–102). Lexington, MA: Lexington Books.

van der Kolk, B. A. (1987). The separation cry and the trauma response: Developmental issues in the psychobiology of attachment and separation. In B. A. van der Kolk (Ed.), *Psychological trauma* (pp. 31–62). Washington, DC: American Psychiatric Press.

van der Kolk, B. A. (1996). The complexity of adaption to trauma: Self-regulation, stimulus, discrimination, and characterological development. In B. A. van der Kolk, A. C. McFarlane, & L. Weisaeth (Eds.), *Traumatic stress: The effects of overwhelming experience on mind, body and society* (pp. 182–213). New York: Guilford Press.

van der Kolk, B. A., Roth, S., Pelcovitz, D., & Mandel, F. (1993). *Complex PTSD: Results of the PTSD field trials for DSM-IV.* Washington, DC: American Psychiatric Press.

Weissman, E., & Bothell, S. (1976). Assessment of patient social adjustment by patient self-report. *Archives of General Psychiatry, 33,* 1111–1115.

Widom, C. S. (1989). The cycle of violence. *Science, 244,* 160–166.

Wilson, A. E., Calhoun, K. S., & Bernat, J. A. (1999). Risk recognition and trauma-related symptoms among sexually revictimized women. *Journal of Consulting and Clinical Psychology, 67,* 705–710.

Wilson, M., Johnson, H., & Daley, M. (1995). Lethal and nonlethal violence against wives. *Canadian Journal of Criminology, 37,* 331–361.

Wind, T. W., & Silvern, L. (1992). Type and extent of child abuse as predictors of adult functioning. *Journal of Family Violence, 7,* 261–281.

Wyatt, G. E. (1985). The sexual abuse of African American and European American women in childhood. *Child Abuse and Neglect, 9,* 507–519.

Wyatt, G. E., Loeb, T. B., Solis, B., & Carmona, J. V. (1999). The prevalence and circumstances of child sexual abuse: Changes across a decade. *Child Abuse and Neglect, 23,* 45–60.

Wyatt, G. E., Guthrie, D., & Notgrass, C. M. (1992). Differential effects of women's child sexual abuse and subsequent sexual revictimization. *Journal of Consulting and Clinical Psychology, 60*(2), 167–173.

CHAPTER FOURTEEN

A Principle-Based Intervention for Couples Affected by Trauma

Leah M. Leonard
Victoria M. Follette
Jill S. Compton

Over the years researchers have presented the individual sequelae as well as the interpersonal consequences of trauma (Beitchman et al., 1992; Browne & Finkelhor, 1986; Polusny & Follette, 1995; Resick, 1993; Resick & Nishith, 1997; Riggs, Byrne, Weathers, & Litz, 1998). In order to address the various impacts of a trauma history, both individual (Foa & Rothbaum, 1998; Krupnick, 2002; Resick & Calhoun, 2001) and couple-based treatments (Buttenheim & Levendosky, 1994; Compton & Follette, 1998; Johnson, 2002; Miller & Sutherland, 1999) for trauma have been developed. Examining the clinical experiences of trauma survivors who have coped more successfully with their trauma, we see that positive, intimate relationships with their partners is frequently how they account for much of their success. Given these accounts and our clinical and research experiences, it is our belief that traumatic experiences have a detrimental impact on close interpersonal relationships and that the formation of a safe and intimate relationship provides many survivors with an enhanced capability for recovery.

In this chapter we present a couple-based approach that we have found useful when working with trauma survivors. The intervention described is intended for couples for whom traumatic experiences are a relevant historical factor for one or both partners. Our model focuses on a principle-based intervention for survivor couples and is applicable to couples who have experienced a wide range of interpersonal traumatic experiences, including trauma arising from childhood sexual abuse (CSA), childhood physical abuse, war and combat, rape, and domestic violence. Although each type of trauma can and does bring different dynamics to be considered, all forms share the potential to elicit intense fear for one's life and helplessness.

Throughout this chapter we refer to trauma survivors and their partners as survivor couples, trauma couples, couples affected by trauma, or couples with a history of trauma. We use all of these terms interchangeably. Given the heterogeneity of this population and the use of all of these terms in the literature, we found it applicable to utilize all of these descriptors to capture the varying phenomenological experiences of these couples. Moreover, our use of the term "couple" is intended to encompass married, cohabitating, dating, and same-sex individuals.

We begin the chapter with a review of the literature on some of the interpersonal difficulties faced by survivor couples as well as a brief summary of the many individual difficulties trauma survivors experience that cannot help but to impact their intimate relationships. Finally, we present a detailed account of a comprehensive, principle-based intervention for survivor couples, grounded in functional contextual philosophy and behavioral theory.

COUPLE FUNCTIONING AMONG TRAUMA SURVIVORS

Relationship distress and dissatisfaction are common complaints among survivor couples. In her early work on incest survivors, Herman (1981) noted clinical examples of the types of relationship problems that can occur. Research shows that relationships of incest survivors tend to be characterized by distress and marital discord, dissatisfaction, difficulties with trust and communication, and violence (DiLillo & Long, 1999; Jehu, 1988; Mullen, Martin, Anderson, Romans, & Herbison 1994; Savarese, Suvak, King, & King, 2001). There is consistent evidence of elevated rates of separation and divorce among trauma couples (Mullen et al. 1994; Riggs et al., 1998; Russell, 1986). In particular, women with a history of CSA are at greater risk of physical mistreatment committed by male partners than are women without such histories (Briere & Runtz, 1987, 1988).

Couples in which one member is a survivor of some type of trauma are vulnerable to a variety of dysfunctional patterns of interacting. The overfunctioning of one partner coupled with the underfunctioning of the other is common. The often well-meaning overfunctioning spouse takes on the additional responsibilities in the relationship (e.g., financial, emotional, practical day-to-day tasks) as a way to decrease the demands on the trauma survivor and avoid or reduce the conflict in the relationship (Rabin & Nardi, 1991). This pattern can eventually lead the overfunctioning partner to feel resentful of his or her spouse and depleted because his or her own wants and needs have not been met (Nelson & Wright, 1996).

Emotional Engagement

A common finding across traumatic experiences in couples in which one or both partners are trauma survivors is a lack of emotional engagement. Emotional withdrawal has been consistently associated with relationship problems. Numbing, which involves restricted affect and detachment from others, has been identified as more difficult to treat than other symptoms of trauma and predicts distress in a survivor's relationships (Riggs et al., 1998). Emotional numbing was found to be significantly related to relationship difficulties, independent of the severity of posttraumatic stress disorder (PTSD) in World War II ex-POWs (Cook, Riggs, Thompson, Coyne, & Sheikh, 2004). Solomon et al. (1992) highlighted the alienation that emotional withdrawal can cause and suggested that combat veterans' withdrawal in their relationships leaves their partners lonely and vulnerable to a wide variety of psychological problems. For couples that have survived a sexual assault, Miller, Williams, and Bernstein (1982) found that partners have difficulties with emotional support and communication. In addition, survivors of CSA and their partners experience decreased emotional expressiveness as well as difficulties in feeling connected (Waltz, 1993).

Sexual Concerns

Individuals who have experienced sexual assault or CSA frequently report problems with sexual functioning and sexual satisfaction (e.g., see Browne & Finkelhor, 1986; Leonard & Follette, 2002; Resick, 1993, for reviews). Many individuals experience a relationship between childhood sexual abuse and later sexual problems, which has been supported by numerous empirical studies and case reports. CSA survivors are reported to have significantly more sexual problems (Becker, Skinner, Abel, Axelrod, & Cichon, 1984; Sarwer & Durlak, 1996; Wenninger & Heiman, 1998), more negative sexual symptoms (Gold, 1986), to be less satisfied with their sexual functioning (Jackson, Calhoun, Amick, Maddever, & Habif, 1990), and to be less satisfied with their present sexual relationship (Gold, 1986) than nonabused women in the control group.

Researchers have investigated the various types of sexual problems experienced by CSA and sexual assault survivors. According to the DSM-IV, there are four types of sexual dysfunctions related to desire, arousal, orgasm, and pain (American Psychiatric Association, 1994). In addition to these areas, a lack of sexual satisfaction is also considered a frequently experienced problem by survivors. Within these parameters, researchers have consistently found that CSA survivors are likely to experience problems with sexual desire and/or sexual arousal (Becker et al., 1984; Jackson et al., 1990; Kirschner, Kirschner, & Rappaport, 1993; Westerlund, 1992). Fear of sexual contact (sexual aversion) is a dysfunction of desire and is also frequently reported by CSA survivors. Clinical experience suggests that women presenting with sexual aversion disorder have almost always been victims of a sexual trauma in childhood and/or as an adult (Wincze & Carey, 1991). Women who were victims of adult sexual assault frequently report decreased sexual satisfaction (Ellis, Calhoun, & Atkeson, 1980), as do CSA survivors (Gold, 1986; Jehu, 1988).

It is difficult to imagine a more open and vulnerable experience than to allow oneself to be close, emotionally and physically, to a spouse or partner. To embrace this degree of vulnerability can be a challenge for anyone. It is a natural tendency to guard oneself from such vulnerability because this is precisely when one can be rejected or hurt the most. The inherent vulnerability associated with sexual intimacy presents individuals with situations that require trust and acceptance of emotional uncertainty. Experiences such as these can be emotionally overwhelming for many trauma survivors.

INDIVIDUAL FACTORS

In addition to the interpersonal correlates of trauma, there are a host of sequelae associated with a trauma history, including depression and substance abuse (Briere, 1988; Resick, 1993). Although these factors are initially associated with individuals, frequently they will impact survivors' intimate relationships, thus adding to the already complex impact trauma can have on relationships. Increased rates of major depression, suicidal ideation, and suicide attempts have all been consistently associated with traumatic experiences (Keane & Wolf, 1990; Polusny & Follette, 1995; Resick, 1993). In addition to the obvious individual impact, evidence suggests that depression may negatively impact relationship satisfaction (e.g., Coyne, 1976). Like depression, substance abuse occurs at high rates among survivors of trauma (Briere, 1988; Kilpatrick, Edmunds, & Seymour, 1992; Lacoursiere, Godfrey, & Ruby, 1980) and may also be a common problem for their partners (Serafin & Follette, 1996). Substance abuse may have several detrimental effects on couples affected by trauma, including use of the substance to maintain a level of emotional distance in the relationship.

Revictimization

It is well known among trauma researchers that revictimization is common among individuals who have already experienced a sexual assault. A sexual assault in childhood has been identified as a risk factor for experiencing a sexual assault in adulthood (Wyatt, Guthrie, & Notgrass, 1992). In addition, research suggests that women who have had more than one sexual assault experience are likely to experience more severe psychological distress. In other words, evidence is mounting that the psychological effects of trauma may be cumulative (Follette, Polusny, Bechtle, & Naugle, 1996). The identification of a sexual assault history as a risk factor, coupled with the cumulative effects of trauma, make the likelihood of revictimization a vital concern in the prevention and treatment of sexual assault. Although a discussion of the abundant literature on revictimization is outside the scope of this chapter, it is imperative that clinicians are aware of revictimization and assess for it (see Cloitre & Rosenberg, Chapter 13, this volume).

INTEGRATIVE BEHAVIORAL COUPLE THERAPY

An important development in behavioral couple treatment has been the development of integrative behavioral couple therapy (IBCT; Christensen, Jacobson, & Babcock, 1995). This approach to the treatment of couple distress is consistent in many ways with the principle-based intervention that we present in this chapter. IBCT is an empirically validated intervention that combines the change-oriented strategies of traditional behavioral couple therapy (TBCT; Jacobson, & Margolin, 1979), including behavioral exchange and communication/problem-solving skills, with newer strategies focused on acceptance.

Christensen and Jacobson developed IBCT in response to a desire to enhance therapy outcomes for couples (Christensen et al., 1995). Although research on TBCT showed couples improving quickly, the percentage of couples that showed reliable improvement directly after treatment was lower than hoped, and there was evidence of deterioration over time (Christensen et al., 2004). IBCT differs from TBCT in that an acceptance component has been added to the change-oriented approach. Three major strategies are used to promote emotional acceptance in IBCT: (1) empathetic joining around the problem, (2) unified detachment from the problem, and (3) building tolerance to some of the responses that the problem can trigger (Christensen et al., 1995).

IBCT incorporates many of the same behavioral principles we use in our approach. Although IBCT is well suited for survivor couples in many ways, it was not developed specifically for use with this population and has not been evaluated as a treatment for trauma.

A PRINCIPLE-BASED INTERVENTION
FOR SURVIVOR COUPLES

Although it is often seen as useful to have a structured treatment package, our experience with these couples suggests that a predetermined structure may interfere with addressing problems as the ongoing functional analysis reveals the underlying dimensions of the situation. We are not suggesting that the therapist should approach the session on a spur-of-the-moment basis, without thoughtful preparation for the general therapeutic approach. Rather, we are advising reliance on principles and not on technique or structure.

It is our firm belief that in the midst of therapy, it is principles derived from personal philosophy and preferred theory that keep therapists from losing a sense of purpose and direction. For clinicians operating from a behavioral orientation, we present an intervention informed by our appreciation of the impact trauma can have on individuals and couples. One of the key functions of a principle-based intervention is flexibility. Although at first it may seem appealing to have a packaged protocol with session-by-session plans, there are two major potential problems in delivering manualized, pre-packaged treatment techniques to survivor couples.

The first problem is that manualized treatment techniques may not provide therapists with guidance when confronted with a new problem outside the scope of the treatment manual. Unfortunately, the norm for treating survivor couples is that things will deviate from the norm. A therapist can find him- or herself off protocol within the first session. When faced with these situations, there are a few likely scenarios. First, a therapist may attempt to press on with the protocol, ignoring the new concern. Second, he or she may attempt to apply different techniques of the treatment haphazardly in an attempt to fix the problem. Finally, he or she may abandon the manual and address the problem in whatever means he or she normally uses in therapy. Whichever scenario occurs, protocols are of little use when novel situations or concerns emerge in treatment.

The second problem, which is related to the first, is that utilizing treatment manuals or prepackaged treatment techniques increases the risk that therapists will cease to remain responsive to new concerns that may become apparent through an ongoing assessment process. The goal in the moment can become getting the couple back on protocol as opposed to listening to and understanding the couple's dynamic in the moment. Treatment manuals can lull therapists into an often-false conviction that they understand the issues, based on initial presentation, and therefore they fail to continually assess throughout treatment. With packaged agendas and session limitations there is often no time or inherent flexibility for continual assessment and possible alterations to the trajectory of treatment.

We are asserting that in order to meet the needs of each individual as well as the couple, a principle-driven intervention is necessary because it provides clinicians with needed flexibility and grounding. Such an approach allows the therapist to handle in-the-moment crises and to listen to and understand the unique presentation of each couple. Advocacy of this approach is in no way an argument for eclecticism. It is about being flexible while simultaneously guided by principles grounded in philosophy and theory. Thus this approach is characterized by philosophical and theoretical consistency, not eclecticism.

Before we introduce the principles on which we rely when conducting therapy, we outline the philosophy and theory from which these principles are derived.

PHILOSOPHY AND THEORY: FUNCTIONAL CONTEXTUALISM, RADICAL BEHAVIORISM, AND EXPERIENTIAL AVOIDANCE

In order to have a coherent and consistent approach to treatment, it must be grounded in an underlying philosophy or worldview. Our principles evolve from a contextual paradigm, which has four core components: (1) focusing on the whole event as the unit of analysis; (2) understanding the fundamental role of context in shaping the nature and function of an event; (3) applying the truth criterion of successful working; and (4) utilizing the goals of prediction and influence (Pepper, 1942). We address each one of these in greater detail.

The unit of analysis in contextualism is the whole event—that is, an event in context that cannot be broken into pieces. This whole event can be anything that a researcher or clinician is interested in, so long as it is an ongoing act in context. For example, a clinician might choose the act of a client sitting in the chair during a therapy session, or the act of a client crying while discussing a recent fight with a friend. In the case of survivor couples, a clinician might choose the act of a trauma survivor saying no to her partner's request for sex, or the act of a partner withdrawing when the trauma survivor begins crying. Each one of these represents an appropriate unit of analysis for contextualism; they all represent ongoing acts in context.

Behavior, for a contextualist, can only be understood in the context in which it occurs; behavior viewed in isolation from its context is meaningless. Thus, in understanding any behavior, we must look to the context. The context can incorporate proximal as well as distal variables. Distal variables can include events that occurred early in an individual's learning history. For trauma survivors this learning history includes experiences involving trauma, such as sexual abuse, that can negatively influence relationships. Proximal variables can include such factors as current stressors, current relationship variables, and other stimuli in the more immediate environment. For example, we can analyze the behavior of a CSA survivor crying in session with her husband in a number of ways. The immediate environment is the therapy session where, just prior to her crying, she and her husband were talking with the therapist about a fight they had had the previous evening concerning sex. Her husband had just expressed a desire to explore ways in which they could be intimate other than sex. Current stressors for the CSA survivor include an upcoming visit from her parents as well as a major presentation she must make at work. She and her husband's most frequent fights concern his request for sex and her withdrawal. Her history, which includes early experiences of forced sex with her stepfather, is negatively influencing her current sexual relationship with her husband. After incorporating the range of variables impacting the client, the therapist can begin to understand and form hypotheses about the meaning of this behavior.

The truth criterion of contextualism is based on outcome: "successful working" or "effective action." Analyses are true only in terms of the accomplishment of particular goals. In other words, you cannot say whether or not you have achieved successful working in a relationship without stating the specific purpose or goal that has been achieved. In the therapy with this couple, for example, it might not be clear whether the goal is to keep the partners together or to support the dissolution of the relationship. If the primary goal is the psychological well-being of the individual, the course of therapy may differ from one in which sustaining the relationship is the primary goal. Ideally these two goals would be congruent. Unfortunately, that is not always the case, and the dilemmas that this kind of discrepancy can produce in treatment is frequently an issue in treating couples in which one member has a significant trauma history. To restate: The therapist must establish a goal in order to ascertain the success of the intervention.

As detailed above, identifying goals is necessary in a contextualist framework because goals are what allow a clinician or researcher to apply the truth criterion of successful working. In order to answer the question "Was this successful?", a researcher or clinician must first answer the question "Successful for *what goals*?" Couples often want to know why their relationship is not working and what they can do about it. Understanding behavior in terms of its function—the purpose it serves—rather than just its form provides a more useful way of understanding the types of problems couples face. For instance, in the example mentioned earlier of a CSA survivor crying in session with her husband, it is important not to assume the meaning of this behavior. Rather, it is necessary to understand what purpose the crying serves for the survivor and how this behavior functions in the relationship. Is the purpose to communicate an emotion? What emotion is being expressed (e.g., sadness, frustration, happiness, confusion, or fear)? Is the survivor attempting to communicate this emotion to herself (self-validate), her partner, or the therapist? Is the purpose to distance herself from her partner or draw her partner closer? Is the purpose to facilitate communication about the topic at hand or to halt communication (e.g., stop her husband from pushing the topic of sex)? Of course, it is possible that the behavior has multiple functions. In addition, the therapist would want to pay particular attention to the outcome of this behavior: Does crying elicit compassion and understanding from her partner, create distance in the relationship, facilitate or block the communication process? Understanding the function of this behavior allows the therapist to accurately conceptualize the issue and intervene according to the goals of prediction and influence.

Given that numerous behaviors can serve the same function, it is often helpful and more efficient to think of certain behaviors in terms of belonging to functional classes. Although behaviors can have various forms, they can be understood to belong to a particular response class. Response classes are hypothetical groupings of individual behaviors that all share the same function, even though the form (topography) of these behaviors may be quite different (Haynes & O'Brien, 2000). To use our same example, the wife's behavior of crying in session may be in the same response class as drinking alcohol, working excessive hours, binge eating, or missing a couple therapy session if each of these behaviors serves the function of avoiding uncomfortable thoughts and feelings (such as those that might arise when the topic is sex). Understanding behaviors in terms of their function and response classes can help therapists working with survivor couples to avoid being swept away by the flood of weekly topics and content that are presented in therapy. Rather than discussing topics that are tangential, therapists can use a functional analysis (see Follette & Naugle, Chapter 2, this volume, for more information on functional analysis) to focus each session around the core interaction patterns that maintain the couple's difficulties. Identifying response classes can also aid therapists in understanding each new behavior that couples enact throughout the course of treatment.

Along with these functional contextual roots we draw from a radical behavioral theory (Skinner, 1974) of human behavior. Contrary to classic conceptualizations or stereotypes of behavioral theory, this approach acknowledges unobservable events such as thoughts and feelings as important forms of behavior. Radical behaviorists seek to identify and understand the variables perceived to be functionally related to the problem behavior in some way.

We use the construct of experiential avoidance in understanding a wide variety of responses in human behavior (Hayes, Wilson, Gifford, Follette, & Strosahl, 1996; see also Walser & Hayes, Chapter 7, this volume). Experiential avoidance occurs when an individual is unwilling to experience painful private events (e.g., bodily sensations, thoughts, feelings, memories) and takes steps to alter the form or frequency of these (Hayes, Strosahl, & Wilson, 1999). This perspective is extremely useful in understanding the experiences of individuals who have undergone a trauma. The diverse outcomes associated with a trauma history can be understood as behaviors employed to minimize, alter, or eliminate the experience of unpleasant internal events. Using the concept of avoidance in understanding reactions to trauma is not unique to behaviorists. A number of researchers and clinicians has noted the importance of avoidance in treating survivors (cf. Briere, 1991; Leitenberg, Gibson, & Novy, 2004; Banyard, 2003).

Here we present principles we have found useful in guiding treatment with survivor couples; by no means do they constitute a comprehensive list of functional contextual behavior principles.

Effectiveness

Perhaps the most ubiquitous principle we rely on is effectiveness or workability. As noted earlier in this chapter, *successful working* is the truth criterion for a contextual-oriented therapist. It is also a principle that guides the in-the-moment decisions made during sessions with survivor couples. During any given session, clients may disclose a whole host of issues and will emit many emotions and overt behaviors that are potential targets for treatment. The principle of effectiveness serves as a filter, a way to identify what to focus on in the moment, what to save for later sessions, and what to set aside because it is unclear how the content or behavior fits into our understanding of the survivor couple or because it is unclear how it is functioning for the couple or individual. There are two necessary questions that must be answered in relation to effectiveness.

The first question is: Is this intervention effective, given our goals? At the outset of treatment the couple and the therapist agree upon a set of goals to address during the course of therapy. For example, many couples describe a desire to be more emotionally connected and physically intimate, to communicate better, and to remove the survivor's abuse history as a barrier between them. These might be the agreed-upon goals between therapist and couple. In addition, as clinicians working with survivor couples, we have several underlying goals that are consistent across couples. These goals include (but are not limited to) developing and maintaining a strong therapeutic relationship with each individual and the couple; managing the therapy process during sessions so that the couple's communication does not become caustic or vengeful, while simultaneously encouraging the couple to be in contact with, but not overwhelmed by, emotion; and continually listening and searching for a more complete understanding of their lives in the service of accurate empathy, continual assessment, and possible alterations to the trajectory of treatment. We are mindful of these goals as therapists and rely on them to help guide our in-the-moment decisions with regard to effectiveness.

The second question involves the current context: Is this intervention effective, given the current context? The current context has many facets, and the therapist must balance each one when making this assessment. Skills that each individual possesses represent part of the context. These skills include an individual's ability to regulate emotions in the moment, to validate his or her partner, to identify and ask for what he or she needs from the partner, and to be emotionally present and willing to hear what his or her partner is saying or requesting. The context also varies from session to session and may involve the presence of vulnerability factors such as lack of sleep or food, level of individual emotional arousal, and how engaged or distant partners are feeling in the relationship. Other important contextual considerations include the amount of time remaining in the session and what each individual must do immediately after session. For example, if the trauma survivor is scheduled to go back to work immediately after the session and does not possess emotion regulation skills, it might not be effective to have him or her disclose abuse-related material to the partner at this time. In fact, it might be effective for the therapist to request that the appointment time be changed so that the context would be more conducive to emotionally charged work. As is the case with treatment goals, the current context involves multiple facets that must be considered when making an in-the-moment decision based on the principle of effectiveness.

Consistency

The second principle we rely on is the importance of consistency, or predictability, in the therapeutic relationship and environment. This principle is the basis for developing therapy as a safe environment. Trauma survivors share an experience in which an environment was not safe, whether it be the home environment in which incest occurred; their adult home, office, or neighborhood in which a rape occurred; or the war zone where the potential for combat was omnipresent. In addition to unsafe historical environments, it is also possible that survivors may feel unsafe in a current relationship or work environment. In this event, the degree of danger and the possibility for revictimization should always be assessed. Even when there is little risk of physical or sexual harm, many survivors and their partners describe their relationships as lacking a foundation of trust necessary for emotional disclosure and intimacy. Thus, in order to effectively discuss trauma-related issues or other problems in the relationship, it is essential to establish and maintain a safe therapy environment. Consistency and predictability of the therapist and therapy environment can provide the foundation for this safety.

Trust can be thought of as predictability of behavior. An individual can trust an environment or individual when he or she can predict what this individual (or individuals) within the environment will do and how he or she will respond. For example, a child who is being abused by her father does not feel safe with him because she cannot predict how he will respond: protectively, as a father, or abusively, as a molestor. There is no consistency in her environment. At certain times her father may respond to her in kind ways and with words of support; at other times, however, he may act sexually abusive toward her. Men and women in combat situations also cannot predict the behavior of certain individuals in their environment. They can be ambushed at any time and essentially cannot trust (i.e., predict) the safety of their environment from one moment to the next. The environment of individuals whose partners are trauma survivors might also lack predictability and consistency, and therefore trust and safety. A partner may not be able to predict when something will trigger a flashback for his or her spouse, or how his or her spouse will respond to a request for intimacy.

When working with survivor couples we strive for consistency and predictability as a way of creating and maintaining a safe and trustworthy environment. There are many ways to demonstrate consistency and predictability, ranging from the basic structure of the therapy environment to maintaining a "peacekeeper" stance to control potentially damaging behavior in session. Maintaining consistency in some of the more basic areas can be extremely beneficial in providing a safe environment (a guideline that is common to most therapeutic orientations). Finding and maintaining a particular day and time for sessions that works for both the therapist and the couple, starting and ending sessions on time, and beginning and ending sessions in a predictable way (e.g., with a mindfulness exercise; by checking in with the couple on thoughts about their previous or current session) are all structural ways of providing consistency.

It is also important that the therapist present as behavior predictable as possible. In couples in which one of the partners is a trauma survivor, it is quite likely that one or both partners may have difficulty with emotion regulation. This deficit may be manifested in session by withdrawal, the picking of fights, verbal attacks, dissociation, or topic changes. The therapist must be able to maintain a peacekeeper stance and stop verbal attacks from one or both partners, reengage a withdrawing partner, and otherwise control and extinguish harmful interactions between partners. This amount of predictability in the therapist's behavior will establish the therapy environment as a place where emotions can be expressed and experienced, concerns can be voiced, and skills can be acquired—all without ineffective or punishing responses from either partner. At the same time, the therapist needs to provide an environment that allows the processing of painful material. Thus a delicate balancing between opening communication and maintaining safety is required.

Contingent Responding

Contingent responding is our third principle. In order to talk about contingent responding effectively, we need to discuss it in relation to the concepts of reinforcement, punishment, and shaping. The premise behind our principles is that behaviors may or may not continue to be part of an individual's or couple's repertoire of behavior. Given this premise, we as therapists work to strengthen and/or introduce behaviors in each individual's or couple's repertoire that are effective (given client goals and the goals of therapy, as described in the first principle). We also work to weaken and/or eliminate behaviors that are ineffective. Reinforcement, punishment, and shaping are the tools we use to accomplish these changes.

Reinforcing stimuli are those stimuli that follow a particular behavior and increase the probability that this behavior will occur in the future. If a male veteran reported feeling vulnerable in the session, the therapist would likely praise him for his self-disclosure, given that self-disclosure of feelings is a behavior that we want to strengthen in his repertoire. Negative reinforcement is also used at times to increase the probability of a behavior recurring. However, as noted by Jacobson and Margolin (1979) in their seminal work on behavioral marital therapy, the use of positive control strategies (vs. aversive control) is highly preferable. Punishment is used, though rarely, to decrease the probability of a behavior occurring through the delivery of an adverse stimulus. If a partner became verbally abusive in session, the therapist would intervene by stopping the behavior and discussing its impact. This discussion would function as a punishment (i.e., given that the partner stops the abusive behavior). The therapist's intervention in this context is sometimes called "traffic-copping"; however, we prefer the term "peacekeeping." Basically, the role of the therapist is to address and punish ineffective behavior immediately. At times we may use traffic-cop-like hand signals to gain the attention of the partner and to achieve the desired effect of decreasing or stopping the behavior. We inform the couple about this technique as a part of our orientation to treatment and informed consent regarding our style and approach. We also process each individual's experience of this traffic-cop behavior when it is used for the first time. The feedback we have received is that by orienting couples to our style and approach, they feel informed and are willing to agree to the rules; furthermore, they find traffic-copping to be an effective way to decrease their ineffective behavior patterns. The goal is to convey the value of therapy as a safe place where verbal abuse is not tolerated. In addition to stopping damaging behavior, it is crucial to provide positive alternatives to the problem behaviors, thereby enhancing the relationship.

Shaping is used by the therapist to identify and reinforce approximations of an effective target behavior toward the goal of gradually strengthening and widening the individual's repertoire. In other words, shaping rewards improvement rather than a preestablished absolute level of performance (Masters, Burish, Hollon, & Rimm, 1987). Shaping is an essential part of therapy with survivor couples. It is our experience that many of these couples lack skills that are necessary for communication and validation; it is not so much an issue of not wanting to communicate with or validate a partner, it is more an issue of not having the skills to do so. Self-disclosure of feelings is often a behavior we want to shape in survivors of trauma. For example, we might reinforce a survivor's disclosure that she is not sure what she is feeling as a beginning step in the process of sharing emotions. The behavior of disclosing uncertainty is closer to the desired behavior of sharing her feelings than the previous behavior of claiming that nothing is wrong. In the future we would cease reinforcing disclosures of uncertainty and reinforce any disclosures involving specific feelings. Typically it is easier for individuals to disclose positive feelings than negative ones; thus we might reinforce all disclosures involving positive feelings, with the knowledge that once the survivor is reinforced for disclosing these types of feelings, he or she will more likely begin to disclose negative feelings over time. It is also imperative that the therapist shape the behavior of the partner. In some cases partners punish their partners self-disclosure unintentionally or intentionally. It is vital to identify this pattern and facilitate a safe environment for this type of disclosure.

Contingent responding, using the principles described above, is a daunting task for any couple therapist; however it is potentially even more difficult when working with survivor couples. Given the complexities of many survivors' histories, it is likely that behaviors considered to be ineffective in their current relationships (and therefore a target for change in session), have been reinforced and even effective in other relationships and contexts. For example, some CSA survivors may have been punished (e.g., yelled at, blamed, ignored by the family) for disclosing that the abuse occurred and expressing feelings about it. Conversely, remaining quiet, pretending that nothing was wrong, and keeping feelings such as sadness, fear, and anger to oneself may have been encouraged and supported by the family. Thus the same behaviors that were praised by the survivor's family now function to create distance in the survivor's intimate relationship and are ineffective. Therefore, it is important for the therapist to be sensitive to small changes in behaviors related to emotions, in order to be able to reinforce the client for gradual changes in being more open and vulnerable, with the goal of enhancing the emotional intimacy between partners.

Modeling

Modeling is frequently used in conjunction with the previous principles. While we were reviewing the principle of contingent responding in relation to couple therapy, we noted that there are a number of clinically relevant behaviors emitted by both partners that represent potential opportunity for intervention by the therapist. Similarly, the therapist's interactions with the couple provide multiple opportunities for modeling new forms of behavior. Again, a thorough and ongoing functional analysis of the couple's problems will serve to make the therapist more mindful of potential opportunities for learning through modeling. At times this modeling will be done explicitly for the couple; however, more important opportunities may occur using a subtler approach. One of the most important forms of behavior that the therapist will work to model consistently is validating behavior. During the first few sessions, the therapist would not draw attention to his or her validating behavior. Orienting the couple to the therapist's approach and style as well as assessing the couple's skills, deficits, and therapy goals is more effective during initial sessions. When an effective time arises for introducing a skill and working toward its incorporation into the couple's repertoire, we discuss the skill, model it directly, and give the partners opportunities to practice it. At times the level of conflict in the couple is too high for partners to engage in this behavior with each other, and the therapist may need to practice with each client. Our approach to and use of validation is adopted from the work of Linehan (see Wagner and Linehan, Chapter 6, this volume).

It is important to be aware that the therapist serves as a model for the couple at all times. Conflict between partners, the raising of difficult questions, expression of intense emotions, and the provision of feedback are all potential opportunities for the therapist to model effective behavior. One important opportunity that should not be overlooked occurs when either one or both of the clients have an issue with the therapist. The ability of the therapist to remain present, validate clients' experience, and work to resolve the issue can be far more important that long tutorials on a topic. The couple's opportunity not only to see the therapist engage in effective behavior but also to experience the feelings associated with being treated in this way can have both short- and long-term benefits. In the short term, the therapist's affective behavior may serve to deescalate a tense clinical situation and clarify any misunderstandings that may be occurring. In the longer term, this behavior can enhance the therapeutic relationship, setting the stage for the difficult work to come. Of course, it is also our hope that the occurrence of this type of interaction in session will help the couple to engage in similar behavior in their private interactions. Thus the therapist's consistent and supportive behavior throughout the couple's time in therapy can provide a powerful modeling experience of a stable, dependable relationship. However, therapist errors can also be useful in this context. For example, when the therapist has missed a session or been inattentive in some way, he or she can use the perceived breach to engage in work to repair the relationship. Responding in this way not only demonstrates the vulnerability of all relationships to difficulties, but also shows clients that the therapist is willing to practice the principles that he or she teaches.

One of the most important opportunities for modeling in therapy with couples in which one member is a survivor involves situations in which a partner is disclosing his or her traumatic experience and/or feelings surrounding the experience. Many survivor couples experience a great deal of difficulty in communicating about the trauma(s). The therapist not only can offer the survivor a safe and validating context within which to disclose his or her feelings and thoughts about the traumatic experience, he or she can also provide the partner with a model of how to listen effectively and validate the survivors feelings. After the survivor has talked about his or her experience and any feelings and thoughts about it, the therapist can ask the survivor what was helpful about the therapist's responses and what he or she would have wanted to be different. By processing this experience, both therapist and partner can gain a greater understanding about what functionally validates the survivor, without putting the partner in the familiar position of ineffectively communicating with his or her partner about the trauma. This interaction also models for the couple the pattern of eliciting feedback from each other regarding what is helpful in their communication and what could be improved. A key factor in this process is acceptance. Being open to the survivor's disclosures and being willing to experience the feelings associated with hearing about these painful events can be critical for both members of the couple. Frequently, partners of survivors can be so overwhelmed with their own pain on hearing about the experience that they try to minimize the event, saying things such as, "It was so long ago, it's over now, can't you let it go?" Of course, this is precisely the type of invalidation that may have occurred in other settings, with the survivor feeling shamed or weak for not having handled the problem. Conversely, the survivor may not want to be seen as fragile and incompetent. Thus a balance of empathic listening, support, and reflection by the therapist can often give the partner guidance on how to respond.

Tacting and Manding

"Tacting" can be thought of as labeling and describing events, feelings, or objects: for example, "I yelled at my husband last night—I'm mad at him," and "That is a pencil." "Manding" refers to the speech involved in requests, commands, and threats: for example, "Stop yelling at me," "If you don't leave me alone, I'll hit you," and "I would like a pencil." The ability to tact and mand effectively is an essential aspect of interpersonal interactions. Couples coming for therapy frequently have deficits in this area. Of course, most people generally have an effective repertoire for dealing with basic instrumental activities. However, we often observe significant difficulties in the area of dealing with complex thoughts and feelings. An inability to label feelings and needs and make requests and demands from a partner will seriously compromise the effectiveness of, and satisfaction with, the relationship. Survivor couples frequently present with deficits in this area. Of course, they do not describe their situation in these terms. Common complaints include, "I never know what she is feeling," "Why can't he just tell me what he wants instead of making me guess all the time?", and "I don't know what I am feeling, so how can I tell him?"

The ability to tact and mand is ideally learned at a young age and effectively shaped by one's environment. When learning to tact (label/describe) an object, a parent or important other in the child's life can point to the object, such as a dog, pronounce the name, and reinforce a response from the child that is "dog" or a close approximation of "dog." After several experiences with the object labeled "dog," sight of the dog elicits the response of "dog." Notice that this activity of teaching tacting involves the principles of reinforcement, shaping, and contingent responding (all discussed under the third principle of contingent responding).

Teaching a child (or anyone, for that matter) to tact an emotion is more complicated. The stimuli to be described are private somatic experiences to which other people do not have access. As a result, a parent or other important person in the child's life looks to the environment and makes a guess as to what the child is experiencing, pronounces the name, and reinforces the name or a close approximation of it. For example, if a young child is crying, the parent may look to the environment and see that the child's knee is scraped and bleeding; perhaps the parent even saw the child fall. At this point the parent guesses that the child is hurt and encourages him or her to say "hurt." Eventually, if the parent was effective, the private experience of pain would be tacted as "I'm hurt." A number of parental difficulties can impact the acquisition of these basic skills. Parents suffering from substance abuse, depression, or other psychological problems may not be sufficiently aware of and responsive to cues from the child that would lead to developing a repertoire for noticing and labeling feelings.

In families where abuse occurs during early developmental periods rather than later in life, tacting and manding can be inappropriately shaped or punished, leaving the individual ineffective at one or both and therefore vulnerable to all kinds of relationship difficulties. Exposure to an abusive environment can lead to confusing and conflicting messages related to tacting and thereby shape the trauma survivor to mistrust his or her own private experiences. For example, a perpetrator might try to convince the child that he or she is enjoying the experience when, in fact, the child is feeling pain, fear, anger, or confusion. The child is then left unsure of how to label his or her private experience. In addition, manding is often punished in an abusive environment. The child requesting (mand) that the abuser stop may be met with threats, ignored, or punished outright. These experiences serve to teach the survivor that manding is ineffective; therefore, this behavior has a high probability of being extinguished from his or her repertoire.

Therapy sessions offer rich opportunities to teach effective tacting and manding. As therapists working with couples, it is important to remain mindful of situations that might induce certain feelings in either or both partners. For example, any conversation that is related to the survivor's abuse experience might evoke feelings of fear, anger, sadness, or confusion. As these situations arise, we have found it effective to highlight the emotions that the survivor and/or partner might be feeling by utilizing environmental cues (e.g., the topic of trauma, body language of the individual) to make educated guesses. It is useful to differentiate between clients who readily identify the emotions and have been punished for expressing them, versus those who cannot label emotions effectively. Teaching emotion labeling skills, as described by Linehan (1993b), is frequently an important part of treatment for any couple. However, it then becomes important to create an environment in which these emotions can be safely discussed. In addition, several of the interpersonal effectiveness skills involve helping clients to ask effectively for what they need and want from their partner (manding) while maintaining the relationship and their own self-respect. The list in Table 14.1 includes several tacts and associated mands that we have found to be difficult for survivors and/or their partners. This list is simply a compilation of our experience with this population and is meant as only a starting point for therapists. An individual assessment of each couple's skills and deficits will allow therapists to generate their own list with each couple and remain mindful of in-session opportunities to work on them.

Exposure

Exposure is not only a technique but also a principle that we believe should be incorporated and acknowledged throughout therapy. Exposure, as a technique, is frequently used in behavior therapies and is especially relevant in the treatment of trauma (see Riggs, Cahill, & Foa, Chapter 4, this volume; Shiperd, Street, & Resick, Chapter 5, this volume). Exposure, as a principle, relies on the explanations offered by both classical and operant conditioning theories, and suggests that by gradually and continually exposing the individual to the feared feelings, topics, objects, and/or thoughts, the learned fear will be extinguished over time. The principle of exposure can be incorporated in a wide variety of ways and perhaps in forms not commonly thought of as exposure. In fact, many of the interventions we incorporate into treatment with couples serve several functions, and one of them is often expo-

TABLE 14.1. Common Tacts and Mands

Tact	Mands
"I am feeling vulnerable."	"Please sit with me," "Please give me a few minutes by myself," or "Please hold me while I cry."
"I am feeling angry."	"Listen to what I am telling you," "Let me tell you about what is bothering me," or "You do not have to fix this situation—all I want is for you to let me talk about it."
"I am feeling scared."	"Please sit with me," "Please let me tell you what I am afraid of," or "Please use a quieter voice when we talk"
"I am feeling happy (excited)."	"Let me tell you about why I am excited," "Celebrate with me," or "Let me be happy."
"I'm not sure what I am feeling."	"Please be patient with me, I am trying," "Help me try and identify what I am feeling," or "Please given me some time to myself."

sure. We include exposure to any topic, thought, feeling, or content that has been avoided. We believe that the avoidance of thoughts and feelings associated with vulnerability are an important factor in a lack of intimacy that many couples in therapy report as a problem.

Psychoeducation about trauma and its potential impact on individuals and couples, emotion regulation skills, and interpersonal effectiveness skills all involve exposure as one of the elements influencing their inclusion in treatment. As we know from generalization and second-order operant conditioning, certain words, phrases, or experiences can come to elicit a fear response even if they were never originally part of the traumatic experience. Including psychoeducation into treatment for survivor couples can function as a low-level form of exposure in addition to its use as a way to assess partners' knowledge about trauma and its impact and their reactivity to trauma-related material. The subject of trauma and its impact can become taboo in relationships, frequently because it has led to arguments, misunderstandings, one or both partner's withdrawing physically or emotionally, and myriad consequences experienced as undesirable. Among other things, psychoeducation exposes the couple to material about the trauma in a contained, safe environment, thus serving at least two functions simultaneously. First, psychoeducation frequently reduces blame, shame, and stigmatization about the trauma and its impact. The survivor and the partner need to know that neither of them is responsible for the trauma or any symptoms that have developed as a result. Second, it also functions to expose the couple to the trauma (e.g., words, phrases, experiences) they may have avoided and therefore begins to reduce their reactivity and avoidance.

When working with trauma survivors and their partners, we often include some skills training, depending on our assessment of the needs of each couple. We select from many of the dialectical behavior therapy skills developed by Marsha Linehan (1993b; see Wagner & Linehan, Chapter 5, this volume). The rationale for including skills training in treatment is based on more than exposure, of course. Skills training is effective for many couples, given their specific treatment goals. Exposure, however, is more influential than perhaps we might think. Emotion regulation skills, interpersonal effectiveness skills, and mindfulness are the most common sets of skills we find useful for survivor couples. Mindfulness can be thought of as a focusing of attention or awareness. As noted earlier, trauma survivors often have difficulty noticing and identifying their emotions; mindfulness is a way to expose clients to emotions and to help them become more aware of them. Learning emotion regulation skills can help survivors and their partners become better at identifying emotions and discriminating between them (as discussed in the section on tacting and manding). Inherent in noticing and identifying emotions is exposure to these emotions. Interpersonal effectiveness skills can also be invaluable for trauma survivors. We have found that acquiring these skills can meaningfully enhance survivor couple's relationships by providing the partners with more effective ways to communicate as well as continually exposing them to situations, topics, and feelings that they have previously avoided. Over time exposure to these situations, topics, and emotions, coupled with a more skillful way of communicating about them, reduces their negative impact while increasing partners' sense of mastery.

Acceptance

Acceptance, the functional alternative to experiential avoidance, is our final principle. Incorporated into numerous treatments (Jacobson, Christensen, Prince, Cordova, & Eldridge, 2000; Orsillo, Roemer, & Barlow, 2003; Wilson, 1996), acceptance continues to be a popular topic for both researchers and clinicians (Hayes, Follette, & Linehan, 2004). Our reliance on acceptance in our work with survivor couples is grounded in acceptance as a treatment principle. Hayes et al. (1999) define acceptance as "an active taking in of an event or situation . . . acceptance involves an abandonment of dysfunctional change agendas and an active process of feeling feelings as feelings, thinking thoughts as thoughts, remembering memories as memories" (p. 77). The principle of acceptance, like all of our other principles, does not operate in isolation; in fact, acceptance is always part of a triad, including effectiveness and exposure. Of course, there are times when acceptance is not even an appropriate strategy. For example, asking a woman in an abusive relationship to accept the beatings she is receiving is not appropriate or ethical. However, being in contact with the feelings associated with the abuse, including her fears associated with leaving a relationship, can lead to more effective behavior—that is, leaving a relationship that continues to be abusive. Given that we are not able to change or alter history, acceptance of a trauma history is an ultimate goal for any survivor. However, survivors or their partners may be ready to be exposed to this principle in the early phases of treatment. Acceptance of our history, whether it be traumatic or not, by definition involves exposure to that experience. A thorough assessment of the couple's strengths and weaknesses will assist the therapist in knowing when to bring the trauma history into the therapy room.

To clarify the role of acceptance in treatment with survivor couples, it may be useful to specify the different domains in which we apply this principle. There is acceptance of internal events, such as thoughts, feelings, or memories; acceptance of one's history; acceptance of self; and acceptance of others (Follette & Pistorello, 1995). We consider each of these domains briefly as it relates to the treatment of survivor couples.

Acceptance of internal events such as thoughts, feelings, or memories is always applicable. The speed, movement, and flow with which we introduce and help survivor couples incorporate acceptance of internal events depends on each couple's ability to tolerate this exposure. For one or both partners in some survivor couples, avoidance of painful thoughts, feelings, and memories is the only tool they posses to keep them emotionally regulated. In these cases it would not be effective to focus on acceptance before first working on emotion regulation skills (as discussed in relation to our fifth and sixth principles) to provide one or both partners with alternative ways of coping. As therapy progresses, we gradually introduce the topic and ask clients to "check their experience" for how effective it is for them to avoid or try to change their thoughts, feelings, and emotions. To illustrate this point, we often incorporate metaphors and exercises outlined in acceptance and commitment therapy (Walser & Hayes, Chapter 7, this volume; Hayes et al., 1999). These metaphors and exercises help clients experience how ineffective attempted control of private events has been in their lives, and the possibility that acceptance may be an effective alternative.

Acceptance of one's history can be most challenging when working with clients who have a trauma history. Survivors frequently want to get rid of or forget their abuse history, and their nonacceptance of the abuse may lead to a range of behaviors aimed at eliminating any thoughts, feelings, or behaviors that serve as reminders of the abuse (Follette & Pistorello, 1995). In the case of CSA survivors, for whom the abuse was of a sexual nature, sexual situations and behaviors with the current partner would serve as reminders of the abuse and therefore would be targeted for avoidance. This could lead the survivor to avoid (through dissociation, substance abuse, or physical avoidance) all sexual intimacy. Enhancing intimacy, both emotional and physical, is at the core of couple therapy and thus this can become a key factor in treatment. In this case, acceptance would be coupled with some traditional sex therapy techniques that are based in behavioral principles. It is important to address not only the survivor's feelings in this regard, but also difficulties the partner may have in dealing with the partner's reactions to sexual intimacy. (For a more complete discussion of modifying sexual dysfunction treatments for CSA survivor couples, see Leonard & Follette, 2002.)

Acceptance of self involves our taking the perspective of the self as an observer of not only external events but also our own thoughts and feelings; seeing ourselves as distinct from our roles, behaviors, emotions, and history (Hayes et al., 1999). By acting from a perspective of self-acceptance, the client can experience events related to the trauma, such as a flashback, without having to engage in familiar patterns of experiential avoidance, such as dissociation (Follette & Pistorello, 1995). Acting from an acceptance of self while experiencing a flashback when touched by his or her partner allows the survivor to break the experiential avoidance pattern and do something differently. The survivor can notice that he or she is having a flashback and choose to talk to his or her partner about it, thus increasing the emotional intimacy between them. Experiencing themselves as more than their thoughts, experiences, and emotions can function to provide distance for survivors between themselves as people and their experiences, thereby allowing them to respond differently.

The acceptance of others entails those private experiences (thoughts and feelings) that at a content level refer to other individuals (Follette & Pistorello, 1995). A piece of this area of acceptance includes the partner's acceptance of the survivor's abuse history. Often the partner is not able to accept his or her own thoughts and feeling about his or her partner's abuse history. This does not mean that the client nonabused partner should condone any behavior that the abused partner emits, but rather that there is an acceptance of the thoughts and feelings that the abused partner brings to the relationship.

The principles described in Table 14.2 are the backbone of our intervention with survivor couples. We incorporate various techniques depending on the needs of each couple, but the principles remain constant. Conducting therapy from this stance allows us to be effective and engaged while appreciating the individuality of each couple and tailoring a treatment specific to partners' needs and abilities.

INDIVIDUAL VERSUS COUPLE TREATMENT AND THE RECOVERY FROM TRAUMA

The impact of trauma, though predicable to some degree, also remains idiographic. As Naugle and Follette (1998) note, "There is no pathognomonic symptom or symptom constellation that always results from a trauma history" (p. 48). We would also argue that the recovery from trauma can be just as idiographic. Although we as clinicians and researchers have learned a great deal from our research and experience with trauma survivors and couples, we must always be mindful of all that we do not yet know and have not yet considered. Recovery from trauma is more of a journey than a destination, and as such, it is likely that both individual and couple treatment will occur on many trauma survivors' journeys. The decision about when each is

TABLE 14.2. Principles and Techniques for Couple Treatment

Principle	Technique	Reference
1. Effectiveness	*Mindfulness practice* is the intentional process of observing, describing, and participating in the moment nonjudgmentally and with effectiveness. To focus attention (be mindful) increases self-knowledge that can manifest in skillful, effective behavior.	Linehan (1993a)
	Chain analyses of problem situations between the couple, or problem behaviors of each partner, involve a step-by-step description of the events leading up to and following a problem situation or behavior; the goal is to identify important antecedents and consequences, which, in turn, guide the therapist's choice of the most effective way to intervene on these problematic behavior patterns.	Linehan (1993b)
2. Consistency	*Validation* is the communication of understanding and acknowledgment of another person's thoughts, emotions, wants, goals, or behavior. This type of communication builds trust and a sense of safety for clients that their experiences and emotions will be acknowledged, understood, and taken seriously.	Fruzzetti & Iverson (2004)
3. Contingent responding	In *behavior exchange* each partner identifies behaviors that he or she would like his or her partner to do more. Each partner then increases the frequency of these desired behaviors and acknowledges the behaviors that the other has done for him or her.	Christensen, Jacobson, & Babcock (1995)
4. Modeling	*In-session role playing* can be used to demonstrate (model) appropriate communication and interpersonal interaction by recreating problematic situations the couple experiences. The therapist enacts the role of one of the partners and demonstrates effective behavior for the given situation.	Masters, Burish, Hollon, & Rimm (1987)
5. Tacting and manding	*Interpersonal effectiveness skills* involve making requests and refusing unwanted requests (manding) skillfully.	Linehan (1993a)
	Emotion regulation skills involve identifying and labeling emotions (tacting) accurately.	
6. Exposure	*Exposure*, in its most structured form involves constructing a hierarchy of feared situations or experiences and then systematically confronting them.	Foa & Rothbaum (1998)
	Emotional exposure is much less structured and involves encouraging and facilitating each partner to experience and tolerate his or her emotions in session, thereby creating experiential awareness of emotions as impermanent and tolerable.	

cont.

TABLE 14.2. *cont.*

Principle	Technique	Reference
7. Acceptance	Identify *controlling strategies as problematic* for internal experiences or private events (i.e., thoughts and feelings) by utilizing metaphors (e.g., Polygraph) and exercises (e.g., Clean vs. Dirty Discomfort Diary) outlined in acceptance and commitment therapy to increase willingness and acceptance.	Hayes, Strosahl, & Wilson (1999); Walser & Hayes, Chapter 7, this volume

appropriate or useful remains more of an art than a science, more a preference than a mandate. We are not arguing for a couple approach as a panacea for all that ails the trauma survivor; quite the contrary. Consistent with the principle-based approach we presented, we believe that what is most effective will depend on each client and the individual context he or she presents. No matter what the context for treatment, we as clinicians and researchers must remain mindful that our collective journey is in the service of improving the lives of trauma survivors.

REFERENCES

American Psychiatric Association. (1994). *The diagnostic and statistical manual of mental disorders* (4th ed.). Washington, DC: Author.

Banyard, V. L. (2003). Explaining links between sexual abuse and psychological distress: Identifying mediating processes. *Child Abuse and Neglect, 27*(8), 869–875.

Baucom, D. H., Shoham, V., Mueser, K. T., Daiuto, A. D., & Stickle, T. R. (1998). Empirically supported couple and family interventions for marital distress and adult mental health problems. *Journal of Consulting and Clinical Psychology, 66,* 53–88.

Becker, J. V., Skinner, L. J., Abel, G. G., Axelrod, R., & Cichon, J. (1984). Sexual problems of sexual assault survivors. *Women and Health, 9,* 5–20.

Beitchman, J. H., Zucker, K. J., Hood, J. E., DaCosta, G. A., Akman, D., & Cassavia, E. (1992). A review of the long-term effects of child sexual abuse. *Child Abuse and Neglect, 16,* 101–118.

Briere, J. (1988). The long-term clinical correlates of childhood sexual victimization. *Annals of the New York Academy of Sciences, 528,* 327–334.

Briere, J., & Runtz, M. (1987). Post-sexual abuse trauma: Data and implications for clinical practice. *Journal of Interpersonal Violence, 2,* 367–397.

Briere, J., & Runtz, M. (1988). Post sexual abuse trauma. In G. E. Wyatt & G. J. Powell (Eds.), *Lasting effects of child sexual abuse* (pp.85–99). Newbury Park, CA: Sage.

Browne, A., & Finkelhor, D. (1986). Impact of child sexual abuse: A review of the research. *Psychological Bulletin, 99,* 66–77.

Buttenheim, M., & Levendosky, A. (1994). Couples treatment for incest survivors. *Psychotherapy: Theory, Research, Practice, Training, 31,* 407–414.

Chambless, D. L., & Hollon, S. D. (1998). Defining empirically supported therapies. *Journal of Consulting and Clinical Psychology, 66,* 7–18.

Christensen, A., Atkins, D. C., Berns, S., Wheeler, J., Baucom, D. H., & Simpson, L. E. (2004). Traditional versus integrative behavioral couple therapy for significantly and chronically distressed married couples. *Journal of Consulting and Clinical Psychology, 72,* 176–191.

Christensen, A., Jacobson, N. S., & Babcock, J. C. (1995). Integrative behavioral couple therapy. In N. S. Jacobson & A. S. Gurman (Eds.), *Clinical handbook of couple therapy* (pp. 31–64). New York: Guilford Press.

Compton, J. S., & Follette, V. M. (1998). Couples surviving trauma: Issues and interventions. In V. M. Follette, J. I. Ruzek, & F. R. Abueg (Eds.), *Cognitive-behavioral therapies for trauma* (pp. 321–352). New York: Guilford Press.

Cook, J. M., Riggs, D. S., Thompson, R., Coyne, J. C., & Sheikh, J. I. (2004). Posttraumatic stress disorder and current relationship functioning among World War II ex-prisoners of war. *Journal of Family Psychology, 18,* 36–45.

Coyne, J. C. (1976). Towards an interactional description of depression. *Psychiatry, 39,* 28–40.

DiLillo, D., & Long, P. J. (1999). Perceptions of couple functioning among female survivors of child sexual abuse. *Journal of Child Sexual Abuse, 7,* 59–76.

Ellis, E. M., Calhoun, K. S., & Atkeson, B. M. (1980). Sexual dysfunctions in victims of rape: Victims may experience a loss of sexual arousal and frightening flashbacks even one year after the assault. *Women and Health, 5,* 39–47.

Foa, E. B., & Rothbaum, B. O. (1998). *Treating the trauma of rape.* New York: Guilford Press.

Follette, V. M., & Pistorello, J. (1995). Couples therapy. In C. Classen & I. D. Yalom (Eds.), *Treating women molested in childhood* (pp. 129–161). San Francisco: Jossey-Bass.

Follette, V. M., Polusny, M. M., Bechtle, A. E., & Naugle, A. E. (1996). Cumulative trauma effects: The impact of child sexual abuse, adult sexual assault, and spouse abuse. *Journal of Traumatic Stress, 9,* 15–25.

Fruzzetti, A. E., & Iverson, K. M., (2004). Mindfulness, acceptance, validation, and "individual" psychopathology in couples. In S. C. Hayes, V. M. Follette, & M. M. Linehan (Eds.), *Mindfulness and acceptance: Expanding the cognitive-behavioral tradition* (pp. 168–191). New York: Guilford Press.

Gold, E. R. (1986). Long-term effects of sexual victimization in childhood: An attributional approach. *Journal of Consulting and Clinical Psychology, 54*(4), 471–475.

Hayes, S. C., Follette, V. M., & Linehan, M. M. (Eds.). (2004). *Mindfulness and acceptance: Expanding the cognitive-behavioral tradition.* New York: Guilford Press.

Hayes, S. C., Strosahl, K. D., & Wilson, K. G. (1999). *Acceptance and commitment therapy: An experiential approach to behavior change.* New York: Guilford Press.

Hayes, S. C., Wilson, K., Gifford, E., Follette, V. M., & Strosahl, K. (1996). Experiential avoidance and behavioral disorders: A functional dimensional approach to diagnosis and treatment. *Journal of Consulting and Clinical Psychology, 64,* 1152–1168.

Haynes, S. N., & O'Brien, W. H. (2000). *Principles and practice of behavioral assessment.* New York: Kluwer Academic/Plenum.

Herman, J. (1981). *Father–daughter incest.* Cambridge, MA: Harvard University Press.

Jackson, J. L., Calhoun, K. S., Amick, A. E., Maddever, H. M., & Habif, V. L. (1990). Young adult women who report childhood intrafamilial sexual abuse: Subsequent adjustment. *Archives of Sexual Behavior, 19*(3), 211–221.

Jacobson, N. S., Christensen, A., Prince, S. E., Cordova, J., & Eldridge, K. (2000).

Integrative behavioral couple therapy: An acceptance-based, promising new treatment for couple discord. *Journal of Consulting and Clinical Psychology, 68,* 351–355.

Jacobson, N. S., & Margolin, G. (1979). *Marital therapy: Strategies based on social learning and behavior exchange principles.* New York: Brunner/Mazel.

Jehu, D. (1988). *Beyond sexual abuse: Therapy with women who were childhood victims.* New York: Wiley.

Johnson, S. M. (2002). *Emotionally focused couple therapy with trauma survivors: Strengthening attachment bonds.* New York: Guilford Press.

Keane, T. M., & Wolfe, J. (1990). Comorbidity in post-traumatic stress disorder: An analysis of community and clinical studies. *Journal of Applied Social Psychology, 20,* 1776–1788.

Kilpatrick, D. G., Edmunds, C. N., & Seymour, A. K. (1992). *Rape in America: A report to the nation.* Arlington, VA: National Victim Center.

Kirschner, S., Kirschner, D. A., Rappaport, R. L. (1993). *Working with adult incest survivors: The healing journey.* New York: Brunner/Mazel.

Krupnick, J. L. (2002). Brief psychodynamic treatment of PTSD. *Journal of Clinical Psychology, 58,* 919–932.

Lacoursiere, R. B., Godfrey, K. E., & Ruby, L. M. (1980). Traumatic neurosis in the etiology of alcoholism: Vietnam combat and other trauma. *American Journal of Psychiatry, 137*(8), 966–968.

Leitenberg, H., Gibson, L. E., & Novy, P. L. (2004). Individual differences among undergraduate women in methods of coping with stressful events: The impact of cumulative childhood stressors and abuse. *Child Abuse and Neglect, 28*(2), 181–192.

Leonard, L. M., & Follette, V. M. (2002). Sexual functioning in women reporting a history of child sexual abuse: Review of the empirical literature and clinical implications. *Annual Review of Sex Research, 13,* 346–389.

Linehan, M. M. (1993b). *Skills training manual for treating borderline personality disorder.* New York: Guilford Press.

Linehan, M. M. (1993a). *Cognitive-behavioral treatment of borderline personality disorder.* New York: Guilford Press.

Masters, J. C., Burish, T. G., Hollon, S. D., & Rimm, D. C. (1987). *Behavior therapy: Techniques and empirical findings* (3rd ed.). New York: Harcourt Brace Jovanovich.

Miller, M. M., & Sutherland, K. J. (1999). Partners in healing: Systemic therapy with survivors of sexual abuse and their partners. *Journal of Family Studies, 5*(1), 97–111.

Miller, W. R., Williams, M., & Bernstein, M. H. (1982). The effect of rape on marital and sexual adjustment. *American Journal of Family Therapy, 10,* 51–58.

Mullen, P. E., Martin, J. L., Anderson, J. C., Romans, S. E., & Herbison, G. P. (1994). The effect of child sexual abuse on social, interpersonal, and sexual functioning in adult life. *British Journal of Psychiatry, 165,* 35–47.

Naugle, A. E., & Follette, W. C. (1998). A functional analysis of trauma symptoms. In V. M. Follette, J. I. Ruzek, & F. R. Abueg (Eds.), *Cognitive-behavioral therapies for trauma* (pp. 48–73). New York: Guilford Press.

Nelson, B. S., & Wright, D. W. (1996). Understanding and treating post-traumatic stress disorder symptoms in female partners of veterans with PTSD. *Journal of Marital and Family Therapy, 22*(4), 455–467.

Orsillo, S. M., Roemer, L., & Barlow, D. H. (2003). Integrating acceptance and mindfulness into existing cognitive-behavioral treatment for GAD: A case study. *Cognitive and Behavioral Practice, 10*, 222–230.

Pepper, S. C. (1942). *World hypotheses: A study in evidence.* Berkeley: University of California Press.

Polusny, M. A., & Follette, V. M. (1995). Long-term correlates of child sexual abuse: Theory and review of the empirical literature. *Applied and Preventive Psychology, 4*, 143–166.

Rabin, C., & Nardi, C. (1991. Treating post-traumatic stress disorder couples: A psychoeducational program. *Community Mental Health Journal, 27*, 209–223.

Resick, P. A. (1993). The psychological impact of rape. *Journal of Interpersonal Violence, 8*, 223–255.

Resick, P. A., & Calhoun, K. S. (2001). Posttraumatic stress disorder. In D. H. Barlow (Ed.), *Clinical handbook for psychological disorders: A step-by-step treatment manual* (3rd ed., pp. 60–113). New York: Guilford Press.

Resick, P. A., & Nishith, P. (1997). Sexual assault. In R. C. Davis, A. J. Lurigio, & W. G. Skogan (Eds.), *Victims of crime* (2nd ed., pp. 27–52). Thousand Oaks, CA: Sage.

Riggs, D. S., Byrne, C., Weathers, F., & Litz, B. (1998). The quality of intimate relationships of male Vietnam veterans: Problems associated with posttraumatic stress disorder. *Journal of Traumatic Stress, 11*, 87–101.

Russell, D. E. H. (1986). *The secret trauma: Incest in the lives of girls and women.* New York: Basic Books.

Sarwer, D. B., & Durlak, J. A. (1996). Childhood sexual abuse as a predictor of adult female sexual dysfunction: A study of couples seeking sex therapy. *Child Abuse and Neglect, 20*(10), 963–972.

Savarese, V. W., Suvak, M. K., King, L. A., & King, D. W. (2001). Relationships among alcohol use, hyperarousal, and marital abuse and violence in Vietnam veterans. *Journal of Traumatic Stress, 14*, 717–732.

Serafin, J. M., & Follette, V. M. (1996, November). *Female survivors of sexual trauma and their partners: Issues in couple functioning.* Paper presented at the annual meeting of the International Society for Traumatic Stress Studies, San Francisco.

Skinner, B. F. (1957). *Verbal behavior.* New York: Appleton-Century-Crofts.

Skinner, B. F. (1974). *About behaviorism.* New York: Random House.

Solomon, Z., Waysman, M., Levy, G., Fried, B., Mikulincer, M., Benbenishty, R., Florian, V., & Bleich, A. (1992). From front line to home front: A study of temporary traumatization. *Family Process, 31*, 289–302.

Waltz, J. (1993). *The long-term effects of childhood sexual abuse on women's relationships with partners.* Unpublished doctoral dissertation, University of Washington, Seattle.

Wenninger, K., & Heiman, J. R. (1998). Relating body image to psychological and sexual functioning in child sexual abuse survivors. *Journal of Traumatic Stress, 11*(3), 543–562.

Westerlund, E. (1992). *Women's sexuality after childhood incest.* New York: Norton.

Wilson, G. T. (1996). Acceptance and change in the treatment of eating disorders and obesity. *Behavior Therapy, 27*, 417–439.

Wincze, J. P., & Carey, M. P. (1991). *Sexual dysfunction: A guide for assessment and treatment.* New York: Guilford Press.

Wyatt, G., Guthrie, D., & Notgrass, C. M. (1992). Differential effects of women's child sexual abuse and subsequent sexual revictimization. *Journal of Consulting and Clinical Psychology, 60*, 167–173.

CHAPTER FIFTEEN

Group Therapies
for Trauma Using
Cognitive-Behavioral Therapy

David W. Foy
Linnea C. Larson

OVERVIEW AND BRIEF HISTORY
OF COGNITIVE-BEHAVIORAL GROUP THERAPY
FOR TRAUMA SURVIVORS

The purpose of this chapter is to present cognitive-behavioral (CB) group therapy methods for use with children, adolescents, and adult survivors of traumatic experiences. We begin by presenting a brief history of the development of group therapy for trauma survivors, followed by reviews of current influential theories and published studies on CB group therapy outcomes. Next we update the current status of our knowledge about CB group psychotherapy for trauma survivors; clinical issues are identified and specific recommendations for addressing these issues are made. Finally, we discuss current limitations in our knowledge of CB group interventions and identify areas that require further investigation and development.

Published reports of group therapy for combat-related trauma date back 60 years to World War II (Dynes, 1945). Two events in the late 1970s greatly accelerated the development of trauma-related group therapy. First, a nationwide network of community-based Vet Centers was established to serve the readjustment needs of Vietnam veterans. "Rap groups," led by counselors who themselves were Vietnam veterans, were featured in these centers (Sipprelle, 1992). Secondly, posttraumatic stress disorder (PTSD) was introduced into the psychiatric diagnostic system in 1980, and was followed by many studies that soon established commonalities in symptom manifestations and pathogenesis across survivors of different traumatic experiences.

Group therapy methods were applied to a variety of trauma populations, ranging from survivors of child sexual abuse to female adults exposed to domestic violence.

The rationale for using group therapy as a treatment for trauma is based on the survivor-acknowledged need for, and advantage of, joining with others in therapeutic work when coping with victimization consequences such as isolation, alienation, shame, and restricted or diminished feelings. Group therapy is especially appropriate because many survivors may feel ostracized from the larger society, or even judged and blamed for their predicament. Bonding with others who have similar histories in the context of a supportive environment can be a critical step toward regaining trust. Beyond its obvious cost advantage, group therapy may be particularly useful for those individuals who fail to hold the common assumptions (e.g., the value of psychological mindedness; responsibility for life choices and outcomes) thought necessary for individual psychotherapy (Klein & Schermer, 2000).

Group therapy methods may differ in their theoretical models of symptom development and therapeutic intervention, but they share a set of key features that builds a therapeutic, safe, and respectful environment. These features include (1) group membership determined by shared type of trauma (e.g., combat veterans or adult survivors of child abuse); (2) disclosure and validation of the traumatic experience; (3) normalization of trauma-related responses; (4) validation of behaviors required for survival during the time of the trauma; and (5) the idea that the nontraumatized therapist cannot be helpful is challenged, because he or she will rely on expert fellow survivors in the group.

INFLUENTIAL THEORIES THAT RELATE TO CB GROUP THERAPY FOR TRAUMA

Mowrer's (1960) two-factor theory is often used to explain the origin and persistence of symptoms of PTSD; that is, the initial trauma reaction becomes a conditioned emotional response (classical conditioning), and subsequent avoidance responses are motivated by fear and reinforced by fear reduction (operant conditioning). Additionally, our CB conceptualization of PTSD (Foy, 1992) is an interactional model that is used to account for the interplay of trauma characteristics, personal factors, and other posttrauma factors in the development of acute or chronic PTSD. Such a model allows for individual differences on other important factors, such as prior trauma exposure, social support, or cognitive attributions about the cause and meaning of the trauma, to be incorporated in case conceptualization.

Currently there are three dominant CB models, effectively summarized and compared by Brewin and Holmes (2003), which are relevant to group therapy for PTSD. These models are Foa and Rothbaum's (1998) emotional processing theory; Brewin, Dalgleish, and Joseph's (1996) dual representation theory; and Ehlers and Clark's (2000) cognitive theory. Although there is a significant amount of common ground among the three models, each also supplies unique nuances that add to the overall understanding of PTSD and its treatment.

All three theories conceptualize memory for traumatic events as being distinctly different from other types of memories. Foa and Rothbaum (1998) conceptualize a single associative network for traumatic events that consists of informational links regarding external stimuli, emotional/physiological responses, and meaning. This "fear network" differs from ordinary memories in that there are increased associations with fear and behavioral/physiological responses. With regard to meaning, Foa and Rothbaum assert that rigid pretrauma views (either positive or negative) increase the likelihood of PTSD, and negative appraisals of one's peritraumatic responses also play an important role. The treatment connected with this model is prolonged exposure therapy; its goal is to activate the fear network and integrate new information into it in order to weaken the associations (Brewin & Holmes, 2003).

Brewin et al. (1996), in contrast, posit that traumatic memory is stored in two different types of systems, verbally accessible memory (or VAM; with regard to trauma, represented by oral or written narratives of the event and accompanying conscious evaluations, including negative appraisals) and situationally accessible memory (or SAM; containing data about the trauma from lower-level perceptual processes that are not under conscious control, are not easily expressed verbally, and are the source of flashbacks). According to Brewin et al., treatment for PTSD must involve two processes: (1) distinctly addressing and modifying negative appraisals in the VAM system; and (2) helping clients to focus conscious attention on memories in the SAM system, so that they can also be encoded in the VAM system. Then, when a person is subsequently exposed to traumatic reminders, the VAM memories compete with the SAM memories and inhibit the fear associated with the SAM memories (Brewin & Holmes, 2003).

Ehlers and Clark's (2000) model emphasizes how the trauma is processed and how that processing impacts traumatic memory. They posit that PTSD occurs when a person's processing of the trauma results in a sense of either internal or external threat. Factors that contribute to a person developing this ongoing sense of threat include negative appraisals during and after the trauma (the likelihood of which are increased by a sense of mental defeat, a pretrauma state of mind in which the person feels unable to affect his or her fate), and the poorly integrated nature of traumatic memory. They distinguish between two types of processing that occur during a trauma and impact the resulting traumatic memory: conceptual processing (centered on meaning, organizing, and contextualizing) and data-driven processing (centered on sensory information). Data-driven processing is considered a risk factor for PTSD due to the difficulty of intentionally retrieving the memories and the difficulty of integrating these memories into the person's autobiographical narrative. In addition to identifying a variety of negative appraisals that contribute to a sense of threat, Ehlers and Clark also identified several maladaptive behavioral strategies that contribute to the maintenance of PTSD (Brewin & Holmes, 2003).

Common treatment elements among the three models include the need to (1) construct a verbal trauma narrative, (2) modify negative appraisals, and (3) activate the sensory or situationally accessible memories associated with the trauma in order to lessen their strength and bring them under conscious control (Brewin & Holmes, 2003). Group therapy lends itself well to the completion of these goals.

In addition to these models concerning the nature of traumatic memories, the theoretical contributions of Yalom's (1995) principles of group process to the conduct of trauma-related group therapy have often been acknowledged. Nevertheless, it is important to note that CB group therapy approaches are not "process-oriented," in that the critical therapeutic ingredient is *not* thought to be the corrective recapitulation of the primary family group nor expression of intense affect between members about their relationship.

EMPIRICAL STUDIES OF CB GROUP THERAPY FOR TRAUMA

To date, the literature on group therapy for trauma survivors contains more than 35 empirical studies, nearly equally divided between adult (Foy, Schnurr, Glynn, et al. 2000) and child/adolescent samples (Reeker, Ensing, & Elliott, 1997). Among these studies, 23 are reports of CB-based or "integrated" model group therapy outcomes. By far, the most widely studied population is that of female sexual assault survivors, both for adult and youth age groups.

Among the 23 studies listed in Table 15.1, there are 15 single-group, pre–post designs, 2 control-group designs, and 6 randomized controlled trials (RCTs). There is an expanding representation of studies with both adult survivors (7 studies) and children/adolescents (16 studies). Within the set of youth studies, 11 were conducted with preteenage children, whereas adolescents were sampled exclusively in 3 studies. Two studies featured "mixed" samples that included both latency-age children and teenagers. In terms of gender representation, most studies featured same-sex samples (females, 9 studies; males, 1 study), but 6 studies reported, primarily with preschool children, included both genders in the group therapies. It is notable that there have been no studies of mixed gender groups with adult survivors.

Each of the studies in Table 15.1 examining the efficacy of CB or "integrated" group treatment demonstrated improvements in group members' distress at the end of treatment. The groups represented a variety of trauma populations (e.g., sexually abused children and adolescents, adult survivors of sexual assault, adult survivors of childhood sexual abuse, and combat vet-

TABLE 15.1. Overview of Current CB Group Therapy for Trauma Studies

Study	Trauma population	Developmental stage (age in years)	Gender (N)	Type of therapy (No. of sessions)	Design rigor
Ashby et al. (1987)	CSA	Teens (13–17)	F (10)	Integrated (10)	Pre-post
Bradley & Follingstad (2003)	CSA/CPA (incarcerated)	Adult	F (49)	CBT/DBT	RCT
Chemtob et al. (2002)	Disaster	Grades 2–6	F/M (248)	CBT individual, group (4)	RCT
Deblinger et al. (2001)	CSA	Children/mothers	F/M (44 pairs)	CBT, supportive (11)	RCT
De Luca et al. (1993)	CSA	Latency (10–11)	F (7)	Integrated (10)	Pre-post
Frueh et al. (1996)	Combat	Adult	M (11)	CBT (10)	Pre-post
Hack et al. (1994)	CSA	Latency (8–11)	M (7)	Integrated (12)	Pre-post
Hall-Marley & Damon (1993)	CSA	(4–7)	F/M (13)	Integrated (13)	Pre-post
Hiebert-Murphy et al. (1992)	CSA	(7–9)	F (5)	Integrated (9)	Pre-post
Hoier et al. (1988)	CSA	(5–15)	F/M (18)	CBT	Pre-post
Kitchur & Bell (1989)	CSA	(11–12)	F (7)	Integrated (16)	Pre-post
Lubin et al. (1998)	Multiple	Adult	F (29)	CBT, trauma focus (16)	Pre-post
McGain & McKinzey (1995)	CSA	(9–12)	F (30)	Integrated (25)	Pre-post
Nelki & Watters (1989)	CSA	(4–8)	F (7)	Integrated (9)	Pre-post
Resick & Schnicke (1992)	SA	Adult	F (39)	CBT, waiting list (12)	CT
Resick et al. (1988)	SA	Adult	F (50)	CBT, supportive (6)	CT
Rust & Troupe (1991)	CSA	(9–18)	F (25)	Integrated (24)	Pre-post
Schnurr et al. (2003)	Combat	Adult	M (360)	CBT, trauma focus, present-centered	RCT
Sinclair et al. (1995)	CSA	Teens	F (43)	CBT (20)	Pre-post
Stauffer & Deblinger (1996)	CSA	(2–6)	F/M (19)	CBT (11)	Pre-post
Stein et al. (2003)	CV	Grade 6	F/M (126)	CBT (10)	RCT
Verleur et al. (1986)	CSA	(13–17)	F (15)	Integrated (24)	Pre-post
Zlotnick et al. (1997)	CSA	Adult	F (43)	CBT affect management (15)	RCT

Note. Trauma populations: CPA, childhood physical abuse; CSA, childhood sexual abuse; CV, community violence; SA, sexual abuse. Therapy type: CBT, cognitive-behavioral therapy; DBT, dialectical behavior therapy. Design type: CT, controlled trial; RCT, randomized controlled trial.

392

erans). The variety of CB techniques used in these groups included the following: exposure therapy, cognitive processing or restructuring, assertiveness training, stress inoculation, affect management, and coping skills. The groups met for a range of 6 to 24 weeks, usually weekly.

Compared to our earlier review (Foy et al., 2000), CB methods have been much more frequently used in recent group studies. Recent RCTs have also addressed the issue of relative effectiveness among the types of trauma group therapies (Deblinger, Stauffer, & Steer, 2001; Schnurr et al., 2003). In these studies, CB trauma focus groups were compared directly to present-centered or supportive groups. Although the Deblinger et al. study found the CB group to be superior, findings were more complex in the Schnurr et al. study, such that there was a significant treatment condition by cohort interaction favoring present-centered therapy in the first cohort. Conversely, the CB trauma focus condition was found to be superior in the second and third cohorts. These findings suggest that there may be a lengthier learning curve for CB trauma group therapists, especially those without previous experience and skills in the CB methods incorporated in the groups. On a positive note, findings from follow-up assessments showed that treatment effects were durable for as long as 1 year posttreatment (e.g., Schnurr et al., 2003).

CLINICAL APPLICATIONS

Evaluation and Assessment

Broadly construed, there are three sets of prerequisites for the intensive trauma work that is outlined in this chapter: psychological symptoms related to the traumatic event, stable living circumstances, and willingness/ability to tolerate intense affect. Thus, to determine if it is the appropriate time for an individual to participate in CB group therapy, these three domains must first be assessed. Typically, this assessment can be conducted in a single meeting with the client; the clinician provides a rationale for the items being assessed and then conducts a clinical interview. For this pregroup screening with adult clients, a brief standard assessment instrument may be useful to determine the severity of trauma-related symptoms. For example, the Impact of Event Scale–Revised (IES-R; Weiss & Marmar, 1996) is a paper-and-pencil measure that can be quickly administered and scored.

As a minimum assessment strategy for CB therapy groups, therapists should collect pre- and posttreatment data from each member that include basic demographic information and a measure of the primary intended outcome of the group. The applicability of findings from the current group to those from other studies is dependent upon similarities in demographics such as age, gender, ethnicity, educational level, and income level. For assessment of intended outcome, the use of a general measure of trauma-related distress, such as the IES-R (Weiss & Marmar, 1996), is encouraged.

Should more extensive documentation of PTSD be required, the Clinician Administered PTSD Scale (CAPS; Blake, Weathers, Nagy, & Kaloupek, 1995) is recommended. Because interview-based and self-report instruments for PTSD usually have a high rate of concordance, many clinicians prefer to utilize a brief self-report tool as part of the documentation of the presence of PTSD and as a foundation for ongoing symptom assessment. The Los Angeles Symptom Checklist (King, King, Leskin, & Foy, 1995) is an example of a useful self-report instrument that gives severity scores for PTSD and more general distress. Other similar scales include the Trauma Symptom Inventory (TSI: Briere, Elliott, Harris, & Cotman, 1995) and the Posttraumatic Stress Diagnostic Scale (PDS; Foa, Cashman, Jaycox, & Perry, 1995).

Guidelines for Client Selection

To date, CB therapy groups for adults have been comprised of same-sex survivors of the same type of traumatic experience. Thus there is no precedent in the literature for selecting adult survivor members on the basis of mixed gender or mixed traumas. As noted, Table 15.1 shows several studies that feature mixed genders for groups with adolescents and younger children. Individuals must, of course, be agreeable to participation in a group; and they must have the capacity to participate in treatment objectives and to interact appropriately with other members. Some group members may require a referral for additional supportive services during participation in the group. In groups with cultural/ethnic diversity, cross-cultural factors must be considered as relevant to group participants; the inclusion of a co-facilitator familiar with these differences is recommended. Table 15.2 summarizes inclusion and exclusion factors to consider. Pending litigation and the activities related to it may compete for the individual's time and attention to the extent that it may be incompatible with full participation in group therapy for trauma.

Overview of Treatment Approach

As applied to chronic PTSD in adults, CB therapy groups are intended to reduce members' current trauma-related distress and provide them with additional skills with which to cope successfully with future exacerbations of their symptoms. CB group therapy uses systematic prolonged exposure and cognitive restructuring techniques to process each group member's trauma experience. In the format we developed for male combat veterans (Foy, Ruzek, Glynn, Riney, & Gusman, 2002; Schnurr et al., 2003), each group member has the opportunity to recount his story as others listen. Group members thereby take part in trauma processing through both direct experi-

TABLE 15.2. Guidelines for Client Selection

Inclusion criteria	Exclusion criteria
Agreeable to participation in a group	Acute psychosis
Can participate in treatment objectives and interact appropriately in a group	Homicidal or suicidal tendencies
Can tolerate high distress and anxiety	Heart disease or severe angina
Accepts rationale for exposure-based therapy	Language difficulties
Willing to share traumatic experiences	Possible: seeking compensation/pending litigation
Stable living arrangements	Consider cross-cultural issues

ence of their own trauma event as well as through the vicarious experiences of others. CB group models emphasize both the strength of personal narrative and the power of group support; members "stand together" and hear each other's experiences without judgment (Foy et al., 2002). Personal narrative involves putting into words the actual sequence of events and reactions in the traumatic experience so that it can be communicated to others and considered therapeutically by the individual.

The use of psychoeducational material regarding relapse prevention and coping skills bolsters group members' resources for responding to current and future PTSD symptoms (Foy et al., 2002). For example, acknowledging the need for support with states of chronic distress takes into account the frequently intractable nature of chronic PTSD, because symptom exacerbation (or "relapse") remains an ongoing challenge for group members.

The rationale for using group therapy methods with children and adolescents is much the same as for adults: It offers advantages over individual therapy in providing a safe, shared therapeutic environment in which children who have survived terrible experiences can normalize their reactions and provide support for each other while processing their traumas. Integrated group therapy for children and adolescents usually involves a collection of techniques (e.g., exploration of feelings, art therapy, play therapy, puppet work, psychoeducation to prevent future sexual abuse) drawn from several theoretical traditions, including CB. Conversely, CB group therapy (e.g., Stauffer & Deblinger, 1996) includes the familiar elements of psychoeducation, coping skills training, exposure therapy, and cognitive restructuring. Groups of both types typically include a series of 8–24 weekly sessions; their composition typically involved children within the same developmental stage, although a few studies included members whose ages ranged across the developmental spectrum from early childhood through late adolescence (Reeker et al., 1997).

Session Design and Clinical Sequence

The format we describe here, termed "trauma focus group therapy" (TFGT), is based upon our work with male veterans receiving outpatient treatment for combat-related trauma (Foy et al., 2002; Schnurr et al., 2003). Group rules are explained to each prospective member in a preliminary individual session. Rules cover expectations in three critical areas: (1) the need for consistent attendance, with prior notice for planned absence; (2) use of positive tone in giving feedback during group participation; and (3) the ability to exercise confidentiality regarding members' identities and the information discussed in group sessions. There are six group members and two group facilitators in each CB trauma group. Each session is organized to include five core elements, listed in Table 15.3.

Homework is considered a crucial part of the treatment described here. In each weekly session, homework tasks are assigned to bridge the gap between group therapy sessions and the challenge of coping with their PTSD-related issues in their home environments.

As outlined in Table 15.4, the group meets weekly for 30 sessions, or about 7 months, then monthly for another 5 months. Trauma focus sessions are planned for 2 hours' duration; other meetings last 90 minutes. Sessions are planned according to the following schedule presented in Table 15.4.

There are three different types of sessions: introductory, trauma focused, and relapse prevention and termination. Introductory sessions have several goals: (1) to provide education about PTSD and the treatment process, (2) to teach and reinforce basic coping skills, (3) to prepare members for their upcoming task of trauma processing by recounting their selected traumatic experiences, and (4) to provide group facilitators and other members with additional background information about each participant. Prepa-

TABLE 15.3. Core Elements: Trauma Focus Group Therapy (TFGT)

Element	Description
Check-in	Members express feelings, concerns, and readiness to engage in group.
Review of homework	Members report on weekly tasks and outcomes; leaders collect homework, shape homework compliance and performance, and problem-solve obstacles to its completion.
Specific topics	Follows session schedule outlined in Table 15.4—majority of group time.
Assignment of homework	Leaders explain homework task and rationale, answer questions, and explore obstacles to completion.
Check-out	Members express reactions to the session; leaders calm distressed members, help plan for the next week, or reinforce individual change.

TABLE 15.4. Session Titles

Introductory sessions

Session 1	Introductions, structure, and group rules
Session 2	PTSD education
Session 3	Coping resources
Session 4	Negative and positive coping
Session 5	PTSD symptoms and self-control
Sessions 6–7	Premilitary autobiographies
Session 8	Pre-warzone military autobiographies

Trauma focus sessions

Sessions 9–10	Trauma scene identification/coping review
Sessions 11–22	Trauma exposure and cognitive restructuring

Relapse prevention and termination

Session 23	Integrating trauma: The three-way mirror
Sessions 24	Improving social support
Sessions 25–26	Anger management
Session 27–28	Risk situations and coping strategies
Sessions 29	Behavioral contracting
Session 30	Transitioning to monthly sessions
Booster sessions (5)	Integration of traumatic experience and relapse prevention

ration for therapeutic exposure is accomplished by setting clear group rules and structure, building member cohesion, discussing realistic expectations for outcome, presenting a clear rationale for exposure treatment, and teaching and supporting coping skills to be consciously employed during the trauma focus section of treatment.

Trauma focus sessions begin with identification of the trauma scene and proceed to systematic exposure to key aspects of the traumatic memories. These sessions are intended to (1) reduce fears of memories of traumatic experiences, (2) improve perceived self-control of memories and accompanying negative emotions, and (3) strengthen adaptive coping responses under conditions of distress. Finally, relapse prevention and termination sessions focus on (1) planning for anticipated difficulties in postdischarge living, (2) identifying individual risk scenarios and positive responses, (3) continued practicing of coping skills, (4) providing a period for consolidation of experiences during exposure, and (5) preparing members for group termination.

Specific content for each session follows these goals. "PTSD education" provides members with a chance to describe their own trauma symptoms and the personal impact of those symptoms. Group facilitators provide didactic education and clarify misperceptions about PTSD. "Coping resources" introduces the concept of coping by having members conduct a personal inventory of their current coping resources, identifying personal strengths, and noting areas in need of development. "Negative and positive coping" continues this theme by examining negative coping behaviors used in the past (e.g., alcohol consumption, social isolation, anger, and violence) and their consequences, and positive alternatives (e.g., finding support from significant others, practicing relaxation). "PTSD symptoms and self-control" emphasizes the importance of responding positively to symptoms; for instance, taking action to manage arousal, control attention, and enlist social support.

"Premilitary autobiographies" provide members with a chance to briefly explore, in a structured way, their childhood and adolescence to help establish their identities before experiencing combat trauma. Key developmental themes are reviewed that are related to early life coping style and response to trauma, including relationships with family members and peers, religious and cultural background, and pre-war traumatic experiences. "Pre-warzone military autobiographies" presents members with a similar opportunity to examine early attitudes toward military life and war, as well as ways in which basic military training affected their responses to war traumas.

"Trauma scene identification/coping review" is designed to help each member select the trauma scene that he will review during his personal trauma focus work. Members are encouraged to select scenes that are especially distressing, related to current symptomatology or vivid imagery, and associated with fear as the predominant affect. "Trauma exposure and cognitive restructuring" sessions are conducted by focusing upon one member at a time to ensure a minimum of 30 minutes of exposure to important trauma-related reminders and to prevent cognitive avoidance. In their narratives of their trauma scenes, members emphasize the sensory perceptions, thoughts, and emotional reactions that occurred during the incident. During recounting of the traumatic experience, minimal prompts are given by the facilitators, because the therapeutic objective is to encourage the member to assume responsibility for "self-exposure." Overall, the task might best be conceptualized as "supported remembering."

After the member describes his traumatic experience, cognitive distortions are identified and challenged, usually by other group members who have also experienced similar traumas. In turn, each member is allocated one session for this work; after each has had a turn, the process is repeated so that members are exposed to the material a second time in group. Following the initial in-session exposure, the member is asked to begin an self-exposure process outside of group as homework. The purpose of the exposure homework is to increase the number of times trauma scenes are reexperienced (exposure "dose") to ensure that fears are effectively reduced. The member is given a cassette recording of his trauma narrative and the related cognitive restructuring, asked to listen to the recording at least once during the next week, note distress levels, and report on coping skills he used to manage any related distress.

Originally, traumatic events may have been so intense that they overwhelmed the member's capacity to comprehend them accurately. Often the simple sequence of events in the scene is not even clear to the survivor. Thus many survivors draw inaccurate inferences from the events that often involve misperceptions about culpability for the tragic outcome. Accordingly, the goal of the self-exposure process is to access painful memories but to prevent overwhelming negative emotion. Facilitators focus attention on key trauma reminders, help prevent avoidance, and assist with management of distress, as necessary. In the cognitive restructuring phase following the member's narrative account of his scene, facilitators and other group members assist the member by carefully and systematically evaluating the "data" supporting the inferences and beliefs the member holds about his scene.

"Integrating trauma: The three-way mirror" is designed to aid the transition of the group from trauma focus work to a current-day perspective, in which integration of traumatic experiences and relapse prevention are emphasized. The mirror metaphor is used to represent each member's life in developmental perspective: premilitary, military, and postmilitary/current time frames.

"Improving social support" focuses on helping veterans recognize the importance of receiving support from significant others to (1) help them achieve relapse prevention, (2) review current key relationships, (3) identify problems in these relationships, and (4) develop (and implement as homework) action plans for improving them.

"Anger management," as the name indicates, directs members' attention to the links between their past traumatic experiences and current anger, and the negative consequences of anger in their present lives. It is intended to help members (1) identify positive anger control strategies, (2) generate individualized plans, and (3) practice some of these strategies in session and as homework. In "risk situations and coping strategies" members complete structured exercises to identify personal high-risk situations and specify steps for constructive coping. They also prepare personalized "emergency cards," which they carry with them to prompt themselves toward more effective coping in emergencies. "Behavioral contracting" further addresses this process of relapse prevention planning by formalizing each member's commitment to coping in a written contract. In "transitioning to monthly sessions" members (1) review lessons learned, (2) develop specific plans for maintaining their treatment gains in the future, and (3) discuss their feelings about moving from weekly to monthly meetings. The five booster sessions are designed to continue the work of trauma integration and relapse prevention within the group while members are weaned gradually from their dependence upon the group. Trouble-shooting the difficulties members encounter in keeping their rehabilitation contracts is the primary focus within these sessions (Foy et al., 2002).

To summarize: The primary treatment elements employed in CB trauma group therapy include PTSD education, prolonged exposure, cognitive restructuring, coping skills training, and relapse prevention training. Groups are structured so that leaders follow a detailed treatment manual, and group members follow instructions in their workbooks for completing weekly homework assignments. Additionally, co-therapists need to plan their roles in advance for each session, and they need to debrief each other after the session.

Common Treatment Obstacles and Possible Solutions

Trauma work often exposes the clinician to profoundly disturbing stories of human suffering and aggression. Much has been written about the necessity of clinician self-care and the need to prevent secondary or vicarious traumatization in view of this ongoing stress. The presence of a co-leader in CB trauma groups is extremely useful concerning the resolution of issues. The co-leaders must work as a team, providing peer supervision and constructive feedback to each other throughout the treatment protocol.

Group members frequently have present-day stressors and crises affecting their lives. The presence of such stressors may interfere with the individual's ability to focus on the content of the group. These issues can be identified during the check-in and a referral for additional services outside the group, if necessary. The identification of these potential distractions remains critical in order for progress to be made during the group, because their presence may elicit avoidance and hamper scheduled work.

As treatment advances to the stage of exposure to traumatic memories, some members may experience exacerbation of PTSD symptoms. Members will need to use the positive coping skills presented during the group to manage their symptoms. It will be important for the group to prepare a plan for symptom flair-ups. It is also useful to review the goals of treatment and the work to be done with members.

Homework is an important element of CB group therapy, and a rationale for implementing treatment at home may be critical to ensure adequate compliance. It is important to explain to group members that progress in treatment may require some of the hardest therapy work that they have ever done. It should be made clear that what they are likely to get out of therapy will be directly related to the work they put into it.

Premature terminations may occur for many reasons. Group members may encounter/experience significant life events such as a death in the family, an unexpected illness, or some other unpredictable circumstance. A group member may also terminate because he or she no longer wishes to continue with the trauma-focused group. A member may be asked to permanently leave when any of the following occur: He or she (1) becomes actively suicidal and cannot be readily stabilized; (2) engages in uncontrolled alcohol or drug use; (3) experiences a psychotic break; or (4) misses more than three consecutive group meetings. Following the member's departure, the group leaders should use the check-in time at the start of each session to review the reactions of the remaining group members to the departure.

CONCLUSION AND RECOMMENDATIONS

There are several unresolved issues in the use of CB group therapy that need empirical attention. For one, future studies should compare the effectiveness of mixed gender groups to single gender groups for adults, especially for types of trauma, such as community disasters, where specific gender issues in the experience are not apparent.

Future studies should extend the posttreatment follow-up period to 6–12 months. In the clinical domain, there is a need to monitor members' progress after weekly sessions are completed, extending the possibility of booster treatment for this period as well. Studies are needed that compare varying lengths of group treatment—for example, brief (< 10 sessions) to extended (> 15 sessions)—so that the design of future groups can be made more efficient.

There is also a need for studies that address matching participants to competing treatments to identify individual factors associated with differential treatment outcomes. One possible matching factor involves assessing the stage of recovery (Herman, 1992) for group prospects. Clients in stage 1 (immediate recovery phase tasks: establishing safety and self-care; reducing intrusion and hyperarousal) or 3 (final recovery phase tasks: giving up survivor identity; repair of relationships with others) may be more appropriate for present-centered groups, whereas clients in stage 2 (intermediate recovery tasks: integration of traumatic memories into general life narrative) may better fit a CB trauma focus approach.

Three of the recent RCTs have been conducted in field settings such as schools (Chemtob, Nakashima, & Hamada, 2002; Stein, et al., 2003) and correctional facilities (Bradley & Follingstad, 2003), all with positive results. These findings give empirical support for future efforts that venture out from traditional clinical research settings and samples when providing CB trauma group therapy.

In regard to dissemination and training, identification of essential therapist competencies for standard delivery of treatment and positive treatment outcomes remains a critical unresolved issue. What are the requisite therapist skills for conducting CB trauma groups? Under ideal circumstances, therapists would have skills in both group therapy and the specialty of trauma assessment and treatment. Additionally, therapists need skills in using common CB techniques (e.g., exposure therapy, cognitive restructuring, SUDs monitoring, thought stopping) used in these groups. When group therapists lack requisite skills and experience in conducting CB trauma groups, they should seek training, ongoing consultation and supervision from a more experienced trauma therapist. They should also obtain and use the empirically tested treatment manuals for group therapists and workbooks for group members. These resources are available for the CB trauma focus approach featured in this chapter (see Authors' Note).

ACKNOWLEDGMENTS

We gratefully acknowledge the extensive contributions of the Veterans Administration Cooperative Study #420 Trauma Focus Group Treatment Workgroup, including F. Gusman, C. Marmar, D. Weiss, J. Ruzek, S. Riney, J. Ford, M. Friedman, P. Schnurr. Contributions included selection of group session topics and sequence; development of the facilitator's manual and the member's workbook; and pilot testing of individual sessions and the exposure therapy homework assignment.

AUTHORS' NOTE

Requests for TFGT leader's manual and member's workbook should be sent to: Josef I. Ruzek, PhD, National Center for PTSD, Education and Clinical Laboratory Division, VA Palo Alto Health Care System, 795 Willow Road, Menlo Park, CA 94025.

REFERENCES

Ashby, M., Gilchrist, L., & Miramontez, A. (1987). Group treatment for sexually abused American Indian adolescents. *Social Work with Groups, 10,* 21–32.

Blake, D. D., Weathers, F. W., Nagy, L. M., & Kaloupek, Danny G. (1995). The development of a Clinician Administered PTSD Scale. *Journal of Traumatic Stress, 8,* 75–90.

Bradley, R. G., & Follingstad, D. R. (2003). Group therapy for incarcerated women who experienced interpersonal violence: A pilot study. *Journal of Traumatic Stress, 16*(4), 337–340.

Brewin, C. R., Dalgleish, T., & Joseph, S. (1996). A dual representation theory of posttraumatic stress disorder. *Psychological Review, 103,* 670–686.

Brewin, C. R., & Holmes, E. A. (2003). Psychological theories of posttraumatic stress disorder. *Clinical Psychology Review, 23,* 339–376.

Briere, J., Elliott, D. M., Harris, K., & Cotman, A. (1995). Trauma Symptom Inventory: Psychometrics and association with childhood and adult victimization in clinical samples. *Journal of Interpersonal Violence, 10,* 387–401.

Chemtob, C. M., Nakashima, J. P., & Hamada, R. S. (2002). Psychosocial intervention for postdisaster trauma symptoms in elementary school children: A controlled community field study. *Archives of Pediatrics and Adolescent Medicine, 156,* 211–216.

Deblinger, E., Stauffer, L. B., & Steer, R. A (2001). Comparative efficacies of supportive and cognitive behavioral group therapies for young children who have been sexually abused and their nonoffending mothers. *Child Maltreatment, 6,* 332–343.

De Luca, R., Hazen, A., & Cutler, J. (1993). Evaluation of a group counseling program for preadolescent female victims of incest. *Elementary School Guidance and Counseling, 28,* 104–114.

Dynes, J. B. (1945). Rehabilitation of war casualties. *War Medicine, 7,* 32–35.

Ehlers, A., & Clark, D. M. (2000). A cognitive model of posttraumatic stress disorder. *Behaviour Research and Therapy, 38,* 319–345.

Foa, E. B., Cashman, L., Jaycox, L., & Perry, K. (1995). The validation of a self-report measure of posttraumatic stress disorder: The Posttraumatic Diagnostic Scale. *Psychological Assessment, 9,* 445–451.

Foa, E. B., & Rothbaum, B. O. (1998). *Treating the trauma of rape: Cognitive-behavioral therapy for PTSD.* New York: Guilford Press.

Foy, D. W. (Ed.) (1992). *Treating posttraumatic stress disorder: Cognitive behavioral strategies.* New York: Guilford Press.

Foy, D. W., Glynn, S. M., Schnurr, P. P., Jankowski, M. K., Wattenberg, M. S., Weiss, D. S., Marmar, C. R., & Gusman, F. D. (2000). Group therapy. In E. Foa, T. Keane, & M. Friedman (Eds.), *Effective treatments for PTSD: Practice guidelines from the International Society for Traumatic Stress Studies* (pp. 155–175, 336–338). New York: Guilford Press.

Foy, D. W., Ruzek, J. I., Glynn, S. M., Riney, S. A., & Gusman, F. D. (2002). Trauma focus group therapy for combat-related PTSD: An update. *In Session: Psychotherapy in Practice, 3,* 59–73.

Frueh, B. C., Turner, S. M., Beidel, D. C., Mirabella, R. F., & Jones, W. J. (1996). Trauma Management Therapy: A preliminary evaluation of a multicomponent behavioral treatment for chronic combat-related PTSD. *Behaviour Research and Therapy, 34,* 533–543.

Hack, T., Osachuk, T., & De Luca, R. (1994). Group treatment for sexually abused preadolescent boys. *Families in Society: Journal of Contemporary Human Services, 4,* 217–228.

Hall-Marley, S., & Damon, L. (1993). Impact of structured group therapy on young victims of sexual abuse. *Journal of Child and Adolescent Group Therapy, 3,* 41–48.

Herman, J. L. (1992). *Trauma and recovery.* New York: Basic Books.

Hiebert-Murphy, D., De Luca, R., & Runtz, M. (1992). Group treatment for sexually abused girls: Evaluating outcome. *Families in Society: Journal of Contemporary Human Services, 3,* 205–213.

Hoier, T., Inderbitzen-Pisaruk, H., & Shawchuck, C. (1988). *Short-term cognitive behavioral group treatment for victims of sexual abuse.* Unpublished manuscript, West Virginia University, Department of Psychology, Morgantown.

King, L. A., King, D. W., Leskin, G. A., & Foy, D. W. (1995). The Los Angeles Symptom Checklist: A self-report measure of posttraumatic stress disorder. *Assessment, 2,* 1–17.

Kitchur, M., & Bell, R. (1989). Group psychotherapy with preadolescent sexual abuse victims: Literature review and description of an inner-city group. *International Journal of Group Psychotherapy, 39,* 285–310.

Klein, R. K., & Schermer, V. L. (2000). *Group psychotherapy for psychological trauma.* New York: Guilford Press.

Lubin, H., Loris, M., Burt, J., & Johnson, D. R. (1998). Efficacy of psychoeducational group therapy in reducing symptoms of posttraumatic stress disorder among multiply traumatized women. *American Journal of Psychiatry, 155,* 1172–1177.

McGain, B., & McKinzey, R. (1995). The efficacy of group treatment in sexually abused girls. *Child Abuse and Neglect, 19,* 1157–1169.

Mowrer, O. H. (1960). *Learning theory and behavior.* New York: Wiley.

Nelki, J., & Watters, J. (1989). A group for sexually abused young children: Unravelling the web. *Child Abuse &Neglect, 13,* 369–377.

Reeker, J., Ensing, D., & Elliott, R. (1997). A meta-analytic investigation of group treatment outcomes for sexually abused children. *Child Abuse and Neglect, 21,* 669–680.

Resick, P. A., Jordan, C. G., Girelli, S. A., Hutter, C. K., & Marhoefer-Dvorak, S. (1988). A comparative outcome study of behavioral group therapy for sexual assault victims. *Behavior Therapy, 19,* 385–401.

Resick, P. A., & Schnicke, M. K. (1992). Cognitive processing therapy for sexual assault victims. *Journal of Consulting and Clinical Psychology, 60,* 748–756.

Rust, J., & Troupe, P. (1991). Relationships of treatment of child sexual abuse with school achievement and self-concept. *Journal of Early Adolescence, 11,* 420–429.

Schnurr, P. P., Friedman, M. F., Foy, D. W., Shea, T. M., Hsieh, F. Y., Lavori, P. W., et al. (2003). Randomized trial of trauma-focused group therapy for posttraumatic stress disorder: Results from a Department of Veterans Affairs cooperative study. *Archives of General Psychiatry, 60,* 481–489.

Sinclair, J. J., Larzelere, R. E., Paine, M., Jones, P., Graham, K., & Jones, M. (1995). Outcome of group treatment for sexually abused adolescent females living in a group home setting. *Journal of Interpersonal Violence, 10,* 533–542.

Sipprelle, R. C. (1992). A Vet Center experience: Multievent trauma, delayed treatment type. In D. Foy (Ed.), *Treating PTSD: Cognitive-behavioral strategies* (pp. 13–38). New York: Guilford Press.

Stauffer, L., & Deblinger, E. (1996). Cognitive behavioral groups for nonoffending mothers and their young sexually abused children: A preliminary treatment outcome study. *Child Maltreatment, 1,* 65–76.

Stein, B. D., Jaycox, L. H., Kataoka, S. H., Wong, M., Tu, W., Elliott, M. N., & Fink, A. (2003). A mental health intervention for schoolchildren exposed to violence: A randomized controlled trial. *Journal of the American Medical Association, 290,* 603–611.

Verleur, D., Hughes, R., & de Rios, M. (1986). Enhancement of self-esteem among female adolescent incest victims: A controlled comparison. *Adolescence, 21,* 843–854.

Weiss, D. S., & Marmar, C. R. (1996). The Impact of Event Scale—Revised. In J. Wilson & T. Keane (Eds.), *Assessing psychological trauma and PTSD* (pp. 399–411). New York: Guilford Press.

Yalom, I. D. (1995). *The theory and practice of group psychotherapy.* New York: Basic Books.

Zlotnick, C., Shea, M. T., Rosen, K. H., Simpson, E., Mulrenin, K., Begin, A., & Pearlstein, T. (1997). An affect-management group for women with posttraumatic stress disorder and histories of childhood sexual abuse. *Journal of Traumatic Stress, 10,* 425–436.

CHAPTER SIXTEEN

Trauma in Childhood

Esther Deblinger
Reena Thakkar-Kolar
Erika Ryan

The term "childhood trauma" encompasses a wide range of traumatic experiences, including exposure to community and domestic violence as well as natural disasters, automobile accidents, neglect, emotional abuse, physical abuse, and sexual abuse. Most of the literature on childhood trauma has focused on the impact and treatment of child sexual abuse and, to a lesser extent, on child physical abuse (Everett & Gallop, 2001). However, child abuse incidence and prevalence rates are difficult to determine due to state-by-state differences in reporting mechanisms and definitions. Furthermore, most abuse remains unreported, and many cases are never investigated. Because of these difficulties, the trend in the literature is to rely on retrospective surveys of adults reporting on their own childhood experiences. In a review of retrospective studies, Finkelhor (1994) found that approximately 20–25% of women and 5–15% of men in North America experienced some form of contact sexual abuse as children. These alarming rates of child sexual abuse may actually underestimate the occurrence of abuse, given the results of research Widom and Morris (1997) and Williams (1994), which demonstrated that over 30% of adults with documented sexual abuse histories failed to report those experiences when questioned. The U.S. Department of Health and Human Services provides prevalence data on child maltreatment collected from child protective service agencies in each state. Out of 2.8 million reports of suspected abuse made to child protective service agencies across the country, 53.5% were related to neglect, 22.7% to physical abuse, 11.5% sexual abuse, and 6.0% to emotional abuse (U.S. Department of Health and Human Services, 2000). Once again, these figures are likely an underestimate of the prevalence of abuse, given that the rates are based on only those cases reported to child protective service agencies (Kolko, 2002). Furthermore, estimates suggest that 3.3 million children and 10 million teens witness violence in their homes each year, and these children tend to be at high risk for suffering child maltreatment (Carlson, 1998; Straus & Gelles, 1996).

In general, the adverse psychosocial impact of childhood trauma, particularly the experience and/or witnessing of sexual or physical violence in childhood, has been well documented. The findings of numerous investigations suggest that children who have suffered these types of traumas are at increased risk for experiencing posttraumatic stress disorder (PTSD), depression, substance abuse, academic difficulties, delinquency, and teenage pregnancy as well as violent revictimization (American Academy of Child and Adolescent Psychiatry [AACAP], 1998; Hill, 2003; Finkelhor, 1995; Kelley, Thornberry, & Smith, 1997). Moreover, recent research suggests that the developing brain may be deleteriously affected by chronic PTSD suffered in childhood (DeBellis et al., 1999). Research also has documented strong long-term associations between adverse childhood experiences and a host of adult emotional and physical health problems (Felitti et al., 1998). Thus, it is imperative to provide early, effective interventions to ameliorate and/or prevent the highly disruptive effects traumatic stress can have on children's emotional, cognitive, behavioral, and psychobiological development.

THEORETICAL ORIENTATION

The trauma-focused cognitive-behavioral therapy approach described in this chapter, is based on principles drawn from social learning and cognitive theories. It is a model that can be applied to children and parents who have suffered a wide array of traumatic experiences, including sexual abuse, physical abuse, traumatic loss, and exposure to domestic violence (Deblinger & Heflin, 1996; Cohen, Mannarino, Berliner & Deblinger, 2000c; Cohen, Mannarino, & Deblinger, 2001). Because the overall approach incorporates several treatment components, including psychoeducation, coping skills training, gradual exposure and processing, and parent training, it should be noted that different psychological theories may explain the effectiveness of these distinct interventions. However, the overall model is based on the notion that behavioral, affective, cognitive, and physiological processes are highly interrelated such that any change in one of these areas of functioning will likely produce change in the other areas as well.

The most direct learning mechanisms—psychoeducation, for example— not only targets misconceptions and faulty thinking, but also often offers new information that may produce change in affective and behavioral patterns. More specifically, when children learn that child sexual abuse happens to many children, they may feel less alone and stigmatized and possibly reduce their tendency to isolate themselves socially, a common behavioral reaction for children who have been sexually abused. Similarly, when parents learn that the vast majority of child sexual abuse survivors do not disclose their abuse in childhood, they may feel less distressed about the fact that their child did not tell immediately.

The mechanisms of learning that lead to the acquisition of stress management skills such as relaxation, regulated emotional expression, and cognitive coping skills include behavior rehearsal and modeling. These skills are taught to both children and parents because parents are usually their children's most influential role models. Thus, not only is it important for therapists to model and practice coping skills with children, but it may be even more important to model them for parents so that they can practice and reinforce these skills in their children.

Interestingly, coping skills training may not only enhance clients' feelings of control and competence in responding to threatening internal and external cues, but also may improve the effectiveness of exposure-based treatments. When children and parents learn how to identify and express their feelings and thoughts regarding everyday events, they are more likely to be able to access and effectively process trauma-related thoughts and feelings during the course of exposure exercises.

Researchers have proposed several different theories to explain the benefits of exposure-based interventions. Mowrer's (1939, 1960) two-factor theory suggests that both classical and operant conditioning underlie the development of fear and anxiety symptoms, and, in turn, these learning mechanisms may explain the effectiveness of exposure. For example, in the case of child sexual or physical abuse, the assaults are unconditioned stimuli that naturally produce unconditioned fear responses in children who are victimized. Conditioned stimuli (CS) may take the form of stimuli present at the time of the assaults (e.g., certain body odors, blood, darkness) as well as abuse-related thoughts and memories. In children suffering PTSD, these conditioned stimuli continue to produce conditioned responses (CR) of anxiety and fear long after the assaultive experiences have ended. Thus, to avoid the distress associated with such reminders, children may avoid stimuli both cognitively (by trying not to think about the abuse experiences) and behaviorally (by avoiding people, places, and things associated with the abuse). Operant conditioning comes into play as avoidant behavior is negatively reinforced by a reduction in anxiety each time the child successfully avoids reminders. In addition, well-meaning parents and others who think it is better for children to "forget" such experiences may model and positively reinforce children's efforts to avoid reminders and/discussion of the traumatic experience(s).

The effectiveness of exposure-based treatment has been traditionally explained by the extinction process. Through the process of extinction, anxiety decreases as a result of repeated exposures to conditioned anxiety-provoking stimuli that ultimately produce less and less distress over time. It has been suggested that exposure ultimately changes clients' expectancies regarding the aversive consequences they anticipate when confronting trauma-related conditioned stimuli (Mackintosh, 1983). For example, a child may be highly avoidant of any attempts to help him or her process the abuse, until discovering through exposure that talking about or writing about traumatic experiences is not nearly as frightening or upsetting as expected—in fact, doing so may even bring relief.

Beyond these more fundamental learning mechanisms, exposure based interventions may provide opportunities for higher-level learning processes by reducing avoidance and encouraging self-confidence. These changes often help children feel more willing to access and confront increasingly anxiety-provoking memories, which, in turn, provide increased opportunities to elicit dysfunctional thoughts and faulty developing beliefs. For example, in describing her exposure to domestic violence, a little girl said that she was scared, thinking, "Daddy hit Mommy because she was bad." Eliciting and correcting this type of faulty thinking may not only be critical for this child and mother, but also may help to prevent the intergenerational transmission of belief systems that justify violence in intimate relationships. Depending on the age of the child, children can be assisted in thinking through these kinds of assumptions with a series of simple questions such as, "What did Mommy do that was bad? Is it OK to make mistakes? Should anyone get beat up because he or she makes a mistake? Is it OK for Daddy to hit Mommy?"

It is important to acknowledge that operant, respondent, and observational learning theories all underlie the effectiveness of the behavior management skills taught to assist parents in learning how to optimally respond to their children's difficulties. For example, parents learn to praise their children for their efforts to confront and address trauma-related issues, thereby reducing the often natural tendency toward avoidance. An individually tailored behavior management plan is generally developed to ameliorate children's behavioral difficulties and/or minimize their risk of developing acting-out behavior problems. Lastly, although this treatment approach is theory driven and structured, therapeutic flexibility, creativity, and a trusting and collaborative therapist–client relationship are central to its successful implementation.

EMPIRICAL RESEARCH

As other chapters in this book demonstrate, the majority of trauma literature focuses on adults. Despite the high prevalence and seriousness of childhood traumatic experiences, the literature on childhood trauma and its sequelae and treatment is somewhat limited. Although adult-focused work has informed and assisted the understanding, assessment, and treatment of childhood trauma (Foa, Rothbaum, Riggs, & Murdock, 1992), it is not sufficient for professionals to extrapolate information from the adult trauma literature to their work with children.

Research with regard to the treatment of various types of childhood trauma is still very much in its infancy. To date, there are only a handful of studies examining the treatment efficacy of treating a range of childhood traumas, such as exposure to community violence, witnessing domestic violence, physical abuse, and traumatic grief. One study, conducted by March, Amaya-Jackson, Murray, and Schulte (1998), found that an intervention based on cognitive-behavioral therapy (CBT) significantly reduced PTSD symptoms in a small group of children exposed to community violence. In a review of treatment for childhood trauma, Cohen, Berliner, and Mannarino (2000a) reported that the available literature addressing domestic violence focused almost exclusively on the battered women or the offenders. Clinical descriptions and reports addressing children's reactions and possible treatment goals are available, but no empirical treatment outcome investigations have been published.

With regard to child physical abuse, several studies have documented significant reductions in PTSD symptoms using a variety of CBT programs. Swenson and Brown (1999) followed children in a 16-week CBT group focused on exposure, social skills, anger management, and relaxation training. Results from this project demonstrated a reduction in the children's level of anxiety, dissociation, anger, and PTSD. In a well-controlled design examining treatment for physically abusive parents, Kolko (1996) demonstrated that individual CBT treatment was superior to family therapy and standard community care in reducing parental anger and use of physical punishment. Both CBT and family therapy led to significant improvements in child behavior problems, parental distress, risk for future abuse, and family conflict. It appears that an integrated child and parent CBT treatment model would lead to greater gains in child and parent functioning (Runyon, Deblinger, Ryan, & Thakkar-Kolar, 2004).

A recent pilot study documents the successful use of CBT-based interventions for treating childhood traumatic grief. Cohen, Mannarino, and Knudsen (2004) examined the efficacy of a 16-week CBT-based program with sequential trauma and grief-focused interventions. Children in the study showed significant improvements in symptoms of depression, anxiety, PTSD, and behavioral problems. The caretakers, who were also included in the treatment program, also showed significant improvement in symptoms of PTSD and depression. In sum, although there are a few empirically based treatment outcome studies focused on a range of childhood traumas, research in the field needs to be expanded.

The treatment outcome literature specifically in regard to the treatment of children who have suffered sexual abuse has grown significantly in the last decade. Empirical treatment outcome data for children who have suffered sexual abuse experiences have received the most attention (Cohen et al., 2000a). Recent reviews of treatment outcome research in this area suggest that trauma-focused CBT has the strongest empirical support for the effective treatment of PTSD and related difficulties with this population of children (AACAP, 1998; Cohen, Berliner, & March 2000b; Saunders, Berliner, &

Hanson, 2003). This chapter offers a description of a trauma-focused treatment model that is rooted in, and supported by, empirical research.

Our trauma-focused CBT treatment model emerged from the assessment research documenting the wide array of difficulties faced by children who have suffered sexual abuse, with the most common diagnosis being PTSD (Finkelhor, 1995; McLeer, Deblinger, Henry, & Orvaschel, 1992). Thus a broad-based approach that could be tailored to children's individual needs and could address difficulties in behavioral, cognitive, affective, and physiological domains was warranted. In addition, research in the field had established the potentially significant influence of nonoffending parents on a child's recovery from the experience of sexual abuse (Conte & Schuerman, 1987; Deblinger, Steer, & Lippmann, 1999). Thus this model was designed to ameliorate the wide array of posttrauma difficulties experienced by children and also assist nonoffending parents in coping with their own distress and optimally responding to their children's difficulties. Toward these goals, this treatment approach involves the participation of the child and nonoffending caregiver in individual therapy sessions that ultimately build toward joint caregiver–child sessions as well as family sessions when appropriate.

Over the past 15 years studies have been conducted that examined the efficacy of trauma-focused CBT models in individual and group contexts with children who have suffered sexual abuse. Deblinger, McLeer, and Henry (1990) first reported the findings of a pilot investigation examining the effectiveness of individual CBT designed for children who had suffered sexual abuse and who met DSM-III-R criteria for PTSD. The results revealed no significant improvement during a 2- to 3-week pretreatment baseline period, but significant improvements on standardized measures of PTSD, anxiety, depression, and behavior problems at posttreatment. However, it was noted that at posttreatment, a significant proportion of the treated children continued to exhibit mild depressive symptoms. This finding led the investigators to combine exposure-based interventions with cognitive therapy techniques that might more effectively target depressive symptoms.

Building on the above preliminary data, a 5-year randomized controlled trial was conducted to evaluate the relative efficacy of the parent and child components of the CBT model with therapy offered in the community (Deblinger, Lippmann, & Steer, 1996). Children between 7 and 13 years of age were randomly assigned to standard community care or one of the following three CBT conditions: (1) a child-only intervention, (2) a parent-only intervention, or (3) a combined child and parent intervention. In the parent-only condition, therapists did not work directly with the children, but rather worked with the nonoffending parents to help them develop skills to serve as their children's therapeutic agents. In the combined parent–child condition, therapists used the same CBT interventions working initially with children and parents individually and later in joint parent–child sessions. The posttreatment results demonstrated significantly greater improvements in parenting practices, children's externalizing behavior problems, and children's self-reported depressive symptoms when nonoffending parents participated in the CBT interventions (i.e., parent-only and parent–child conditions). On the other hand, children's PTSD symptoms were significantly more likely to improve when children received treatment directly from the CBT therapist (i.e., child-only or parent–child condition). Finally, the significant improvements children made in PTSD symptoms, depression, and externalizing behavior problems following treatment were maintained throughout a 2-year follow-up period (Deblinger et al., 1999).

Several investigations have documented the efficacy of this CBT model in group therapy settings as well (Stauffer & Deblinger, 1996; Deblinger, Stauffer, & Steer, 2001). Most recently, the findings of a group treatment investigation, examining the comparative efficacies of supportive and CBT groups designed for very young survivors of sexual abuse (ages 2–8) and their nonoffending mothers, demonstrated that children assigned to the CBT group exhibited greater improvements in body safety skills compared to those in the support group (Deblinger et al., 2001). That no differences were found in children's PTSD symptoms across conditions may be due to the fact that gradual exposure and processing interventions were not utilized in the CBT group with the children because of their young age and the group format. On the other hand, mothers assigned to the CBT group did participate in exposure and processing exercises, and they did demonstrate significantly greater reductions in intrusive, abuse-related thoughts and negative parental emotional reactions compared to mothers assigned to the support groups.

Simultaneous with the work of Deblinger and her colleagues, Cohen and Mannarino developed and tested a very similar CBT approach that also included an individual parent component. Cohen and Mannarino (1996a, 1997) first evaluated the efficacy of this trauma-focused CBT model in comparison to nondirective supportive therapy, another well-defined alternative treatment, with preschool children and their nonoffending parents. The results of this investigation demonstrated the superior effectiveness of the CBT model over the nondirective model with regard to general behavior problems, sexual behavior problems and trauma-related emotional difficulties. These differences were sustained over a 1-year follow-up.

Cohen and Mannarino (1998) used a similar randomized controlled design to evaluate the efficacy of CBT versus nondirective supportive therapy with school-age children. This study also demonstrated the superior effectiveness of CBT over the nondirective approach in reducing self-reported depressive symptoms and improving social competence. The 1-year follow-up findings revealed superior improvement in PTSD and dissociative symptoms for those children who had completed trauma-focused CBT compared to nondirective therapy. In addition, the findings of intent-to-treat analyses indicated superior response in depression, state and trait anxiety, and in sexual concerns among children assigned to CBT from pretreatment to 12-month follow-up (Cohen, Mannarino, & Knudsen, 2003).

A recent study conducted in Australia with children who had been sexually abused utilized the above described CBT model and documented its replicability: Superior outcomes were reported for children randomly assigned to the CBT as opposed to the waiting-list control condition (King et al., 2000). These investigators also compared children who received CBT with or without caregiver involvement (i.e., family CBT vs. child CBT) and found no differences at posttreatment, but one important difference emerged at follow-up: 3 months after completing treatment, children who had participated in family CBT reported significantly less fear related to the sexual abuse as compared to those who received child-only CBT.

Recognizing the similarities of their treatment models, Cohen and Mannarino collaborated with Deblinger and her colleagues (Cohen, Deblinger, & Mannarino, 2005; Cohen, Deblinger, Mannarino, & Steer, 2004) in conducting the largest and first two-site randomized treatment outcome trial in the field. In this investigation, children 8–14 years of age and their nonoffending parents were randomly assigned to receive CBT or client-centered treatment. The results of posttreatment analyses demonstrated that children assigned to trauma-focused CBT, as compared to client-centered treatment, showed significantly greater reductions in PTSD, depression, behavior problems, abuse-related attributions, and shame. Similarly, parents who received CBT, as compared to client-centered treatment, exhibited significantly greater improvement in depression, abuse-specific emotional distress, support of the child, and positive parenting practices. Thus these findings seem to replicate and expand on the results of earlier investigations that have supported the superior efficacy of the CBT model over less-focused approaches to treatment. The case study described later in the chapter focuses on the application of trauma-focused CBT with a child who has suffered sexual abuse.

CLINICAL APPLICATIONS

Client Selection

Before initiating abuse-specific treatment, the therapist should have clarity regarding the sexual abuse allegations. Investigation of a child's allegations of sexual abuse by child protective services and/or law enforcement agencies is a prerequisite for initiating this trauma-focused treatment model. Credible evidence of the alleged sexual abuse can also originate from a medical evaluation or a forensic psychological evaluation. Although many components of the treatment model are appropriate for a variety of clients, gradual exposure and processing should not be used if it is unclear whether the child has experienced abuse.

The treatment model described below is not intended to treat significant psychological problems that predate the trauma, such as psychosis or active suicidality. The model was developed to assist children with a history of sexual abuse and their nonoffending caregivers; therefore, it includes components aimed at targeting common presenting problems among this population. The model focuses, in part, on alleviating symptoms such as avoidance, increased arousal, and distress regarding reminders of the abuse, commonly experienced symptoms of PTSD, as well as other problems often present in children with a history of sexual abuse, including depressive symptoms, generalized anxiety, and externalizing behavior problems.

Research with children who have a history of sexual abuse suggests that support from a nonoffending caregiver is associated with less severe symptomatology, compared to children who do not receive support from a caregiver. Furthermore, research studies have demonstrated that the way the nonoffending caregiver copes with the sexual abuse is related to the child's adjustment following the abuse (Conte, & Schuerman, 1987; Deblinger, Steer, & Lippmann, 1999; Everson, Hunter, Runyon, Edelson, & Coulter, 1989). Based on these findings, a caregiver's active participation in the child's treatment is highly beneficial. However, individual child treatment is an option when the nonoffending caregiver is not available or is not supportive of the child's disclosure.

Assessment

Prior to beginning therapy, therapists should conduct a thorough pretreatment assessment to develop an individualized treatment plan. This type of assessment is not intended to serve as an investigative sexual abuse evaluation. An investigative evaluation is warranted prior to beginning therapy in the following situations: (1) Sexual abuse is suspected but has not been substantiated by child protection, law enforcement agencies, or medical professionals; (2) children are unable to provide a clear disclosure, or they provide an ambiguous disclosure; (3) allegations emerge in the context of a custody dispute; or (4) allegations are recanted after the original disclosure (Lippmann, 2002). The reader is referred to "Psychological Issues" in *Medical Evaluation of Child Sexual Abuse: A Practical Guide* (Lippmann, 2002) for an overview of the unique and specialized aspects of forensic sexual abuse evaluations.

The pretreatment assessment process is designed to assess for PTSD-related symptoms, sexually reactive behaviors, depression, anxiety, and behavior problems in the child. Several standardized measures used to assess symptomatology specific to the effects of sexual abuse are available. The current standard for diagnosing PTSD in children is to use a structured interview format such as the Kiddie Schedule for Affective Disorders and Schizophrenia (K-SADS) (Kaufman, Birmaher, & Brent, 1996). The K-SADS should be administered separately to the child and parent, with a consensus response obtained for each item. The Children's Attributions and Perceptions Scale (CAPS; Mannarino, Cohen, & Berman, 1994) is a structured interview that can be used to assess abuse-specific attributions and perceptions in children. This measure is comprised of four subscales, including Feeling Different from Peers, Interpersonal Trust, Personal Attributions for Negative Events, and Perceived Credibility.

Feiring, Taska, and Lewis (1999) developed a brief self-report measure for children to tap feelings of shame related to sexual abuse. This shame measure includes items such as "What happened to me makes me feel dirty" and "I'm ashamed because I think that people can tell from looking at me what happened." The Children's Depression Inventory (CDI; Kovacs, 1985) is a widely used self-report measure to assess depressive symptomatology in children between 7 and 17 years of age. This measure assesses the affective, cognitive, and behavioral symptoms associated with depression in children. A useful measure to assess anxiety in children is the Multidimensional Anxiety Scale for Children (MASC; March, 1997). The MASC is a self-report instrument that taps the dimensions of anxiety in individuals ages 8–19 years old. It is also important to assess for the presence and frequency of sexual behaviors in the child. Friedrich et al. (1992) developed the Child Sexual Behavior Inventory (CSBI), a standardized caregiver report questionnaire that measures normative as well as problematic sexual behaviors in children (ages 2–12 years old). Internalizing and externalizing behavior problems in children can be assessed by having the caregiver complete the Child Behavior Checklist (CBCL; Achenbach & Edelbrock, 1991), a widely used, well-established measure that provides normative data by age and gender.

An equally important part of the pretreatment assessment process involves evaluating the caregiver's level of emotional distress in relation to the sexual abuse. The Impact of Event Scale–Revised (IES-R; Weiss & Marmar, 1997) can be utilized to measure PTSD-related symptoms in caregivers. The IES-R taps responses to traumatic experiences, such as intrusive thoughts, avoidance, and hyperarousal. The caregiver's level of depression should also be assessed. The Beck Depression Inventory–2 (BDI-2; Beck, Steer, & Brown, 1996) is a revised version of the BDI, the most widely used self-report measure of depressive symptomatology in adults. Additional instruments that are useful in assessing the caregiver's emotional reactions and behaviors in response to the sexual abuse are the Parent Emotional Reaction Questionnaire (PERQ; Cohen & Mannarino, 1996b) and the Parental Support Questionnaire (PSQ; Cohen & Mannarino, 1996b). The PERQ taps into caregiver reactions of fear, guilt, anger, and embarrassment. The PSQ was developed to assess caregivers thoughts and perceptions regarding their own behavior in reaction to their child's experience of sexual abuse. The PSQ also measures caregivers' perceptions of the support they provided to the child as well as their attributions regarding responsibility for the sexual abuse. Based on the results of these pretreatment assessment measures, combined with information gathered from child and caregiver interviews, an individually tailored treatment plan should be developed to address the clients' specific needs and symptoms.

Treatment Model

For a more thorough explanation of the following treatment model, as it is applied to children who have suffered sexual abuse, the reader is referred to *Treating Sexually Abused Children and Their Nonoffending Parents: A Cognitive Behavioral Approach* (Deblinger & Heflin, 1996) as well as to other descriptive articles regarding children who have suffered a wide array of traumatic experiences, such as physical abuse, traumatic loss, and exposure to domestic and community violence (Cohen & Mannarino, 1993; Cohen et al., 2005, in press).

In general, the approach described here is based on a short-term model that generally involves 12–18 sessions subsequent to a pretreatment assessment. However, depending on the needs of the family (e.g., multiple diagnoses, legal complexity, reunification with the perpetrator), treatment may be extended. Treatment begins by dividing session time into two separate 30- to 45-minute individual sessions for the child and the participating nonoffending caregiver. These initial individual sessions are important for children because therapists may be more effective than caregivers in helping them overcome their avoidance and take those initial steps toward talking about the abuse (Deblinger et al., 1996). Individual sessions for caregivers are designed to help them cope with their own distress so that when joint sessions begin, they can be more effective coping models for their children. Generally, after four to six sessions, a portion of the session time is devoted to joint caregiver–child work. Joint sessions provide a forum for caregivers and children to rehearse skills (e.g., giving/receiving praise, practicing personal safety skills) and to participate in activities that are designed to facilitate positive interactions and open communication, particularly with regard to the traumatic experiences and related issues. These session lay the groundwork on which caregivers and children can continue to discuss and process the traumatic experiences outside of the therapeutic environment and beyond the termination of therapy. Therapists may choose to assign homework to caregivers that involves rehearsal of skills learned in treatment. In this homework the caregiver is generally asked to apply a behavior management technique; the caregiver practices his or her skills at home and receives corrective feedback later from the therapist. Additionally, homework designed to facilitate more open communication between the child and caregiver is also recommended. Caregivers can be referred to books, videos, games, and other aids that are often useful in assisting children to engage in discussions about sexual abuse as well as healthy sexuality (e.g., Mayle, 1977; Cole, 1988; Staufler & Deblinger, 2003).

The treatment model consists of three broad intervention components that can be viewed as distinct treatment goals; coping skills training, gradual exposure and processing, and psychoeducation about child sexual abuse, healthy sexuality, and body safety skills (see Figure 16.1). Although the components are presented in a specific order and discussed as such, in practice a

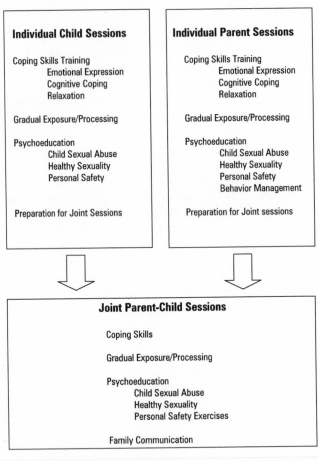

FIGURE 16.1. Synopsis of therapeutic model.

therapist can adjust the focus and timing of each component to best meet the needs of a particular client. Parents are also offered behavior management skills training to assist them in responding optimally to their children's difficulties.

The initial goals of treatment may be focused on helping children and caregivers acquire effective coping skills, including emotional expression, cognitive coping, and relaxation. Emotional expression skills training involves assisting caregivers and children in accurately identifying, labeling, and communicating their feelings. For example, children may benefit from the use of posters that depict feelings, charade games, and role plays to facilitate their ability to identify emotions in themselves and others, and to more effectively communicate their emotions. Cognitive coping skills training begins with teaching the interrelationships among thoughts, feelings, and behaviors. The goal of cognitive coping exercises is to help clients understand that they can change their thoughts and, in turn, change their feelings.

Additionally, cognitive coping skills include the ability to dispute dysfunctional abuse-related thoughts and replace them with more accurate and productive thoughts. For example, a caregiver may be experiencing distress related to thoughts that she should have known that her child was being sexually abused. Using cognitive coping skills, the therapist would assist the caregiver in disputing her thoughts through educational material and discussion related to the dysfunctional thoughts. In this example, the therapist could point out that there are no specific characteristics of sexual offenders and that even experts cannot identify sexual offenders; therefore, the caregiver had no way of knowing about the sexual abuse. Relaxation skills training is particularly helpful with those clients (both children and adults) who experience physical tension or high levels of anxiety surrounding the sexual abuse. Relaxation training needs to be aimed at children's developmental levels and should include imagery (e.g., "Pretend you are a tin soldier/a wet noodle") to facilitate progressive muscle relaxation (Deblinger & Heflin, 1996).

Gradual exposure and trauma processing are the foundation of this treatment model. The skills discussed above help prepare children for this phase of therapy, in which they are gradually exposed to their own thoughts, feelings, memories, and reminders of their abuse until they can tolerate all of these without significant distress. This component of treatment may be anxiety-provoking for children, caregivers, and therapists alike, perhaps making it difficult for therapists to implement. However, it may be a critical skill for children to learn to tolerate and cope with trauma-related distress, as opposed to avoiding or suppressing negative emotions, in general. A rationale for why gradual exposure is important should be given to both child and caregiver. A useful analogy is to compare gradually talking about sexual abuse to easing oneself into a cold swimming pool (Deblinger & Heflin, 1996):

> "When you first put your foot in the water, it might feel really cold and uncomfortable, but if you get in the water a little bit at a time, it starts to feel better. Once you're fully in the pool, you can swim around, and the water starts to feel good."

Over time, the child's experience of discomfort with talking about the sexual abuse will diminish and become disconnected from the abuse-related cues. The overall goal of gradual exposure for both child and caregiver is to help them confront and become comfortable with abuse-related reminders and memories. It is important for the therapist to be creative in providing materials and options for the child to use in the process of gradual exposure. There are a variety of therapeutic games and books about child sexual abuse that may help the child engage in general discussions about topic, which then can be related to his or her specific experiences. The gradual exposure process often takes the form of helping the child create a book with chapters describing the abuse, the disclosure, and the repercussions in detail. However, sometimes children prefer to engage in the exposure process by writing a poem or song, drawing a picture, or visualizing and reporting their abusive experiences.

Following the process of gradual exposure, therapists should engage the child and caregiver in cognitive and affective processing of the abuse experiences. This processing provides an opportunity for child and caregiver to further explore the experience of abuse as well as to clarify and correct any remaining dysfunctional abuse-related beliefs by applying the cognitive coping skills and general knowledge learned earlier in treatment. One useful tool with which to engage clients in cognitive and affective processing is role playing. For example, the child can play a therapist who is helping another child deal with sexual abuse. The therapist plays the child and makes statements related to concerns this particular child raised earlier, during the gradual exposure. This role reversal allows the child to rehearse positive statements and to dispute problematic thoughts while simultaneously allowing the therapist to assess progress.

The third component of treatment involves psychoeducation about a variety of issues, including general information about child sexual abuse, healthy sexuality, personal safety skills, and behavior management principles. Education with regard to child sexual abuse is generally offered early in treatment because it may help to dispute dysfunctional thoughts that may be expressed during gradual exposure and processing. The therapist may provide information about what child sexual abuse is, who abuses children, how children might feel when they are sexually abused, and some reasons why most children do not reveal the sexual abuse. Personal safety skills training is incorporated later in treatment, in an effort to reduce the child's risk of revictimization. Children should acquire skills that enable them (1) to successfully differentiate between acceptable and unacceptable types of touching, (2) to say "no" to unwanted touches, and (3) to seek assistance from a trusted adult if unwanted touching occurs. Given that children who experience sexual abuse may have many questions and misconceptions about sexuality, age-appropriate sex education may be provided by both the therapist and the caregiver during joint parent–child sessions.

Education regarding principles of behavior management and their application to parenting situations is often an essential component of treatment for nonoffending caregivers. Children who have experienced sexual abuse are at increased risk of developing emotional and/or behavioral problems. To prevent and/or ameliorate such problems, caregivers are taught to increase their focus on positive behaviors through the use of praise. Both global and specific forms of praise are used not only as a behavioral tool but also to improve the relationship between child and caregiver. Additionally, caregivers are also taught to handle maladaptive behaviors such as opposition, whininess, tantrums, and sleep problems by applying principles of differential attention, effective instructions, and negative consequences.

It should be noted that the therapist–client relationship in the context of CBT is critical and intended to be collaborative. The cognitive-behavioral therapist listens and educates, sharing specific rationales underlying cognitive-behavioral interventions and encouraging collaboration in the implementation of treatment. This type of empathic and empowering therapist–client relationship may be healing and restorative, in and of itself, for children and caregivers who not only have been betrayed by the perpetrator of the abuse, but also may feel they have limited influence over child protection and legal decisions that are being made on their behalf.

CASE EXAMPLE

Presenting Problem

The client, Danielle, was a 10-year-old girl who lived with her 28-year-old single mother, Ms. Williams, and her 6-year-old sister, Charlene. Danielle's biological father, Jack, had little contact with the family, with the exception of providing child support payments. Maternal grandparents lived nearby and were involved in the daily care of the children.

Danielle began displaying behavioral problems at home, such as temper tantrums, talking back, and frequent mood changes, that resulted in problematic interactions with her family members. Ms. Williams was concerned about the changes in Danielle's behavior and repeatedly asked Danielle if something were wrong. Eventually, Danielle disclosed having experienced inappropriate sexual contact from a 17-year-old named Jon. Ms. Williams was shocked and became highly distraught; she immediately contacted the local police, who notified the prosecutor's office. At the time of the referral, the prosecutor's office was pursuing prosecution of the perpetrator. The prosecutor's office initially referred Danielle for a medical evaluation to diagnose and treat any potential medical concerns related to the sexual abuse.

According to the medical report, Danielle disclosed that the abuse included fondling of her breasts and vagina and penile vaginal penetration. The abuse allegedly occurred during several overnight visits at the home of the perpetrator, who was the older brother of Danielle's best friend. Consistent with recommendations from the medical examination, Danielle was referred for sexual-abuse-specific treatment to address the psychological impact of the trauma. Ms. Williams agreed to accompany Danielle to the sessions and to actively participate in her daughter's treatment.

Assessment and Case Formulation

A pretreatment assessment was conducted over the course of two sessions. The therapist gathered information regarding Danielle's current emotional and behavioral functioning as well as details regarding her experience of sexual abuse in order to formulate a treatment plan. This information was gathered through the administration of semistructured diagnostic and background interviews as well as standardized measures tapping symptoms of PTSD, depression, anxiety, and behavior problems. Ms. Williams also completed various self-report measures to assess her emotional distress related to her daughter's sexual abuse.

Results of the pretreatment assessment indicated that Danielle met full diagnostic criteria for PTSD, characterized primarily by symptoms of avoidance and intrusive thoughts related to the sexual abuse. Danielle was also exhibiting moderate levels of anxiety, including fear of men, difficulty falling asleep, and difficulty separating from her mother and grandparents. Similarly, Ms. Williams's responses to standardized measures revealed that she was experiencing moderate symptoms of depression, such as excessive guilt and self-blame, PTSD-related symptoms such as intrusive thoughts and avoidance of topics related to the sexual abuse, and excessive anger about the sexual abuse.

Based on these results, the following plan was developed for Danielle and her mother. Both Danielle and Ms. Williams met individually with the therapist for approximately 30–45 minutes on a weekly basis for the first five treatment sessions. During the remaining seven sessions, briefer individual sessions with Danielle and Ms. Williams were followed by joint parent–child sessions. Treatment goals for Danielle included (1) assisting her in the development of emotional expression and cognitive coping skills and (2) providing gradual exposure to, and processing of, abuse-related thoughts and feelings; and (3) learning about child sexual abuse, personal safety skills, and healthy sexuality. Treatment goals for Ms. Williams included (1) assisted processing of, and coping with, her own feelings about the abuse; (2) increasing her ability to support Danielle, through open communication, as she dealt with the sexual abuse; and (3) aiding her in the utilization of behavior management skills to address Danielle's problematic behavior at home.

Course of Treatment

Initial sessions with Danielle focused on establishing rapport, building a trusting relationship, and obtaining a baseline for her ability to discuss abuse-related information. Danielle was specifically asked to talk about why she was coming to therapy. She stated, "Because of what happened with Jon." During this statement, she did not make eye contact with the therapist and appeared more withdrawn, revealing her avoidance of the topic of sexual abuse. The therapist acknowledged Danielle's response and informed her that another reason she was coming to therapy was to learn more about expressing feelings and coping with experiences like "what happened with Jon." The therapist used a variety of techniques to engage Danielle in emotional expression skills, such as playing feeling-oriented charades and reading a book about feelings (Curtis, 1998).

To assess Danielle's ability to provide a detailed narrative, she was asked to talk about a recent positive event, including details of what had occurred as well as her thoughts and feelings about the experience. Sternberg and colleagues (1997; Sternberg, Lamb, Esplin, & Baradaran, 1999) suggested that using open-ended questions and encouraging spontaneous narratives about neutral events facilitates rapport building and sets an expectation for the child to provide detailed information when describing traumatic experiences.

During the first session, Danielle had mentioned that she recently went to the toy store with her grandmother. The therapist used this opportunity to ask Danielle to describe everything that occurred during her trip to the store, starting with what happened when she first arrived and ending with what happened when she left. Danielle was encouraged to share as many details as possible. The therapist prompted additional information by using statements such as, "Tell me what happened next. . . . Then what happened? . . . and I wasn't there, so tell me more about that." Additionally, Danielle was asked to talk about her thoughts and feelings during various points in the story. She was able to provide many details about her trip to the store, including the toys she saw, what she and her grandmother had talked about, the other children she saw, and the clerks with whom she interacted. She reported feeling happy upon entering the store and feeling sad when she was not able to buy the toy she wanted. However, she did not understand how to describe what she was thinking.

Based on this narrative, the therapist was able to determine that Danielle had an extensive ability to recall and describe events from her past. In addition, though she seemed to have an adequate understanding of emotions, she had a limited vocabulary with which to describe feelings. Thus the therapist was made aware that Danielle would require additional skills related to identifying thoughts and more complex emotions. The therapist was very enthusiastic about Danielle's ability to talk about her feelings, and she praised Danielle for providing detail in her story. The therapist provided feedback to Danielle with comments such as, "You did such a good job describing the toy store that I felt like I was there" and "I really liked that you told me how you felt sad when you couldn't buy that toy." The therapist then asked Danielle to provide a disclosure of the abuse, using Danielle's own words, by saying, "Now, tell me everything you can about *what happened with Jon,* just like you told me everything about going to the toy store." This segue from a neutral topic to the abuse topic set an example for how the abuse would be discussed in future sessions, and Danielle's response provided the therapist with an understanding of Danielle's level of comfort when discussing the abuse.

In contrast to Danielle's detail-filled story about going to the toy store, her narrative about the sexual abuse was limited. She initially stated that she did not remember. The therapist responded by praising Danielle for doing such a good job when telling all about the toy store. She then encouraged

Danielle to do the same thing about all that happened with Jon. Danielle reluctantly began talking about a time when she was at her friend's house for a sleep-over. She talked about her friend, shared some feelings, then ended by stating, "My friend's brother, Jon, did something bad. That's pretty much it." Given that this was an initial baseline assessment, the therapist did not push for further details but simply reflected back what Danielle had managed to share and appreciatively acknowledged her effort.

Over the course of the next few sessions, Danielle and the therapist reviewed emotional expression skills and practiced identifying and discussing abuse-related feelings. For example, Danielle reported feeling guilty, embarrassed, and scared about the sexual abuse. Cognitive coping was introduced to help Danielle learn to monitor and share her thoughts. The therapist taught Danielle that her thoughts, feelings, and behaviors are all related, emphasizing that by changing her thoughts she could change her feelings and behaviors. To help Danielle understand the concept of thoughts and self-talk, the therapist asked her to say out loud the things she says to herself inside her head. The therapist began with neutral examples, such as, "What did you say to yourself when you first woke up this morning?" This process was continued until Danielle could spontaneously provide her own examples. Danielle was then asked to describe the thoughts behind her abuse-related feelings. For example, Danielle reported feeling guilty because she had not told her mother about the abuse right away. This disclosure provided the therapist with an opportunity to dispute Danielle's thoughts in this area by introducing education about child sexual abuse, such as the fact that most children never tell about sexual abuse. Danielle was praised for being brave and smart for having told her mother about the abuse when she did. Additionally, Danielle was also taught that by using positive or helpful self-talk, she could replace her negative or hurtful thought that she should have told her mother sooner by stating, "I'm brave that I told—most kids never tell."

After Danielle learned about emotional expression and cognitive coping skills, she was introduced to the treatment rationale for talking about sexual abuse. The therapist explained that even though Danielle might initially feel upset talking about it, doing so would gradually become easier. Danielle stated, "I just want to forget about it." The therapist used an analogy about how "the first time you see a scary movie, it can be really scary, but if you keep watching the same movie over and over again it isn't that scary anymore." To further prepare her for the process, the therapist read Danielle a story about a little girl who had been sexually abused (Jesse, 1991). The therapist then suggested that it might be helpful for Danielle to write and/or illustrate her own book about sexual abuse. She offered Danielle a choice between starting with a page about the day when she told her mother about the abuse or the day when the abuse first occurred. By providing a choice, Danielle was given some control over the content of the session, but she was not given the option to avoid the topic of sexual abuse all together. Danielle opted to draw a picture about the day "Jon did something bad at a sleep-over." Although this was an unusual choice, in that many children prefer to share the experience of disclosing the abuse first, for Danielle, it made sense because she had reported a great deal of distress related to her mother's reaction to her disclosure.

After Danielle had drawn a picture, the therapist told her to imagine that she was back at the sleep-over and to talk about everything that had happened, including the thoughts, feelings, and sensations she experienced during the sexual abuse. To facilitate a detailed description, the therapist waited for lengthy pauses in Danielle's narrative and then used prompts such as, "Tell me more about that. . . . What happened next? . . . Tell me what you said. . . . Tell me what he said. . . . How were you feeling? . . . What were you thinking?" While Danielle provided a narrative, the therapist wrote down everything she said. This procedure allowed the therapist to keep a record for future processing exercises without interrupting Danielle's experience of exposure.

In future sessions Danielle's work on the book progressed as she was given options of drawing pictures depicting additional episodes of sexual abuse, the investigation by the prosecutor's office, the medical examination, her disclosure to her mother, and her experience of coming to therapy. At the beginning of each session, Danielle's work from the previous session was reviewed. Reviewing her book provided another opportunity for exposure and allowed the therapist to assist Danielle in processing her abuse-related thoughts and feelings further. For example, Danielle's narratives repeatedly included statements such as "I let him touch my private parts." The therapist used Socratic questioning to help dispute the belief that Danielle "let him" abuse her. Additionally, the therapist continued to provide education about sexual abuse, including the fact that it is *never* the child's fault, and that just because Danielle did not say "no," she did not give Jon permission to touch her.

Throughout these sessions, Danielle became more comfortable discussing specific details of the sexual abuse, but she remained very avoidant about discussing how and when she disclosed the abuse to her mother. When Danielle did complete her narrative about the disclosure to her mother, it became evident that she felt very guilty about her mother's extremely strong emotional reaction. Danielle reported that her mother was very angry with her for not telling her about the abuse after the first time it had happened, and that her mother made her feel bad for continuing to go over to her friend's house for sleep-overs and "allowing" Jon to sexually abuse her repeatedly.

In conjunction with Danielle's individual sessions, the therapist also met individually with Danielle's mother, Ms. Williams. The focus of Ms. Williams's sessions paralleled those of her daughter's sessions and included the same therapeutic strategies. The therapist helped Ms. Williams identify and process her abuse-related feelings and thoughts and provided education about child sexual abuse to help dispute her dysfunctional thoughts. For example, Ms. Williams felt guilty for letting her daughter go to the sleep-overs. The therapist engaged Ms. Williams in a role play to help her understand that sleep-overs are a normal part of childhood, and that she had no way of knowing that the sexual abuse would take place during the sleep-over. Ms. Williams realized that she had many reasons to trust that her daughter would be safe in this home, because she was friends with the mother and knew the children in the home.

Ms. Williams also participated in gradual exposure exercises as the therapist, with Danielle's permission, shared Danielle's pictures and narratives about the abuse. In these private sessions the therapist helped Ms. Williams process her own reactions to Danielle's experiences and also prepared her to provide supportive responses in their joint sessions to allay Danielle's fears and concerns. Specifically, the therapist worked with Ms. Williams about her anger toward her daughter for not disclosing the abuse sooner. Reading Danielle's narrative about the disclosure helped Ms. Williams realize that her own reactions were negatively impacting Danielle. The therapist also educated Ms. Williams about the many reasons children may not disclose abuse ever (e.g., threats, fear, embarrassment, trying to forget about it) and how a parent's responses can influence the child's recovery.

After the process of gradual exposure began, the therapist also initiated joint sessions with Danielle and her mother. Initially focusing on strengthening the relationship between Ms. Williams and Danielle, the therapist guided them in learning to exchange specific and global praise and engage in open communication about neutral topics. Eventually, joint sessions focused on abuse-related material, beginning with general information about child sexual abuse and then gradually moving toward the process of having Danielle share pages from her book with her mother. One very important component for Ms. Williams and Danielle was to address Danielle's belief that the abuse was her fault because she did not tell her mother immediately and because she enjoyed sleeping over at her friend's house. The therapist helped Ms. Williams prepare praise for her daughter for telling her about the abuse. Ms. Williams was also encouraged to emphasize that it is never too late to tell about sexual abuse and that the abuse was not Danielle's fault. Toward the end of treatment, joint parent–child sessions were focused on the topic of healthy sexuality and the practice of personal safety skills. For homework, the therapist encouraged mother and daughter to read an age-appropriate sex education book and an interactive personal safety skills book together (Mayle, 1977; Stauffer & Deblinger, 2003). As they prepared for termination, the therapist reviewed the skills they had learned and encouraged them to continue to their practice and to maintain their openness, particularly with regard to talking about difficult subjects such as sexual abuse, sexuality, peer pressure, bullying, etc.

When asked what she had gained from treatment, Danielle immediately responded that it was a lot easier to talk about the sexual abuse, especially with her mom. Similarly, Ms. Williams indicated that she had become closer to her daughter and felt more confident as a parent. However, she was still not sure she would have the courage to let her daughter go to sleep-overs again. The therapist pointed out that sleep-overs are a common activity for children and reminded Ms. Williams of the many times Danielle had slept over at friends' homes and nothing bad happened.

Ms. Williams was then asked to share her feelings about the strengths and skills that her daughter had demonstrated during the course of therapy. Danielle was similarly encouraged to express that the efforts her mom had made to help her cope with the sexual abuse had been so helpful to her. To further mark the end of therapy as a graduation celebration, the therapist presented certificates of achievement to both mother and daughter.

COMMON TREATMENT OBSTACLES AND POSSIBLE SOLUTIONS

It is not uncommon for children to display some level of avoidance or anxiety in response to the gradual exposure process. Therapists are encouraged to be creative in their selection of gradual exposure exercises that may appeal to children's particular interests and preferences. For example, flexibility can always be offered in terms of giving the child a choice of activities, such as drawing, writing, or reading about sexual abuse. The choice allows the child some control over the session but does not allow him or her to avoid the topic completely. In many cases, a general discussion about child sexual abuse can be used as a low-level gradual exposure exercise until the child can tolerate discussing specific details of his or her own experience. Parents should also be forewarned that children may begin to complain about treatment as therapy focuses increasingly on their traumatic experiences. If and when this happens, parents should be reminded of this forewarning and encouraged to maintain a firm commitment to attending sessions on a weekly basis. Not surprisingly, more consistent attendance greatly facilitates children's abilities to work through their trauma-related avoidance and/or anxiety.

Another common obstacle may stem from the therapist's own level of avoidance. For example, if a child displays anxiety or distress during session, a natural empathic response for the therapist would be to take a break from discussing the abuse for some time. However, this response may reinforce the child's avoidance and is counterproductive to the gradual exposure process. Another obstacle of using a model that encourages detailed descriptions of abuse is the risk of the therapist experiencing vicarious trauma. For this reason, it is important for therapists to be aware of their own feelings and reactions to hearing about trauma and the inadvertent impact of their responses on the child's progress. Supervision, case consultation, continuing education, and a balance between professional and personal endeavors can alleviate some of the stress a therapist may experience.

Supportive caregiver involvement is the ideal for the model described above; however, this involvement may not always be possible. Although the model can be applied to children individually, it is best to find some outside source of adult support. If a caregiver is not available, other adults in the child's life, such as a caseworker, relative, or family friend, may be able to participate in some aspects of treatment. In cases where a caregiver is present but does not believe the child's allegations of abuse and is clearly standing by the perpetrator, it may be best to recommend individual therapy for the caregiver. A long-term goal could be to reunite the child and caregiver for joint sessions, once the caregiver is able to provide more appropriate levels of support to the child. On the other hand, nonoffending parents who are trying to be supportive but are struggling with initial feelings of shock, disbelief, and/or ongoing feelings for the perpetrator may respond well to this treatment model, though extended sessions may be necessary.

Children often present with complex problems, demonstrate a broad constellation of symptoms, and have histories that include multiple traumas. Although the treatment model outlined in this chapter focuses primarily on reducing PTSD symptoms resulting from child sexual abuse, it can be modified to treat PTSD symptoms resulting from other types of traumas, including exposure to domestic violence, physical abuse, traumatic bereavement, and community violence. A critical step in addressing each of these traumas is that of providing education to both children and parents about the identified trauma in terms of its prevalence, characteristics, psychosocial impact, etc. For example, it is important for mothers to be made aware of the dramatic behavioral impact that exposure to domestic violence can have on children, despite the fact that the children may have never been physically harmed by the batterer. Educational information can be shared and explored with children, using question-and-answer games as well as educational books. There are, in fact, quite a few books available that can help children cope with exposure to family and/or community violence. Similarly, psychoeducation in treatment of traumatic grief might involve reading a book about death and discussing the family's beliefs about death and dying.

The other components of this treatment model can also be applied to children who have suffered a wide array of traumatic experiences. Coping skills training, for example, can help reduce anxiety and distress surrounding any traumatic experience. Coping skills exercises for a child who has witnessed community violence might focus on facilitating the child's affective reactions to the crime witnessed and its aftermath. The gradual exposure and cognitive processing component for children who have experienced violence or a traumatic loss would follow the same procedure outlined above, with a focus on encouraging children to recount the traumatic experiences as well as their associated thoughts and feelings. It is important to note that different traumas may produce highly distinct emotional reactions that are likely to be driven by unique developing beliefs that may be dysfunctional. For example, therapists may find that children who have lost a loved one may experience guilt because they are inappropriately making a connection between the loved one's death and something they said or did. During exposure and processing exercises, children exposed to domestic violence may also reveal that they believe that they were the cause of their parents' fighting, perhaps describing ongoing feelings of guilt and sadness long after the exposure to the violence has ended.

Education and cognitive coping exercises can help children develop more accurate conclusions about "why" the traumas happened. It is important to note, however, that additional treatment components may need to be added to the model described in this chapter, depending on the nature of the trauma. For example, in cases of domestic violence and physical abuse, the development and rehearsal of a personal safety plan is essential (Runyon, Basilio, Van Hasselt, & Hersen, 1998) to reduce the risk of future harm. Children should role-play and rehearse responses to potentially dangerous situations, such as a caregiver coming home intoxicated, and identify concrete steps to help ensure their safety (e.g., go to a neighbor's home, call 911, go to a safe place in their home). The treatment of childhood traumatic grief should help children incorporate components of the normal grieving process, such as accepting the reality of the loss, expressing pain associated with the death, adjusting to daily life without the presence of the individual, honoring the memory of the individual, and developing new relationships (Worden, 1996; Wolfelt, 1996; Cohen et al., in press).

Ultimately, regardless of the type of trauma, this treatment model is designed to help children and parents cope more effectively. The education, skill building, and exposure/processing exercises are all designed to help children make sense of their experience(s) in ways that allow them to feel empowered rather than victimized. Thus it is important for children to develop narratives that incorporate cognitive corrections as well as positive experiences that help them place their traumatic experience(s) in a context that encourages realism as well as optimism about the future.

CONCLUSIONS AND RECOMMENDATIONS

There is increasing evidence supporting the efficacy of the trauma-focused CBT treatment model described in this chapter. Based on the treatment comparisons made thus far, the findings suggest at least two important general guidelines for working with children who have suffered trauma. First, findings across several of the treatment outcome investigations highlight the value of involving a nonoffending parent-figure in treatment. This person may be a supportive mother, father, grandparent, foster parent, or other individual serving in a guardian role. Helping a caregiver to function as a supportive resource for a child has value that may exceed what a therapist can offer in weekly sessions and may produce therapeutic benefits that last long after therapy has terminated. Thus, when possible, it behooves therapists to engage both nonoffending maternal and paternal figures in the therapy process. Second, it appears that the structure and directive nature of the CBT model enables parents and children to focus effectively on skills and/or information relevant to overcoming the traumatic experience(s). The results from several studies in which nondirective and/or client-centered approaches were utilized indicate that children are not likely to focus on the abuse without the structured and directive guidance of a skilled therapist.

Given the mounting evidence that the aftereffects of abuse may not only disrupt children's emotional, behavioral, and social development but also may negatively impact brain development, it is critical that effective treatment models, such as the one described here, be identified and utilized as early as possible. However, there is much work to be done in terms of enhancing the availability and utilization of evidence-based treatment models in community settings. Most children who have suffered abuse either never receive treatment or receive services at agencies where up-to-date training is limited. Recently, however, several organizations, including the Kauffman Foundation, the National Child Traumatic Stress Network, and the U.S. Department of Health and Human Services Substance Abuse and Mental Health Services Administration, have recognized the efficacy and/or supported efforts to further training and dissemination of this evidence-based treatment model. Additionally, as noted, this model has been modified and expanded for use with children who have suffered traumatic loss, children exposed to domestic violence, and children who have experienced physical abuse (Cohen et al., in press; Runyon et al., 2004; Cohen et al., 2004).

Although these developments are exciting, much remains to be learned about the effective treatment of children who have suffered abuse and/or other traumas. For example, current treatment practices may be enhanced by research efforts aimed at identifying important underlying psychological processes as well as "critical therapy ingredients." In addition, research may help us better understand differential treatment responses as a function of cultural background, gender, developmental stage, coping style, and other child and family characteristics. Finally, there is a critical need for continued development of innovative treatment approaches for less responsive youngsters as well as high-risk adolescents, such as those engaging in self-destructive behaviors. Continued research efforts in these areas will not only help to improve general practice, but most importantly, may help us to individually tailor treatment approaches to achieve optimal outcomes for all children and families who have suffered traumatic experiences.

REFERENCES

Achenbach, T. M., & Edelbrock, C. S. (1991). *Manual for the Child Behavior Checklist and Revised Child Behavior Profile.* Burlington: University of Vermont.

American Academy of Child and Adolescent Psychiatry [AACAP]. (1998). Practice parameters for the assessment and treatment of children and adolescents with PTSD. *Journal of the American Academy of Child and Adolescent Psychiatry, 37*(Suppl.), 4S–26S.

Beck, A. T., Steer, R. A., & Brown, G. K. (1996). *Manual for the Beck Depression Inventory–Second Edition.* San Antonio, TX: Psychological Corporation.

Carlson, B. E. (1998). Children's observations of interparental violence. In A. R. Roberts (Ed.), *Battered women and their families.* New York: Springer.

Cohen, J. A., Berliner, L., & Mannarino, A. P. (2000a). Treatment of traumatized children: A review and synthesis. *Journal of Trauma, Violence, and Abuse, 1,* 29–46.

Cohen, J. A., Berliner, L., & March, J. S. (2000b). Treatment of children and adolescents. In E. B. Foa, T. M. Keane, & M. J. Friedman (Eds.), *Effective treatments for PTSD* (pp. 106–138). New York: Guilford Press.

Cohen, J. A., Deblinger, E., & Mannarino, A. P. (2005). Trauma-focused, cognitive behavioral therapy for sexually abused children. In E. Hibbs & P. Jensen (Eds.), *Psychosocial treatments for child and adolescent disorders: Empirically based strategies for clinical practice* (2nd ed., pp. 743–765). Washington, DC: American Psychological Association.

Cohen, J. A., Deblinger, E., Mannarino, A. P., & Steer, R. A. (2004). A multisite, randomized controlled trial for sexually abused children with PTSD symptoms. *Journal of the American Academy of Child and Adolescent Psychiatry, 43,* 393–402.

Cohen, J. A., & Mannarino, A. P. (1993). A treatment model for sexually abused preschoolers. *Journal of Interpersonal Violence, 8,* 115–131.

Cohen, J. A., & Mannarino, A. P. (1996a). A treatment outcome study for sexually abused preschool children: Initial findings. *Journal of the American Academy of Child and Adolescent Psychiatry 35,* 42–50.

Cohen, J. A., & Mannarino, A. P. (1996b). Factors that mediate treatment outcome of sexually abused preschool children. *Journal of the American Academy of Child and Adolescent Psychiatry, 35,* 1402–1410.

Cohen, J. A., & Mannarino, A. P. (1997). A treatment study of sexually abused preschool children: Outcome during one year follow-up. *Journal of the American Academy of Child and Adolescent Psychiatry, 36,* 1228–1235.

Cohen, J. A., & Mannarino, A. P. (1998). Interventions for sexually abused children: Initial treatment findings. *Child Maltreatment, 3,* 17–26.

Cohen, J. A., Mannarino, A. P., Berliner, L., & Deblinger, E. (2000c). Trauma-focused cognitive behavioral therapy for children and adolescents: An empirical update. *Journal of Interpersonal Violence, 15,* 1202–1223.

Cohen, J. A., Mannarino, A. P., & Knudsen, K. (2004). Treating childhood traumatic grief: A pilot study. *Journal of the American Academy of Child and Adolescent Psychiatry, 43,* 1225–1233.

Cohen, J. A., Mannarino, A. P., & Deblinger, E. (in press). *Treating trauma and traumatic grief in children and adolescents: A clinician's guide.* New York: Guilford Press.

Cole, J. (1988). *Asking about sex and growing up.* New York: Morrow.

Conte, J. R., & Schuerman, J. R. (1987). Factors associated with an increased impact of child sexual abuse. *Child Abuse and Neglect, 11,* 201–211.

Curtis, J. L. (1998). *Today I feel silly and other moods that make my day.* New York: HarperCollins.

DeBellis, M. D., Baum, A., Birmaher, B., Keshavan, M. S., Eccard, C. H., Boring, A.M., et al. (1999). Developmental traumatology. Part I: Biological stress systems. *Biological Psychiatry 45,* 1259–1270.

Deblinger, E., & Heflin, A. H. (1996). *Treating sexually abused children and their nonoffending parents: A cognitive behavioral approach.* Thousand Oaks, CA: Sage.

Deblinger, E., Lippmann, J., & Steer, R. (1996). Sexually abused children suffering posttraumatic stress symptoms: Initial treatment outcome findings. *Child Maltreatment, 1,* 310–321.

Deblinger, E., McLeer, S. V., & Henry, D. (1990). Cognitive behavioral treatment for sexually abused children suffering post-traumatic stress: Preliminary findings. *Journal of the American Academy of Child and Adolescent Psychiatry, 29,* 747–752.

Deblinger, E., Stauffer, L. B., & Steer, R. A. (2001). Comparative efficacies of supportive and cognitive behavioral group therapies for young children who have been sexually abused and their nonoffending mothers. *Child Maltreatment, 6,* 332–343.

Deblinger, E., Steer, R., & Lippmann, J. (1999). Maternal factors associated with sexually abused children's psychosocial adjustment. *Child Maltreatment, 4,* 13–20.

Everett, B., & Gallop, R. (2001). *The link between childhood trauma and mental illness: Effective interventions from mental health professionals.* Thousand Oaks, CA: Sage.

Everson, M. D., Hunter, W. M., Runyon, D. K., Edelson, G. A., & Coulter, M. L. (1989). Maternal support following disclosure of incest. *American Journal of Orthopsychiatry, 59,* 197–207.

Feiring, C., Taska, L., & Lewis, M. (1999). Age and gender differences in children's and adolescents' adaptation to sexual abuse. *Child Abuse and Neglect, 23,* 115–128.

Felitti, V. J., Anda, R. F., Nordenberg, D., Williamson, D. F., Spitz, A.M., Edwards, V., Koss, M. P., & Marks, J. S. (1998). Relationship of childhood abuse and household dysfunction to many of the leading causes of death in adults: The Adverse Childhood Experiences (ACE) study. *American Journal of Preventive Medicine, 14*(4), 245–258.

Finkelhor, D. (1994). Current information on the scope and nature of child sexual abuse. *Future of Children, 4,* 31–53.

Finkelhor, D. (1995). The victimization of children: A developmental perspective. *American Journal of Orthopsychiatry, 65,* 177–193.

Foa, E. B., Rothbaum, B. O., Riggs, D. S., & Murdock, T. B. (1992). Treatment of posttraumatic stress disorder in rape victims: A comparison between cognitive behavioral procedures and counseling. *Journal of Consulting and Clinical Psychology, 59,* 715–723.

Friedrich, W. N., Grambsch, P., Damon, L., Hewitt, S. K., Koverola, C., Lang, R., Wolf, V., & Broughton, D. (1992). The child sexual behavior inventory: Normative and clinical comparisons. *Psychological Assessment, 4,* 303–311.

Hill, J. (2003). Childhood trauma and depression. *Current Opinion in Psychiatry, 16,* 3–6.

Jesse, N. (1991). *Please tell! A child's story about sexual abuse.* Center City, MN: Hazelden Foundation.

Kaufman, J., Birmaher, B., & Brent, D. A. (1996). Schedule for Affective Disorders and Schizophrenia for school-age children: Present and lifetime version (K-SADS-PL): Initial reliability and validity data. *Journal of the American Academy of Child and Adolescent Psychiatry, 36,* 980–988.

Kelley, B. T., Thornberry, T. P., & Smith, C. A. (1997, August). In the wake of childhood maltreatment. *Juvenile Justice Bulletin,* pp. 1–15.

King, N., Tonge, B. J., Mullen, P., Myerson, N., Heyne, D., Rollings, S., et al. (2000). Treating sexually abused children with post-traumatic stress symptoms: A randomized clinical trial. *Journal of the American Academy of Child and Adolescent Psychiatry, 59,* 1347–1355.

Kolko, D. J. (1996). Individual cognitive-behavioral treatment and family therapy for physically abused children and their offending parents: A comparison of clinical outcomes. *Child Maltreatment, 1,* 322–342.

Kolko, D. J. (2002). Child physical abuse. In J. E .B. Myers, L. Berliner, J. Briere, C. T. Hendrix, C. Jenny, & T. A. Reed (Eds.), *The APSAC handbook on child maltreatment* (2nd ed., pp. 21–54). Thousand Oaks, CA: Sage.

Kovacs, M. (1985). The Children's Depression Inventory (CDI). *Psychopharmacology Bulletin, 21,* 995–998.

Lippmann, J. (2002). Psychological issues. In M. A. Finkel & A. P. Giardino (Eds.), *Medical evaluation of child sexual abuse: A practical guide* (2nd ed., pp. 193–213). Thousand Oaks, CA: Sage.

Mackintosh, N. (1983). *Conditioning and associative learning.* New York: Oxford University Press.

Mannarino, A. P., Cohen, J. A., & Berman, S. R. (1994). The Children's Attributions and Perceptions Scale: A new measure of sexual abuse-related factors. *Journal of Clinical Child Psychology, 23,* 204–211.

March, J. S. (1997). *Multidimensional Anxiety Scale for Children: Technical Manual.* North Towanda, NY: Multi-Health Systems.

March, J. S., Amaya-Jackson, L., Murray, M., & Schulte, A. (1998). Cognitive-behavioral psychotherapy for children and adolescents with posttraumatic stress disorder following a single incident stressor. *Journal of the American Academy of Child and Adolescent Psychiatry, 37,* 585–593.

Mayle, P. (1977). *"Where did I come from?" The facts of life without any nonsense and with illustrations.* New York: Kensington.

McLeer, S. V., Deblinger, E., Henry, D., & Orvaschel, H. (1992). Sexually abused children at high risk for PTSD. *Journal of the American Academy of Child and Adolescent Psychiatry, 31,* 875–879.

Mowrer, O. H. (1939). A stimulus response analysis of anxiety and its role as a reinforcing agent. *Psychological Review, 46,* 553–565.

Mowrer, O. H. (1960). *Learning theory and behavior.* New York: Wiley.

Runyon, M., Basilio, I., Van Hasselt, V. B., & Hersen, M. (1998). Child witnesses of interparental violence: A manual for child and family treatment. In V. B. Van Hasselt & M. Hersen (Eds.), *Sourcebook of psychological treatment manuals for children and adolescents* (pp. 203–278). Hillsdale, NJ: Erlbaum.

Runyon, M. K., Deblinger, E., Ryan, E. E., & Thakkar-Kolar, R. (2004). An overview of child physical abuse: Developing an integrated parent–child cognitive-behavioral treatment approach. *Trauma, Violence, and Abuse: A Review Journal, 5,* 65–85.

Saunders, B. E., Berliner, L., & Hanson, R. F. (Eds.). (2003). *Child physical and sexual abuse: Guidelines for treatment* (final report: January 15, 2003). Charleston, SC: National Crime Victims Research and Treatment Center.

Stauffer, L., & Deblinger, E. (1996). Cognitive behavioral groups for nonoffending mothers and their young sexually abused children: A preliminary treatment outcome study. *Child Maltreatment, 1,* 65–76.

Stauffer, L., & Deblinger, E. (2003). *Let's talk about taking care of you!* Hatfield, PA: Hope for Families.

Sternberg, K. J., Lamb, M. E., Esplin, P. W., & Baradaran, L. P. (1999). Using a scripted protocol in investigative interviews: A pilot study. *Applied Developmental Science, 3,* 70–76.

Sternberg, K. J., Lamb, M. E., Hershkowitz, I., Yudilevitch, L., Orbach, Y., Esplin, P. W., & Hovav, M. (1997). Effects of introductory style on children's abilities to describe experiences of sexual abuse. *Child Abuse and Neglect, 21,* 1133–1146.

Straus, M. A., & Gelles, R. J. (1996). *Physical violence in American families.* New Brunswick, NJ: Transaction.

Swenson, C. C., & Brown, E. J. (1999). Cognitive-behavioral group treatment for physically abused children. *Cognitive and Behavioral Practice, 6,* 212–220.

U.S. Department of Health and Human Services, Administration on Children, Youth, and Families. (2000). *Child maltreatment, 1998: Reports from the states to the National Child Abuse and Neglect Data System.* Washington, DC: Government Printing Office.

Weiss, D. S., & Marmar, C.R. (1997). The Impact of Event Scale—Revised. In J. Wilson & T. M. Keane (Eds.), *Assessing psychological trauma and PTSD* (pp. 399–411). New York: Guilford Press.

Widom, C., & Morris, S. (1997). Accuracy of adult recollection of childhood victimization: Part 2. Childhood sexual abuse. *Psychological Assessment, 9,* 34–46.

Williams, L. (1994). Recall of childhood trauma: A prospective study of women's memories of child sexual abuse. *Journal of Consulting and Clinical Psychology, 62,* 1167–1176.

Wolfelt, A. D. (1996). *Healing the bereaved child: Grief gardening, growth through grief and other touchstones for caregivers.* Fort Collins, CO: Companion Press.

Worden, J. W. (1996). *Children and grief: When a parent dies.* New York: Guilford Press.

CHAPTER SEVENTEEN

Bringing Cognitive-Behavioral Psychology to Bear on Early Intervention with Trauma Survivors

Accident, Assault, War, Disaster, Mass Violence, and Terrorism

Josef I. Ruzek

Increasing recognition of the potential impact of trauma exposure, coupled with humanitarian concern about responding to victims, has led to widespread implementation of trauma-related services in recent years. In particular, interest in working with trauma survivors in the first weeks and months following their traumatic experiences has grown, with goals that include reducing acute distress, limiting suffering, maintaining functioning, and reducing rates of chronic problems. Several systems of early posttrauma intervention have evolved, relatively independently, to serve survivors of diverse traumas, including physical and sexual assault, natural and technological disaster, terrorism and mass violence, war, and the exposure to life threat, human suffering, and loss often associated with emergency response work and peacekeeping operations. Scrutiny of existing early intervention efforts has increased as the field of traumatic stress studies has developed, and has gained greater urgency due to recent terrorist attacks (e.g., September 11, 2001), the Iraq war, and widespread ethnic conflicts. In parallel with an increasing availability of posttrauma services, researchers are beginning to test the efficacy and effectiveness of existing interventions and to design and test new ones. In this context, studying cognitive-behavioral interventions designed to reduce problems associated with traumatic stress has become of increased importance.

In this chapter I look at the trauma resulting from these sources in order to (1) describe the potential for cognitive-behavioral psychology to inform the efforts to help survivors in established domains of post-trauma care; (2) explore the implications of cognitive-behavioral theory and research in relation to the goals and practices embodied in conventional early intervention efforts; (3) outline several key issues that must be confronted during the development of new approaches; and (4) draw attention to the need to plan, at the outset in what is a developing field, for the dissemination of new concepts and methods to the real-world settings where professionals work with trauma survivors.

DOMAINS OF EARLY POSTTRAUMA CARE

Established domains of early trauma care include efforts to serve individuals seeking emergency medical care (e.g., as a result of motor vehicle accidents or violent assault), survivors of disaster and terrorist attacks, survivors of sexual assault, and those traumatized during military deployment (e.g., combat, peacekeeping). In the past, cognitive-behavioral theory and intervention methods have had relatively little impact on development of these response services. More recently, however, cognitive-behavioral practitioners have become increasingly active in these settings, cognitive-behavioral interventions are being applied, and demonstration projects are being developed and evaluated.

Hospital Trauma Care: Accident and Assault Survivors

A primary environment for the early application of cognitive-behavioral interventions is the hospital, where a major opportunity to reach trauma survivors soon after their traumatic experience can be found (Ruzek & Cordova, 2003). Very large numbers of individuals who have experienced life-threatening motor vehicle and industrial accidents, physical and sexual assaults, unexpected losses of loved ones, and traumatic life-threatening illness present in hospital trauma centers and other medical settings. Also, in circumstances of mass violence and disasters that affect larger numbers of people, hospitals constitute a primary element of community response (Ruzek, Young, Cordova, & Flynn, 2004). To date, hospitals do not routinely provide preventive services that address the mental health consequences of traumatic events.

At the present time, the best-developed cognitive-behavioral approach to secondary prevention of posttraumatic stress disorder (PTSD) has been applied and tested with accident and assault survivors. Foa, Hearst-Ikeda, and Perry (1995) delivered a four-session intervention that used, in abbreviated form, the same helping procedures—education, breathing/relaxation, training, imaginal and *in vivo* exposure, and cognitive restructuring—that have been used successfully in the treatment of chronic PTSD to help female victims of sexual and nonsexual assault. Subjects were assessed within 3 weeks of the assault, and treatment was begun immediately following assessment. Compared with a matched control group, individuals receiving the cognitive-behavioral intervention were significantly less depressed and reported fewer reexperiencing symptoms 5 months postassault. None of the treated participants showed depression or more than six PTSD symptoms; 56% of the control group reported moderate-to-severe depression, and 33% had more than six PTSD symptoms.

Bryant and colleagues developed and validated a procedurally similar four-to-five session cognitive-behavioral approach to intervention with accident and nonsexual assault survivors diagnosed with acute stress disorder. In two randomized controlled trials (Bryant, Harvey, Dang, Sackville, & Basten, 1998; Bryant, Sackville, Dang, Moulds, & Guthrie, 1999), this approach has been shown to reduce posttraumatic stress symptoms and prevent development of PTSD (see Bryant, Chapter 9, this volume, for a more detailed account of this work). Furthermore, Bryant, Moulds, and Nixon (2003) reported that, four years after being helped, participants who had received the intervention showed a lower intensity of PTSD symptoms than those receiving education and support.

Demonstration projects have shown the feasibility of mounting traumatic stress services that include similar interventions in emergency medical settings (e.g., Shepherd & Bisson, 2004). Bisson, Shepherd, Joy, Probert, and Newcombe (2004) examined an intervention similar to that employed by Bryant with patients who visited an accident and emergency department following a physical injury that resulted in psychological distress. Patients receiving the cognitive-behavioral intervention showed significantly greater decrease in PTSD symptoms at 13-month follow-up, but did not differ from standard care on anxiety or depression. Symptoms in both groups decreased significantly over time. It is notable that this study differed from those of Bryant in several respects. Bryant and colleagues intervened with individuals diagnosed with acute stress disorder, whereas this study focused on those with high initial levels of posttraumatic stress symptoms. The intervention procedure was similar but was somewhat less intensive (i.e., four hour-long sessions compared with four-to-five 1.5 hour sessions), and it was initiated later after a greater lapse of time from the traumatic event (5–10 weeks after injury, as opposed to approximately 2 weeks). The treatment providers may also have been less experienced with the intervention methods.

Zatzick and colleagues have developed and tested a model of stepped collaborative care for acutely injured trauma survivors (Zatzick et al., 2001b). Collaborative care aims to integrate mental health care into general medical care, and here consisted of ongoing postinjury case management, motivational interviewing targeted at alcohol abuse or dependence, and evidence-based pharmacotherapy or cognitive-behavioral therapy for those with PTSD at the 3-month period. Zatzick et al. (2004) recruited injured surgical inpatients who indicated clinically significant levels of posttraumatic stress symptoms or depression. Compared with a usual care control, patients who received the collaborative care intervention showed significantly less alcohol abuse/dependence at 6 and 12 months after the injury. At 12-month followup, a significantly lower percentage receiving collaborative care met criteria for PTSD. Collaborative care patients showed little change in PTSD symptoms over the year, whereas usual care patients showed significant worsening. The authors speculated that the relatively weak impact on PTSD may have been due to the fact that some patients with minimal PTSD symptoms were recruited into the study. Importantly, cognitive-behavioral methods were integrated into this effort, modeled after those developed by Bryant and colleagues to treat persons diagnosed with PTSD (Wagner, 2003). Early evaluation and supportive care were not associated with a reduction in PTSD, which was only observed at the 3-month period when pharmacotherapy or cognitive-behavioral treatments were implemented.

A different cognitive-behavioral intervention embedded in emergency medical care was described by Cordova, Ruzek, Benoit, and Brunet (2003). This one- or two-session intervention is delivered by hospital personnel to both the patient and a significant other. The approach includes elements of coping skills training and motivational interviewing and targets communication between the patient and significant other, aiming to facilitate support, promote disclosure by the patient, reduce disclosure-constraining behavior by the other, and improve coping.

Although work on early delivery of cognitive-behavioral interventions to accident and assault survivors is promising, the Bisson et al. (2004) and Zatzick et al. (2004) findings highlight the need for delineation of the conditions under which the interventions may be effective as well as replication in multiple laboratories.

Mental Health Response to Terrorism and Disaster

As disaster response systems have matured, they have increasingly included explicit attention to the mental health consequences of exposure to natural and technological disaster and terrorist attack. This development has accelerated as a result of the terrorist attacks of September 11, 2001 and heightened concern about future attacks. Historically, disaster mental health response has not included services explicitly informed by a cognitive-behavioral perspective. This state is now beginning to change (e.g., Walser et al., 2004), driven by increased interest in delivery of evidence-based interventions on the part of organizations charged with disaster mental health response (Gibson et al., in press).

An important initial demonstration of the utility of cognitive-behavioral treatment for those with PTSD associated with terrorist attack and disaster was provided in efforts to help survivors of a 1998 terrorist bombing in Omagh, Northern Ireland. Gillespie, Duffy, Hackmann, and Clark (2002) conducted an open trial of a cognitive-behavioral therapy delivered between 1 and 34 months (median 10 months) postattack with survivors who had developed PTSD. Ninety-one patients who met criteria for PTSD resulting from the bombing received 2–78 sessions (with a mean of 8) of a treatment that combined imaginal exposure with cognitive therapy; 37% of survivors were treated in five or less sessions. Seventy-eight patients demonstrated significant pre–post improvement on standardized measures of symptoms, with an effect size for improvement in PTSD symptoms of 2.47, a magnitude of change comparable to, or larger than, controlled trials of cognitive-behavioral therapy for PTSD.

The terrorist attacks on the World Trade Center and the Pentagon set into motion a number of initiatives to apply cognitive-behavioral methods of care for survivors (Neria, Suh, & Marshall, 2003; Levitt, Davis, Martin, & Cloitre, 2003). A cognitive-behavioral intervention (Hamblen et al., 2003) was delivered to some survivors of the World Trade Center attacks, beginning approximately 18 months after 9/11, as part of an "enhanced" service offered under the auspices of Project Liberty crisis counseling programs. Comprised of psychoeducation, coping skills training, and cognitive restructuring, the treatment was delivered in 9–12 sessions to users of crisis counseling services who had screened positive on a paper-and-pencil selection tool. Clinicians reported that this intervention was well received by clients (Norris et al., in press), but no formal outcome assessment has been conducted, to date. Cognitive-behavioral interventions have also been delivered to emergency workers who responded to the 9/11 attacks (Difede, Roberts, Jayasinghe, & Leck, in press).

Fear of terrorism often is the fear of traumatic events that may happen in the future; thus, a cognitive-behavioral approach has been tested that helps those who fear potential attacks. Somer, Tamir, Maguen, and Litz (2005) found that a 15-minute cognitive-behavioral telephone-administered anxiety management intervention was more effective than standard hotline counseling in reducing distress, anxiety, and worry about missile attack among Israeli citizens (see below).

Rape Crisis Services

Rape crisis centers are now established in many communities and provide a range of services, including telephone hotline counseling, hospital-based sexual assault nurse examiner programs (that link with individuals in the hospital setting where they come immediately following the assault), individual counseling, and group support. Although these services have largely not been informed by research in cognitive-behavioral psychology, cognitive-behavioral perspectives may have much to offer in these contexts. As noted above, the possibility that PTSD can be prevented was signaled by cognitive-behavioral work with survivors of sexual assault (Foa et al., 1995). More generally, cognitive-behavioral treatments set the standard for evidence-based care for individuals with rape-related PTSD (for detailed accounts of these treatments, see Riggs, Cahill, Foa, Chapter 4, this volume, and Shipherd, Street, & Resick, Chapter 5, this volume). Foa and colleagues (Foa, Cahill, & Hembree, 2001) demonstrated that exposure therapy for PTSD, shown to be effective in efficacy trials, could be similarly effective when delivered by rape crisis counselors who received systematic training and supervision.

In a rather different demonstration, Resnick, Acierno, Holmes, Kilpatrick, and Jager (1999) showed that simple education, informed by a cognitive-behavioral conceptual framework, is capable of producing some important benefits for sexual assault survivors. They showed a 17-minute educational videotape to women survivors of recent assault, to prepare them for forensic rape examinations. The video, which included information about and modeling of examination procedures, advice about ways of engaging in self-exposure to rape-related cues, information about cognitive and physiological reactions to rape, and ways of managing mood, resulted in significant decreases in postexamination distress ratings and anxiety symptoms.

The Military

For much of the 20th century, there have been efforts to reduce emotional breakdown during combat, to prevent decreased troop capability. These approaches are variously known as "frontline psychiatry," "combat and operational stress control," and so on. They emphasize the need to deliver services as close as possible to the front lines, as soon as possible after traumatization, in the context of a strong expectation that personnel will be able to return to functioning and their military role; and that this will take place as simply as possible—hence the well-known acronym PIES (proximity, immediacy, expectancy, simplicity). A recent report provided some support for the impact of these principles (Solomon, Shklar, & Mikulincer, 2004). Because there have been few methodologically sound studies of the impact of these services, however, the evidence as a whole does not demonstrate, at present, their utility in preventing mental health problems (Jones & Wessely, 2003).

Although these efforts have developed largely independent of cognitive-behavioral psychology, combat stress control and, more generally, Department of Defense (DoD) mental health care are beginning to include practices that have been informed by cognitive-behavioral intervention methods. For example, the *U.S. Army Combat Stress Control Handbook* (Department of the Army, 2003) includes reference to stress-control methods such as abdominal breathing, visual imagery relaxation techniques, positive self-talk, and progressive muscular relaxation. The recently constructed and approved joint *VA–DoD Clinical Practice Guideline for the Management of Traumatic Stress* (VA–Department of Defense Clinical Practice Guideline Working Group, 2003) includes significant reference to cognitive-behavioral practices. Some military mental health providers, searching for effective ways of intervening with affected personnel returning from the Iraq and Afghanistan Wars, have been delivering cognitive-behavioral treatments for PTSD (e.g., cognitive processing therapy; Resick & Schnicke, 1993), and cognitive-behavioral treatments figure prominently in the *Iraq War Clinician Guide* designed to help prepare the Veterans Administration Health Care System for returning service men and women (Ruzek et al., 2003).

Comment

Broad concern about the effectiveness of early posttrauma services and a desire to move toward evidence-based care are leading to increased adaptation of cognitive-behavioral interventions with varying populations of trauma survivors. As is evident above, most such adaptation is in its infancy. Cognitive-behavioral approaches to early intervention require conceptual development, practical formulation and "packaging," and empirical study in a range of settings with varying trauma survivor populations. In the next section, components of cognitive-behavioral intervention that may be brought to bear are outlined.

COGNITIVE-BEHAVIORAL INTERVENTIONS: IMPLICATIONS FOR CURRENT PRACTICES IN EARLY INTERVENTION

Cognitive-behavioral psychology includes an extensive array of behavior change principles and intervention methods that are relevant to the care of trauma survivors. To date, they have not been extensively adapted for early delivery to the major trauma populations and have not seen wide application within the delivery systems considered above. Because of the randomized controlled trials conducted by Bryant and colleagues as well as the larger body of evidence supporting cognitive-behavioral therapy as a treatment for chronic PTSD, there is much interest in early interventions based on cognitive-behavioral priciples. But the Bryant package has not yet been adequately replicated, and it is not clear how easily and effectively the approach can be generalized across types of trauma and delivery contexts. Bryant (Chapter 9, this volume) has described a range of circumstances in which the treatment may require modification or not be appropriate. There is also a widespread reluctance to employ exposure therapy methods soon after traumatization out of a concern, not yet systematically tested, that such methods may exacerbate symptoms or be used ineffectively by inexperienced providers. But cognitive-behavioral early intervention should not be equated with this application, which represents one possible approach. In fact, early intervention incorporates a broad range of activities that have received relatively little attention by cognitive-behavioral psychologists but that require conceptual development, practical formulation, and empirical study.

Survivor Education

Education is a primary component of all efforts to provide early mental health response, including cognitive-behavioral interventions. It is provided via verbal interactions between helper and survivor, individually and in groups, and via written or media communications. It is intended to change beliefs by "normalizing" the experience of the survivor and making stress reactions seem more predictable and less frightening. It is intended to change behavior by instigating and reinforcing adaptive coping, reducing negative forms of coping (e.g., alcohol or drug use, social withdrawal, extreme emotional avoidance), and instructing survivors about when to seek additional counseling.

Early trauma-related education is often provided in single contacts between survivor and practitioner, although evidence does not support the efficacy of single-session interventions with trauma survivors (Bisson, 2003). The limitations of brief information giving or verbal instruction are well known. Most of the methodology of behavior change relies on more intensive multisession interventions that harness known learning processes (e.g., reinforcement contingencies, classical conditioning, modeling). In fact, the utility of early educational activities in changing trauma-related beliefs and behaviors has received almost no research attention. The only study of a self-help manual treatment for PTSD was reported by Ehlers et al. (2003), who found that an educational manual was ineffective in reducing PTSD symptoms, possibly because of difficulties in inducing self-managed exposure to feared situations. In studies reported by Bryant and colleagues, even multisession education and support were insufficient to significantly reduce risk of development of PTSD in accident and assault survivors diagnosed with acute stress disorder (e.g., Bryant et al., 1998, 1999).

Despite the problems with simple instruction, there are reasons to continue exploring the utility of brief advice in posttrauma situations. First, brief advice is easily disseminated and currently represents perhaps the primary means of reaching trauma survivors in some types of events (e.g., mass violence). Second, it is possible that even if such approaches are relatively ineffective in changing the behavior of significant percentages of those impacted by trauma, a brief intervention that helps only 5% of recipients might nonetheless effect significant results if it could be delivered easily to thousands of people. Finally, if brief advice interventions are shown to be ineffective, then such a finding might precipitate a change in current practices to incorporate more robust behavior change methods.

In some behavioral domains, however, research has suggested that brief advice may sometimes be as effective as more intensive interventions. For example, research on alcohol problems has shown that relatively brief treatments can reduce consumption (e.g., Moyer, Finney, Swearingen, & Vergun, 2002). This work is important in the context of traumatic stress because many trauma survivors have preexisting alcohol problems and/or increase

their consumption to problem levels following traumatization. Some research does suggest that trauma survivors will respond to brief interventions targeting their drinking. Working with patients admitted to a hospital trauma center for treatment of injury, who screened positive for excessive alcohol use, Gentilello et al. (1999) demonstrated that a single 30-minute interview can reduce alcohol consumption in those with existing alcohol problems. Another study, of an intervention based on motivational enhancement (Miller & Rollnick, 1992), which addressed substance use problems in patients seeking emergency medical care, suggested that more than one contact may be important. Longabaugh et al. (2001) found that a 40- to 60-minute intervention, plus booster session, reduced consumption and was more effective in reducing alcohol-related negative consequences than standard care or a single-session intervention. In addition to these brief one-to-one interventions, it is possible that education to reduce consumption by trauma survivors can be supplied by media. Acierno, Resnick, Flood, and Holmes (2003) reported that their 17-minute educational video reduced likelihood of marijuana abuse at 6 weeks, and there was a trend for the video to be associated with less alcohol abuse among women with a prior history of alcohol or marijuana use.

In addition to indicating the potential of brief educational interventions, such studies also suggest that cognitive-behavioral methods may be used to increase their effectiveness. The Gentilello et al. (1999) intervention included individualized feedback about drinking habits, comparison to national norms, discussion of personal negative consequences of alcohol, consideration of a menu of strategies for change, and other motivational enhancement tools. Additional ways of magnifying the impact of brief advice include use of written self-help materials, instruction in self-monitoring activities, telephone follow-up, and supplementing face-to-face care using Internet services.

Normalization

An important goal of early intervention, as practiced in most settings, is "normalization" of stress reactions. According to the thinking underlying this practice, negative interpretation of acute stress responses (e.g., "I'm going crazy," "There's something wrong with me," "I must be weak") may lead survivors to pathologize their own common responses and increase their anxiety associated with these reactions. There has been little effort to investigate this hypothesis, but an emphasis on reducing misinterpretation and fear of acute stress responses is consistent with some current theories of PTSD (e.g., Ehlers & Clark, 2003). It is also consistent with research that suggests that attributing dysfunctional meanings to posttraumatic intrusions is a determinant of PTSD severity (e.g., Steil & Ehlers, 2000) and findings of high levels of anxiety sensitivity among trauma survivors with PTSD (Taylor, 2003). At present, it is not clear whether individuals who interpret their

acute stress reactions in negative ways will be at risk for posttrauma problems or whether intervention can change those interpretations and thereby improve outcomes. In most posttrauma care, helpers try to normalize acute stress reactions by simply telling survivors that these are common, normal, and not dangerous. But among those at risk for development of PTSD, such simple instruction may be insufficient. Again, cognitive-behavioral methods might be used profitably to accomplish normalization; cognitive therapy methods might be used to address negative interpretations of reactions, breathing training methods might help reduce the intensity of hyperarousal symptoms or increase their controllability, and interoceptive exposure might be used to reduce fear of anxiety sensations.

Ensuring Utilization of Services

Concepts of normalization should also include normalization of help-seeking behavior, because research suggests that many individuals with significant levels of posttraumatic stress symptoms do not use mental health services, even when they are available. For example, following terrorist attacks, this nonutilization of services appears to be the case with direct survivors (Delisi et al., 2003), family members who lose loved ones (Smith, Kilpatrick, Falsetti, & Best, 2002), emergency workers (e.g., North et al., 2002), and medical staff (e.g., Luce & Firth-Cozens, 2002). Indeed, 3–6 months after the World Trade Center attacks in New York City, only 27% of those reporting severe psychiatric symptoms had obtained mental health treatment (Delisi et al., 2003). This reluctance to use services may characterize many trauma populations. Hoge et al. (2004) found that only 23–40% of those recently returned from combat duty in Iraq or Afghanistan, who met screening criteria for a mental disorder (PTSD, major depression, or general anxiety), sought professional help, and only 38–45% indicated an interest in receiving help. Jaycox, Marshall, and Schell (2004) showed low use of mental health services despite high need among men injured through community violence. Weisaeth (2001) reported significant levels of nonacceptance of early intervention in industrial accident survivors.

Identifying the reasons for reluctance to utilize available services requires more investigation, but we do know that many factors may contribute. Lack of help-seeking behavior may sometimes reflect an awareness that some stress symptoms are to be expected, an acceptance of posttrauma distress, and an intention to "get on with life" nonetheless. Some individuals who endorse high levels of PTSD symptoms may not label themselves as significantly distressed or disabled (Shalev, Tuval, Frenkiel, & Hadar, 2004). Other reasons may be more problematic. Families experiencing grief following the Lockerbie bombing reported thinking that they could handle it on their own, with help from family, friends, and their religious faith; that accessing mental health counseling would be a sign of weakness or stigma; that they could not afford it financially; or that they could not admit to hav-

ing a problem (Smith et al., 2002). In the Hoge et al. (2004) study of Iraq or Afghanistan War returnees, concern about stigma as a result of seeking help was greatest among those most in need of help. Although most of those screening positive for a mental health problem acknowledged having a problem (78%), many indicated that they "don't trust mental health professionals," that "mental health care doesn't work," that they would be "seen as weak" if they sought help (65%), that participation in mental health services would harm their career, or that seeking help would be "too embarrassing" (41%). Difede et al. (in press) reported that, among emergency services workers who responded to the World Trade Center collapse, distress at trauma reminders was seen as a normal reaction to the events and not a reason to seek treatment. Rather, anger, irritability, and sleep problems were seen as reasons to seek help. Zatzick et al. (2001a) conducted an open-ended assessment of the concerns expressed by hospitalized survivors of motor vehicle accidents and assaults, who were most concerned with physical health (73%), psychological concerns (58%), work and financial issues (53%), social concerns (40%), and legal and medical concerns (10% each). Generally, a failure to assess and address the concerns of survivors will affect use of services and intervention compliance (Zatzick & Wagner, 2004). More research that systematically explores the perspectives of the potential users of early intervention services is clearly needed.

Pragmatic approaches to increasing the accessibility of services have been developed for various survivor populations, but these approaches have not been evaluated. Relatively little is known about how survivors make decisions about self-referral, how to encourage use of services, or how to increase the acceptance of referral for more intensive counseling. It is possible that a cognitive-behavioral framework might be usefully applied to these issues. For example, the motivational interviewing methods (Miller & Rollnick, 1992) that have become widely accepted might be adapted to the contexts of disaster outreach (in which helpers make contact with survivors at places where they congregate, such as emergency shelters, shopping malls, on doorsteps, in workplaces, at religious gatherings), and peer counseling programs, now very common in professions with expectable trauma exposure (e.g., police, military, emergency response). It may be especially important to regard environments in which recently traumatized individuals naturally present as "capture" sites that can be used to initiate processes that reduce the likelihood of disappearance from the system of care.

Finally, in some trauma populations, development of posttrauma problems may be associated with a dysfunctional withdrawal from family and other social interaction, increased irritability and anger, or increased use of alcohol or drugs. In such circumstances, trauma survivors may be unlikely to avail themselves of care opportunities at the same time that they create significant problems for those close to them. This pattern of behavior was commonly observed among Vietnam veterans and may be a possible pattern among some returning Iraq or Afghanistan war veterans. One useful response may be to develop and test a cognitive-behavioral intervention similar to that developed by Smith and Meyers (2004) that works with family members of substance abusers to increase likelihood of treatment entry.

Return to Functional Roles and Reinforcing Activities

One piece of coping advice that is often given to survivors of disaster/terrorism is to, at the appropriate time, resume involvement in important personal work, school, and family roles. Similarly, combat and operational stress-control doctrine emphasizes the importance of preventing military personnel from adopting a sick role and instead keeping them actively engaged in work activities. Wagner (2003) has described an ongoing project that uses a cognitive-behavioral approach to achieving similar goals. In this work, behavioral activation, a component of cognitive-behavioral treatments for depression, has been modified to be used in the prevention of PTSD and depression in injured trauma survivors. Behavioral activation includes a review of daily activities, identification of personal values and goals, selection of personally meaningful and enjoyable activities, and activity scheduling. It focuses on blocking avoidance and withdrawal in trauma survivors and increasing involvement in reinforcing activities. This approach to "guided activity" is supplemented with ongoing self-monitoring of the relationship between activity and mood. Factors related to avoidance are identified to initiate problem solving. Because behavioral activation is a relatively simple, time-limited intervention, it is conceptualized as an initial service in a stepped-care approach, such that those who do not improve can be referred for more intensive evidence-based treatments.

Coping Support

The recognition that most trauma survivors cope relatively well with trauma and do not develop PTSD or other problems has led those providing early care to seek to support the natural coping efforts of survivors. Helpers discuss coping with survivors, encourage adaptive efforts, and seek to provide additional instrumental support. These actions are consistent with models that emphasize perceived coping self-efficacy (Benight & Bandura, 2004). However, although coping styles have been found to be related to development of chronic PTSD, there has been little investigation of how survivors cope with acute stress reactions and the various other challenges of the early posttrauma period. That early interventions affect coping behaviors and that these behaviors are related to outcome have not been demonstrated.

Skills training involves a set of systematic methods used by cognitive-behavioral practitioners to develop new repertoires of behavior in patients. There are many skills that might conceivably benefit survivors of recent trauma, including those related to problem solving, social support seeking and giving, assertion, and parenting. A prime example of a skills set relevant to survivors of recent trauma is that of anxiety management. Stress inoculation training has been found effective in treating people with chronic PTSD (Foa et al., 1999), and anxiety management skills (e.g., breathing retraining, relaxation) are part of the intervention package used by Bryant and colleagues to successfully treat acute stress disorder. Although the addition of anxiety management training to exposure and cognitive therapy as an early treatment for acute stress disorder did not result in improved outcomes over and above the effects of cognitive therapy and exposure (Bryant et al., 1999), anxiety management was not tested as an intervention in its own right in this study. Echeburua, de Corral, Sarasua, & Zubizarreta (1996) randomly assigned 20 treatment-seeking female survivors of recent (< 90 days) sexual assault to either a cognitive-behavioral package intervention or to progressive muscular relaxation training alone. Results indicated that both groups improved in global severity of PTSD and other areas (anxiety, depression, daily life functioning).

In another demonstration of the utility of anxiety management skills, a single session of telephone-delivered anxiety management training was shown to decrease anxiety among Israeli citizens worried about the possibility of a SCUD missile attack (Somer et al., 2005). When citizens called a hotline due to SCUD-related distress, they were randomized to either cognitive-behavioral intervention or a standard hotline counseling (unconditional positive regard, empathic listening, validation, social support) control group. The intervention lasted around 15 minutes and included normalization of stress responses, instruction in diaphragmatic breathing and cognitive restructuring, phone practice of the latter techniques, and assignments to practice at home. Compared with standard hotline practice, the experimental intervention was associated with significantly less distress, anxiety, and worry about missile attack three days after the intervention. More research is needed to evaluate the impact of anxiety management skills training as an early posttrauma intervention, and also to establish the effects of training in skills for managing intense acute anxiety. For example, "grounding" techniques (e.g., Najavits, 2002) in which survivors are taught coping responses (e.g., washing face and hands, verbally describing their environment, feeling the chair on which they are sitting) that are intended to help them remain aware of their surroundings may reduce overwhelming anxiety, limit panic, and prevent dissociation. Such techniques should be examined to determine their impact on control of acute stress reactions.

Social Support

"Social support" is an umbrella term that is used to describe a multitude of helping activities (e.g., practical help with problems, emotional understanding and acceptance, normalization of reactions and experiences, mutual instruction about coping). Perceived lack of social support posttrauma is a risk factor for PTSD (Brewin, Andrews, & Valentine, 2000), and negative reactions from others have been found to predict PTSD symptomatology among several groups of survivors, including those exposed to physical assault, sexual assault, and military peacekeeping duties (e.g., Zoellner, Foa, & Brigidi, 1999; Ullman & Filipas, 2001; Bolton, Glenn, Orsillo, Roemer, & Litz, 2003). Declines in social support among disaster survivors have been associated with declines in mental health (Norris et al., 2002).

Little is known about naturally occurring support behaviors that take place during the first weeks and months following traumatization. Little is known, as well, about the impact of efforts to promote posttrauma social support on perceptions of support, actual support behaviors/interactions, or subsequent outcomes. The possibility exists that support can be influenced and that individuals may be trained to better support one another more effectively. The work of Lepore and colleagues (e.g., Lepore, Silver, Wortman, & Wayment, 1996) on the social constraints on disclosure—that the reactions of other persons may impede or "constrain" efforts to talk about a traumatic experience—suggests one direction for such intervention. Following this idea, Cordova et al. (2003) recently described the development of a one- or two-session cognitive-behavioral intervention that works with trauma survivors and a significant other to increase supportive communication and disclosure and reduce constraints on disclosure within the dyad. Goals of the intervention include (1) to improve patient and family knowledge of the process of adjustment to stressful experiences, such as illness/injury; (2) to increase tolerance for negative emotions (e.g., anxiety, fear, anger); (3) to increase rates of initiation of talking about the illness/injury; and (4) to decrease social constraint behaviors (e.g., changing the subject, criticizing, ignoring) by both patients and families in response to others' disclosure of thoughts and feelings.

Social support research suggests another important conceptual and practical dimension of early help for trauma survivors. Early interventions have focused largely on the individual trauma survivor. It may be useful, however, to conceptualize trauma as affecting a dyad or family group, and to encourage the development of interventions that target the evolving reactions among the group itself. Obviously, the family represents, for many survivors, an important environment in which recovery must occur and which can be expected to affect the trajectory of that recovery in many ways. Moreover, the traumatization of a family member is a family stressor that potentially has great impact on the well-being of the other family members. For more chronic posttrauma problems, cognitive-behavioral interventions focusing on parent–child (e.g., Deblinger, Thakkar-Kolar, & Ryan, Chapter 16, this volume) and adult couple dyads (Leonard, Follette, & Compton, Chapter 14, this volume; Monson, Schnurr, Guthrie, & Stevens, 2004) have been developed. Similarly conceived early interventions for trauma survivors require development.

Assessment

Most forms of help for trauma survivors involve some kind of assessment, and the assessment process itself may sometimes influence behavior. Assessment involves validation of concerns and may provide education about stress reactions, direct attention to reactions, reduce emotional avoidance, and so on. Some research with trauma survivors has suggested that assessment and self-monitoring may engender sustained reduction in PTSD symptoms in some trauma survivors (Tarrier, Sommerfield, Reynolds, & Pilgrim, 1999; Ehlers et al., 2003). Self-monitoring is, of course, a behavior change procedure that is used as a component of many cognitive-behavioral treatments. However, little is known about the effect of formal self-monitoring on acute traumatic stress reactions, coping responses, posttrauma alcohol consumption, or other trauma-related behaviors.

Assessment also represents an opportunity for a helper to present the survivor with individualized feedback on his or her behavior and reactions. With regard to alcohol problems, assessment results are sometimes provided to the drinker as part of motivational enhancement to reduce drinking (Gentilello et al., 1999) or seek treatment. It is possible that such an exercise may also increase motivation to change trauma-related behaviors or accept referral for treatment.

Group Interventions

In many posttrauma environments, group-administered early intervention activities are a staple element of care. This is especially true when (1) large numbers of persons are exposed to the same traumatic event (e.g., terrorist attacks, industrial accidents, mass violence, community disasters), (2) preexisting groups are exposed to trauma (e.g., a workplace exposed to a violent assault), and (3) workgroups are exposed to trauma as part of their job duties (e.g., military personnel, emergency response workers, police, forensic investigators). Groups would appear to be well-suited to challenging common distressing perceptions of survivors (e.g., feeling alone, different, misunderstood by those around them), reducing social isolation, and providing social support and may also be useful in helping survivors address the worries associated with traumas that are particularly difficult to talk about with family and friends (e.g., sexual assault), due to perceived social stigma, embarrassment or shame, guilt, or fear of negative reactions from others. In the case of work-related trauma exposure, work groups can continue to function as a unit so that group interventions will potentially affect the ongoing recovery environment.

Although little is known about the effectiveness of early group services in preventing PTSD and other trauma-related problems, we do know that group treatment is beneficial for those with chronic PTSD (Foy et al., 2000;

Foy & Larsen, Chapter 15, this volume). The primary current model of early group intervention to reduce the impact of trauma is group stress debriefing (Raphael & Wilson, 2000). There are several variations of group debriefing, but in all, groups of persons affected by a common event are gathered together and led through a structured protocol intended to provide education to help normalize stress reactions, give advice about coping, facilitate the verbal sharing of experiences, mobilize mutual support, and give information about available services. Most debriefings start with a focus on factual information and move toward discussion of feelings associated with the trauma. Outcome studies have indicated that individual stress debriefing does not prevent development of PTSD, and these findings, together with a relative absence of methodologically sound studies of group debriefing, have led to widespread questioning of the effectiveness of this procedure (e.g., McNally, Bryant, & Ehlers, 2003). From a cognitive-behavioral perspective, the lack of support for debriefing is not unexpected. Debriefing, like brief psychoeducation more generally, employs few powerful behavior change procedures, and relies instead on a one-time combination of simple advice and group discussion to change complex behaviors.

Groups, however, will remain important in posttrauma care, albeit with a need to rethink their design. Debriefing remains a common practice at the current time, in part, because no viable alternative group interventions have been developed and tested. New cognitive-behavioral models of structured early interventions with groups that better harness effective change technologies are required (e.g., skills training with instruction, practice, and coaching; modeling; self-monitoring or recording of key behaviors; use of task assignments). When verbal presentation of information is expanded to include opportunities to observe and practice coping behaviors, likelihood of behavior change may increase. Wherever possible, groups should involve multisession contact so that key messages can be repeated, supportive relationships among members can be developed, skills can be learned, and recovery behaviors can be shaped and reinforced.

ISSUES IN EARLY INTERVENTION

Posttrauma Screening

Fundamental to early posttrauma care are effective systems of matching survivor to intervention. Most survivors will improve without help, and given resource constraints and concerns about "pathologization," more formal interventions should be delivered only to those likely to need them. Screening and assessment to identify those at risk for chronic problems can, in principle, be used to help accomplish this objective. Wessely (2003) has argued that such screening should meet a variety of conditions, including the following:

- Spontaneous recovery is unlikely.
- Those who are screened would not have presented for care in the absence of screening efforts.
- There is a proven intervention for those detected.
- The anticipated benefits of screening outweigh the negative consequences.
- Screening and treatment are acceptable to those screened.
- A validated screening tool is available.
- Evidence indicates that early treatment will lead to better outcomes than late treatment.

At the current time, most of these conditions are not met. We are not yet able to identify with adequate precision those who will go on to develop significant problems. Bryant (2003) suggested that it may be premature to identify individuals for intervention before 2 weeks posttrauma, that active cognitive-behavioral intervention should not be offered earlier than 2 weeks, and that survivors will need to deal with practical problems before seeking care. However, counselors may have more confidence in initiating intervention after a few months because remission rates decline with the passage of time. For example, motor vehicle accident survivors who continue to have PTSD at 6 months following their crash are relatively unlikely to remit without treatment (Blanchard & Hickling, 2004). More of Wessely's conditions are met when screening is implemented after several months following the trauma; for example, validated screening tools and evidence-based treatment for PTSD are available.

Screening for PTSD and other posttrauma difficulties is beginning to be used routinely for returning military personnel and has been tried as well in the context of disaster and hospital trauma care. Following the World Trade Center attacks in New York, Project Liberty created a range of services intended to help the community, and in its second year of operation, a paper-and-pencil screening tool was used to identify those who might benefit from a referral for more specialized cognitive-behavioral care. Also in New York, Difede et al. (in press) developed a screening program for emergency relief workers responding to the attacks. With regard to screening for excessive alcohol consumption, screening tools exist and brief interventions are effective, but there is a need to implement screening protocols more widely with recently traumatized persons.

Selected Follow-Up with Survivors

Some of the potential limitations of early screening efforts are no longer evident if positive screens are used to initiate routine telephone follow-up monitoring, not treatment, of survivors judged to be at elevated risk for continuing posttrauma problems (cf. Brewin, 2003). Screening can be used to identify those who should be monitored, not those who require early intervention. This process may be less likely to be associated with stigmatization, and those who do not wish to be followed up can simply deny permission. In the hospital trauma center, most victims of assault will indicate, if asked, an interest in receiving counseling (Roy-Byrne, Berliner, Russo, Zatzick, & Pitman, 2003) and are receptive to case management (Zatzick et al., 2004). Because individuals may be expected to differ in their receptivity to offers of counseling at different points in time, this approach may provide the survivor with multiple opportunities to seek services.

Early Intervention Contexts Involving Continued Threat

Interventions designed for the treatment of PTSD are almost always applied under conditions of relative safety, in which threat of continued harm is minimal. In some environments (e.g., war zones, terrorist threat situations), however, these conditions do not apply. Realistic threats of ongoing exposure to continued attacks may form part of the environment in which traumatic stress reactions must be managed. Shalev et al. (2003) described modifications in delivery of cognitive-behavioral treatment for terrorism-related PTSD in Israel, designed to reflect these changed circumstances. During *in vivo* exposure assignments, survivors were encouraged to expose themselves to situations that were clearly safe, but not to those widely considered dangerous and avoided by most of the populace (e.g., city centers where repeated bombings had occurred). Their appropriate avoidance was characterized as "positive safety behaviors" and their goal as achieving "normal fear." Cognitive therapy was applied to help the PTSD group modify their beliefs, but differences between cognitions underlying avoidance by the general population and those related to avoidance by those with PTSD were noted. The latter group was thinking, "If I go there will definitely be another attack, and this time I will definitely die," whereas individuals without PTSD were thinking, "The risk is very small, but I really don't need to go and buy a book—it is not worth the risk" (Shalev et al., 2003, p. 182).

Cost-Effective Delivery

In most posttrauma environments, resource limitations inhibit the delivery of individual assessment and intervention to all survivors who might benefit. This limitation is especially apparent in situations involving large numbers of affected persons (e.g., terrorist attacks, large-scale disaster). It is also true in countries or communities with few available mental health resources. But it is also a limitation in hospital emergency medicine, in which staffing levels do not encourage routine screening and brief intervention with those showing high levels of acute traumatic stress (Zatzick et al., 2000).

Ways of delivering cost-effective cognitive-behavioral services require more development. One possibility is increased use of bibliotherapy. Written materials are routinely provided to trauma survivors, but their impact is not known. Certainly, cognitive-behavioral self-help interventions have been demonstrated to be effective for treatment of anxiety problems in a number of controlled treatment outcome studies (e.g., Lidren et al., 1994; Gould & Clum, 1995) and require more investigation with survivors of recent trauma.

Telephone delivery represents another potential way of reaching early trauma survivors. In New York after the 9/11 attacks, a LifeNet hotline established as part of Project Liberty received heavy use; it provided 24-hour mental health counseling, information, and referral, offering assistance in multiple languages. A study by Gidron et al. (2001) reported on an innovative effort to use the telephone to intervene with motor vehicle accident survivors soon after discharge from emergency room care. Survivors were called twice (24 and 48 hours following discharge), using either a two-session telephone-based memory structuring intervention (MSI) or a control intervention consisting of supportive listening by a counselor who also provided information about available treatment services. In the first session of MSI, the therapist listened to and clarified the details of the accident, repeated back the narrative in an organized manner, and then asked the survivor to do a subsequent retelling. As a between-session task, the patient was instructed to practice telling friends and family the structured account. In the second session with the therapist, the survivor was asked to once again disclose the details in a structured manner. Greater reductions in PTSD symptoms at 3- to 4-month follow-up were noted in the MSI group. And as noted earlier, the telephone has also been used to reduce anxiety levels among individuals fearing future terrorist attacks (Somer et al., 2005).

Finally, the Internet represents a delivery system with significant potential that has yet to be effectively harnessed to meet the needs of trauma survivors. Websites were a significant information resource after the terrorist attacks of 9/11. They have also been used to provide information to returning military personnel and their families, and to rape survivors. Hypothetical advantages of Internet-facilitated services include (1) an ability to reach large numbers of people in a cost-effective manner; (2) potential delivery in hospital and home settings; (3) an ability to reach people who might not otherwise have any mental health contact (e.g., those affected by perceived stigma or concerned about confidentiality concerns; those unable to travel to face-to-face services due to distance, acute injury, ongoing environmental risk, or quarantine); and (4) an ability to place survivors in contact with one another to facilitate mutual aid and support. From a cognitive-behavioral perspective, Web-delivered care has significant potential, because it can include task assignments, self-monitoring, interactive individualized content, and skills instruction such as modeling, personalized assessment, and feedback.

There has been little systematic effort to use the Internet as a medium through which to help trauma survivors. A writing-based cognitive-behavioral protocol delivered to students over the Internet—"Interapy"—was associated with significantly lower intrusion and avoidance symptoms, lower general psychopathology scores, and more improvement in mood, compared to a waiting-list control, and gains were maintained or improved upon at a 6-week follow-up (Lange, van den Ven, Schrieken, & Emmelkamp, 2001). Lange et al. (2003) provided the 5-week Web-delivered writing treatment to a sample of Dutch Internet users with significant post-traumatic stress symptoms, and found greater reduction among treated subjects in PTSD symptoms, anxiety, depression, somatization, and sleep problems than among those assigned to a waiting-list control condition. These studies provide an early demonstration of the feasibility of delivering Web-based interventions to traumatized populations. Litz, Williams, Wang, Bryant, and Engel (2004) have described a cognitive-behavioral therapist-assisted Internet-based self-help intervention designed to enable the treatment of large numbers of traumatized individuals, that uses a form of stress inoculation training for both secondary prevention of PTSD and treatment of the chronic disorder.

Related to this issue of cost-effectiveness is a question about the "boundary conditions" of cognitive-behavioral interventions. The work of Bryant and colleagues together with research on treatment of patients with chronic PTSD suggests that cognitive therapy and exposure therapy methods are effective in reducing traumatic stress symptomatology. However, in research studies these procedures are usually delivered by relatively expert, well-trained and supervised practitioners in ways that will maximize intervention impact (e.g., 5–12+ individual sessions). Although there have been some early demonstrations that indigenous helpers can deliver effective care for survivors who have developed PTSD as a result of terrorist attack (Gillespie et al., 2002; Levitt et al., 2003) or sexual assault (Foa et al., 2001), it is also important to determine the degree to which cognitive-behavioral interventions may be "degraded" and still affect outcome. Will abbreviated versions of interventions have measurable impact on behaviors of importance?

My colleague and I (Prins & Ruzek, 1999) worked with rape crisis centers to identify a means of applying principles derived from cognitive-behavioral evidence-based interventions in ways that would "fit" the existing rape crisis counseling service delivery context. We designed a set of "counseling tools" to be used by rape crisis counselors as appropriate to the situation. Although it may take 10–30 minutes to deliver all of the modular tools, pieces of any module can be "dropped into" the conversation, as needed. These mini-tools can be delivered in 2–5 minutes, even if the conversation is largely concerned with other matters. Examples of such brief tools include ways of explaining the relationship between beliefs and distress, identifying negative trauma-related beliefs and encouraging alternative beliefs, identifying sources of social support, assessing past disclosure experiences, and encouraging participation in follow-up (e.g., provide a rationale for participating, make a plan for how this can happen).

"Psychopathology" versus "Resilience" Perspectives

It could be argued that much current thinking in the field of early intervention has been shaped by research grounded in concepts of posttrauma psychopathology. Research on development of PTSD informs secondary prevention efforts, and methods of intervention have been adapted from
treatments designed to treat chronic PTSD. Bonanno (2004) has suggested
that most research on coping with trauma has focused on treatment seekers
and those experiencing psychological problems and argued that it is important to distinguished between "resilience" (characterized by low initial and
continuing levels of trauma reactions) and "recovery," in which individuals
show PTSD or subclinical stress reactions that remit over the course of several months. In practice, those working with recent trauma survivors have
been concerned to avoid defining acute stress reactions as abnormal or
reflective of psychopathology. In most settings that provide services for combat stress, disaster mental health, and rape crisis, there is active avoidance of
the language of "disorder" and little application of diagnostic labels, along
with a corresponding effort to acknowledge the strength and resilience of
survivors. Certainly, those showing Bonnano's pattern of resilient response
require more systematic study, and the implications of a resilience perspective require more exploration. Such work might lead to different ideas about
helping, as when Shalev and Ursano (2003) suggested conceptualizing the
task of the helper as that of helping the survivor identify and manage obstacles to self-regulation.

It is not yet clear how best to integrate the strengths of these somewhat
different approaches to early trauma response. There is some concern that
provision of "mental health" services or associated activities (e.g., screening
for problems, education about mental health consequences of trauma)
might have potential for worsening the outcome of some survivors, perhaps
by increasing their expectancies of developing psychological symptoms or
increasing their awareness of psychological distress (Rose, Bisson, &
Wessely, 2003). Against this concern must be weighed the problems associated with failing to ensure that individuals with clinically significant problems require adequate, evidence-supported care. In some ways, cognitive-
behavioral psychology is well placed to draw upon research into the etiology
and treatment of PTSD and, at the same time, avoid some of the pitfalls of
an emphasis on psychopathology. In addition to its strong theoretical and
empirical grounding, cognitive-behavioral psychology has a tradition of viewing problem behaviors as adaptive responses to the environment, emphasizing the training of skills for coping with specific problem situations, viewing
the client–therapist relationship as one of collaboration, and embracing a
model of care in which therapists act as teachers and coaches for their clients. These and other elements of the cognitive-behavioral orientation are
good "fits" with the resilience perspective and with the environments in
which recent trauma survivors may be offered support.

DISSEMINATION

Most mental health providers have not been trained in evidence-based treatments for PTSD and other trauma-related problems. Consequently, as cognitive-behavioral early interventions are developed, it will be a challenge to disseminate them to those who serve the various populations of trauma survivors, many of whom are volunteers, paraprofessionals, or professionals who are unfamiliar with cognitive-behavioral interventions. Recent evidence and experience does suggest, however, that mental health professionals can be rapidly trained in the delivery of these treatments. As noted previously, rape crisis counselors trained to deliver an evidence-based treatment for chronic PTSD (exposure therapy) demonstrated a clinical impact similar to that shown in efficacy trials (Foa et al., 2001). In their successful open trial of cognitive therapy with survivors of the 1998 Omagh terrorist bombing, Gillespie et al. (2002) provided an important initial demonstration of the feasibility of training indigenous mental health providers in evidence-based treatments for traumatic stress problems. Therapists were National Health Service mental health providers with no previous experience in treating trauma.

Following 9/11, several efforts to train mental health providers in evidence-based treatments were undertaken. Neria et al. (2003) described their efforts to provide New York City trauma therapists with systematic training and supervision in prolonged exposure treatment for people with PTSD (Foa & Rothbaum, 1998). Training was initiated approximately 2 months after the attacks, and over a 12-month period, more than 500 local clinicians were trained. Levitt et al. (2003) reported on an effort to train community-based counselors to deliver the skills training in affective and interpersonal regulation/narrative trauma processing intervention (see Cloitre & Rosenberg, Chapter 13, this volume) to New York City survivors who were experiencing psychological distress as a result of 9/11 and reported some symptoms of PTSD (not necessarily fulfilling a diagnosis of PTSD). Treatment was provided 1 year after the attack and consisted of a mean of 18 individual sessions that targeted emotion management skills (e.g., self-monitoring, distress tolerance), interpersonal skills (e.g., communicating feelings with others, enlisting social support), and imaginal exposure. Seven providers (including master's level social workers and clinical psychologists) were trained in the intervention in a 2-day workshop, followed by weekly group supervision. Data indicated that the treatment was effective in reducing symptoms of PTSD and depression, hostility, interpersonal sensitivity, and use of alcohol/drugs to cope, and in improving overall social–occupational functioning; effect sizes were comparable to those obtained in an earlier efficacy study with child abuse survivors with PTSD (Cloitre, personal communication, September 15, 2004).

This work is especially significant for its demonstration that evidence-based treatments may be applied in flexible ways that allow providers to adapt treatments to their own delivery preferences and situational constraints. Providers were permitted to "adjust the dose" by repeating protocol sessions, as needed, to eliminate sessions perceived as inappropriate, and to spend time attending to issues that were not the focus of the manualized intervention. In Israel, also in a terrorism context, Somer et al. (2005) demonstrated the feasibility of training paraprofessional hotline counselors in a telephone-administered anxiety reduction intervention via a single 5-hour training workshop.

Planning for Dissemination

Those engaged in development and testing of early intervention approaches might benefit from consideration of the exigencies of eventual dissemination. Current community standards of care do not reflect the evidence from treatment outcome research in too many domains of behavioral problems. There are many reasons for this state of affairs, but it is possible that design of interventions might benefit from incorporating dissemination considerations early in the development process.

Therapeutic interventions must be acceptable to the groups expected to use them. Too often, interventions are developed by psychologists and other researchers who then attempt to persuade established communities of providers to adopt their approaches. As an alternative, the intervention development process could include early collaboration partnerships with likely providers. This kind of teamwork would help ensure that interventions are designed in ways that can be easily integrated into existing structures and repertoires. Further, these partners might facilitate eventual efforts to disseminate the methods to other similar settings. Collaborative design will be important if innovative services are to be adopted by the practitioners who must deliver them within prevailing cultures of care. In addition, helping approaches must be acceptable to another major consumer group: survivors and their families. And given the general reluctance to seek help, successful interventions will be ones that have been designed to be attractive to consumers by addressing their perceived needs and preferences.

Another consideration that may affect rates of utilization by practitioners is choice of intervention target. Much of the research related to posttrauma problems has a disorder-specific focus (e.g., PTSD), which may represent an impediment to adoption of methods. In fact, there are many appropriate, and sometimes necessary, targets of early posttrauma intervention, including posttraumatic stress reactions, alcohol and drug consumption, anxiety and panic, depression, family problems, and difficulties with returning to work or other functional roles. Often, these difficulties are co-occurring. For example, among traumatic injury survivors, 23% screened positive for high levels of posttraumatic stress reactions and/or depression and alcohol/stimulant intoxication at the time of hospital acute care admission (Zatzick et al., 2002). Methods of prevention of PTSD must be developed that are compatible with the need in most settings to also intervene with other psychosocial problems and to address interacting problem behaviors efficiently. Given the heterogeneity of presentations and multiple problems faced by survivors of recent trauma, Wagner (2003) has suggested that ways of promoting behavioral assessment/functional analysis leading to individualized case formulation should be explored.

CONCLUSION

Historically, there have been relatively few settings in which cognitive-behavioral practitioners and researchers worked with recent trauma survivors. This past reality is changing as cognitive-behavioral practitioners and scientists become more active in military mental health, rape crisis centers, hospital behavioral medicine settings, and disaster relief settings, and as these settings become increasingly more concerned about the evidence base for their services. Very important in this regard is hospital emergency medicine. The fact that trauma centers and other hospital settings serve large numbers of trauma survivors contains several important implications. First, it is in such settings that methodologically strong outcome research can most readily be conducted. Second, the lack of existing services, coupled with increasing recognition by medical staffs that their trauma patients will experience mental health difficulties, means that practitioners may be welcomed if they propose delivery of services to a population in need. Finally, these settings may serve as training environments for those who wish to develop skills in working with recent trauma survivors.

The application of cognitive-behavioral perspectives to early posttrauma intervention has much to offer. The best supported psychosocial treatments for PTSD have emerged from cognitive-behavioral psychology, and many aspects of cognitive-behavioral intervention, including anxiety management, skills training, therapeutic exposure, cognitive therapy, functional assessment, self-monitoring, and goal setting, might be of value to patients in the first weeks and months posttrauma. Methods developed to change a variety of behaviors—to reduce alcohol and drug consumption, manage depression, reduce social anxiety, increase participation in rewarding activities, treat panic disorder, manage anger problems, improve assertion and conflict resolution, and manage pain, among others—may have useful application in the aftermath of trauma. Significant challenges include the development of cognitive-behavioral group- and family-administered early interventions, brief but effective forms of helping, and, in the context of multiple posttrauma problems, systems for matching survivors to brief cognitive-behavioral interventions.

REFERENCES

Acierno, R., Resnick, H. S., Flood, A., & Holmes, M. (2003). An acute post-rape intervention to prevent substance use and abuse. *Addictive Behaviors, 28*, 1701–1715.

Benight, C. C., & Bandura, A. (2004). Social cognitive theory of posttraumatic recovery: The role of perceived self-efficacy. *Behaviour Research and Therapy, 42*, 1129–1148.

Bisson, J. I. (2003). Single-session early psychological interventions following traumatic events. *Clinical Psychology Review, 23*, 481–499.

Bisson, J. I., Shepherd, J. P., Joy, D., Probert, R., & Newcombe, R. G. (2004). Early cognitive-behavioural therapy for post-traumatic stress symptoms after physical injury: Randomised controlled trial. *British Journal of Psychiatry, 184*, 63–69.

Blanchard, E. B., & Hickling, E. J. (2004). *After the crash: Psychological assessment and treatment of survivors of motor vehicle accidents* (2nd edition). Washington, DC: American Psychological Association.

Bolton, E. E., Glenn, D. M., Orsillo, S., Roemer, L., & Litz, B. T. (2003). The relationship between self-disclosure and symptoms of posttraumatic stress disorder in peacekeepers deployed to Somalia. *Journal of Traumatic Stress, 16*, 203–210.

Bonanno, G. A. (2004). Loss, trauma, and human resilience: Have we underestimated the human capacity to thrive after extremely aversive events? *American Psychologist, 59*, 20–28.

Brewin, C. R. (2003). *Post-traumatic stress disorder: Malady or myth?* London: Yale University Press.

Brewin, C. R., Andrews, B., & Valentine, J. D. (2000). Meta-analysis of risk factors for posttraumatic stress disorder in trauma-exposed adults. *Journal of Consulting and Clinical Psychology, 68*, 748–766.

Bryant, R. A. (2003). Cognitive behaviour therapy of acute stress disorder. In R. Orner & U. Schnyder (Eds.), *Reconstructing early intervention after trauma: Innovations in the care of survivors* (pp. 159–168). Oxford, UK: Oxford University Press.

Bryant, R. A., Harvey, A. G., Dang, S. T., Sackville, T., & Basten, C. (1998). Treatment of acute stress disorder: A comparison of cognitive-behavioral therapy and supportive counseling. *Journal of Consulting and Clinical Psychology, 66*, 862–866.

Bryant, R. A., Moulds, M. L., & Nixon, R. D. V. (2003). Cognitive behaviour therapy of acute stress disorder: A four-year follow-up. *Behaviour Research and Therapy, 41*, 489–494.

Bryant, R. A., Sackville, T., Dang, S. T., Moulds, M., & Guthrie, R. (1999). Treating acute stress disorder: An evaluation of cognitive behavior therapy and supportive counseling techniques. *American Journal of Psychiatry, 156*, 1780–1786.

Cordova, M. J., Ruzek, J. I., Benoit, M., & Brunet, A. (2003). Promotion of emotional disclosure following illness and injury: A brief intervention for medical patients and their families. *Cognitive and Behavioral Practice, 10*, 359–372.

Delisi, L. E., Maurizio, A., Yost, M., Papparozzi, C. F., Fulchino, C., Katz, C. L., Altesman, J., Biel, M., Lee, J., & Stevens, P. (2003). A survey of New Yorkers after the Sept. 11, 2001, terrorist attacks. *American Journal of Psychiatry, 160*, 780–783.

Department of the Army. (2003). *U.S. Army combat stress control handbook.* Guilford, CT: Lyons Press.

Difede, J., Roberts, J., Jayasinghe, N., & Leck, P. (in press). Evaluation and treatment of emergency services personnel following the World Trade Center attack. In Y.

Neria, R. Gross, R. Marshall, & E. Susser (Eds.), *September 11, 2001: Treatment, research and public mental health in the wake of a terrorist attack*. New York: Cambridge University Press.

Echeburua, E., deCorral, P., Sarasua, B., & Zubizarreta, I. (1996). Treatment of acute posttraumatic stress disorder in rape victims: An experimental study. *Journal of Anxiety Disorders, 10*, 185–199.

Ehlers, A., & Clark, D. M. (2003). Early psychological interventions for adult survivors of trauma: A review. *Biological Psychiatry, 53*, 817–826.

Ehlers, A., Clark, D. M., Hackmann, A., McManus, F., Fennell, M., Herbert, C., & Mayou, R. A. (2003). A randomized controlled trial of cognitive therapy, self-help, and repeated assessment as early interventions for PTSD. *Archives of General Psychiatry, 60*, 1024–1032.

Foa, E. B., Cahill, S. P., & Hembree, E. (2001). *Effectiveness of prolonged exposure with and without cognitive restructuring for PTSD in community and expert clinics.* Paper presented at the Association for Advancement of Behavior Therapy, Philadelphia, Pennsylvania.

Foa, E. B., Dancu, C. V., Hembree, E. A., Jaycox, L. H., Meadows, E. A., & Street, G. P. (1999). A comparison of exposure therapy, stress inoculation training, and their combination for reducing posttraumatic stress disorder in female assault victims. *Journal of Consulting and Clinical Psychology, 67*, 194–200.

Foa, E. B., Hearst-Ikeda, D., & Perry, K. J. (1995). Evaluation of a brief cognitive-behavioral program for the prevention of chronic PTSD in recent assault victims. *Journal of Consulting and Clinical Psychology, 63*, 948–955.

Foa, E. B., & Rothbaum, B. O. (1998). *Treating the trauma of rape: Cognitive-behavioral therapy for PTSD*. New York: Guilford Press.

Foy, D. W., Glynn, S. M., Schnurr, P. P., Jankowski, M. K., Wattenberg, M. S., Weiss, D. S., Marmar, C. R., & Gusman, F. D. (2000). Group therapy. In E. B. Foa, T. M. Keane, & M. J. Friedman (Eds.), *Effective treatments for PTSD: Practice guidelines from the International Society for Traumatic Stress Studies* (pp. 155–175). New York: Guilford Press.

Fredrickson, B. L., Tugade, M. M., Waugh, C. E., & Larkin, G. R. (2003). What good are positive emotions in crisis? A prospective study of resilience and emotions following the terrorist attacks on the United States on September 11th, 2001. *Journal of Personality and Social Psychology, 84*, 365–376.

Gentilello, L. M., Rivara, F. P., Donovan, D. M., Jurkovich, G. J., Daranciang, E., Dunn, C. W., Villaveces, A., Copass, M., & Ries, R. R. (1999). Alcohol interventions in a trauma center as a means of reducing the risk of injury recurrence. *Annals of Surgery, 230*, 473–483.

Gibson, L., Ruzek, J. I., Naturale, A., Bryant, R. A., Hamblen, J., Jones, R., Rynearson, T., Watson, P. J., & Young, B. H. (in press). *Early intervention.* Paper developed for SAMHSA/NIMH Screening and Assessment, Outreach, and Intervention for Mental Health and Substance Abuse Needs Following Disasters and Mass Violence meeting, August 26–28, 2003, Bethesda, Maryland.

Gidron, Y., Gal, R., Freedman, S. A., Twiser, I., Lauden, A., Snir, Y., & Benjamin, J. (2001). Translating research findings to PTSD prevention: Results of a randomized-controlled pilot study. *Journal of Traumatic Stress, 14*(4), 773–780.

Gillespie, K., Duffy, M., Hackmann, A., & Clark, D. M. (2002). Community based cognitive therapy in the treatment of post-traumatic stress disorder following the Omagh bomb. *Behaviour Research and Therapy, 40*, 345–357.

Gould, R. A., & Clum, G. A. (1995). Self-help plus minimal therapist contact in the treatment of panic disorder: A replication and extension. *Behavior Therapy, 26,* 533–546.

Hamblen, J., Gibson, L. E., Mueser, K., Rosenberg, S., Jankowski, K., Watson, P., & Friedman, M. (2003). *The National Center for PTSD's brief intervention for continuing postdisaster distress.* White River Junction, VT: National Center for PTSD.

Hoge, C. W., Castro, C. A., Messer, S. C., McGurk, D., Cotting, D. I., & Koffman, R. L. (2004). Combat duty in Iraq and Afghanistan, mental health problems, and barriers to care. *New England Journal of Medicine, 351,* 13–22.

Jaycox, L. H., Marshall, G. N., & Schell, T. (2004). Use of mental health services by men injured through community violence. *Psychiatric Services, 55,* 415–420.

Jones, E., & Wessely, S. (2003). "Forward psychiatry" in the military: Its origins and effectiveness. *Journal of Traumatic Stress, 16,* 411–419.

Lange, A., Rietdijk, D., Hudcovicova, M., van den Ven, J. P., Schrieken, B., & Emmelkamp, P. M. G. (2003). Interapy: A controlled randomized trial of the standardized treatment of posttraumatic stress through the Internet. *Journal of Consulting and Clinical Psychology, 71,* 901–909.

Lange, A., van den Ven, J. P., Schrieken, B., & Emmelkamp, P. M. G. (2001). Treatment of posttraumatic stress disorder through the Internet: A controlled trial. *Journal of Behavior Therapy and Experimental Psychiatry, 32,* 73–90.

Lepore, S. J., Silver, R. C., Wortman, C. B., & Wayment, H. A. (1996). Social constraints, intrusive thoughts, and depressive symptoms among bereaved mothers. *Journal of Personality and Social Psychology, 70,* 271–282.

Levitt, J. T., Davis, L., Martin, A., & Cloitre, M. (2003). *Bringing a manualized treatment for PTSD to the community in the aftermath of 9/11.* Paper presented at Association for Advancement of Behavior Therapy, Boston, Massachusetts.

Lidren, D. M., Watkins, P. L., Gould, R. A., Clum, G. A., Asterino, M. A., & Tulloch, H. L. (1994). A comparison of bibliotherapy and group therapy in the treatment of panic disorder. *Journal of Consulting and Clinical Psychology, 62,* 865–869.

Litz, B. T., Williams, L., Wang, J. L., Bryant, R. A., & Engel, C. C. (2004). A therapist-assisted Internet self-help program for traumatic stress. *Professional Psychology: Research and Practice, 35,* 628–634.

Longabaugh, R., Woolard, R. E., Nirenberg, T. D., Minugh, A. P., Becker, B., Clifford, P. R., Carty, K., Sparadeo, F., & Gogineni, A. (2001). Evaluating the effects of a brief motivational intervention for injured drinkers in the emergency department. *Journal of Studies on Alcohol, 62,* 806–816.

Luce, A., & Firth-Cozens, J. (2002). Effects of the Omagh bombing on medical staff working in the local NHS trust: A longitudinal survey. *Hospital Medicine, 63,* 44–47.

McNally, R., Bryant, R. A., & Ehlers, A. (2003). Does early psychological intervention promote recovery from posttraumatic stress? *Psychological Science in the Public Interest, 4,* 45–79.

Miller, W. R., & Rollnick, S. (2002). *Motivational interviewing: Preparing people for change* (2nd ed.). New York: Guilford Press.

Monson, C. M., Schnurr, P. P., Guthrie, K. A., & Stevens, S. P. (2004). Cognitive-behavioral couple's treatment for posttraumatic stress disorder: Initial findings. *Journal of Traumatic Stress, 17,* 341–344.

Moyer, A., Finney, J. W., Swearingen, C. E., & Vergun, P. (2002). Brief interventions for alcohol problems: A meta-analytic review of controlled investigations in treatment-seeking and non-treatment-seeking populations. *Addiction, 97,* 279–292.

Najavits, L. M. (2002). *Seeking safety: A treatment manual for PTSD and substance abuse.* New York: Guilford Press.

Neria, Y., Suh, E. J., & Marshall, R. D. (2003). The professional response to the aftermath of September 11, 2001 in New York City: Lessons learned from treating victims of the World Trade Center attacks. In B. Litz (Ed.), *Early intervention for trauma and traumatic loss* (pp. 201–215). New York: Guilford Press.

Norris, F. H., Friedman, M. J., Watson, P. J., Byrne, C. M., Diaz, E., & Kaniasty, K. (2002). 60,000 disaster victims speak: Part I. An empirical review of the empirical literature, 1981–2001. *Psychiatry, 65,* 207–239.

Norris, F. H., Hamblen, J. L., Watson, P. J., Ruzek, J. I., Gibson, L. E., Price, J. L., Stevens, S. P., Young, B. H., Friedman, M. J., & Pfefferbaum, B. J. (in press). Toward understanding and creating systems of postdisaster care: Findings and recommendations from a case study of New York's response to the World Trade Center disaster. In E. C. Ritchie, P. J. Watson, & M. J. Friedman (Eds.), *Mental health intervention following disasters or mass violence.* New York: Guilford Press.

North, C. S., Tivis, L., McMillen, J. C., Pfefferbaum, B., Spitznagel, E. L., Cox, J., Bunch, K., Schorr, J., & Smith, E. (2002). Coping, functioning, and adjustment of rescue workers after the Oklahoma City bombing. *Journal of Traumatic Stress, 15,* 171–175.

Prins, A., & Ruzek, J. I. (1999). Crisis counseling for sexual assault survivors. In *Rape crisis counseling model manual.* Oakland, CA: California Coalition Against Sexual Assault (CalCASA).

Raphael, B., & Wilson, J. P. (2000). *Psychological debriefing: Theory, practice and evidence.* Cambridge, UK: Cambridge University Press.

Resick, P. A., & Schnicke, M. K. (1993). *Cognitive processing therapy for rape victims: A treatment manual.* Newbury Park, CA: Sage.

Resnick, J., Acierno, R., Holmes, M., Kilpatrick, D. G., & Jager, N. (1999). Prevention of post-rape psychopathology: Preliminary findings of a controlled acute rape treatment study. *Journal of Anxiety Disorders, 13,* 359–370.

Rose, S., Bisson, J., & Wessely, S. (2003). A systematic review of single psychological interventions ("debriefing") following trauma: Updating the Cochrane review and implications for good practice. In R. Orner & U. Schnyder (Eds.), *Reconstructing early intervention after trauma: Innovations in the care of survivors* (pp. 24–39). Oxford, UK: Oxford University Press.

Roy-Byrne, P., Berliner, L., Russo, J., Zatzick, D., & Pitman, R. K. (2003). Treatment preferences and determinants in victims of sexual and physical assault. *Journal of Nervous and Mental Disease, 191,* 161–165.

Ruzek, J.I., & Cordova, M. J. (2003). The role of hospitals in delivering early intervention services following traumatic events. In R. Orner & U. Schnyder (Eds.), *Reconstructing early intervention after trauma: Innovations in the care of survivors* (pp. 228–235). Oxford, UK: Oxford University Press.

Ruzek, J. I., Curran, E., Friedman, M. J., Gusman, F. D., Southwick, S., Swales, P., Walser, R. D., Watson, P. J., & Whealin, J. (2003). Treatment of the returning Iraq War veteran. *The Iraq War clinician guide* (2nd ed.). White River Junction, VT: Department of Veterans Affairs, National Center for PTSD, and Walter Reed Army Medical Center. Available online at www.ncptsd.org/war/guide/index.html

Ruzek, J. I., Young, B. H., Cordova, M. J., & Flynn, B. W. (2004). Integration of disaster mental health services with emergency medicine. *Prehospital and Disaster Medicine, 19,* 46–53.

Shalev, A. Y., Adessky, R., Boker, R., Bargai, N., Cooper, R., Freedman, S., Hadar, H., Peri, T., & Tuval-Mashiach, R. (2003). Clinical intervention for survivors of prolonged adversities. In R. J. Ursano, C. S. Fullerton, & A. E. Norwood (Eds.), *Terrorism and disaster: Individual and community mental health interventions* (pp. 162–188). Cambridge, UK: Cambridge University Press.

Shalev, A. Y., Tuval, M. R., Frenkiel, S., & Hadar, H. (2004). Posttraumatic stress disorder as a result of mass trauma. *Journal of Clinical Psychiatry, 65*(Suppl.), 4–10.

Shalev, A. Y., & Ursano, R. J. (2003). Mapping the multidimensional picture of acute responses to traumatic stress. In R. Orner & U. Schnyder (Eds.), *Reconstructing early intervention after trauma: Innovations in the care of survivors* (pp. 118–129). Oxford, UK: Oxford University Press.

Shepherd, J. P., & Bisson, J. I. (2004). Towards integrated health care: A model for assault victims. *British Journal of Psychiatry, 184,* 3–4.

Smith, D. W., Kilpatrick, D. G., Falsetti, S. A., & Best, C. L. (2002). Postterrorism services for victims and surviving family members: Lessons from Pan Am 103. *Cognitive and Behavioral Practice, 9,* 280–286.

Smith, J. E., & Meyers, R. J. (2004). *Motivating substance abusers to enter treatment: Working with family members.* New York: Guilford Press.

Solomon, Z., Shklar, R., & Mikulincer, M. (2004). *A window of opportunity for psychological first-aid: PIE revised 20 years after the Lebanon War.* Paper presented at the annual meeting of the International Society for Traumatic Stress Studies, New Orleans, Louisiana.

Somer, E., Tamir, E., Maguen, S., & Litz, B. T. (2005). Brief cognitive-behavioral phone-based intervention targeting anxiety about the threat of attack: A pilot study. *Behaviour Research and Therapy, 43,* 669–679.

Steil, R., & Ehlers, A. (2000). Dysfunctional meaning of posttraumatic intrusions in chronic PTSD. *Behaviour Research and Therapy, 38,* 537–558.

Tarrier, N., Sommerfield, C., Reynolds, M., & Pilgrim, H. (1999). Symptom self-monitoring in the treatment of post-traumatic stress disorder. *Behavior Therapy, 30,* 597–605.

Taylor, S. (2003). Anxiety sensitivity and its implications for understanding and treating PTSD. *Journal of Cognitive Psychotherapy, 17,* 179–186.

Ullman, S. E., & Filipas, H. H. (2001). Predictors of PTSD symptom severity and social reactions in sexual assault victims. *Journal of Traumatic Stress, 14,* 369–389.

VA–Department of Defense Clinical Practice Guideline Working Group, Veterans Health Administration, Department of Veterans Affairs and Health Affairs, Department of Defense. (2003). *Management of post-traumatic stress* (publication 10Q-CPG/PTSD-04). Washington, DC: Office of Quality and Performance.

Wagner, A. W. (2003). Cognitive-behavioral therapy for posttraumatic stress disorder: Applications to injured trauma survivors. *Seminars in Clinical Neuropsychiatry, 8,* 175–187.

Walser, R. D., Ruzek, J. I., Naugle, A. E., Padesky, C., Ronell, D. M., & Ruggiero, K. (2004). Disaster and terrorism: Cognitive-behavioral interventions. *Prehospital and Disaster Medicine, 19,* 54–63.

Weisaeth, L. (2001). Acute posttraumatic stress: Nonacceptance of early intervention. *Journal of Clinical Psychiatry, 62*(Suppl. 17), 35–40.

Wessely, S. (2003). The role of screening in the prevention of psychological disorders arising after major trauma: Pros and cons. In R. J. Ursano, C. S. Fullerton, & A. E. Norwood (Eds.), *Terrorism and disaster: Individual and community mental health interventions* (pp. 121–145). Cambridge, UK: Cambridge University Press.

Zatzick, D. F., Kang, S. M., Hinton, W. L., Kelly, R. H., Hilty, D. M., Franz, C. E., Le, L., & Kravitz, R. L. (2001a). Posttraumatic concerns: A patient-centered approach to outcome assessment after traumatic physical injury. *Medical Care, 39*, 327–339.

Zatzick, D. F., Kang, S., Kim, S., Leigh, P., Kravitz, R., Drake, C., Sue, S., & Wisner, D. (2000). Patients with recognized psychiatric disorders in trauma surgery: Incidence, inpatients length of stay, and cost. *Journal of Trauma, 49*, 487–495.

Zatzick, D. F., Kang, S. M., Mueller, H. G., Russo, J. E., Rivara, F. P., Katon, W., Jurkovich, G. J., & Roy-Byrne, P. (2002). Predicting posttraumatic distress in hospitalized trauma survivors with acute injuries. *American Journal of Psychiatry, 159*, 941–946.

Zatzick, D., Roy-Byrne, P., Russo, J., Rivara, F., Droesch, R., Wagner, A., Dunn, C., Jurkovich, G., Uehara, E., & Katon, W. (2004). A randomized effectiveness trial of stepped collaborative care for acutely injured trauma survivors. *Archives of General Psychiatry, 61*, 498–506.

Zatzick, D. F., Roy-Byrne, P., Russo, J., Rivara, F. P., Koike, A., Jurkovich, G. J., & Katon, W. (2001b). Collaborative interventions for physically injured trauma survivors: A pilot randomized effectiveness trial. *General Hospital Psychiatry, 23*, 114–123.

Zatzick, D. F., & Wagner, A. W. (2004). Evaluating and treating injury trauma survivors in trauma care systems. In B. T. Litz (Ed.), *Early intervention for trauma and traumatic loss in children and adults*. New York: Guilford Press.

Zoellner, L. A., Foa, E. B., & Brigidi, B. D. (1999). Interpersonal friction and PTSD in female victims of sexual and nonsexual assault. *Journal of Traumatic Stress, 12*, 689–700.

Index

T-U